Third Edition

CURRENT
CARDIOVASCULAR
DRUGS

Third Edition

CURRENT CARDIOVASCULAR DRUGS

Edited by

William H. Frishman
Professor of Medicine and Pharmacology
Chairman of Medicine
New York Medical College
Director of Medicine
Westchester Medical Center
Valhalla, New York

Angela Cheng-Lai
Clinical Pharmacy Manager, Adult Medicine
Montefiore Medical Center
Assistant Professor of Medicine
Albert Einstein College of Medicine
Bronx, New York

Julie Chen
Clinical Pharmacy Manager, Critical Care
Montefiore Medical Center
Assistant Professor of Medicine
Albert Einstein College of Medicine
Bronx, New York

Springer Science+Business
Media, LLC

ISBN 978-1-57340-135-7   ISBN 978-1-4615-6767-7 (eBook)
DOI 10.1007/978-1-4615-6767-7
ISSN: 1070-4345

Managing editor: Mary Kinsella
Developmental editors: Susan L. Hunsberger and Ira Smiley
Art director: Jerilyn Kauffman
Design and layout: Christine Keller-Quirk
Illustration director: Debra Wertz
Illustrators: Nicole Mock, Anne Rains, and Paul Schiffmacher
Production manager: Lori Holland
Production assistant: Peter O'Steen

Although every effort has been made to ensure that drug doses and other information are presented accurately in this publication, the ultimate responsibility rests with the prescribing physician. Neither the publishers nor the authors can be held responsible for errors or for any consequences arising from the use of information contained herein. Products mentioned in this publication should be used in accordance with the prescribing information prepared by the manufacturers. No claims or endorsements are made for any drug or compound at present under clinical investigation.

Manufactured in the United States of America

5 4 3 2 1

One hundred years ago, not a single chapter heading in this book on cardiovascular drug therapy would have been recognized. Over the past 35 years, there have been major advances in our understanding of cardiovascular pharmacology related, in part, to the contributions of basic science and clinical investigation. These advances are occurring now at such a rapid pace that it is difficult, if not impossible, for the healthcare professional to integrate all of this new knowledge into clinical practice. Of immediate relevance has been the introduction of a large number of new drugs for the treatment of patients with ischemic heart disease, arrhythmias, systemic hypertension, myocardial failure, and for the primary and secondary prevention of cardiovascular disease. For each new drug that becomes available, physicians must become familiar with its pharmacokinetic profile, especially when prescribing drugs to patients having various medical conditions. The clinician must also be aware of potential drug-drug interactions.

Current Cardiovascular Drugs is a practical compendium of current knowledge of cardiovascular drug therapy and, in a concise, easily readable format, provides the most updated information on the major cardiovascular drug classes, detailing the pharmacologic characteristics of specific agents. The clinical efficacy and limitations of the various drug therapies are discussed using information from the most authoritative sources.

This book is not designed to replace traditional textbooks of cardiology and pharmacology, or to resolve ongoing controversies in patient management. Rather, its purpose is to provide the most updated information on the drugs used to treat cardiovascular disease in clinical practice. Innovative approaches to pharmacotherapy are also presented in specific chapters. Since many of the cardiovascular drugs can also be used for multiple conditions, this information is highlighted in the different chapters. Suggested readings from the medical literature are provided at the end of each chapter.

This book discusses only those drugs that are available for use in the United States. This edition also includes a chapter on Drugs in Development, which highlights ongoing clinical investigations of the future. Some of these investigational agents will become available in the year 2000 and some in subsequent years. In addition, Appendices are included that summarize drug use recommendations regarding gender and in specific clinical situations— pregnancy, old age, hepatic and renal diseases. The final Appendix includes a list of hundreds of cardiovascular drug trial acronyms that stretch the imagination in their innovation and uniqueness in medical research. This book will be updated frequently to provide the most current information to practicing physicians, physicians-in-training, pharmacists, nurses, physician assistants, and medical students.

The authors acknowledge the editorial contribution of Mrs. Joanne Pyror to both this and previous editions of the book, and Ms. Susan Hunsberger of Current Medicine for her editorial guidance. Finally, the authors wish to thank our colleagues and students for the inspiration to prepare this book, and our respective families whose love, support, and encouragement have provided the impetus to complete this work.

William H, Frishman, M.D.
Angela Cheng-Lai, Pharm.D.
Julie Chen, Pharm.D.

DEDICATION

To our families

CONTENTS

CONTRIBUTORS

Julie Chen, Pharm.D., BCPS

Clinical Pharmacy Manager, Critical Care
Montefiore Medical Center
Assistant Professor of Medicine
Albert Einstein College of Medicine
Bronx, New York

Angela Cheng-Lai, Pharm.D.

Clinical Pharmacy Manager, Adult Medicine
Montefiore Medical Center
Assistant Professor of Medicine
Albert Einstein College of Medicine
Bronx, New York

William H. Frishman, M.D.

Professor of Medicine and Pharmacology
Chairman of Medicine
New York Medical College
Valhalla, New York
Director of Medicine
Westchester Medical Center
Valhalla, New York

James Nawarskas, Pharm.D.

Assistant Professor of Clinical Pharmacy
College of Pharmacy
University of New Mexico
Albuquerque, New Mexico

Hieu T. Tran, Pharm.D.

Assistant Professor
School of Pharmacy
Wilkes University
Wilkes-Barre, Pennsylvania

Current Cardiovascular Drugs is a quick and easy reference for the prescriber. The information in it is drawn from a number of sources, chiefly the manufacturers' data sheets and the international published literature. The recommendations also reflect current prescribing practice among physicians.

The information has been rigorously checked by the authors, the publishers, the manufacturers, and qualified pharmacists. However, the book is intended as a memory aid rather than a substitute for the data sheets. **The information in this book must always be used in conjunction with the manufacturers' prescribing information.**

Each chapter is devoted to a different drug class. The first pages of the chapter, the introductory pages, briefly describe the development of drugs in that class, report the results of recent major clinical trials, and provide tabular summaries of the current use and actions of the drugs.

INTRODUCTORY PAGES

The tables on the introductory pages bring together the information given on the individual drug pages in that chapter and give additional guidelines: the reasons for contraindications and warnings, the nature of drug interactions, and the action to be taken in the event of adverse reactions.

INDIVIDUAL DRUG PAGES

Note: There are apparent differences in the incidence of adverse reactions and interactions between drugs of the same class. These differences are due to factors such as variations in the level of reporting by different manufacturers. Many effects are not well validated and a causal connection between drug use and effect has not always been proved.

Doses reflect the manufacturers' data sheets and the authors' recommendations, based on current clinical practice. Dosage requirements for special patient groups may be listed separately.

Guidelines for treating overdosage are given but the prescriber should always consult the data sheet.

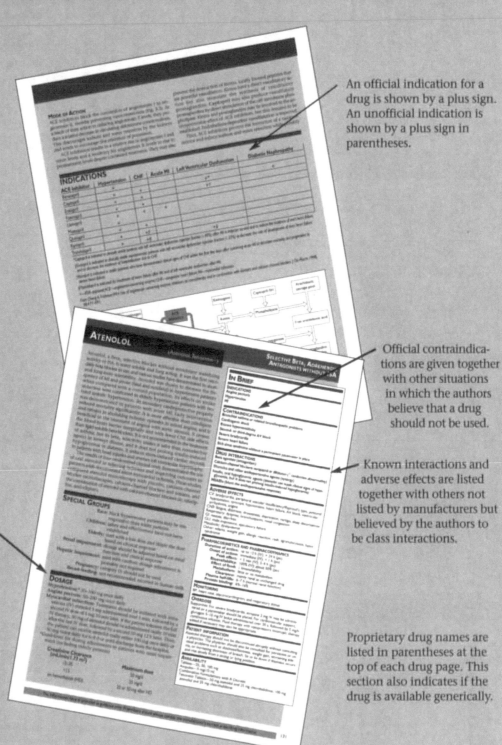

An official indication for a drug is shown by a plus sign. An unofficial indication is shown by a plus sign in parentheses.

Official contraindications are given together with other situations in which the authors believe that a drug should not be used.

Known interactions and adverse effects are listed together with others not listed by manufacturers but believed by the authors to be class interactions.

Proprietary drug names are listed in parentheses at the top of each drug page. This section also indicates if the drug is available generically.

The information here is provided as guidance only. Prescribers should always consult the manufacturer's current prescribing information.

I

ALPHA-ADRENERGIC BLOCKERS (PERIPHERALLY ACTING ANTIHYPERTENSIVE AGENTS)

The alpha-receptor blockers were the first adrenergic receptor antagonists to be developed for cardiovascular therapy. This occurred shortly after Alquist suggested the alpha/beta classification scheme to explain differences between the pharmacologic actions of adrenergic agonists. The alpha blockers, **phenoxybenzamine** and **phentolamine** (now recognized as antagonists for both alpha$_1$ and alpha$_2$ receptors), have been in use since the 1960s, primarily for management of massive catecholamine excess in pheochromocytoma. Subsequently, the quinazolines were found to have antagonism for a set of alpha receptors, primarily found on postsynaptic sites, thus characterized as alpha$_1$. In the cardiovascular system, alpha$_1$ receptors are found in vascular smooth muscle. These receptors mediate the action of norepinephrine released from presynaptic adrenergic nerve terminals, thus causing vasoconstriction, as shown in Figure 1.1. There may be two subtypes of the alpha$_1$ receptors—alpha$_{1a}$ and alpha$_{1b}$. The former regulates transmembrane calcium entry channels, whereas the latter, through its intracellular action on phospholipase-C and the phosphoinositol system, controls intracellular sequestration of free calcium.

Alpha$_2$ receptors are located within the regulatory centers of the central nervous system (CNS) that control outflow of the autonomic nervous system. These receptors are also found on presynaptic autonomic nerve terminals where, when activated by a released neurotransmitter, they inhibit neurosecretion. Other locations for alpha$_2$ receptors include platelets, pancreatic islet cells, and nonsynaptic locations of vascular smooth muscle. In vascular tissue, alpha$_2$ receptors mediate the effect of circulating catecholamines. The major actions and characteristics of the alpha receptors are shown in Table 1.1.

The alpha receptor antagonists may be divided into two categories—those drugs that block both the alpha$_1$ and alpha$_2$ receptors (**phenoxybenzamine** and **phentolamine**), and the quinazoline-type specific alpha$_1$ blockers (**doxazosin, prazosin,** and **terazosin**). Most adrenergic receptor blocking drugs are competitive antagonists that bind reversibly to their specific receptors and can be displaced by high concentrations of competing agonists. **Phenoxybenzamine** is the exception, as it bonds irreversibly to alpha receptors as an alkylating agent. Both **phenoxybenzamine** and **phentolamine** reduce vasoconstriction and decrease blood pressure. However, these drugs cause tachycardia. This is probably because of their antagonism of inhibitory presynaptic alpha$_2$ receptors, which leads to increased release of norepinephrine to postsynaptic cardiac beta receptors, increasing the heart rate. The effectiveness of these two drugs in pheochromocytoma may be a result of their ability to antagonize both postsynaptic alpha$_1$ and nonsynaptic alpha$_2$ receptors on vascular tissue.

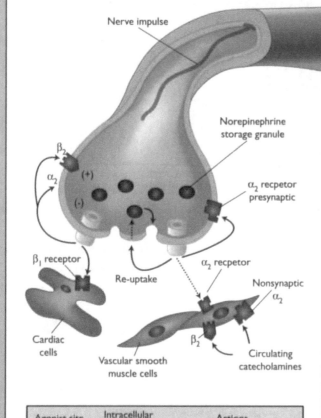

FIGURE 1.1 Site of action of alpha-blockers.

TABLE 1.1 COMPARISON OF THE ALPHA RECEPTORS		
	Alpha$_1$ receptors	Alpha$_2$ receptors
Prototype agonist	Norepinephrine	Clonidine
Prototype antagonist	Prazosin	Yohimbine
Presynaptic location	No	Yes
Postsynaptic location	Yes	No
Nonsynaptic location	?	Yes
In the CNS cardio vascular centers	?	Yes
Vascular smooth muscle location	Yes	Yes
Pancreatic islet cells	No	Yes
Platelets	?	Yes
Intracellular signaling system	Alpha$_{1a}$-calcium entry via channels; alpha$_{1b}$-phospholipase-C system- intracellular calcium	Inhibition of adenylcyclase

CNS—central nervous system.

Phentolamine is available for intravenous bolus injection or infusion to be used in controlling the hypertensive crises of pheochromocytoma. The major use of **phenoxybenzamine** is as an oral agent for the treatment of hypertension in pheochromocytoma.

EFFICACY OF ALPHA₁ ANTAGONISTS

The quinazoline alpha₁ antagonists—**prazosin, terazosin,** and **doxazosin**—have become widely accepted as effective antihypertensive agents (other alpha₁ antagonists not available in the United States include **indoramine** and **bunazosin**). They reduce systemic vascular resistance with little change in heart rate, fluid retention, or activation of the renin-angiotensin system. The differences among these drugs are primarily related to their pharmacokinetic profiles and duration of action, as shown in Table 1.2. **Prazosin** has the shortest half-life and must be given 2–3 times daily for effective reduction of arterial pressure. **Terazosin** and **doxazosin** have longer half-lives; **terazosin** can be given once or twice daily, and **doxazosin** is usually given once daily. The alpha₁ antagonists are metabolized almost entirely by hepatic routes, and so are unaffected by renal insufficiency.

Doxazosin was compared with other once daily agents from other antihypertensive drug classes in the Trial of Mild Hypertension Study (TOMHS). Daily **doxazosin** (1–2 mg) was found to be as effective as either **chlorthalidone, enalapril, acebutolol,** or **amlodipine** in reducing arterial pressure over 4 years, when compared with a placebo-treated group in this randomized controlled trial. Although the pattern of morbidity was favorable for all those on drug treatment, compared with the placebo group, no difference between the drug classes was found in this study.

OTHER EFFECTS

All three quinazoline alpha₁ blockers have similar and favorable effects on serum lipid fractions, tending to reduce total and low-density lipoprotein cholesterol, and slightly increasing high-density lipoprotein cholesterol fractions (Table 1.3). **Prazosin** and **doxazosin** have been shown to reduce resistance to insulin action. This effect has potential, but unproven, benefit for noninsulin-dependent diabetic hypertensive patients or those with the insulin-resistance syndrome. One action of the alpha₁ antagonists, unique among the antihypertensive agents, is their ability to antagonize urethral alpha receptors and thus decrease resistance to urinary outflow. This has been the basis for their successful use (**terazosin,** in particular) in treating the symptoms of benign prostatic hypertrophy (BPH). **Tamsulosin** (Flomax [Boehringer Ingelheim]), an alpha₁ receptor antagonist with selectivity for the alpha₁ₐ receptors in prostatic tissue, is indicated only for alleviating symptoms associated with benign prostatic hypertrophy. **Tamsulosin** is not recommended for use as an antihypertensive drug because of its specificity for prostatic tissue and limited systemic effect. However, orthostatic hypotension remains a problem with **tamsulosin** therapy, especially when higher doses are administered.

The vasodilating effect of alpha₁ receptor antagonists reduces afterload in patients with reduced left ventricular systolic function. On that basis, **prazosin** was studied in a randomized clinical trial for possible efficacy in advanced congestive heart failure (CHF). However, when compared with placebo, **prazosin** had no effect, whereas a combination of **hydralazine** and **isosorbide** was beneficial in decreasing cumulative mortality. At present, CHF is not considered an indication for use of the alpha₁ receptor antagonists.

TABLE 1.2 PHARMACOKINETICS AND USUAL DOSE RANGE FOR THE ALPHA₁-RECEPTOR ANTAGONISTS		
Drug	Approximate half-life	Usual initial dose and dose range
Prazosin	2–4 h	1 mg orally at bedtime; 1–5 mg 2–3 times daily
Terazosin	10–12 h	1 mg daily; 1–5 mg twice daily
Doxazosin	20–22 h	1 mg daily; 1–10 mg daily

TABLE 1.3 EFFECTS OF ALPHA BLOCKERS ON PLASMA LIPID PROFILE	
	Effect
Total cholesterol	↓
High-density lipoprotein cholesterol	↑
Low-density lipoprotein cholesterol	↓
Triglycerides	↓
Lipoprotein lipase activity	↑

It has been suggested that the effects of alpha blockers may be attributable to their stimulation of lipoprotein lipase activity.

The information here is provided as guidance only. Prescribers should always consult the manufacturer's current prescribing information.

3

ADVERSE EFFECTS

All three alpha$_1$ antagonists share the same adverse effects profile. Most often mentioned is first-dose orthostatic hypotension, defined as dizziness or syncope caused by a sudden reduction in blood pressure when upright, shortly after either the initial dose or the first time a higher dose is taken. It is suggested, but not thoroughly evaluated, that this effect is less likely with those drugs having a slower onset and longer half-life (**terazosin** and **doxazosin**). First-dose hypotension should be anticipated when an alpha$_1$ antagonist is given to older patients or those already taking other antihypertensive agents, especially diuretics and angiotensin-converting enzyme (ACE) inhibitors. A variety of adverse effects have been reported in those taking alpha$_1$ antagonists. Some, such as fatigue, asthenia, or dizziness, are nonspecific and difficult to relate to specific drug action. Postural hypotension can be understood as a cause of reduced activation of normal alpha$_1$-adrenergic receptor function. Patients receiving alpha antagonists should be routinely monitored for postural changes in blood pressure. This is particularly important in elderly hypertensive patients. Nasal congestion is probably a specific adverse effect of alpha receptor blockade. Other reported adverse effects are listed with each agent.

COMBINATION THERAPY WITH OTHER ANTIHYPERTENSIVE AGENTS

Caution is urged when alpha$_1$ antagonists are prescribed with other antihypertensive agents; there is increased likelihood of first-dose or postural hypertension. Diuretics at high dose, centrally acting agents, or sympatholytics are to be avoided. When used cautiously, alpha$_1$ receptor antagonists may be effective in combination with beta receptor antagonists. For example, the combination of **doxazosin** and **atenolol** can be effective as a once daily alpha/beta receptor blockade in selected patients. **Labetalol**, a nonselective beta blocker with alpha$_1$ receptor antagonism, is as effective as an oral or intravenous agent. This drug also may be used intravenously for treatment of hypertensive emergencies. Combinations of ACE inhibitors and alpha$_1$ receptor antagonists, when used carefully, may be useful in the absence of reduced blood volume or impaired cardiovascular reflexes. Theoretically, alpha$_1$ blockers might add to the antihypertensive action of either **verapamil** or **diltiazem**, the calcium-channel blockers with cardiac effects. Whether alpha$_1$ antagonists may be additive in combination with the dihydropyridine calcium-channel blockers has not been adequately studied. There may be some degree of overlap in the actions of these two classes because of the effect of alpha$_1$ receptors on transmembrane calcium entry channels.

INDICATIONS

	Doxazosin	Prazosin	Terazosin
Benign prostatic hypertrophy	+	—	+
Hypertension	+	+	+

+—FDA approved; —not FDA approved

DOXAZOSIN (Cardura®)

Doxazosin is structurally related to prazosin. Its long half-life, however, enables it to be used once daily. It is highly selective for alpha$_1$ adrenoceptors, with a ratio of affinities for alpha$_1$/alpha$_2$ of < 600. Interestingly, it does not appear to be characteristically associated with a first-dose effect, but this may reflect the more careful dose titration in the clinical studies. It has the beneficial effect on plasma lipid values characteristic of its class (Table 1.3). With its long duration of action, doxazosin once daily appears to be as effective as prazosin given twice daily and as beta blockers, ACE inhibitors, and calcium-channel blockers given once daily.

By blocking the alpha$_1$ receptors in the urinary bladder neck and prostatic urethra, doxazosin is effective in increasing urinary flow rates and alleviating outflow obstruction and irritation symptoms associated with benign prostatic hypertrophy (BPH) in both hypertensive and normotensive males. It is important to remember that doxazosin does not reverse the underlying pathophysiology of the disease. Also, prior to initiating doxazosin therapy for BPH, the patient should be examined to rule out the presence of prostatic malignancy.

SPECIAL GROUPS

Race: no differences in response
Children: safety and effectiveness have not been established
Elderly: more sensitive to hypotensive effect; dose should be titrated based on clinical response
Renal impairment: use with caution; dose should be titrated based on clinical response
Hepatic impairment: use with caution; dose should be titrated based on clinical response
Pregnancy: category C; should only be used if clearly indicated
Breast-feeding: use with caution; not known if the drug is excreted in human milk

DOSAGE

Benign prostatic hypertrophy: 1–8 mg once daily
Hypertension: 1–16 mg once daily
Doxazosin should be initiated at 1 mg/d (0.5 mg/d for the elderly) with blood pressure (BP) monitoring. The dose may be increased every 1–2 wk based on response. Careful BP monitoring for hypotension and orthostasis is recommended especially for the elderly. Maintenance dose may be divided and administered twice daily to reduce excessive BP response. If the therapy is discontinued for several days, therapy should be reinstituted with low dose and slowly increased based on the clinical response.

IN BRIEF

INDICATIONS
Benign prostatic hyperplasia (BPH)
Hypertension

CONTRAINDICATIONS
Known hypersensitivity to quinazolines, such as prazosin and terazosin

DRUG INTERACTIONS
Alcohol and any agents that may affect vascular tone or sodium/water homeostasis in the body:
Antihypertensive agents
Corticosteroids
Estrogen
Nonsteroidal anti-inflammatory drugs (NSAIDs)
Sympathomimetics

ADVERSE EFFECTS
CV: orthostatic or postural hypotension, syncope, palpitation, chest pain, edema, dyspnea
CNS: dizziness, drowsiness, fatigue, headache, vertigo
GU: impotence, priapism, urinary frequency
Skin: rash, pruritus, facial edema
Other: leukopenia/neutropenia, flu-like syndrome, hypersensitivity reaction

PHARMACOKINETICS AND PHARMACODYNAMICS
Duration of action: 24 h
Onset of action: 1–2 h
Peak effect: 5–6 h
Bioavailability: 65%
Effect of food: decrease peak concentration by 18% and the extent of absorption by 12%
Metabolism: metabolized by liver extensively; several active metabolites
Excretion: 9% in the urine and 63% in the feces; mainly as metabolites (4.8% unchanged)
Plasma half-life: 19-22 h
Protein binding: 98%–99%

MONITORING
Supine and sitting/standing BP, pulse function, complete blood count (CBC) with differential, urinary flow and dysuria (for BPH).

OVERDOSE
Supportive—consider fluid therapy with vasopressor added if necessary for profound hypotension.

PATIENT INFORMATION
Doxazosin can cause syncope, orthostatic problems, and drowsiness; avoid driving or performing hazardous tasks, especially within 24 h after the first dose or a dosage increment. Sit or lie down if dizziness occurs and rise slowly from a sitting or lying position.

AVAILABILITY
Tablets—1, 2, 4, 8 mg

PRAZOSIN

(Prazosin, Minipress®)

Prazosin is a selective alpha1-adrenoceptor blocker. Because its bioavailability varies and its half-life is relatively short, twice daily dosing is required for the conventional formulation. Sustained-release formulations may eventually be available. It is an effective antihypertensive agent, but its first-dose effect, its frequency of administration, and the difficulty of titration has limited its clinical usage.

The failure of the VHeFT study to demonstrate a beneficial effect of prazosin on mortality when compared with placebo in the treatment of CHF is supported by other trials. It is suspected that prazosin may induce tachyphylaxis in patients with CHF, even after short periods of treatment.

SPECIAL GROUPS

Race: no differences in response

Children: safety and effectiveness have not been established

Elderly: more sensitive to hypotensive effect; dose should be titrated based on clinical response

Renal impairment: use with caution; dose should be titrated based on clinical response

Hepatic impairment: use with caution; dose should be titrated based on clinical response

Pregnancy: category C; should only be used if clearly indicated

Breast-feeding: use with caution; excreted in human milk

DOSAGE

Prazosin should be initiated at 1 mg two to three times daily and slowly increased to the usual maintenance dose of 6–15 mg daily in divided doses. Most patients can be maintained on twice daily dosing after initial titration.

Maximum daily dose—40 mg; limited gain in efficacy for dose above 20 mg/d.

When adding a new antihypertensive agent or a diuretic, the dose of prazosin should be reduced to 1–2 mg 3 times daily and slowly increased based on blood pressure response.

If the therapy is discontinued for several days, therapy should be reinstituted with low dose and slowly increased based on the clinical response.

IN BRIEF

INDICATIONS
Hypertension

CONTRAINDICATIONS
Known hypersensitivity to quinazolines, such as doxazosin and terazosin

DRUG INTERACTIONS
Alcohol and any agents that may affect vascular tone or sodium/water homeostasis in the body:
 Antihypertensive agents
 Corticosteroids
 Estrogen
 NSAIDs
 Sympathomimetics

ADVERSE EFFECTS
CV: orthostatic or postural hypotension, syncope, palpitation, chest pain, edema, dyspnea
CNS: dizziness, drowsiness, fatigue, headache, vertigo, depression
GI: nausea, vomiting, diarrhea
GU: impotence, priapism, urinary frequency
Skin: rash, pruritus
Other: fever, positive antinuclear antibody (ANA) titer, hypersensitivity reaction

PHARMACOKINETICS AND PHARMACODYNAMICS
Duration of action: <24 h
Onset of action: <2 h
Peak effect: 2–4 h
Bioavailability: 43%–82% (mean 60%)
Effect of food: delayed absorption but no effect on the extent of absorption
Metabolism: metabolized in liver extensively, several active metabolites
Excretion: mainly via bile and feces as metabolites
Plasma half-life: 2–4 h
Protein binding: 97%

MONITORING
Supine and sitting/standing BP, pulse rate.

OVERDOSE
Supportive—consider fluid therapy with vasopressor added if necessary for profound hypotension.

PATIENT INFORMATION
Prazosin can cause syncope, orthostatic problems, and drowsiness; avoid driving or performing hazardous tasks, especially within 24 h after the first dose or a dosage increment. Sit or lie down if dizziness occurs and rise slowly from a sitting or lying position.

AVAILABILITY
Capsules—1, 2, 5 mg

TERAZOSIN   (HYTRIN®)

Terazosin is a selective alpha$_1$-adrenoceptor blocker with an alpha$_1$/alpha$_2$ affinity ratio of 200. Compared to prazosin, terazosin is approximately 25 times more water soluble and has 25 times less affinity for alpha$_1$ receptors. Similar to other alpha$_1$ blockers, terazosin reduces both resistance and capacitance vessel tone, which results in a concurrent afterload and preload reduction. When administered once or twice daily, it is an effective antihypertensive agent with the potential for advantageous effect on the plasma lipid profile. In clinical practice, terazosin is preferred to prazosin because of its more gradual onset of action and potential for once daily dosing. Orthostatic hypotension remains a problem. Terazosin is also effective in the management of symtomatic BPH and is the preferred antihypertensive agent in patients with BPH.

SPECIAL GROUPS

Race: no differences in response

Children: safety and effectiveness have not been established

Elderly: more sensitive to hypotensive effect; dose should be titrated based on clinical response

Renal impairment: use with caution; dose should be titrated based on clinical response

Hepatic impairment: use with caution; dose should be titrated based on clinical response

Pregnancy: category C; should only be used if clearly indicated

Breast-feeding: use with caution; not known if the drug is excreted in human milk

DOSAGE

BPH: Usual dose range—up to 10 mg/d at bedtime. Starting with 1 mg at bedtime, slowly increase the dose to achieve desired response, dose of 10 mg should be continued for a minimum of 4–6 wk to assess/determine the response.

Hypertension: Usual dose range—1–5 mg/d at bedtime. Starting with 1 mg at bedtime, slowly increase the dose to achieve desired BP response. Maximum daily dose is 40 mg; limited gain in efficacy for dose above 20 mg/d.

If the therapy is discontinued for several days, therapy should be re-instituted with low dose (1 mg) and slowly increased based on the clinical response. Maintenance dose may be divided and administered twice daily to reduce excessive BP response.

IN BRIEF

INDICATIONS
BPH

Hypertension

CONTRAINDICATIONS
Known hypersensitivity to quinazolines, such as doxazosin and prazosin

DRUG INTERACTIONS
Alcohol and any agents that may affect vascular tone or sodium/water homeostasis in the body:

Antihypertensive agents

Corticosteroids

Estrogen

NSAIDs

Sympathomimetics

ADVERSE EFFECTS
CV: orthostatic or postural hypotension, syncope, palpitation, tachycardia, chest pain, edema

CNS: dizziness, headache, drowsiness, fatigue, vertigo, paresthesia, depression

GI: nausea

GU: impotence, priapism, urinary frequency

Other: weight gain, fever, nasal congestion/rhinitis, flu-like syndrome, hypersensitivity reaction

PHARMACOKINETICS AND PHARMACODYNAMICS
Duration of action: >24 h

Onset of action: 15 min

Peak effect: 2–3 h

Bioavailability: 100%

Effect of food: delayed absorption, but no effect on the extent of absorption

Metabolism: mainly metabolized in the liver

Excretion: urine—40% (10% as unchanged drug); feces—60% (20% as unchanged drug)

Plasma half-life: 12 h

Protein binding: 90%–94%

MONITORING
Supine and sitting/standing BP, pulse rate, urinary flow or dysuria (for BPH).

OVERDOSE
Supportive—consider fluid therapy with vasopressor added if necessary for profound hypotension.

PATIENT INFORMATION
Terazosin can cause syncope and orthostatic problems; avoid driving or performing hazardous tasks, especially within 12–24 h after the first dose or a dosage increment. Sit or lie down if dizziness occurs and rise slowly from a sitting or lying position.

AVAILABILITY
Capsules—1, 2, 5, 10 mg

PHENOXYBENZAMINE (Dibenzyline®)

Phenoxybenzamine is a long-acting alpha-adrenergic blocker which can produce a "chemical sympathectomy" with oral use. It is used in patients with pheochromocytoma to control episodes of hypertension and sweating. It is also used in the preoperative management of patients with pheochromocytoma who are being prepared for surgery, and in chronic management of patients with malignant pheochromocytoma. The drug can induce a tachycardia, which requires the concomitant use of a beta blocker. The possibility of a tachycardia prohibits the routine use of phenoxybenzamine for systemic hypertension. Phenoxybenzamine has also been used to treat dysuria associated with neurogenic bladder, functional outlet obstruction, BPH, and postoperative urinary retention associated with the use of epidural morphine.

SPECIAL GROUPS

Race: no differences in response
Children: safety and effectiveness have not been established
Elderly: use with caution; dosage is adjusted based on clinical response
Renal impairment: use with caution; dosage is adjusted based on clinical response
Hepatic impairment: use with caution, dosage is adjusted based on clinical response
Pregnancy: category C; should only be used if clearly indicated
Breast-feeding: use with caution; not known if the drug is excreted in human milk

DOSAGE

Initial dose is 10 mg twice daily. Dose should be increased every other day by 10 mg until the desired response is achieved without significant side effects. Usual dose range is 20–40 mg 2–3 times daily.
Note: May be used concurrently with a beta-blocker if troublesome tachycardia coexists.

IN BRIEF

INDICATIONS
Pheochromocytoma to control hypertensive episodes and excessive sweating

CONTRAINDICATIONS
Hypersensitivity
Any conditions when a decrease in BP is undesirable

DRUG INTERACTIONS
Any agents that may affect BP or heart rate, such as sympathomimetic agents (excessive hypotension or tachycardia)

ADVERSE EFFECTS
CV: hypotension, tachycardia, arrhythmias, orthostatic problem
CNS: drowsiness, fatigue
GI: irritation, dyspepsia
GU: inhibition of ejection
Other: nasal congestion, miosis

PHARMACOKINETICS AND PHARMACODYNAMICS
Duration of action: 3–4 d (single dose)
Onset of action: few hours
Peak effect: 7 d after repeated dosing
Bioavailability: 20%–30%
Effect of food: not known
Metabolism: mainly in the liver
Excretion: urine and bile
Plasma half-life: 24 h
Protein binding: not known

MONITORING
BP, pulse rate, sweat reduction.

OVERDOSE
Supportive—fluid therapy or norepinephrine may be used in severe hypotension. Other vasopressors are not effective, and epinephrine is contraindicated.

PATIENT INFORMATION
Phenoxybenzamine may cause a significant lowering of BP. Sit or lie down if dizziness occurs and rise slowly from a sitting or lying position.

AVAILABILITY
Capsules—10 mg

PHENTOLAMINE (Regitine®)

Phentolamine is a short-acting, nonselective alpha-adrenergic blocking agent. Its effect is derived by antagonizing the effects of circulating epinephrine or norepinephrine. Phentolamine causes peripheral vasodilation and a reduction in peripheral vascular resistance. It also exhibits some beta-adrenergic activity that contributes to its positive inotropic and chronotropic effect. Phentolamine is used mainly in the management of pheochromocytoma to control or prevent paroxysmal hypertension prior to and during pheochromocytomectomy. It is also used to prevent or treat extravasation associated with intravenous norepinephrine. In addition, phentolamine may be used to treat hypertensive crises caused by sympathomimetic amines or catecholamine excess associated with monoamine oxidase inhibitors. A mixture of phentolamine and papaverine injected into the corpus cavernosum of the penis has been effective in patients with erectile dysfunction.

SPECIAL GROUPS

Race: no differences in response

Children: use safely in children with pheochromocytoma (reduced dose)

Elderly: no dosage adjustment is required

Renal impairment: use with caution; dose adjustment is not required

Hepatic impairment: use with caution; dose adjustment is not required

Pregnancy: category C; should only be used if clearly indicated

Breast-feeding: use with caution; not known if the drug is excreted in human milk

DOSAGE

Prevention/Control of hypertensive episodes associated with pheochromocytoma:

Preoperative—5 mg administered intravenously (IV) or intramuscularly (IM) 1–2 h before surgery and repeated if indicated.

Intraoperative—5 mg IV and repeat as indicated to prevent or control hypertension, tachycardia, respiratory depression, convulsions, or other effects related to epinephrine intoxication.

Prevention/Treatment of dermal necrosis and sloughing associated with IV norepinephrine:

Prevention—10 mg of phentolamine is added to each liter of norepinephrine solution.

Treatment—initiate within 12 h (as soon as possible) of extravasation; 5–10 mg of phentolamine in 10 mL of saline is infiltrated into the area using a small needle syringe.

Diagnosis of pheochromocytoma (not the first test of choice; all nonessential medications should be withheld for at least 24 h prior to the test): 5 mg IV (preferred) or IM is administered; after the IV dose, BP should be monitored immediately, every 30 s for the first 3 min, and every minute for the next 7 min; after IM dose, BP should be monitored every 5 min for 30–45 min. A BP decrease of at least 35 mm Hg systolic and 25 mm Hg diastolic within 2 min after IV or 20 min after IM administration of phentolamine is considered a positive test for pheochromocytoma.

IN BRIEF

INDICATIONS
Pheochromocytoma—prevention or control of hypertensive episodes; diagnostic test

Prevention or treatment of dermal necrosis and sloughing associated with intravenous administration or extravasation of norepinephrine

CONTRAINDICATIONS
Coronary artery disease

Hypersensitivity

Myocardial infarction

DRUG INTERACTIONS
Any agents that may affect BP or heart rate.

ADVERSE EFFECTS
CV: hypotension, tachycardia, arrhythmias, orthostatic problem

CNS: weakness, dizziness

GI: nausea, vomiting, diarrhea

Other: nasal congestion

PHARMACOKINETICS AND PHARMACODYNAMICS
Duration of action: 15–30 min (IV); 30–45 min (IM)

Onset of action: immediate

Peak effect: < 2 min (IV); 20 min (IM)

Bioavailability: 100%

Effect of food: not applicable

Clearance: metabolized in liver; 13% is excreted in urine unchanged

Plasma half-life: 19 min (IV)

Protein binding: not known

MONITORING
BP, pulse rate and specific clinical response as per indication.

OVERDOSE
Supportive—phentolamine has short duration of action. Fluid therapy or norepinephrine may be used in severe hypotension. Other vasopressors are not effective and epinephrine is contraindicated.

PATIENT INFORMATION
Phentolamine may cause a significant lowering of BP. Sit or lie down if dizziness occurs and rise slowly from a sitting or lying position.

AVAILABILITY
Vials—5 mg

The information here is provided as guidance only. Prescribers should always consult the manufacturer's current prescribing information.

9

SUGGESTED BIBLIOGRAPHY

Axelrod FB, Krey L, Glickstein JS, *et al.*: Preliminary observations on the use of midodrine in treating orthostatic hypotension in familial dysautonomia. *J Auton Nerv Syst* 1995, 55:29–35.

Baba T, Tomiyama T, Takebe K: Enhancement by an ACE inhibitor of first-dose hypotension caused by an alpha-1 blocker. *N Engl J Med* 1990, 322:1237.

Cohn JN, Archibald DG, Ziesche S, *et al.*: Effect of vasodilator therapy on mortality in chronic congestive heart failure: results of a Veterans Administration Cooperative Study. *N Engl J Med* 1986, 314:1547–1552.

Fouad-Tarazi FM, Okabe M, Goren J: Alpha sympathomimetic treatment of autonomic insufficiency with orthostatic hypotension. *Am J Med* 1995, 90:604–610.

Frishman WH: Alpha- and beta-adrenergic blocking drugs. In *Cardiovascular Pharmacotherapeutics Companion Handbook*. Edited by Frishman WH, Sonnenblick EH. New York: McGraw Hill; 1998, 23–64.

Frishman WH, Kotob F: α-Adrenergic blocking drugs in clinical medicine. *J Clin Pharmacol* 1999, 39:7–16.

Frishman WH, Shevell T: Drug therapy for orthostatic hypotension and vasovagal syncope. In *Cardiovascular Pharmacotherapeutics*. Edited by Frishman WH, Sonnenblick EH. New York: McGraw Hill; 1997:1231–1246.

Hoffman BB, Lefkowitz RJ: Adrenergic receptor antagonists. In *Goodman and Gilman's The Pharmacologic Basis of Therapeutics*. Edited by Gilman AG, Rall TW, Nies AS, Taylor P. New York: Pergamon Press; 1990:221–228.

Lepor H, Meretyk S, Knapp-Maloney G: The safety, efficacy and compliance of terazosin therapy for benign prostatic hypertrophy. *J Urol* 1992, 147:1554–1557.

Minneman KP: Alpha 1-adrenergic receptor subtypes, inositol phosphates and sources of cell Ca^{2+}. *Pharm Rev* 1988, 40:87–119.

Mobley DF, Dias N, Levenstein M: Effects of doxazosin in patients with mild, intermediate and severe benign prostatic hyperplasia. *Clin Ther* 1998, 20:101–109.

Mobley DF, Kaplain SA, Ice K, *et al.*: Effect of doxazosin on the symptoms of benign prostatic hyperplasia: results from three double-blind placebo-controlling studies. *Int J Clin Pract* 1997, 51:282–288.

Neaton JD, Grimm RH Jr, Prineas RJ, *et al.*: Treatment of mild hypertension study: final results. *JAMA* 1993, 207:713–724.

Pllare T, Lithell H, Selinus I, Berne C: Application of prazosin is associated with an increase of insulin sensitivity in obese patients with hypertension. *Diabetologia* 1988, 31:415–420.

Shieh S-M, Sheu WH-H, Shen DD-C, *et al.*: Glucose, insulin and lipid metabolism in doxazosin-treated patients with hypertension. *Am J Hypertens* 1992, 5:827–831.

Terazosin for benign prostatic hyperplasia. *Medical Letter* 1994, 36:15–16.

ALPHA$_2$-ADRENERGIC AGONISTS (CENTRALLY ACTING ANTIHYPERTENSIVE AGENTS)

Centrally acting inhibitors of the sympathetic nervous system have been available for the treatment of hypertension for nearly 40 years. This clinical use has been limited because of the central sedative and depressive effects associated with the antihypertensive action of these drugs. The search continues for similar acting drugs that do not produce these unwanted effects.

EFFICACY AND USE

The centrally acting antihypertensive agents can be highly effective when used alone. They are equally effective in treating hypertension in the young and in the elderly. They are especially effective in treating isolated systolic hypertension, which usually occurs in the elderly. The agents appear to be equally effective in treating hypertension in black and white patients. Their record is good in the treatment of hypertensive patients with coexisting diabetes or renal dysfunction. They appear to have little or no deleterious effect on glucose tolerance or renal function, with no effect on the lipid profile of treated patients. Thus, the range of patients suitable for these drugs is broad and specific, and contraindications to their use are few. Table 2.1 shows the relative differences between the centrally acting drugs and the first-line antihypertensive agents.

The centrally acting agents appear to reduce left ventricular hypertrophy and to enhance diastolic function to some extent. The main limitation to their use is their unwanted central effects, which may impair quality of life for some patients.

These agents work synergistically with diuretics when an additional antihypertensive effect is required. They have been used successfully with beta blockers. However, abrupt drug withdrawal, especially with clonidine, can cause blood pressure exacerbation due to rebound hypertension and should be avoided. Their hemodynamic effects are shown in Table 2.2.

TABLE 2.1 CLINICAL EFFECTS OF THREE TYPES OF ANTIHYPERTENSIVE THERAPY

	Centrally acting agents	Beta blockers	Diuretics
Young patients	Effective	Effective	Somewhat less effective
Elderly patients	Effective	Somewhat less effective	Effective
Black patients	Effective	Somewhat less effective	Effective
White patients	Effective	Effective	Somewhat less effective
Patients with concurrent diabetes mellitus	Well tolerated and effective	Caution required with non-selective drugs in insulin-dependent patients	May influence concurrent diabetes therapy- increased insulin required
Patients with concurrent plasma lipid abnormalities	Cholesterol decreased	Possible increase in plasma triglycerides and decrease in HDL (greatest with non-selective drugs)	Increase in total cholesterol and LDL. Decrease in serum potassium and impaired glucose tolerance

HDL—high-density lipoprotein; LDL—low-density lipoprotein.

TABLE 2.2 HEMODYNAMIC EFFECTS OF CENTRALLY ACTING AGENTS

Agent	Cardiac output	Plasma volume	Glomerular filtration rate	Orthostasis	Total peripheral vascular resistance	Plasma renin activity
Clonidine	↑	← →	← →	no	↓	↓ or ← →
Guanabenz	↓	← →	← →	mild	↓	↓ or ← →
Guanfacine	↓	← →	← →	mild	↓	↓ or ← →
Methyldopa	—	↑	← →	mild	↓	↓

↑—increase; ↓—decrease; ← →—no change.

MODE OF ACTION

Clonidine, methyldopa, guanabenz, and guanfacine appear to have a common mechanism of action. By various means, they stimulate the $alpha_2$ adrenoceptors in the vasomotor center of the medulla oblongata, with the result that sympathetic out-flow from the brain is inhibited (Fig. 2.1). In the case of methyl-dopa, this does not occur directly. Instead, methyldopa is me-tabolized to alpha methylnoradrenaline, in the brain. The pro-duction of this false neurotransmitter from methyldopa at peripheral sites in the body may explain some of its antihyper-tensive effects. The other drugs in this group do not appear to require biotransformation for activity, but are rather direct-act-ing central $alpha_2$-adrenoceptor stimulants. Stimulation of presy-naptic $alpha_2$ receptors on peripheral adrenergic neurons may make some contribution to the antihypertensive action.

After the bolus intravenous administration, clonidine tends to produce a transient rise in blood pressure (BP). This response is a result of stimulation of peripheral $alpha_2$ recep-tors on blood vessels. Thereafter, BP falls as central $alpha_2$ receptors are stimulated.

INDICATIONS

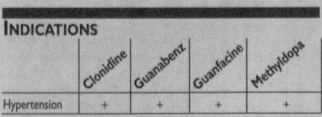

	Clonidine	Guanabenz	Guanfacine	Methyldopa
Hypertension	+	+	+	+

+—FDA approved.

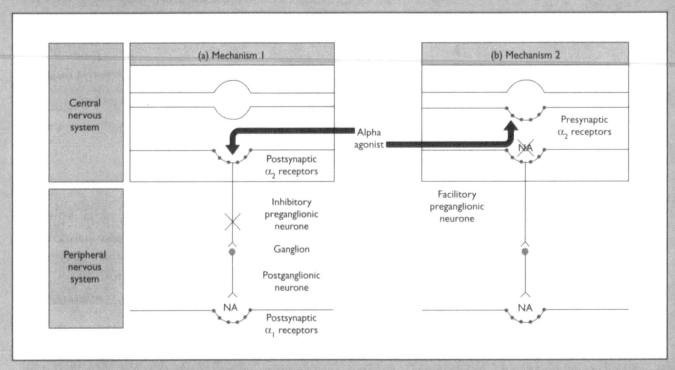

FIGURE 2.1 The interaction of clonidine and related drugs with post- and presynaptic alpha receptors in the brainstem as a basis for their central hypotensive effect. Two possible mechanisms are shown: (a) Clonidine stimulates postsynaptic $alpha_2$-receptors; the inhibitory bul-bospinal neuron is activated and peripheral sympathetic nervous activ-ity is diminished, which causes a hypotensive effect: (b) Clonidine stim-ulates presynaptic $alpha_2$-receptors, diminishing release of central no-radrenaline (NA); the facilitatory neuron is activated less and peripheral sympathetic activity is diminished, causing a hypotensive effect. The first mechanism (a) is most likely correct. (*Adapted from* Van Zwieten PA: The role of adrenoceptors in circulatory and metabolic regulation. *Am Heart J* 1988; 116:1384-92.)

CLONIDINE (Clonidine, Catapres®, Duraclon®)

Clonidine stimulates alpha₂-adrenergic receptors in the central nervous system (CNS), which results in a decrease in sympathetic outflow from the brain. This, in turn, results in reduced peripheral sympathetic nervous system activity, reduction of BP, and bradycardia. The alpha₂-agonist activity of clonidine is also responsible for its side effects, such as sedation and dry mouth. Clonidine has been used as an adjunct to alleviate withdrawal symptoms in individuals with opioid or nicotine dependence. By stimulating central presynaptic alpha₂-adrenergic receptors, clonidine causes a reduction in adrenergic activity in the CNS, which may be responsible for the withdrawal symptoms. Clonidine is usually administered as oral tablets or the transdermal system. The latter formulation is applied to the skin once weekly, which may provide more consistent BP control and improve patient compliance. Clonidine is also available as an injectable for the management of severe cancer pain only. For this indication, clonidine is used in combination with an opiate and is administered via an epidural infusion device.

SPECIAL GROUPS

Race: no differences in response
Children: safety and effectiveness have not been established
Elderly: use with caution; start with low dose and titrate based on response
Renal impairment: dosage reduction by 25%–50% is recommended in severe renal impairment (creatinine clearance <10 mL/min)
Hepatic impairment: no dosage adjustment is required
Pregnancy: category C; should only be used if clearly indicated
Breast-feeding: not recommended; drug is excreted in human milk

DOSAGE

Oral: Usual dose range: 0.2–2.4 mg/d in two to three divided doses.
Initial dose is 0.5–1 mg twice a day; the dose may be increased by 0.1–0.2 mg daily every few days until the desired response is achieved. For rapid BP reduction in patients with severe hypertension, clonidine 0.1–0.2 mg may be given, followed by 0.05–0.2 mg every hour until a total dose of 0.5–0.7 mg or adequate BP control is achieved. Then, maintenance dose of clonidine is administered and adjusted based on clinical assessment.
Transdermal: 0.1–0.6 mg/d, applied weekly to a hairless area of intact skin on the upper outer arm or chest. There is no predictable relationship between the effective oral dose and transdermal dose of clonidine. All patients, including those who have been receiving oral clonidine, should be started with one 0.1 mg/d system applied to a hairless skin area on the upper outer arm or chest every 7 d. If the desired BP control is not achieved, the dose may be increased every 1–2 wk by 0.1 mg/d up to a maximum of 0.6 mg/d (two transdermal 0.3 mg/d systems). Each new transdermal system should be applied to a different site from the previous location. *Note:* For patients who are already on oral clonidine, it is recommended that the oral dose be continued for 1–2 d after the first transdermal system is applied.
Intravenous: For hypertensive crisis (not an FDA-approved indication), clonidine 0.15–0.3 mg has been given intravenously over 5 min* with an initial goal of reducing mean arterial BP by ≤ 25% within the first 2 hours, followed by further reduction toward the target BP of 160/100 mm Hg within 2–6 h.
* Slow intravenous administration can minimize the possible hypertension that may precede its hypotensive effect.

IN BRIEF

INDICATIONS
Hypertension (oral and transdermal)
Severe cancer pain not adequately relieved by opioid analgesics alone (continuous epidural infusion)

CONTRAINDICATIONS
Known hypersensitivity

DRUG INTERACTIONS
CNS depressants, such as alcohol, opiates, barbiturates
Tricyclic antidepressants, such as imipramine, desipramine
Monoamine oxidase (MAO) inhibitors
Digoxin
Calcium channel blockers
Beta blockers
Other antihypertensive agents

ADVERSE EFFECTS
CV: hypotension, tachycardia, bradycardia, Raynaud's symptoms, heart failure, AV block, arrhythmias, orthostatic symptoms, syncope, rebound hypertension
CNS: sedation, dizziness, headache, nervousness, agitation, depression, sleep disturbances, hallucinations, delirium
GI: dry mouth, constipation, nausea, vomiting, anorexia, liver function abnormality
GU: impotence, ↓ libido, urinary frequency
Skin: rash, pruritus, hives, angioedema, contact dermatitis (transdermal system only)
Other: ↑ sensitivity to alcohol, dry eyes, blurred vision, dry nasal mucosa, weight gain

PHARMACOKINETICS AND PHARMACODYNAMICS
Duration of action: (po) >8–12 h; (IV) 4 h; (topical) few days
Onset of action: (po/IV) 30–60 min
Peak effect: (po/IV) 2–4 h; (topical) 2–3 d
Bioavailability: (po) 75%–100%
Effect of food: not known
Metabolism: (po) 50% metabolized in liver
Excretion: renal—65%–72% (32%–36% unchanged); feces—20%
Plasma half-life: 12–16 h (up to 41 h in endstage renal disease)
Protein binding: 20%–40%

MONITORING
BP and drug intolerance.

OVERDOSE
Supportive-atropine for bradycardia; fluid therapy and vasopressor therapy, such as dopamine for profound hypotension; vasodilators, such as phentolamine, as needed for severe hypertension.

PATIENT INFORMATION
Clonidine therapy should not be discontinued abruptly without consulting a physician. Sedation associated with the therapy may impair the ability to perform hazardous activities requiring mental alertness or physical coordination. Concurrent alcohol intake may enhance the sedative effect. Sit or lie down if dizziness occurs and rise slowly from a sitting or lying position.

AVAILABILITY
Tablets—0.1, 0.2, 0.3 mg
Transdermal System—
  TTS-1: 0.1 mg/24 h (2.5 mg/3.5 cm²)
  TTS-2: 0.2 mg/24 h (5 mg/7 cm²)
  TTS-3: 0.3 mg/24 h (7.5 mg/10.5 cm²)
Vials–1 mg/10 mL (100 µg/mL), preservative free
Combination Formulations (with a diuretic):
  Combipres Tablets—
    0.1 mg clonidine and 15 mg chlorthalidone
    0.2 mg clonidine and 15 mg chlorthalidone
    0.3 mg clonidine and 15 mg chlorthalidone

GUANABENZ (Guanabenz, Wytensin®)

Guanabenz, similar to clonidine, is a central alpha$_2$-adrenergic agonist. Its antihypertensive effect is mediated via stimulation of alpha$_2$-adrenergic receptors in the central nervous system which results in a decrease in sympathetic outflow. Chronic guanabenz therapy is associated with a decrease in peripheral resistance and heart rate while cardiac output and left ventricular ejection fraction remain unchanged. Similar BP reduction is observed in both supine and standing positions. This may account for less orthostatic problems reported with guanabenz therapy.

SPECIAL GROUPS

Race: no differences in response

Children: safety and effectiveness have not been established

Elderly: use with caution; start with low dose and titrate based on clinical response

Renal impairment: use with caution; titrate based on clinical response

Hepatic impairment: use with caution; start with low dose and titrate based on clinical response

Pregnancy: category C; should only be used if clearly indicated

Breast-feeding: not recommended; not known if the drug is excreted in human milk

DOSAGE

Usual dose range: 8–32 mg/d, in two divided doses.

The initial dose is 2–4 mg twice daily. The dosage may be increased in increments of 4–8 mg/d every 1–2 wk (or longer) based on BP response.

IN BRIEF

INDICATIONS
Hypertension

CONTRAINDICATIONS
Known hypersensitivity

DRUG INTERACTIONS
CNS depressants, such as alcohol, opiates, barbiturates

Tricyclic antidepressants, such as imipramine, desipramine

MAO inhibitors

Digoxin

Calcium channel blockers

Beta blockers

Other antihypertensive agents

ADVERSE EFFECTS
CV: hypotension, tachycardia, bradycardia, chest pain, heart failure, edema, AV block, arrhythmias, orthostatic symptoms, rebound hypertension

CNS: sedation, dizziness, weakness, headache, nervousness, agitation, depression, tremor, sleep disturbances, confusion

GI: dry mouth, constipation, nausea, vomiting, anorexia, abnormal liver function test

GU: urinary frequency, sexual dysfunction

Skin: rash, pruritus

Other: ↑ sensitivity to alcohol, dry eyes, blurred vision, nasal congestion, weight gain

PHARMACOKINETICS AND PHARMACODYNAMICS
Duration of action: 10–12 h or longer

Onset of action: < 1 h

Peak effect: 2–7 h

Bioavailability: 70%–80%

Effect of food: not known

Metabolism: extensively metabolized in liver

Excretion: urine— 70%–80% (1% unchanged)
feces— 10%–30%

Plasma half-life: 12–14 hours

Protein binding: 90%

MONITORING
BP and drug intolerance.

OVERDOSE
Supportive—atropine for bradycardia; fluid therapy and vasopressor therapy, such as dopamine for profound hypotension if necessary.

PATIENT INFORMATION
Guanabenz therapy should not be discontinued abruptly without consulting a physician. Sedation associated with the therapy may impair the ability to perform hazardous activities requiring mental alertness or physical coordination. Concurrent alcohol intake may enhance the sedative effect. Sit or lie down if dizziness occurs and rise slowly from a sitting or lying position.

AVAILABILITY
Tablets—4, 8 mg

GUANFACINE (Guanfacine, Tenex®)

Guanfacine is a long-acting, central alpha$_2$-adrenergic agonist. Its mechanism of action is similar to clonidine and guanabenz. With chronic guanfacine therapy, peripheral vascular resistance is reduced and heart rate is slightly decreased with minimum effect on cardiac output. Abrupt withdrawal of guanfacine therapy has been associated with less rebound hypertension secondary to its long half-life and longer duration of action. The BP usually increases slowly back to pretreatment baseline level over 2–4 d after discontinuation of guanfacine.

SPECIAL GROUPS

Race: no differences in response

Children: safety and effectiveness have not been established

Elderly: use with caution; start with low dose and titrate based on clinical response

Renal impairment: use with caution; start with low dose and titrate based on clinical response

Hepatic impairment: use with caution; start with low dose and titrate based on clinical response

Pregnancy: category B; should only be used if clearly indicated

Breast-feeding: use with caution; not known if the drug is excreted in human milk

DOSAGE

Usual dose range: 1–3 mg once daily at bedtime.

The initial dose is 1 mg administered at bedtime to minimize somnolence. The dose may be increased in 1 mg increments every 3–4 wk if adequate BP control is not achieved, up to the maximum of 3 mg/d.

IN BRIEF

INDICATIONS
Hypertension

CONTRAINDICATIONS
Known hypersensitivity

DRUG INTERACTIONS
CNS depressants, such as alcohol, opiates, barbiturates
Tricyclic antidepressants, such as imipramine, desipramine
MAO inhibitors
Digoxin
Calcium channel blockers
Beta blockers
Other antihypertensive agents
Phenytoin
Phenobarbital

ADVERSE EFFECTS
CV: hypotension, tachycardia, bradycardia, chest pain, heart failure, edema, AV block, arrhythmias, orthostatic symptoms, rebound hypertension
CNS: sedation, dizziness, weakness, headache, nervousness, agitation, depression, tremor, sleep disturbances, confusion
GI: dry mouth, constipation, nausea, vomiting, anorexia, abnormal liver function test, taste alteration
GU: urinary incontinence/ frequency, sexual dysfunction
Skin: rash, pruritus, dermatitis, conjunctivitis
Other: ↑ sensitivity to alcohol, dry eyes, blurred vision, weight gain

PHARMACOKINETICS AND PHARMACODYNAMICS
Duration of action:	24 h or longer
Onset of action:	2 h
Peak effect:	6 h
Bioavailability:	80%
Effect of food:	not known
Metabolism:	50% metabolized
Excretion:	urine (40%–75% as unchanged)
Plasma half-life:	17 h (10–30 h)
Protein binding:	70%

MONITORING
BP and drug intolerance.

OVERDOSE
Supportive—atropine for bradycardia; fluid therapy and vasopressor therapy, such as dopamine for profound hypotension if necessary.

PATIENT INFORMATION
Guanfacine therapy should not be discontinued abruptly without consulting a physician. Sedation associated with the therapy may impair the ability to perform hazardous activities requiring mental alertness or physical coordination. Concurrent alcohol intake may enhance the sedative effect. Sit or lie down if dizziness occurs and rise slowly from a sitting or lying position.

AVAILABILITY
Tablets—1, 2 mg

The information here is provided as guidance only. Prescribers should always consult the manufacturer's current prescribing information.

15

METHYLDOPA, METHYLDOPATE HCL

(Methyldopa, Methyldopate HCl, Aldomet®)

Methyldopa is converted to alpha-methylnorepinephrine, an alpha$_2$-adrenergic agonist, in the CNS. This indirect central alpha$_2$-adrenergic stimulation has been proposed as the major mechanism responsible for the antihypertensive effect of chronic methyldopa therapy. In addition, methyldopa inhibits decarboxylase, which is responsible for the conversion of norepinephrine and serotonin from their precursors in the CNS and peripheral tissues. Plasma methyldopa concentrations do not correlate well with its therapeutic effect. The onset and maximum decrease in blood pressure occurs in 3–6 h after oral administration. Similar to oral methyldopa, intravenous methyldopate has a relatively slow onset of hypotensive action (3–6 h). Although intravenous methyldopate has been used in hypertensive emergencies, other antihypertensive agents with more rapid onset of action are preferred when a rapid blood pressure reduction is indicated. Methyldopa has been used effectively for the management of hypertension during pregnancy with minimum adverse effects on the fetus.

SPECIAL GROUPS

Race: no differences in response
Children: safety and effectiveness have been established
Elderly: use with caution; start with low dose and titrate based on clinical response
Renal impairment: use with caution; start with low dose and titrate based on clinical response
Hepatic impairment: use with caution; start with low dose and titrate based on clinical response
Pregnancy: category B (IV) and C (po); although it has been used safely in the third trimester, used only if clearly indicated
Breast-feeding: use with caution; excreted in human milk in negligible amounts.

DOSAGE

Oral (methyldopa): Usual dose range: 500–3000 mg/d in 2 to 4 divided doses. The initial dose is 250 mg 2 to 3 times daily for 2 d. The dose is then adjusted at intervals of at least 2 d until a desired response is achieved.
Intravenous (methyldopate): Usual dose range: 250–500 mg every 6 h Maximum dose: 1000 mg every 6 h

IN BRIEF

INDICATIONS
Hypertension

CONTRAINDICATIONS
Active hepatitis/ cirrhosis
Known hypersensitivity to methyldopa or sulfites
Concurrent MAO inhibitor therapy

DRUG INTERACTIONS
Other antihypertensive agents	Lithium carbonate	Norepinephrine
Phenothiazine	MAO inhibitors	General anesthetics
Tricyclic antidepressant agents	Iron supplements	Levodopa

ADVERSE EFFECTS
CV: hypotension, orthostatic symptoms, syncope, bradycardia, chest pain, heart failure, edema, rebound hypertension
CNS: sedation, ↓ mental acuity, paresthesia, Parkinsonism, sleep disorders, psychosis, depression, abnormal choreoathetotic movements
GI: dry mouth, nausea, vomiting, diarrhea, constipation, abnormal liver function test, drug-induced hepatitis, pancreatitis, tongue ulceration
GU: sexual dysfunction
Blood: positive Coombs' test, hemolytic anemia (rare), hemolysis (in glucose-6-phosphate dehydrogenase deficiency)
Skin: rash, urticaria, eczema, ulceration
Other: weight gain, drug-induced fever, flu-like syndrome, nasal congestion

PHARMACOKINETICS AND PHARMACODYNAMICS
Duration of action: (po) 24–48 h; (IV)10–16 h
Onset of action: 3–6 h
Peak effect: 4–6 h
Bioavailability: (po) 25%–50%; (IV) 100%
Effect of food: not known
Metabolism: extensively metabolized, liver–50%
Excretion: urine—70% as metabolites
feces—30%–50%
Plasma half-life: 90–127 min
Protein binding: negligible

MONITORING
BP (both supine and sitting/standing);
Lab—CBC, liver function test, and direct Coombs' test.

OVERDOSE
Supportive—fluid therapy and vasopressor therapy, such as norepinephrine or dopamine, for profound hypotension and atropine for bradycardia; methyldopa is dialyzable.

PATIENT INFORMATION
Methyldopa therapy should not be discontinued abruptly without consulting a physician. Sedation associated with the therapy may impair the ability to perform hazardous activities requiring mental alertness or physical coordination (especially within the first 2–3 d of therapy or dose increase). Concurrent alcohol intake may enhance the sedative effect. Sit or lie down if dizziness occurs and rise slowly from a sitting or lying position.

AVAILABILITY
Tablets—125, 250, 500 mg
Suspension—250 mg/5 mL, 473 mL
Vials—250 mL/5 mL, injectable (methyldopate HCl)
Combination formulations (with a diuretic):
Aldoclor® Tablets—
250 mg methyldopa
250 mg chlorothiazide
Aldoril® Tablets—
250 mg methyldopa
15 mg hydrochlorothiazide
250 mg methyldopa
25 mg hydrochlorothiazide
Aldoril® D Tablets—
500 mg methyldopa
30 mg hydrochlorothiazide
500 mg methyldopa
50 mg hydrochlorothiazide

SUGGESTED BIBLIOGRAPHY

Cressman MD, Vlasses PH: Recent issues in antihypertensive drug therapy. *Med Clin North Am* 1988; 72:373–98.

Croog SH, Levine S, Testa MA, *et al*: The effects of antihypertensive therapy on the quality of life. *N Engl J Med* 1986; 314:1657–64.

Farsang CS: Update on methyldopa. *Ther Hung* 1986; 34:139–49.

Frishman WH, Katz B: Controlled-release drug delivery system in cardiovascular disease treatment. In *Cardiovascular Pharmacotherapeutics*. Edited by Frishman WH, Sonnerblick EH. New York: McGraw Hill; 1997,1363–1373.

Kaplan NM: Treatment of hypertension: drug therapy. In Kaplan NM (ed): *Clinical Hypertension*. Baltimore: Williams &Wilkins; 1994: 211–16.

Krakoff LR: Antiadrenergic drugs with central action, ganglionic blockers, and neuron depletors. In *Cardiovascular Pharmacotherapeutics*. Edited by Frishman WH, Sonnenblick EH. New York: McGraw Hill; 1997, 220–227.

Leonetti G: Centrally acting antihypertensive agents. *J Cardiovasc Pharmacol* 1988; 12 (Suppl 8):S68–73.

Lowenthal DT, Matzek KM, MacGregor TR: Clinical pharmacokinetics of clonidine. *Clin Pharmacokinet* 1988; 14:287–310.

Sorkin BM, Heel RC: Guanfacine. *Drugs* 1986; 31:301–306.

Struthers AD, Dollery CT: Central nervous system mechanism in blood pressure control. *Eur J Clin Pharmacol* 1985; 28 (Suppl):3–11.

Van Zwieten PA: The role of adrenoceptors in circulatory and metabolic regulation. *Am Heart J* 1988; 116:1384–92.

Weber MA: Clinical pharmacology of centrally acting antihypertensive agents. *J Clin Pharmacol* 1989; 29:698–602.

Weber MA, Draye JIM: Centrally acting antihypertensive agents: a brief overview. *J Cardiovasc Pharmacol* 1984; 6 (Suppl):S803–07.

Weber MA, Graethinger WF, Cheung DG: Centrally acting antihypertensive agents. In Kaplan NM, Brenner BM, Laragh JH (eds): *New Therapeutic Strategies in Hypertension*. New York: Raven Press; 1989: 33–50.

Angiotensin-converting enzyme (ACE) inhibitors have been available for more than a decade for clinical use to treat hypertension and congestive heart failure (CHF). An intravenous agent, **enalaprilat**, has been approved by the Food and Drug Administration (FDA) for use in hypertension, and ten oral agents—**benazepril, captopril, enalapril, fosinopril, lisinopril, moexipril, perindopril, quinapril, ramipril, and trandolapril**—are approved and available in the United States. **Spirapril** has also been approved by the FDA for the treatment of hypertension; however, this agent has not been marketed by the pharmaceutical industry at press time. All ACE inhibitors are similar in their effects, differing principally in their pharmacokinetics and approved indications.

EFFICACY AND USE
Hypertension
ACE inhibitors offer an important therapeutic option for hypertension, either as first-line treatment or when other more established drugs are contraindicated or do not have the desired effect (Table 3.1). Repeated clinical studies have demonstrated the efficacy of ACE inhibitors in lowering blood pressure (BP) and their ability to reduce left ventricular hypertrophy. They are effective and particularly well tolerated in mild to moderate hypertension (both primary and secondary). They do not disturb plasma lipid concentration and may improve insulin sensitivity and glucose tolerance.

As monotherapy, ACE inhibitors have similar efficacy to beta blockers and diuretics, but large-scale studies tend to show some narrow superiority of ACE inhibitors, usually with regard to systolic blood pressure and possibly as a result of improved arterial compliance. Long-acting ACE inhibitors may provide better blood pressure control than short-acting ones. ACE inhibitors are particularly effective when combined with a low dose of a thiazide diuretic, in which case they offset hypokalemia; however, they may increase potassium levels in the presence of potassium-sparing agents. They have additive antihypertensive effects with calcium antagonists, but less so with beta blockers.

Heart Failure
ACE inhibitors are also used to treat CHF. By removing renin-angiotensin–mediated vasoconstriction (which frequently underlies the increased afterload on the heart associated with this syndrome), they produce favorable and sustained hemodynamic changes. The CONSENSUS I study demonstrated that the addition of **enalapril** to the treatment of patients with severe heart failure (New York Heart Association class IV) who were already treated with digitalis, diuretics, and (in some cases) other vasodilators produced a significant reduction in mortality compared with addition of placebo (Fig. 3.1). ACE inhibition reduced death caused by progression of heart failure but had no impact on the rate of sudden death.

ACE inhibitors also benefit patients with mild to moderate CHF (class II–III). The treatment arm of the SOLVD study showed

TABLE 3.1 COMPLICATED HYPERTENSIVE PATIENTS PARTICULARLY SUITED TO TREATMENT WITH ANGIOTENSIN-CONVERTING ENZYME INHIBITORS	
Concurrent condition	**Reason for use of angiotensin-converting enzyme inhibitor**
Asthma	No effect on airway resistance
Diabetes	No important effect on glycemic control or insulin resistance; reduces signs of progression of diabetic nephropathy
Gout	Reduces uric acid levels
Chronic heart failure	Improves symptoms, hemodynamics, and survival
Post myocardial infarction	Reduces morbidity and mortality caused by cardiovascular events

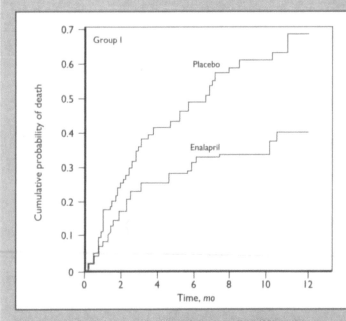
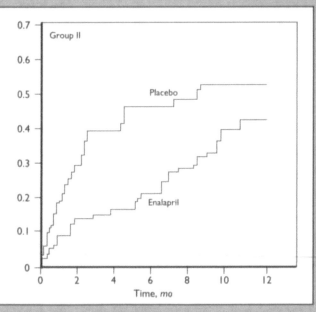

FIGURE 3.1 Cumulative probability of death in CONSENSUS I in patients not taking vasodilators (group I) and those taking vasodilators (group II) at the time of random assignment. (*Adapted from* the CON-SENSUS Trial Study Group: Effects of enalapril on mortality in severe congestive heart failure: results of the cooperative New Scandanavian Enalapril Survival Study [CONSENSUS II]. *N Engl J Med* 1987, 316:1429–1435).

that **enalapril** significantly reduced all-cause mortality by 16%, with a 22% reduction in deaths due to progressive heart failure and a significant reduction in hospital admissions (Fig. 3.2). In addition, the SOLVD-Prevention and SAVE studies showed that intervention with **enalapril** and **captopril** reduced the development of severe heart failure and hospital admissions in patients with asymptomatic left ventricular dysfunction. Favorable findings with the use of ACE inhibitor in patients with heart failure were also observed in the V-Heft II study, where **enalapril** was shown to reduce both total mortality and sudden death over the combination of **hydralazine** and **isosorbide dinitrate**.

Although the benefits associated with ACE inhibition mostly have been illustrated with **captopril** and **enalapril** in patients with CHF, this is probably a class effect. **Ramipril** reduced mortality when therapy was initiated between 3 and 10 days after an acute myocardial infarction in patients with heart failure in the AIRE study. **Quinapril** and **fosinopril** have been demonstrated to improve exercise tolerance and symptoms in patients with heart failure. At this time, seven of ten ACE inhibitors available in the United States possess FDA-approved labeling for heart failure: **captopril, enalapril, fosinopril, lisinopril, quinapril, ramipril, and trandolapril. Captopril, enalapril, lisinopril, ramipril, and trandolapril** have been studied for their impacts on mortality in patients with heart failure.

Unless contraindicated, ACE inhibitor therapy is recommended for all patients with significantly reduced left ventricular ejection fraction. If possible, the dosage should be titrated to the dosage used in major clinical trials. Once ACE inhibitor therapy is started for the treatment of heart failure, it should be continued for an indefinite period of time unless unbearable side effects occur.

Postmyocardial Infarction

Immediately following myocardial infarction (MI), the renin-angiotensin system is activated and progression of ventricular dysfunction (ventricular remodeling) begins to take place. Based on this observation, investigations were initiated to evaluate the possible benefits of ACE inhibitor therapy on mortality and progression to heart failure in patients after myocardial infarction. Favorable effects from ACE inhibitor therapy

were found when **captopril, ramipril, and trandolapril** were started at least 3 days after MI in the SAVE, AIRE, and TRACE trials, respectively.

The SAVE trial recruited patients with an ejection fraction of 40% or less but without overt heart failure or symptoms of myocardial ischemia after MI. Patients were assigned in randomized fashion to begin treatment with either **captopril** or placebo on days 3 through 16 after MI. Follow-up evaluation for a mean of 3.5 years revealed a reduction in morbidity and mortality caused by major cardiovascular events in the **captopril** group. The AIRE trial enrolled patients with clinical evidence of heart failure after MI; **ramipril** or placebo was initiated in these patients 3–10 days after myocardial infarction. Treatment with **ramipril** was associated with a 27% reduction in all cause mortality. In the TRACE trial, patients with left ventricular dysfunction on echocardiogram after acute MI were recruited. **Trandolapril** or placebo was randomly assigned to patients 3–7 days after the onset of MI. After a follow-up period of 24–50 months, an 18 % reduction in overall mortality was demonstrated in the **trandolapril** group.

Trials of ACE inhibitors as early intervention after MI have shown conflicting results. The CONSENSUS II study involving the use of **enalapril** early postinfarction (within 24 hours) was stopped prematurely, with a 10% excess in deaths in the treatment group. In contrast, ACE inhibitor therapy with **lisinopril** started within 24 hours of acute infarction produced a small but statistically significant reduction in overall mortality in the GISSI-3 study. Similar benefits were observed when **captopril** was initiated within 24 hours of acute MI in the ISIS-4 study.

For many patients who have an acute MI, evidence from clinical trials has confirmed that ACE inhibitors are a valuable addition to standard therapy. Following timely and careful observation of the patient's hemodynamic and clinical status and following administration of routinely recommended treatments (thrombolysis, aspirin, and beta-blockers), ACE inhibitor therapy may be initiated in patients within 24 hours of acute MI. Because simple criteria of efficacy (especially in the early phase) are not available, the starting dose of ACE inhibitor may be individualized on the basis of safety measures, such as hemodynamic response. The target dose should be that used in the clinical trials (Table 3.2).

In patients with left ventricular dysfunction or heart failure after acute MI, therapy should be continued indefinitely; however, based on clinical experience from the GISSI-3 and ISIS-4 studies, treatment can be stopped safely after 4–6 weeks if a patient does not show signs or symptoms of left ventricular dysfunction. Investigations are now in progress to evaluate the effects of long-term ACE inhibition in survivors of acute MI who have minimal impairment of ventricular function. Because different ACE inhibitors have demonstrated favorable effects in post-MI patients in clinical trials, it would be reasonable to speculate that this is a class effect. On the basis of the SAVE, AIRE, and TRACE studies, the ACE inhibitors **captopril, ramipril, and trandolapril** have received FDA approval for the management of patients with left ventricular dysfunction and/or heart failure after sustaining MI. **Lisinopril** is FDA approved for the treatment of hemodynamically stable patients within 24 hours of acute MI to improve survival.

Diabetic Nephropathy

ACE inhibitors have been shown to reduce intraglomerular pressure in diabetic patients, resulting in a reduction in proteinuria and a slight but important reduction in the rate of decline in glomerular filtration rate and prevention of nephropa-

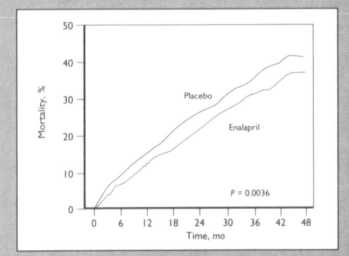

FIGURE 3.2 Cumulative mortality in the SOLVD treatment study. (*Adopted from* the SOLVD Investigators: Effects of enalapril on survival in patients with reduced left ventricular ejection fractions and congestive heart failure. *N Engl J Med* 1991, 327: 293–302).

thy. In a randomized placebo-controlled trial of **captopril** (25 mg three times daily) in patients with insulin-dependent diabetes and diabetic nephropathy (proteinuria ≥ 500 mg/d and serum creatinine ≤ 2.5 mg/dL or 221 μmol/L), it was demonstrated that **captopril** could protect against deterioration in renal function and was significantly more effective than in blood pressure control alone. **Captopril** treatment was associated with a 50% reduction in the risk of combined end points of death,

TABLE 3.2 SUMMARY OF RANDOMIZED CLINICAL TRIALS OF ANGIOTENSIN-CONVERTING ENZYME INHIBITORS IN PATIENTS WITH ACUTE MYOCARDIAL INFARCTION

Trial	No. randomized/no. screened, (%)*	Population	Exclusion criteria	Drug initiation from MI
Trials in High-Risk Acute MI Patients				
SAVE	2231/36,630 (6)	MI, EF ≤ 40%	ACE inhibitor for CHF or HBP, age > 80 yr, Cr > 221 μmol/L	3–16 d (mean, 11 d)
AIRE	2006/30,717 (6.5)	MI, clinical HF	NYHA IV, clinical severe RF	3–10 d (mean, 5.4 d)
TRACE	1749/7010 (25)	MI, WMI ≤ 1.2	0.5 mg trandolapril not tolerated, Cr > 200 μmol/L	3–7 d (median, 4 d)
SMILE	1556/20,261 (8)	Anterior MI, nonthrombolyzed	SBP <100 mmHg, Killip 4, Cr > 221 μmol/L	6–24 h (mean, 15 h)
CATS	298	Anterior MI, thrombolyzed	BP < 100/55 mmHg, > 200/120 mmHg, RF	≤ 6 h
CONSENSUS-II	6090/10,387 (59)	MI	BP < 100/60 mmHg, <105/65 mmHg, clinical severe RF	≤ 1 d
Trials in Relatively Unselected Acute MI Patients				
GISSI-3	19,394/43,047 (45)	MI	Severe heart failure, Killip 4, SBP ≤ 100 mmHg, Cr >177 μmol/L	≤ 1 d
ISIS-4	58,050	MI	SBP < 90–100 mmHg, Killip 4	≤ 1 d
CCS-1	13,634	MI	SBP < 90 mmHg, chronic diuretic	≤ 36 h

continued on next page

INDICATIONS

ACE Inhibitor	Hypertension	HF	Acute MI	Left Ventricular Dysfunction	Diabetic Nephropathy
Benazepril	+				
Captopril	+	+		+*	+
Enalapril	+	+		+†	
Fosinopril	+	+			
Lisinopril	+	+	+		
Moexipril	+				
Perindopril	+				
Quinapril	+	+			
Ramipril	+	+‡			
Trandolapril	+	+§		+§	

*Captopril is indicated in clinically stable patients with left ventricular dysfunction (ejection fraction ≤ 40%) after MI to improve survival and to reduce the incidence of overt heart failure.

†Enalapril is indicated in clinically stable asymptomatic patients with left ventricular dysfunction (ejection fraction ≤ 35%) to decrease the rate of development of overt heart failure and to decrease the incidence of hospitalization due to congestive heart failure (CHF).

‡Ramipril is indicated in stable patients who have demonstrated clinical signs of CHF within the first few days after sustaining acute MI to decrease mortality and progression to severe heart failure.

§Trandolapril is indicated for treatment of heart failure after MI and of left ventricular dysfunction after MI.

+—FDA approved; ACE—angiotensin-converting enzyme; HF—heart failure; MI—myocardial infarction.

Adapted from Cheng A, Frishman WH: Use of angiotensin converting enzyme inhibitors as monotherapy and in combination with diuretics and calcium channel blockers. J Clin Pharm 1998, 38:477–491.

need for dialysis, or renal transplantation. Based on this study, **captopril** was approved for use in the treatment of diabetic nephropathy (proteinuria ≥ 500 mg/d) to slow the progression of diabetic kidney disease.

VASCULAR DISEASE

Preliminary results of the >4 year HOPE study in 9541 patients age ≥55 years with previous manifest cardiovascular disease, or at high risk, showed that ramipril (5 mg bid) significantly reduced mortality and cardiovascular events.

MODE OF ACTION

ACE inhibitors block the conversion of angiotensin I to angiotensin II, thereby preventing vasoconstriction (Fig. 3.3). As a result of their action in reducing angiotensin II levels, they produce a relative decrease in circulating aldosterone concentrations.

TABLE 3.2 SUMMARY OF RANDOMIZED CLINICAL TRIALS OF ANGIOTENSIN-CONVERTING ENZYME INHIBITORS IN PATIENTS WITH ACUTE MYOCARDIAL INFARCTION (*CONTINUED*)

Drug and dose (mg)	Follow-up duration	Overall mortality (control/treated), %	Reduction in mortality, %	p
Captopril 12.5—50 tid	24–60 mo (mean, 42 mo)	24.6/20.4	19	0.019
Ramipril 2.5—5 bid	6–30 mo (mean, 15 mo)	23/17	27	0.002
Trandolapril 1—4/d	24–50 mo	42.3/34.7	18	0.001
Zofenopril 7.5–30 bid	12 mo	14.1/10.0	29	0.011
Captopril 6.25–25 tid	3 mo	4.0/6.0	—	—
Enalaprilat IV, oral 2.5 bid–20 daily	41–180 d (mean, 6 mo; 2952 patients)	9.4/10.2	—	0.26
Lisinopril 2.5–10 once daily	6 wk	7.1/6.3	11	0.03
Captopril 6.25–50 bid	5 wk	7.7/7.2	7.0	0.02
Captopril 6.25–12.5 tid	4 wk	9.6/9.1	6.0	0.3

*Figures are not comparable with post-acute MI trials because of different screening procedures.

ACE—angiotensin-converting enzyme; AIRE—Acute Infarction Ramipril Efficacy Study; bid—twice a day; CATS—Captopril and Thrombolysis Study; CCS—Chinese Cardiac Study; CHF—congestive heart failure; CONSENSUS—Cooperative New Scandinavian Enalapril Survival Study; Cr—serum creatinine; EF—ejection fraction; GISSI-3—Gruppo Italiano per lo Studio della Sopravvivenza nell'Infarto Miocardico-3; HBP—high blood pressure; ISIS-4—International Study of Infarct Survival-4; IV—intravenous; MI—myocardial infarction; NYHA—New York Heart Association class; RF—renal failure; SAVE—Survival and Ventricular Enlargement Trial; SBP—systolic blood pressure; Smile—Survival of Myocardial Infarction: Long-term Evaluation; tid—three times a day; TRACE—Trandolapril Cardiac Evaluation Study; WMI—wall motion index.

Adapted from Latini R, Maggioni AP, Flather M, et al. for the meeting participants: ACE inhibitor use in patients with myocardial infarction: summary of evidence from clinical trials. Circulation 1995, 92:3132–3137.

The information here is provided as guidance only. Prescribers should always consult the manufacturer's current prescribing information.

21

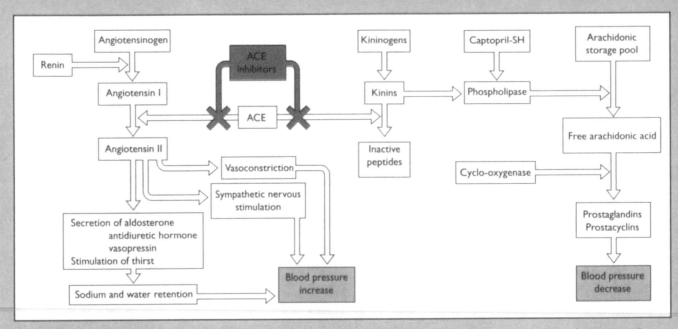

FIGURE 3.3 ACE inhibitors block the formation of vasoconstrictive sodium-retaining factors, while enhancing accumulation of vasodilatory factors.

Tissue	Effect of angiotensin-converting enzyme inhibitor
TABLE 3.3	**TISSUE EFFECTS OF ANGIOTENSIN-CONVERTING ENZYME INHIBITORS**
Lung	High concentration of ACE. It is possible that ACE inhibitor–induced cough is related to marked ACE inhibition in this tissue
Central nervous system	Reduced sympathetic outflow with ACE inhibitors could be due to an effect in the CNS
Arterial wall	Increased arterial compliance and decreased myointimal proliferation, and reduced adverse effects of hypertension on vascular wall structure
Heart	Possible reduction in hypertrophy, partly by direct action on cardiac ACE as well as by blood pressure reduction. Possible reduction in cardiac arrhythmias by direct cardiac action
Kidney	Reduces intraglomerular pressure mainly by dilatation of the efferent arteriole. Reduced albuminuria in patients with nephropathy and also slowing of progressive decline in glomerular filtration rate regardless of cause (although acute renal failure can occur in the presence of low renal perfusion and high plasma renin activity eg, renal artery stenosis or severe heart failure). The antiproteinuric effect of ACE inhibitors may be additive to that of aspirin.

ACE—angiotensin-converting enzyme; CNS—central nervous system; NSAIDs—nonsteroidal anti-inflammatory drugs.

This discourages sodium and water retention by the kidneys and tends to encourage the retention of potassium.

ACE inhibition results in a relative rise in angiotensin I and renin levels and a tendency for angiotensin II levels to rise to pretreatment levels despite continued treatment. Alternative pathways, including chymase, also result in angiotensin II formation during treatment with ACE inhibitors. They may also prevent the destruction of kinins, locally formed peptides that are powerful vasodilators. Kinins have a direct vasodilatory action but also stimulate the synthesis of vasodilatory prostaglandins. **Captopril** may also produce vasodilatory prostaglandins by direct stimulation of the cell membrane phospholipase. Kinins and prostaglandins may be involved in the antihypertensive effect of ACE inhibitors, but this remains to be established. Endothelium-dependent vasodilatation is improved.

Thus, ACE inhibitors prevent the formation of a vasoconstrictor and reduce sodium and water retention while possibly enhancing the activity of natural vasodilators. A central mechanism has also been postulated because naloxone blunts the antihypertensive effects of ACE inhibitors.

ACE appears to be almost ubiquitous, found in many if not all body tissues. All ACE inhibitors appear capable of inhibiting the enzyme in all tissues, but their effects in different tissues (Table 3.3) may reflect their relative tissue penetration and the relative concentration of ACE in that tissue. ACE inhibition in different tissues may account for some of the effects of these drugs over and above their vasodilatory activity.

Clinical pharmacologic studies suggest that the reason why ACE inhibitors do not induce a reflex increase in heart rate may be either a decrease in sympathetic tone or a rise in vagal activity. In uncomplicated hypertension there appears to be no adverse effects on organ perfusion; indeed, renal blood flow characteristically increases. In heart failure, renal perfusion pressure may decline to critical levels, particularly in patients with severe forms of the syndrome.

BENAZEPRIL (Lotensin®)

Benazepril belongs to the largest group of ACE inhibitors, which contains the carboxyl group. It is a prodrug that is metabolized in the liver and other tissues to produce the active metabolite benazeprilat. The effective accumulation half-life of benazeprilat is estimated to be about 10 to 11 h, thus allowing for once daily dosing. Benazepril is currently indicated for the treatment of hypertension. It can be used alone or in combination with other antihypertensive agents.

SPECIAL GROUPS

Race: whites may respond better than blacks due to lower renin levels usually found in blacks; however, racial differences in BP responses are greatly reduced by the concurrent use of diuretics

Children: safety and effectiveness have not been established

Elderly: no dosage adjustment is required

Renal impairment: reduction of daily dose is required in patients with CrCl < 30 mL/min/1.73m^2

Patients on hemodialysis: anaphylactoid reactions have been reported in patients dialyzed with high-flux membranes and treated concurrently with an ACE inhibitor. A different type of dialysis membrane or a different class of medication should be considered

Pregnancy: category C (first trimester); category D (second and third trimesters). Use of ACE inhibitors in the second and third trimesters of pregnancy has been associated with fetal skeletal abnormalities, neonatal renal failure, and neonatal death. Benazepril should be discontinued as soon as possible when pregnancy is detected

Breast-feeding: not recommended; may be excreted in breast milk

IN BRIEF

INDICATIONS
Treatment of hypertension. Benazepril can be used alone or in combination with other antihypertensive agents.

CONTRAINDICATIONS
Hypersensitivity, pregnancy, history of angioedema related to ACE inhibitors, patients dialyzed with high-flux membranes, severe aortic stenosis or outflow obstruction.

DRUG INTERACTIONS
Adrenergic-blocking agents
Allopurinol
Anesthetics
Antacids
Digoxin
Diuretics
NSAIDS (indomethacin)
Potassium supplements
Potassium-sparing diuretics
Lithium

ADVERSE EFFECTS
Cardiovascular: hypotension (< 1%), orthostatic hypotension (< 1%)
CNS: headache (6%), dizziness (4%), fatigue (2%–3%), somnolence/drowsiness (1%–2%)
GI/GU: abdominal pain (<1%), nausea (1%–2%), pancreatitis (<1%), UTI (<1%)
Respiratory: cough (2%–4%), dyspnea (<1%)
Dermatologic: rash, pruritus, photosensitivity (<1%), flushing (<1%)
Renal: increased BUN and serum creatinine (< 1%), increased serum creatinine to > 150% of baseline values (2%)
Others: angioedema (0.5%), neutropenia (rare), anemia, syncope (0.1%), asthenia (<1%), impotence (<1%), elevations of liver function tests, hyperkalemia (1%)

PHARMACOKINETICS AND PHARMACODYNAMICS
Duration of action: up to 24 h
Onset of action: 1 h
Peak effect: 2–4 h
Bioavailability: ≈ 37%
Effect of food: none
Metabolism: cleavage of the ester group (primarily in the liver) converts benazepril to its active metabolite, benazeprilat
Elimination: mostly renal, nonrenal (biliary): 11%–12%
Effective half-life of accumulation: 10–11 h (benazeprilat)
Protein binding: 96.7% benazepril; 95.3% benazeprilat

MONITORING
BP—observe carefully for first-dose hypotension, especially in patients with heart failure, renovascular hypertension, and in patients who are sodium or volume depleted.
Renal function—Acute renal failure may occur on initiation of ACE inhibitor therapy if the kidneys are dependent on angiotensin II for perfusion. This affects patients with bilateral renal artery stenosis or stenosis of the artery to a solitary kidney, patients with heart failure, or patients who are in hypovolemic states. Rises in serum creatinine or BUN should be an indication to reduce diuretic or benazepril dosage. Suspect renal artery stenosis.
Electrolytes, CBC.

OVERDOSE
Treatment should be symptomatic and supportive. The patient's BP may be maintained with infusion of normal saline solution. Benazepril is only slightly dialyzable, but dialysis may be considered in overdosed patients with severe renal impairment.

BENAZEPRIL (CONTINUED)

DOSAGE

Usual initial dose is 10 mg once daily. Dose can be titrated up to 40 mg/d (in one or two divided doses.) A dose of 80 mg gives an increased response, but experience with this dose is limited. Lower initial dose of 5 mg once daily should be given to patients with renal impairment (CrCl of < 30 mL/min/1.73m^2) or in patients in whom diuretics have not been discontinued.

PATIENT INFORMATION

Benazepril may be taken with or without food. Benazepril may cause dizziness, fainting or lightheadedness, especially during the first few days of therapy; avoid abrupt changes in posture. Use caution when driving or doing other things that require alertness. Consult with physician immediately if pregnancy is detected. Notify physician if persistent or unusual side effects occur. Do not discontinue therapy without your physician's advice. Do not use salt substitute unless advised by physician.

AVAILABILITY

Tablets—5 mg, 10 mg, 20 mg, 40 mg
Combination formulations:
Lotensin HCT—benazepril hydrochloride/hydrochlorothiazide combination tablets
  5 mg/6.25 mg
  10 mg/12.5 mg
  20 mg/12.5 mg
  20 mg/25 mg
Lotrel—amlodipine/benazepril hydrochloride combination capsules
  2.5 mg/10 mg
  5 mg/10 mg
  5 mg/20 mg

CAPTOPRIL (Capoten®)

Captopril was the first clinically useful ACE inhibitor. Early severe reactions were related to the very high doses used in high-risk patients. It is directly active and rapidly absorbed. It is about as effective as beta blockers and diuretics and combines well with diuretics and calcium antagonists (and to a lesser extent with beta blockers) to lower BP. Quality of life was reported to be good with captopril. Captopril seems to be as effective as digoxin in controlling heart failure in patients without atrial fibrillation. It modifies postinfarction heart enlargement (remodeling). In the SAVE study, intervention with captopril started on days 3 through 16 after MI demonstrated a reduction of all-cause mortality by 19%. Recurrent MI, development of severe heart failure, and CHF requiring hospitalization were also reduced significantly. Similarly, early intervention with captopril in the ISIS-IV study showed a slight but significant reduction in postinfarction mortality. Captopril also benefits patients with diabetic nephropathy. It is associated with a 51% reduction in the risk of end-stage renal disease or death compared to placebo.

SPECIAL GROUPS

Race: whites may respond better than blacks due to lower renin levels usually found in blacks; however, racial differences in BP responses are greatly reduced by the concurrent use of diuretics

Children: there is limited experience reported in the literature with the use of captopril in the pediatric population. Captopril should be used in children only if other measures for controlling BP have not been effective

Elderly: usually respond well. Dose should allow for age-related reduction in renal function

Renal impairment: reduce initial dosage and use smaller or less frequent doses

Patients on hemodialysis: anaphylactoid reactions have been reported in patients dialyzed with high-flux membranes and treated concurrently with an ACE inhibitor. A different type of dialysis membrane or a different class of medication should be considered

Pregnancy: category C (first trimester); category D (second and third trimesters). Use of ACE inhibitors in the second and third trimesters of pregnancy has been associated with fetal skeletal abnormalities, neonatal renal failure, and neonatal death. Captopril should be discontinued as soon as possible when pregnancy is detected

Breast-feeding: not recommended; captopril has been detected in breast milk

IN BRIEF

INDICATIONS
Hypertension
Heart failure
Left ventricular dysfunction after MI
Diabetic nephropathy

CONTRAINDICATIONS
Hypersensitivity, pregnancy, history of angioedema related to ACE inhibitors, patients dialyzed with high-flux membranes, severe aortic stenosis or outflow obstruction.

DRUG INTERACTIONS
Allopurinol
Adrenergic-blocking agents
Anesthetics
Antacids
Digoxin
Diuretics
Lithium
NSAIDs (indomethacin)
Phenothiazines
Potassium sparing diuretics
Potassium supplements
Probenecid
Vasodilators

ADVERSE EFFECTS
Cardiovascular: hypotension, orthostatic hypotension, chest pain (1%), tachycardia (1%)
CNS: headache (0.5%–2%), dizziness (0.5%–2%), fatigue (0.5%–2%), somnolence/drowsiness, insomnia (0.5%–2%), paresthesias (0.5%–2%)
GI/GU: abdominal pain (0.5%–2%), nausea (0.5%–2%), diarrhea (0.5%–2%), dysgeusia (2%–4%), dry mouth (0.5%–2%), hepatitis, pancreatitis
Respiratory: cough (0.5%–2%), dyspnea (0.5%–2%)
Dermatologic: rash (4%–7%), pruritus (2%), photosensitivity, flushing.
Renal: proteinuria (< 1%), nephrotic syndrome (< 0.5%), elevations of BUN or serum creatinine
Others: angioedema (0.1%), anemia, eosinophilia, neutropenia (rare), impotence, syncope, elevations of liver function tests, hyperkalemia

PHARMACOKINETICS AND PHARMACODYNAMICS
Duration of action: 6–12 h
Onset of action: 15 min to 1 h
Peak effect: 1–1.5 h
Bioavailability: 70%
Effect of food: the bioavailability of captopril can be reduced as much as 40% when taken with food. It is not known whether the effects of food on the pharmacokinetics of captopril translate into effects on its clinical efficacy
Metabolism: mainly uncharacterized; protein-captopril conjugates formed
Elimination: mostly renal (95%); 40%–50% as unchanged drug; remainder as metabolites
Half-life: 2 h
Protein binding: 25%–30%

MONITORING
BP—Observe carefully for first-dose hypotension, especially in patients with heart failure, renovascular hypertension, and in patients who are sodium or volume depleted.
Renal function—Acute renal failure may occur on initiation of ACE inhibitor therapy if the kidneys are dependent on angiotensin II for perfusion. This affects patients with bilateral renal artery stenosis or stenosis of the artery to a solitary kidney, patients with heart failure, or patients who are in hypovolemic states. Rises in serum creatinine or BUN should be an indication to reduce diuretic or captopril dosage.
Suspect renal artery stenosis.
Electrolytes, CBC.

The information here is provided as guidance only. Prescribers should always consult the manufacturer's current prescribing information.

25

CAPTOPRIL (CONTINUED)

DOSAGE

Hypertension: Initially 12.5–25 mg, usually as two divided doses. Increased if necessary to 150 mg/d (given as 3 divided doses) depending on severity of hypertension and clinical response. In renovascular hypertension, when diuretics have not been discontinued or in renal impairment, initial dose should be 6.25 mg, titrated cautiously according to response.

Children: Initiate with 0.3 mg/kg of body weight three times daily. Dosage may be increased in increments of 0.3 mg/kg at intervals of 8–24 h to the minimum effective dose if necessary.

Elderly: Initiate with the lowest dose possible and titrate according to clinical response.

Congestive heart failure: Initially, 6.25–12.5 mg 3 times a day, increased according to clinical response. The usual daily dose is 50–150 mg in two or three divided doses.

Diabetic nephropathy: 25 mg 3 times daily.

Left ventricular dysfunction after MI: Initially, 6.25 mg, followed by 12.5 mg 3 times daily. Then increase dose to 25 mg 3 times a day during the next several days. Target dose of 50 mg 3 times a day may be achieved over the next several weeks.

OVERDOSE

Treatment should be symptomatic and supportive.

The patient's BP may be maintained with infusion of normal saline solution. Although captopril may be removed from the adult circulation by hemodialysis, there is inadequate data concerning the effectiveness of hemodialysis for removing captopril from the circulation of neonates or children.

PATIENT INFORMATION

Take captopril 1 h before meals. Captopril may cause dizziness, fainting, or lightheadedness, especially during the first few days of therapy; avoid abrupt changes in posture. Use caution when driving or doing other things that require alertness. Consult with physician immediately if pregnancy is detected. Notify physician if persistent or unusual side effects occur. Do not discontinue therapy without your physician's advice. Do not use salt substitute unless advised by physician.

AVAILABILITY

Tablets—12.5 mg, 25 mg, 50 mg, 100 mg
Combination formulations:
  Capozide—captopril/ hydrochlorothiazide combination tablets
    25 mg/15 mg
    25 mg/25 mg
    50 mg/15 mg
    50 mg/25 mg

ENALAPRIL (Vasotec®)

Enalapril was the first nonsulfhydryl prodrug. It is rapidly absorbed and converted relatively slowly to enalaprilat, the active ACE inhibitor. It has a long duration of action and has been demonstrated to reduce left ventricular hypertrophy. Enalapril reduces systolic blood pressure to a slightly greater extent than do beta blockers. It has an antihypertensive effect similar to that of the calcium antagonists but is generally better tolerated. In mild to moderate heart failure, enalapril significantly reduced mortality by 16% and death from progressive heart failure by 22% (SOLVD). The prevention arm of SOLVD resulted in delay in the onset of overt heart failure and reduced hospital admissions. Early intervention with enalapril post-MI did not benefit patients in the CONSENSUS II study.

An intravenous form is available (enalaprilat) that is the metabolite of the prodrug enalapril. It is approved for the parenteral treatment of hypertension but should be used with caution in patients with renovascular hypertension.

SPECIAL GROUPS

Race: whites may respond better than blacks due to lower renin levels usually found in blacks; however, racial differences in BP responses are greatly reduced by the concurrent use of diuretics

Children: safety and effectiveness have not been established

Elderly: usually respond well. Dose should allow for age-related reduction in renal function

Renal impairment: dose must be adjusted according to renal function

Patients on hemodialysis: anaphylactoid reactions have been reported in patients dialyzed with high-flux membranes and treated concurrently with an ACE inhibitor. A different type of dialysis membrane or a different class of medication should be considered

Pregnancy: category C (1st trimester); category D (second and third trimesters). Use of ACE inhibitors in the second and third trimesters of pregnancy has been associated with fetal skeletal abnormalities, neonatal renal failure, and neonatal death. Enalapril should be discontinued as soon as possible when pregnancy is detected

Breast-feeding: not recommended; enalapril and enalaprilat have been detected in breast milk

IN BRIEF

INDICATIONS
Hypertension
Heart failure
Asymptomatic left ventricular dysfunction

CONTRAINDICATIONS
Hypersensitivity, pregnancy, history of angioedema related to ACE inhibitors, patients dialyzed with high-flux membranes, severe aortic stenosis or outflow obstruction.

DRUG INTERACTIONS
Adrenergic-blocking agents
Anesthetics
Antacids
Allopurinol
Digoxin
Diuretics
NSAIDs (indomethacin)
Lithium
Potassium sparing diuretics
Potassium supplements
Rifampin

ADVERSE EFFECTS
Cardiovascular: hypotension (1%–7%), orthostatic hypotension (1%–3%), chest pain (2%), angina pectoris (1%–2%)
CNS: headache (2%–5%), dizziness (4%–7%), fatigue (1%–3%), somnolence/drowsiness, insomnia, paresthesias
GI/GU: abdominal pain (1%–2%), nausea (1%–2%), diarrhea (1%–2%), dysgeusia (≤ 1%), dry mouth, hepatitis, pancreatitis, UTI (1%–2%)
Respiratory: cough (1%–3%), dyspnea (1%–2%), bronchitis (1%–2%)
Dermatologic: rash (1%–2%), pruritus, photosensitivity, flushing
Renal: elevations of BUN or serum creatinine
Others: angioedema (0.2%), syncope (0.5%–2%), impotence, anemia, eosinophilia, neutropenia (rare), thrombocytopenia (rare), elevations of liver function tests, hyperkalemia (1%)

PHARMACOKINETICS AND PHARMACODYNAMICS
Duration of action:	up to 24 h
Onset of action:	within 1 h, IV: 15 min
Peak effect:	4–6 h, IV: 1–4 h
Bioavailability:	60%
Effect of food:	none
Metabolism:	converted to enalaprilat in the liver; no further metabolism known
Elimination:	enalapril: 60% renal, 33% fecal; enalaprilat: 100% renal (as unchanged drug)
Half-life:	1.3 h, enalapril; 11 h, enalaprilat
Protein binding:	50%–60%, enalaprilat

MONITORING
Blood pressure—Observe carefully for first-dose hypotension, especially in patients with heart failure, renovascular hypertension, and in patients who are sodium or volume depleted.
Renal function—Acute renal failure may occur on initiation of ACE inhibitor therapy if the kidneys are dependent on angiotensin II for perfusion. This affects patients with bilateral renal artery stenosis or stenosis of the artery to a solitary kidney, patients with heart failure, or patients who are in hypovolemic states. Rises in serum creatinine or BUN should be an indication to reduce diuretic or enalapril dosage.
Suspect renal artery stenosis.
Electrolytes, CBC.

OVERDOSE
Treatment should be symptomatic and supportive. The patient's BP may be maintained with infusion of normal saline solution. Enalaprilat may be removed from general circulation by hemodialysis.

The information here is provided as guidance only. Prescribers should always consult the manufacturer's current prescribing information.

27

DOSAGE

Hypertension: Adult—Initial oral dose is 2.5 to 5 mg/d. Increased to the usual effective maintenance dose of 10–20 mg/d (maximum, 40 mg/d can be given in two divided doses) as needed and as tolerated. In renovascular hypertension or in patients in whom diuretics have not been discontinued, the starting dose should be 2.5 mg/d. The usual IV dose in hypertension is 1.25 mg every 6 h administered intravenously over a 5-min period. An initial dose of 0.625 mg over 5 min should be used in patients who are sodium and volume depleted or who have renal impairment (CrCl < 30 mL/min). Patients should be observed 1 h after dose to watch for hypotension. If response is inadequate after 1 h, the 0.625 mg dose can be repeated and therapy continued at a dose of 1.25 mg every 6 h. For conversion from intravenous to oral therapy, the recommended initial dose of enalapril tablets is 5 mg once a day for patients with creatinine clearance > 30 mL/min and 2.5 mg once daily for patients with creatinine clearance ≤ 30 mL/min. Dosage should then be adjusted according to BP response.

Elderly—Initially 2.5 mg by mouth. Titrated according to clinical response.

Renal impairment—In patients with moderate to severe renal impairment (CrCl < 30 mL/minute), the starting oral dose should be 2.5 mg daily, adjusted according to response.

Heart failure: Initially, 2.5 mg by mouth once daily. Titrated according to clinical response. The usual maintenance dose is 5–40 mg/d given in two divided doses.

Asymptomatic left ventricular dysfunction: Initially, 2.5 mg by mouth once or twice daily. Titrated according to clinical response. Targeted daily dose is 20 mg/d given in 2 divided doses.

PATIENT INFORMATION
Enalapril may be taken with or without food. Enalapril may cause dizziness, fainting or lightheadedness, especially during the first few days of therapy; avoid abrupt changes in posture. Use caution when driving or doing other things that require alertness. Consult with physician immediately if pregnancy is detected. Notify physician if persistent or unusual side effects occur. Do not discontinue therapy without your physician's advice. Do not use salt substitute unless advised by physician.

AVAILABILITY
Tablets—2.5 mg, 5 mg, 10 mg, 20 mg
Injection—1.25 mg enalaprilat/mL, in 1 and 2 mL vials
Combination formulations:
Vaseretic—enalapril maleate/ hydrochlorothiazide combination tablets
5 mg/12.5 mg
10 mg/25 mg
Teczem—enalapril maleate/ diltiazem malate ER (extended-release) combination tablets
5 mg/180 mg
Lexxel—enalapril maleate/felodipine ER (extended-release) combination tablets
5 mg/5 mg

FOSINOPRIL

(Monopril®)

Fosinopril is a nonsulfhydryl prodrug ACE inhibitor, containing a phosphinic acid rather than a carboxylic acid group. Fosinopril is metabolized by the liver and other tissues to produce the active diacid metabolite fosinoprilat. The published values for the elimination half-life of fosinoprilat are longer than those of captopril, but similar to those of enalapril. This allows for once daily dosing in the management of hypertension. Fosinopril has also demonstrated to improve exercise tolerance and symptoms in patients with heart failure. Fosinoprilat is excreted to equal degrees by the liver and kidneys. This feature allows compensatory clearance in either hepatic or renal impairment or old age, suggesting that little dosage adjustment is required in the general population.

SPECIAL GROUPS

Race: whites may respond better than blacks due to lower renin levels usually found in blacks; however, racial differences in BP responses are greatly reduced by the concurrent use of diuretics

Children: safety and effectiveness have not been established

Elderly: usually respond well. Dose reduction generally not required

Renal impairment: due to partial compensatory clearance by the liver, dose reduction is not required

Patients on hemodialysis: anaphylactoid reactions have been reported in patients dialyzed with high-flux membranes and treated concurrently with an ACE inhibitor. A different type of dialysis membrane or a different class of medication should be considered

Pregnancy: category C (first trimester); category D (second and third trimesters). Use of ACE inhibitors in the second and third trimesters of pregnancy has been associated with fetal skeletal abnormalities, neonatal renal failure, and neonatal death. Fosinopril should be discontinued as soon as possible when pregnancy is detected

Breast-feeding: not recommended; fosinoprilat has been detected in breast milk

IN BRIEF

INDICATIONS
Hypertension
Heart failure

CONTRAINDICATIONS
Hypersensitivity, pregnancy, history of angioedema related to ACE inhibitors, patients dialyzed with high-flux membranes, severe aortic stenosis or outflow obstruction.

DRUG INTERACTIONS

Adrenergic-blocking agents	Phenothiazines
Allopurinol	Diuretics
Anesthetics	Lithium
Antacids	NSAIDS (indomethacin)
Digoxin	Potassium sparing diuretics
	Potassium supplements

ADVERSE EFFECTS
Cardiovascular: hypotension ($\leq$ 1%–4.4%), orthostatic hypotension (1%–2%), chest pain (1%–2%), rhythm disturbances ($\leq$ 1%–1.4%)
CNS: headache ($\geq$ 1%), dizziness (1%–12%), fatigue ($\geq$ 1%), somnolence/drowsiness ($\leq$ 1%), insomnia ($\leq$ 1%), paresthesias ($\leq$ 1%)
GI/GU: abdominal pain ($\leq$ 1%), nausea (1%–2%), diarrhea (> 1%), hepatitis ($\leq$ 1%), pancreatitis ($\leq$ 1%), dry mouth ($\leq$ 1%)
Respiratory: cough (2%–10%), dyspnea ($\geq$ 1%), upper respiratory infection (2%)
Dermatologic: rash ($\leq$ 1%), pruritus ($\leq$ 1%), photosensitivity ($\leq$ 1%), flushing ($\leq$ 1%)
Renal: elevations of BUN or serum creatinine
Others: angioedema ($\leq$ 1%), syncope ($\leq$ 1%), neutropenia (rare), elevations of liver function tests, hyperkalemia (2%–3%)

PHARMACOKINETICS AND PHARMACODYNAMICS
Duration of action: 24 h
Onset of action: 1 h
Peak effect: 2–6 h
Bioavailability: 36%
Effect of food: decreased rate of absorption, unknown clinical significance
Metabolism: converted to fosinoprilat in the liver; fosinoprilat is also conjugated to the beta-glucuronide.
Elimination: cleared equally by renal and hepatic routes
Half-life: 12 h (fosinoprilat)
Protein binding: 97%–98% (fosinoprilat)

MONITORING
BP—Observe carefully for first-dose hypotension, especially in patients with heart failure, renovascular hypertension, and in patients who are sodium or volume depleted.
Renal function—Acute renal failure may occur on initiation of ACE inhibitor therapy if the kidneys are dependent on angiotensin II for perfusion. This affects patients with bilateral renal artery stenosis or stenosis of the artery to a solitary kidney, patients with heart failure, or patients who are in hypovolemic states. Rises in serum creatinine or BUN should be an indication to reduce diuretic or fosinopril dosage.
Suspect renal artery stenosis.
Electrolytes, CBC.

OVERDOSE
Treatment should be symptomatic and supportive. The patient's BP may be maintained with infusion of normal saline solution. Fosinoprilat is poorly removed from the body by both hemodialysis and peritoneal dialysis.

The information here is provided as guidance only. Prescribers should always consult the manufacturer's current prescribing information.

29

DOSAGE

Hypertension: Initial dose is 10 mg/d, increased to the usual effective dose of 20–40 mg/d. Some patients appear to have a further response to 80 mg. Total daily doses may be divided into two if trough effect is inadequate. In renovascular hypertension or in patients in whom diuretics have not been discontinued, the starting dose should be 5 mg.

Heart failure: The usual initial dose is 10 mg/d. Following the initial dose of fosinopril, the patient should be observed under medical supervision for at least 2 h for the presence of hypotension or orthostasis and, if present, until BP stabilizes. An initial dose of 5 mg is preferred in patients with moderate to severe renal failure or in those who have been vigorously diuresed. Dosage should be increased, over a period of several weeks, to a dose that is maximal and tolerated but not exceeding 40 mg/d. The usual effective dosage range is 20–40 mg once daily.

PATIENT INFORMATION

Fosinopril may be taken with or without food. Fosinopril may cause dizziness, fainting, or lightheadedness, especially during the first few days of therapy; avoid abrupt changes in posture. Use caution when driving or doing other things that require alertness. Consult with physician immediately if pregnancy is detected. Notify physician if persistent or unusual side effects occur. Do not discontinue therapy without your physician's advice. Do not use salt substitute unless advised by physician.

AVAILABILITY

Tablets—10 mg, 20 mg, 40 mg

LISINOPRIL
(Prinivil®, Zestril®)

Lisinopril is not a prodrug and is a close analogue of enalaprilat, the active metabolite of enalapril. Because lisinopril does not undergo metabolism and is excreted unchanged entirely in the urine, it can be selected for patients with hepatic impairment. Lisinopril has been shown to be effective in both hypertension and CHF when given once daily. It reduces systolic and diastolic pressure more than diuretics and reduces systolic blood pressure more than atenolol or metoprolol. Lisinopril has similar antihypertensive efficacy when compared to nifedipine, but is associated with a lower incidence of side effects. It has an additive antihypertensive effect when added to either hydrochorothiazide or nifedipine, but less so when added to a beta blocker.

In a study comparing the use of lisinopril with captopril in 189 patients with class II to IV CHF, lisinopril 5 to 20 mg/d produced significantly greater improvements in left ventricular ejection fraction than captopril 37.5 to 150 mg/d. Furthermore, lisinopril (but not captopril) was shown to improve exercise duration in patients with impaired renal function. In addition to its established efficacy in the treatment of hypertension and heart failure, lisinopril has been demonstrated to reduce mortality and cardiovascular morbidity in patients with MI when given as early treatment.

SPECIAL GROUPS

Race: whites may respond better than blacks because of lower renin levels usually found in blacks; however, racial differences in BP responses are greatly reduced by the concurrent use of diuretics

Children: safety and effectiveness have not been established

Elderly: usually respond well. Dose should allow for age-related reduction in renal function

Hepatic impairment: lisinopril is not metabolized, hepatic impairment is unlikely to be of any clinical importance

Renal impairment: dose must be adjusted according to renal function

Patients on hemodialysis: anaphylactoid reactions have been reported in patients dialyzed with high-flux membranes and treated concurrently with an ACE inhibitor. A different type of dialysis membrane or a different class of medication should be considered

Pregnancy: category C (first trimester); category D (second and third trimesters). Use of ACE inhibitors in the second and third trimesters of pregnancy has been associated with fetal skeletal abnormalities, neonatal renal failure, and neonatal death. Lisinopril should be discontinued as soon as possible when pregnancy is detected

Breast-feeding: not recommended; lisinopril may be excreted in breast milk

IN BRIEF

INDICATIONS
Hypertension
Heart failure
Acute MI

CONTRAINDICATIONS
Hypersensitivity, pregnancy, history of angioedema related to ACE inhibitors, patients dialyzed with high-flux membranes, severe aortic stenosis or outflow obstruction.

DRUG INTERACTIONS
Adrenergic-blocking agents
Allopurinol
Anesthetics
Antacids
Digoxin
Diuretics
Lithium
NSAIDS (indomethacin)
Potassium sparing diuretics
Potassium supplements

ADVERSE EFFECTS
Cardiovascular: hypotension (1%–4.4%), orthostatic hypotension (1%–2%), chest pain (3%–4%), angina pectoris (>1%), rhythm disturbances (≤1%)
CNS: headache (4%–5%), dizziness (5%–11%), fatigue (2%–3%), somnolence/drowsiness (≤1%), insomnia (≤1%), paresthesias (≤1%) depression (>1%)
GI/GU: abdominal pain (2%–3%), nausea (1%–2%), diarrhea (2%–4%), hepatitis (≤1%), pancreatitis (≤1%), dry mouth (≤1%), UTI (≤1%)
Respiratory: cough (>1%), dyspnea (>1%), upper respiratory infection (1%–2%)
Dermatologic: rash (1%–2%), pruritus (>1%), photosensitivity (≤1%), flushing (≤1%)
Renal: elevations of BUN or serum creatinine.
Others: angioedema (0.1%), neutropenia (rare), syncope, impotence (1%), asthenia (>1%), myalgia (>1%), elevations of liver function tests (rare), hyperkalemia (2%)

PHARMACOKINETICS AND PHARMACODYNAMICS
Duration of action: 24 h
Onset of action: 1 h
Peak effect: 6 h
Bioavailability: ≈ 25%, widely variable between individuals
Effect of food: no effect
Metabolism: no significant metabolism
Elimination: 100% in urine as unchanged drug
Half-life: 12 h
Protein binding: none

MONITORING
BP—Observe carefully for first-dose hypotension, especially in patients with heart failure, renovascular hypertension, and in patients who are sodium or volume depleted.
Renal function—Acute renal failure may occur on initiation of ACE inhibitor therapy if the kidneys are dependent on angiotensin II for perfusion. This affects patients with bilateral renal artery stenosis or stenosis of the artery to a solitary kidney, patients with heart failure, or patients who are in hypovolemic states. Rises in serum creatinine or BUN should be an indication to reduce diuretic or lisinopril dosage.
Suspect renal artery stenosis.
Electrolytes, CBC.

OVERDOSE
Treatment should be symptomatic and supportive. The patient's BP may be maintained with infusion of normal saline solution. Lisinopril can be removed by hemodialysis.

DOSAGE

Hypertension: Initial dose is 10 mg/d, adjusted to usual effective dose range of 10–40 mg/d according to response (maximum daily dose is 40 mg). In elderly patients, patients with hyponatremia, patients with renal impairment (CrCl ≤ 30 mL/min), or in patients in whom diuretics have not been discontinued, the starting dose should be 2.5 mg/d.

Heart failure: The usual initial dose is 5 mg/d, administered under close medical observation, especially in patients with low BP. The usual effective dosage range is 5–20 mg once daily. Preliminary results of the ATLAS trial found that high dose lisinopril (35 mg once daily) was more effective than a low dose (5 mg once daily)

Acute MI: In hemodynamically stable patients within 24 h of the onset of acute MI, the first dose of lisinopril is 5 mg, followed by 5 mg after 24 h, 10 mg after 48 h, and then 10 mg once daily. Dosing should be continued for 6 wk. Patients should receive, as appropriate, the standard recommended treatments, such as thrombolytics, aspirin, and beta blockers. Patients with a low systolic blood pressure (≤ 120 mmHg) when treatment is initiated or during the first 3 days after the infarct should be given a lower dose of 2.5 mg. If hypotension occurs (systolic blood pressure ≤ 100 mmHg), a daily maintenance dose of 5 mg may be given with temporary reductions to 2.5 mg if needed.

PATIENT INFORMATION

Lisinopril may be taken with or without food. Lisinopril may cause dizziness, fainting or lightheadedness, especially during the first few days of therapy. Avoid abrupt changes in posture. Use caution when driving or doing other things that require alertness. Consult with physician immediately if pregnancy is detected. Notify physician if persistent or unusual side effects occur. Do not discontinue therapy without your physician's advice. Do not use salt substitute unless advised by physician.

AVAILABILITY

Tablets—2.5 mg, 5 mg, 10 mg, 20 mg, 40 mg
Combination formulations:
Prinzide—lisinopril/ hydrochlorothiazide combination tablets
  10 mg/12.5 mg
  20 mg/12.5 mg
  20 mg/25 mg
Zestoretic—lisinopril/ hydrochlorothiazide combination tablets
  10 mg/12.5 mg
  20 mg/12.5 mg
  20 mg/25 mg

MOEXIPRIL (Univasc®)

Moexipril is a nonsulfhydryl prodrug that is hydrolyzed after oral administration to its active metabolite moexiprilat. Moexipril has an oral bioavailability of about 13%. Food can affect the rate and extent of absorption of moexipril. The peak concentration (C_{max}) and area under the concentration-time curve (AUC) of moexipril are reduced by approximately 70% and 40%, respectively, after a low-fat breakfast. Greater reductions of C_{max} and AUC have been observed after a high-fat meal. Moexipril has an elimination half-life of about 12 hours, allowing for once daily dosing in the management of hypertension.

Moexipril administered at 7.5 to 15 mg once daily has demonstrated similar efficacy in BP control to those of atenolol 25–50 mg once daily, metoprolol 100 mg once daily, verapamil sustained release 180–240 mg once daily, nitrendipine 20 mg once daily, or captopril 25–50 mg twice daily. Further reductions in BP were achieved when moexipril was added to either hydrochlorothiazide or nifedipine in patients who were inadequately controlled with monotherapy.

SPECIAL GROUPS

Race: the antihypertensive effect is considerably smaller in black patients because of lower renin levels usually found in blacks; however, racial differences in BP responses with ACE inhibitors are greatly reduced by the concurrent use of diuretics

Children: safety and effectiveness have not been established

Elderly: usually respond well. Dose should allow for age-related reduction in renal function

Hepatic impairment: dosage adjustment is generally not necessary. However, a lower initial dose should be considered

Renal impairment: dose must be adjusted according to renal function

Patients on hemodialysis: anaphylactoid reactions have been reported in patients dialyzed with high-flux membranes and treated concurrently with an ACE inhibitor. A different type of dialysis membrane or a different class of medication should be considered

Pregnancy: category C (first trimester); category D (second and third trimesters). Use of ACE inhibitors in the second and third trimesters of pregnancy has been associated with fetal skeletal abnormalities, neonatal renal failure, and neonatal death. Moexipril should be discontinued as soon as possible when pregnancy is detected

Breast-feeding: not recommended; moexipril may be excreted in breast milk

IN BRIEF

INDICATIONS
Hypertension

CONTRAINDICATIONS
Hypersensitivity, pregnancy, history of angioedema related to ACE inhibitors.

DRUG INTERACTIONS
Anesthetics
Diuretics
Lithium
Potassium-sparing diuretics
Potassium supplements

ADVERSE EFFECTS
Cardiovascular: hypotension (< 1%), orthostatic hypotension (< 1%), chest pain (> 1%), angina pectoris (< 1%), rhythm disturbances (< 1%), peripheral edema (> 1%)
CNS: headache (> 1%), dizziness (4%), fatigue (2%–3%), somnolence/drowsiness (< 1%), insomnia (< 1%)
GI/GU: abdominal pain (< 1%), nausea (> 1%), diarrhea (3%), hepatitis (< 1%), pancreatitis (< 1%), dry mouth (< 1%)
Respiratory: cough (6%), dyspnea (< 1%), upper respiratory infection (> 1%)
Dermatologic: rash (1%–2%), pruritus (< 1%), photosensitivity (< 1%), flushing (1%–2%)
Renal: elevations of BUN or serum creatinine
Others: angioedema (<1%), anemia (< 1%), syncope (< 1%), myalgia (1%–2%), elevations of liver function tests, hyperkalemia (1%)

PHARMACOKINETICS AND PHARMACODYNAMICS
Duration of action: up to 24 h
Onset of action: 1 h
Time to peak plasma concentration: 1.5 h (moexiprilat)
Bioavailability: 13% as moexiprilat
Effect of food: C_{max} and AUC are markedly reduced when moexipril is taken with food. Therefore, this agent should be taken in a fasting state
Metabolism: both moexipril and moexiprilat are converted to diketopiperazine derivatives and unidentified metabolites
Elimination: 13% in urine (7% as moexiprilat, 1% as moexipril, 5% as other metabolites); 53% in feces (52% as moexiprilat, 1% as moexipril)
Half-life: 12 h (moexiprilat)
Protein binding: 50% (moexiprilat)

MONITORING
BP—Observe carefully for first-dose hypotension, especially in patients with heart failure, renovascular hypertension, and in patients who are sodium or volume depleted.
Renal function—Acute renal failure may occur on initiation of ACE inhibitor therapy if the kidneys are dependent on angiotensin II for perfusion. This affects patients with bilateral renal artery stenosis or stenosis of the artery to a solitary kidney, patients with heart failure, or patients who are in hypovolemic states. Rises in serum creatinine or BUN should be an indication to reduce diuretic or moexipril dosage.
Suspect renal artery stenosis.
Electrolytes, CBC.

OVERDOSE
Treatment should be symptomatic and supportive. The patient's BP may be maintained with infusion of normal saline solution. The dialyzability of moexipril is not known.

DOSAGE

Hypertension: Usual initial dose of Univasc in patients not receiving diuretics is 7.5 mg once daily, increased gradually to a maximum of 30 mg/d according to response, given as a single dose or two divided doses. In renovascular hypertension or in patients in whom diuretics have not been discontinued, the starting dose should be 3.75 mg once daily with close medical supervision. For patients with creatinine clearance ≤ 40 mL/min/1.73 m², the initial dose should also be 3.75 mg once daily given cautiously.

PATIENT INFORMATION

Moexipril should be taken 1 h before meals. Moexipril may cause dizziness, fainting, or lightheadedness, especially during the first few days of therapy; avoid abrupt changes in posture. Use caution when driving or doing other things that require alertness. Consult with physician immediately if pregnancy is detected. Notify physician if persistent or unusual side effects occur. Do not discontinue therapy without your physician's advice. Do not use salt substitute unless advised by physician.

AVAILABILITY

Tablets—7.5 mg, 15 mg
Combination formulations:
Uniretic—moexipril hydrochloride/ hydrochlorothiazide combination tablets
7.5 mg/12.5 mg
15 mg/25 mg

PERINDOPRIL (Aceon®)

Perindopril, a carboxyl-containing ACE inhibitor structurally related to enalapril, is the 10th ACE inhibitor to become available for treatment of hypertension in the United States. Perindopril is a prodrug that is hydrolyzed in the liver to its active metabolite perindoprilat. Unlike enalapril, perindopril's molecular structure includes a lipophilic perhydroindole group, which may contribute to its longer duration of action. Furthermore, perindoprilat has a high affinity for ACE, which appears to contribute to perindopril's longer ACE inhibitory activity, compared with enalapril.

Clinical trials have found perindopril to be effective for the treatment of essential hypertension when given once daily. Several clinical trials also demonstrated that perindopril was as effective as captopril, atenolol, and the combination of amiloride and hydrochlorothiazide for the reduction of blood pressure. Perindopril appears to provide other ACE inhibitor–related advantages, such as reduction of left ventricular hypertrophy, reduction of proteinuria in diabetic renal impairment, and improvement of arterial structure and function. According to a study performed by Reid *et al.* in elderly patients with heart failure, the initial doses of both oral enalapril (2.5 mg) and oral captopril (6.25 mg) significantly decreased blood pressure compared with placebo, whereas the initial dose of oral perindopril (2 mg) did not. Thus, the lack of first-dose hypotension may be an advantage that perindopril has over other ACE inhibitors. Treatment with perindopril was shown to improve functional and clinical status in patients with mild, moderate, and severe congestive heart failure in several small and short-term clinical trials. Further studies are required to clarify perindopril's role in the treatment of heart failure. In addition, further study (PROGRESS) will define the role of perindopril in the prevention of cerebrovascular disease.

IN BRIEF

INDICATIONS
Hypertension

CONTRAINDICATIONS
Hypersensitivity, pregnancy, history of angioedema related to ACE inhibitors, patients dialyzed with high-flux membranes.

DRUG INTERACTIONS
Anesthetics
Diuretics
Potassium sparing diuretics
Potassium supplements
Lithium

ADVERSE EFFECTS
Cardiovascular: hypotension, chest pain, abnormal ECG
CNS: headache, dizziness, somnolence, insomnia, paresthesias, depression
GI: dyspepsia, nausea, vomiting, pancreatitis
Respiratory: cough (12%), upper respiratory infection, sinusitis, pneumonitis
Dermatologic: rash
Renal: elevations of BUN or serum creatinine
Others: small decreases in hemoglobin and hematocrit, hyperkalemia (< 2%), tinnitus, low extremity pain, asthenia, impotence (1%), elevation of liver function tests, neutropenia, angioedema (0.1%)

PHARMACOKINETICS AND PHARMACODYNAMICS
Duration of action: ≈ 24 h
Time to peak plasma concentration: 1 h (perindopril), 3–7 h (perindoprilat)
Peak effect: 6 h
Bioavailability: ≈ 75% (perindopril), 25% (perindoprilat)
Effect of food: food does not affect the rate or extent of absorption of perindopril but decreases bioavailability of perindoprilat by about 35%.
Metabolism: perindopril is extensively hydrolyzed in the liver to its active metabolite, perindoprilat
Elimination: perindopril and its metabolites are excreted mostly in the urine with approximately 4%–12% excreted as unchanged drug
Half-life: 1.5–2.9 h (perindopril), 3–10 h (apparent plasma half-life of perindoprilat), 30–120 h (terminal elimination half-life of perindoprilat)
Protein binding: 60% (perindopril), 10%–20% (perindoprilat)

MONITORING
Blood pressure.
Renal function—Acute renal failure may occur on initiation of ACE inhibitor therapy if the kidneys are dependent on angiotensin II for perfusion. This affects patients with bilateral renal artery stenosis or stenosis of the artery to a solitary kidney, patients with heart failure, or patients who are in hypovolemic states. Rises in serum creatinine or blood urea nitrogen should be an indication to reduce diuretic or perindopril dosage.
Suspect renal artery stenosis.
Electrolytes, CBC.

SPECIAL GROUPS

Race: whites may respond better than blacks because of lower renin levels usually found in blacks; however, racial differences in blood pressure responses are greatly reduced by the concurrent use of diuretics

Children: safety and effectiveness have not been established

Elderly: lower dose is required. Dose should also allow for age-related reduction in renal function

Hepatic impairment: dose adjustments may not be necessary in patients with compensated hepatic cirrhosis. Further studies are required to evaluate the need for dose reductions in patients with more severe forms of liver disease

Renal impairment: dose must be adjusted according to renal function

Patients on hemodialysis: anaphylactoid reactions have been reported in patients dialyzed with high-flux membranes and treated concurrently with an ACE inhibitor. A different type of dialysis membrane or a different class of medication should be considered

Pregnancy: category C (first trimester); category D (second and third trimesters). Use of ACE inhibitors in the second and third trimesters of pregnancy has been associated with fetal skeletal abnormalities, neonatal renal failure, and neonatal death Perindopril should be discontinued as soon as possible when pregnancy is detected

Breast-feeding: not recommended. Perindopril may be excreted in breast milk

DOSAGE

The recommended initial dose as monotherapy for hypertension is 4 mg once daily. This dose can be titrated according to response to a maximum of 16 mg per day. The usual maintenance dose is 4 to 8 mg once daily. For patients over age 70 and for patients with CrCl of 30–60 mL/min, initiate with 2 mg once daily and titrate according to response to a maximum of 8 mg daily. The safety and efficacy of perindopril have not been established for patients with CrCl of < 30 mL/min.

OVERDOSE

Treatment should be symptomatic and supportive. Blood pressure may be maintained with infusion of normal saline solution. Perindopril can be removed by hemodialysis.

PATIENT INFORMATION

Perindopril may be taken with or without food. Perindopril may cause headache, dizziness, or lightheadedness. Use caution when driving or doing other things that require alertness. Consult with physician immediately if pregnancy is detected. Notify physician if persistent or unusual side effects occur. Do not discontinue therapy without your physician's advice. Do not use salt substitute unless advised by physician.

AVAILABILITY

Tablets: 2 mg, 4 mg, 8 mg

QUINAPRIL (Accupril®)

Quinapril is a nonsulfhydryl prodrug ACE inhibitor. Although quinapril has a short elimination half-life of 2 h, its ability to bind strongly with tissue ACE enables this agent to give an antihypertensive effect for as long as 24 h. Similar to other ACE inhibitors, quinapril reduces left ventricular hypertrophy. In patients with mild to severe hypertension, quinapril 10 to 40 mg/d given as a single dose or in two divided doses daily appeared to have similar efficacy to enalapril 10 to 40 mg/d. A further increase in antihypertensive effect was observed when quinapril was combined with hydrochlorothiazide. Administration of quinapril 2.5 to 30 mg/d to patients with CHF improved New York Heart Association class, symptoms of heart failure, exercise tolerance, and workload in these patients. Similar to most of the other agents in this class, quinapril is FDA approved for the treatment of hypertension and heart failure.

SPECIAL GROUPS

Race: whites may respond better than blacks because of lower renin levels usually found in blacks; however, racial differences in BP responses are greatly reduced by the concurrent use of diuretics

Children: safety and effectiveness have not been established

Elderly: usually respond well. Dose should allow for age-related reduction in renal function

Hepatic impairment: conversion of parent drug into active metabolite may be impaired depending on degree of liver impairment. However, dose adjustment may not be needed

Renal impairment: dose must be adjusted according to renal function

Patients on hemodialysis: anaphylactoid reactions have been reported in patients dialyzed with high-flux membranes and treated concurrently with an ACE inhibitor. A different type of dialysis membrane or a different class of medication should be considered

Pregnancy: category C (first trimester); category D (second and third trimesters). Use of ACE inhibitors in the second and third trimesters of pregnancy has been associated with fetal skeletal abnormalities, neonatal renal failure, and neonatal death. Quinapril should be discontinued as soon as possible when pregnancy is detected

Breast-feeding: not recommended; quinapril is secreted in breast milk

IN BRIEF

INDICATIONS
Hypertension
Heart failure

CONTRAINDICATIONS
Hypersensitivity, pregnancy, history of angioedema related to ACE inhibitors, patients dialyzed with high-flux membranes, severe aortic stenosis or outflow obstruction

DRUG INTERACTIONS
Adrenergic-blocking agents
Allopurinol
Anesthetics
Antacids
Digoxin
Diuretics

Drugs that interact with magnesium
Lithium
NSAIDS (indomethacin)
Potassium supplements
Potassium sparing diuretics
Tetracycline

ADVERSE EFFECTS
Cardiovascular: hypotension (3%), orthostatic hypotension (< 1%), chest pain (2%–3%), angina pectoris (< 1%), rhythm disturbances (< 1%)
CNS: headache (1%–6%), dizziness (4%–8%), fatigue (2%–3%), somnolence/drowsiness (≤ 1%), insomnia (≤ 1%)
GI/GU: abdominal pain (1%), nausea (1%–3%), diarrhea (1%–2%), hepatitis (< 0.5%), pancreatitis (< 0.5%), dry mouth (≤ 1%)
Respiratory: cough (2%–5%), dyspnea (2%)
Dermatologic: rash (1%–2%), pruritus (≤ 1%), photosensitivity (< 0.5%), flushing (≤ 1%)
Renal: elevations of BUN or serum creatinine
Others: angioedema (0.1%), neutropenia (rare), anemia (< 0.5%), syncope (≤ 1%), impotence (≤ 1%), myalgia (1%–2%), elevations of liver function tests, hyperkalemia (2%)

PHARMACOKINETICS AND PHARMACODYNAMICS
Duration of action: up to 24 h
Onset of action: 1 h
Peak effect: 2–4 h
Bioavailability: 60%
Effect of food: the rate and extent of quinapril absorption are diminished moderately (about 25%–30%) when administered with a high-fat meal
Metabolism: converted to quinaprilat and two minor metabolites in the liver
Elimination: 61% renal; 37% fecal
Effective accumulation half-life: ≈ 3 h (quinaprilat)
Protein binding: 97%

MONITORING
BP—Observe carefully for first-dose hypotension, especially in patients with heart failure, renovascular hypertension, and in patients who are sodium or volume depleted.
Renal function—Acute renal failure may occur on initiation of ACE inhibitor therapy if the kidneys are dependent on angiotensin II for perfusion. This affects patients with bilateral renal artery stenosis or stenosis of the artery to a solitary kidney, patients with heart failure, or patients who are in hypovolemic states. Rises in serum creatinine or blood urea nitrogen should be an indication to reduce diuretic or quinapril dosage. Suspect renal artery stenosis.
Electrolytes, CBC.

OVERDOSE
Treatment should be symptomatic and supportive. The patient's BP may be maintained with infusion of normal saline solution. Hemodialysis has little effect on the elimination of quinapril and quinaprilat.

DOSAGE

Hypertension: The recommended initial dosage of Accupril in patients not on diuretics is 10 or 20 mg once daily. Dosage adjustments should be made at intervals of at least 2 weeks. Most patients require dosages of 20, 40, or 80 mg/d given as a single dose or in two equally divided doses. In renovascular hypertension, or in patients in whom diuretics have not been discontinued, the starting dose should be 2.5–5 mg/d. For patients with creatinine clearance of 31–60 mL/min, the initial dose should be 5 mg daily. For patients with creatinine clearance of 10–30 mL/min, the initial dose should be 2.5 mg daily.

Heart failure: The usual initial dose is 5 mg twice daily, administered under close medical observation, especially in patients with low BP. If the initial dosage is well tolerated, patients should then be titrated as tolerated at weekly intervals until an effective dose, usually 20–40 mg daily given in two equally divided doses, is reached. For patients with creatinine clearance of 31–60 mL/min, the initial dose should be 5 mg daily. For patients with creatinine clearance of 10–30 mL/min, the initial dose should be 2.5 mg daily. If the initial dose is well tolerated, quinapril may be given as a twice-daily regimen on the following day.

PATIENT INFORMATION

Quinapril may be taken with or without food. Quinapril may cause dizziness, fainting, or lightheadedness, especially during the first few days of therapy. Avoid abrupt changes in posture. Use caution when driving or doing other things that require alertness. Consult with physician immediately if pregnancy is detected. Notify physician if persistent or unusual side effects occur. Do not discontinue therapy without your physician's advice. Do not use salt substitute unless advised by physician.

AVAILABILITY

Tablets—5 mg, 10 mg, 20 mg, 40 mg

RAMIPRIL
(Altace®)

Ramipril is a nonsulfhydryl prodrug, that is hydrolyzed after absorption to form the active metabolite ramiprilat. Ramiprilat has a long elimination half-life of 13–17 h, thus permitting once daily administration. In patients with mild to moderate essential hypertension, ramipril 10 mg administered once daily demonstrated similar antihypertensive efficacy as atenolol 100 mg once daily and captopril 50 mg twice daily. In addition, ramipril 5 to 10 mg given once daily was shown to be comparable to enalapril 10 to 20 mg once daily. The addition of hydrochlorothiazide may yield adequate BP reduction in those patients who did not respond to ramipril alone. Ramipril has also exhibited beneficial effects in patients with moderate to severe CHF. A significant reduction in mortality was observed when ramipril was initiated between 3 and 10 days after an acute MI in patients with heart failure in the AIRE study. Ramipril presents as a useful alternative ACE inhibitor for use in patients with hypertension and CHF. Preliminary results of the HOPE study found that ramipril (5 mg bid) significantly reduced mortality and cardiovascular events in patients with cardiovascular disease or at high risk.

SPECIAL GROUPS

Race: whites may respond better than blacks because of lower renin levels usually found in blacks; however, racial differences in BP responses are greatly reduced by the concurrent use of diuretics

Children: safety and effectiveness have not been established

Elderly: usually respond well. Dose should allow for age-related reduction in renal function

Hepatic impairment: conversion of parent drug into active metabolite may be impaired, depending on degree of liver impairment

Renal impairment: dose must be adjusted according to renal function

Patients on hemodialysis: anaphylactoid reactions have been reported in patients dialyzed with high-flux membranes and treated concurrently with an ACE inhibitor. A different type of dialysis membrane or a different class of medication should be considered

Pregnancy: category C (first trimester); category D (second and third trimesters). Use of ACE inhibitors in the second and third trimesters of pregnancy has been associated with fetal skeletal abnormalities, neonatal renal failure, and neonatal death. Ramipril should be discontinued as soon as possible when pregnancy is detected

Breast-feeding: not recommended; ramipril may be excreted in breast milk

IN BRIEF

INDICATIONS
Hypertension
Heart failure post MI

CONTRAINDICATIONS
Hypersensitivity, pregnancy, history of angioedema related to ACE inhibitors, patients dialyzed with high-flux membranes, severe aortic stenosis or outflow obstruction.

DRUG INTERACTIONS
Adrenergic-blocking agents
Allopurinol
Anesthetics
Antacids
Digoxin
Diuretics
NSAIDS (indomethacin)
Potassium sparing diuretics
Potassium supplements
Lithium

ADVERSE EFFECTS
Cardiovascular: hypotension (0.5%–10%), orthostatic hypotension (2%), chest pain (≤ 1%), angina pectoris (< 1%–3%)
CNS: headache (1%–5%), dizziness (2%–4%), fatigue (2%), somnolence/drowsiness (< 1%), insomnia (< 1%), vertigo (< 1%–1.5%)
GI/GU: abdominal pain (< 1%), nausea (<1%–2%), diarrhea (≤ 1%), hepatitis (< 1%), pancreatitis (< 1%), dry mouth (< 1%)
Respiratory: cough (7%–12%), dyspnea (< 1%) upper respiratory infection
Dermatologic: rash, pruritus, photosensitivity(< 1%)
Renal: elevations of BUN or serum creatinine
Others: angioedema (0.3%), asthenia (< 1%–2%) neutropenia (rare), anemia (< 1%), syncope (< 1%–2%), impotence (< 1%), myalgia (< 1%), elevations of liver function tests, hyperkalemia (1%)

PHARMACOKINETICS AND PHARMACODYNAMICS
Duration of action: up to 24 h
Onset of action: 1–2 h
Peak effect: 4–6 h
Bioavailability: up to 60%
Effect of food: the rate, but not extent, of absorption is reduced.
Metabolism: ramipril is almost completely metabolized to ramiprilat, which has about six times the ACE inhibitory activity of ramipril, and to the diketopiperazine ester, the diketopiperazine acid, and the glucuronides of ramipril and ramiprilat, all of which are inactive.
Elimination: 60% renal; 40% fecal
Effective accumulation half-life: 13–17 h (ramiprilat)
Protein binding: 73%, ramipril; 56%, ramiprilat

The information here is provided as guidance only. Prescribers should always consult the manufacturer's current prescribing information.

39

DOSAGE

Hypertension: Usual initial dose is 2.5 mg/d, increased gradually to a maximum of 20 mg/d according to response, given in a single dose or two equally divided doses. In renovascular hypertension or in patients in whom diuretics have not been discontinued, the starting dose should be 1.25 mg/d. For patients with creatinine clearance of < 40 mL/min/1.73m^2, the initial dose should be 1.25 mg/d. Dosage may be titrated upward until BP is controlled or to a maximum of 5 mg/d.

Heart failure: The usual initial dose is 2.5 mg twice daily. Patients who become hypotensive at this dose may be switched to 1.25 mg twice daily, but all patients should then be titrated toward a target dose of 5 mg twice daily if tolerated. For patients with creatinine clearance of < 40 mL/min/1.73m^2, the initial dose should be 1.25 mg daily. Dosage may then be increased to 1.25 mg twice daily up to a maximum dose of 2.5 mg twice daily, depending on clinical response and tolerance.

MONITORING

BP—Observe carefully for first-dose hypotension, especially in patients with heart failure, renovascular hypertension, and in patients who are sodium or volume depleted.

Renal function—Acute renal failure may occur on initiation of ACE inhibitor therapy if the kidneys are dependent on angiotensin II for perfusion. This affects patients with bilateral renal artery stenosis or stenosis of the artery to a solitary kidney, patients with heart failure, or patients who are in hypovolemic states. Rises in serum creatinine or BUN should be an indication to reduce diuretic or ramipril dosage.

Suspect renal artery stenosis.

Electrolytes, CBC.

OVERDOSE

Treatment should be symptomatic and supportive. The patient's BP may be maintained with infusion of normal saline solution. It is not known if ramipril or ramiprilat can be usefully removed from the body by hemodialysis.

PATIENT INFORMATION

Ramipril may be taken with or without food. Capsule usually is swallowed whole but may be sprinkled on applesauce or mixed in water or apple juice. The mixture should be consumed in its entirety. Ramipril may cause dizziness, fainting, or lightheadedness, especially during the first few days of therapy; avoid abrupt changes in posture. Use caution when driving or doing other things that require alertness. Consult with physician immediately if pregnancy is detected. Notify physician if persistent or unusual side effects occur. Do not discontinue therapy without your physician's advice. Do not use salt substitute unless advised by physician.

AVAILABILITY

Capsules—1.25 mg, 2.5 mg, 5 mg, 10 mg

TRANDOLAPRIL (Mavik®)

Trandolapril is a nonsulfhydryl prodrug and is hydrolyzed in the liver to its active metabolite trandolaprilat after oral administration. Trandolaprilat has a high affinity for ACE, which results in a slow dissociation and a long biological half-life. Near total ACE inhibition 24 h after a single dose and significant ACE inhibition 72 h following drug withdrawal after long-term therapy have been observed with trandolapril. The trough:peak ratio with once-daily administration of trandolapril was found to be higher than 50% (50%–100%). In patients with essential hypertension, trandolapril administered once daily can effectively reduce systolic and diastolic BP throughout the 24-h post-dose period.

The antihypertensive efficacy of trandolapril 0.5–4 mg/d has demonstrated to be comparable to those of enalapril 2.5–20 mg/d and lisinopril 10 mg/d. Concomitant therapy with a thiazide diuretic or calcium antagonist further enhances the antihypertensive efficacy of trandolapril. In addition, trandolapril 2–4 mg/d appeared to be as effective as atenolol 100–200 mg/d, hydrochlorothiazide 25 mg/d or sustained release nifedipine 40 mg/d in BP control. Trandolapril has also exhibited beneficial effects in patients with left ventricular dysfunction. A significant decrease in mortality was observed when trandolapril was initiated between 3– 7 d after an acute MI in patients with left ventricular dysfunction.

Trandolapril is indicated for the treatment of hypertension and for the management of patients with heart failure or left ventricular dysfunction post MI.

SPECIAL GROUPS

Race: whites may respond better than blacks because of lower renin levels usually found in blacks; however, racial differences in BP responses are greatly reduced by the concurrent use of diuretics

Children: safety and effectiveness have not been established

Elderly: usually respond well; dose should allow for age-related reduction in renal function

Hepatic impairment: lower doses should be considered in patients with hepatic insufficiency

Renal impairment: dose must be adjusted according to renal function

Patients on hemodialysis: anaphylactoid reactions have been reported in patients dialyzed with high-flux membranes and treated concurrently with an ACE inhibitor. A different type of dialysis membrane or a different class of medication should be considered

Pregnancy: category C (first trimester); category D (second and third trimesters). Use of ACE inhibitors in the second and third trimesters of pregnancy has been associated with fetal skeletal abnormalities, neonatal renal failure, and neonatal death. Trandolapril should be discontinued as soon as possible when pregnancy is detected

Breast-feeding: not recommended. Trandolapril may be excreted in breast milk

IN BRIEF

INDICATIONS
Hypertension
Heart failure post-MI
Left ventricular dysfunction post-MI

CONTRAINDICATIONS
Hypersensitivity, pregnancy, history of angioedema related to ACE inhibitors, patients dialyzed with high-flux membranes, severe aortic stenosis or outflow obstruction.

DRUG INTERACTIONS
Adrenergic-blocking agents
Allopurinol
Anesthetics
Antacids
Digoxin
Diuretics
Lithium
NSAIDS (indomethacin)
Potassium sparing diuretics
Potassium supplements

ADVERSE EFFECTS
Cardiovascular: hypotension (0.3%–11%), chest pain (≤ 1%), palpitations (≤ 1%)
CNS: headache (> 1%), dizziness (1%–23%), fatigue (> 1%), somnolence/drowsiness (≤ 1%), insomnia (≤ 1%)
GI/GU: abdominal pain (≤ 1%), vomiting (≤ 1%), diarrhea (≤ 1%), dyspepsia (≤ 5%) pancreatitis (≤ 1%), UTI (1%)
Respiratory: cough (2%–35%), dyspnea (≤ 1%), upper respiratory infection (≤ 1%)
Dermatologic: rash (≤ 1%), pruritus (≤ 1%), flushing (≤ 1%)
Renal: elevations of BUN or serum creatinine
Others: angioedema (0.1%), neutropenia (rare), asthenia (3%–4%), syncope (≤ 6%), impotence (≤ 1%), myalgia (4%–5%), elevations of liver function tests, hyperkalemia (0.4%).

PHARMACOKINETICS AND PHARMACODYNAMICS
Duration of action: ≥ 24 h
Onset of action: 4 h
Time to peak plasma concentration: 1 h, trandolapril; 4–10 h, trandolaprilat
Bioavailability: 10% as tradolapril, 70% as trandolaprilat
Effect of food: food slows absorption of trandolapril, but does not affect AUC or C_{max} of trandolaprilat or C_{max} of trandolapril
Metabolism: in addition to trandolaprilat, at least seven other metabolites have been found, principally glucuronides or deesterification products
Elimination: 33% in urine (mostly as trandolaprilat); 66% in feces
Half-life: 6 h, trandolapril; 10 h, trandolaprilat
Protein binding: 80%, trandolapril; 65%–94%, trandolaprilat

DOSAGE

Hypertension: Usual initial dose is 1 mg/d in nonblack patients and 2 mg/d in black patients. Increased (at ≥ 1wk intervals) to a maximum of 8 mg/d according to response. Most patients have required dosages of 2–4 mg/d. There is little experience with doses more than 8 mg/d. Patients inadequately treated with once-daily dosing at 4 mg may be treated with twice-daily dosing. In renovascular hypertension or in patients in whom diuretics have not been discontinued, the starting dose should be 0.5 mg/d. For patients with a creatinine clearance < 30 mL/min or with hepatic cirrhosis, the recommended initial dose is also 0.5 mg/d.

Heart failure or left-ventricular dysfunction post MI: The usual initial dose is 1 mg/d. Following the initial dose, titrate as tolerated toward a target dose of 4 mg/d. If a 4 mg dose is not tolerated, patients can continue therapy with the greatest tolerated dose. For patients with a creatinine clearance < 30 mL/min or with hepatic cirrhosis, the recommended initial dose is 0.5 mg/d.

MONITORING

BP—Observe carefully for first-dose hypotension, especially in patients with heart failure, renovascular hypertension, and in patients who are sodium or volume depleted.

Renal function—Acute renal failure may occur on initiation of ACE inhibitor therapy if the kidneys are dependent on angiotensin II for perfusion. This affects patients with bilateral renal artery stenosis or stenosis of the artery to a solitary kidney, patients with heart failure, or patients who are in hypovolemic states. Rises in serum creatinine or BUN should be an indication to reduce diuretic or trandolapril dosage. Suspect renal artery stenosis.

Electrolytes, CBC.

OVERDOSE

Treatment should be symptomatic and supportive. The patient's BP may be maintained with infusion of normal saline solution. Trandolaprilat is removed by hemodialysis.

PATIENT INFORMATION

Trandolapril may be taken with or without food. Trandolapril may cause dizziness, fainting, or lightheadedness, especially during the first few days of therapy; avoid abrupt changes in posture. Use caution when driving or doing other things that require alertness. Consult with physician immediately if pregnancy is detected. Notify physician if persistent or unusual side effects occur. Do not discontinue therapy without your physician's advice. Do not use salt substitute unless advised by physician.

AVAILABILITY

Tablets—1 mg, 2 mg, 4 mg
Combination formulations:
Tarka—trandolapril/verapamil hydrochloride ER tablets—
2 mg/180 mg
1 mg/240 mg
2 mg/240 mg
4 mg/240 mg

SELECTED BIBLIOGRAPHY

ASHP Commission on Therapeutics: ASHP therapeutic guidelines on angiotensin-converting-enzyme inhibitors in patients with left ventricular dysfunction. *Am J Health Syst Pharm* 1997, 54:299–313.

Binder SB: ACE inhibitors: review of four new agents. *Am Fam Physician* 1993, 48:851–857.

Björck S, Nyberg G, Mulec H, *et al.*: Beneficial effects of angiotensin converting enzyme inhibition on renal function in patients with diabetic nephropathy. *Br Med J* 1986, 293:471–474.

Brogden RN, Wiseman LR: Moexipril: A review of its use in the management of essential hypertension. *Drugs* 1998, 55:845–860.

Burris JF: The expanding role of angiotensin converting enzyme inhibitors in the management of hypertension. *J Clin Pharmacol* 1995, 35:337–342.

Cheng A, Frishman WH: Use of angiotensin-converting enzyme inhibitors as monotherapy and in combination with diuretics and calcium channel blockers. *J Clin Pharmacol* 1998, 38:477–491.

Cohn JN, Johnson G, Ziesche S, *et al.*: A comparison of enalapril with hydralazine-isosorbide dinitrate in the treatment of chronic congestive heart failure. *N Engl J Med* 1991, 325:303–310.

CONSENSUS Trial Study Group: Effects of enalapril on mortality in severe congestive heart failure. Results of the Cooperative North Scandinavian Enalapril Survival Study (CONSENSUS). *N Engl J Med* 1987, 316:1429–1435.

Croog SM, Levine S, Testa MA, *et al.*: The effects of antihypertensive therapy on the quality of life. *N Engl J Med* 1986, 314:1657–1664.

Dunn A, Chow MSS: Focus on perindopril: a long-acting ACE inhibitor for hypertension that improves arterial distensibility and compliance. *Formulary* 1998, 33:33–43.

Frishman WH, Cheng A: Secondary prevention of myocardial infarction: the role of β-adrenergic blockers and angiotensin converting enzyme inhibitors. *Am Heart J* 1999, 137:S25–S34.

Giles TD: Clinical experience with lisinopril in congestive heart failure: focus on the older patient. *Drugs* 1990, 39(suppl 2):17–22.

Goa KL, Balfour JA, Zuanetti G: Lisinopril: a review of its pharmacology and clinical efficacy in the early management of acute myocardial infarction. *Drugs* 1996, 52:564–588.

Gosse P, Dallocchio M, Gourgon R: ACE inhibitors in mild to moderate hypertension: comparison of lisinopril and captopril administered once daily. *J Human Hypertens* 1989, 3:23–28.

Gruppo Italiano per lo Studio della Sopravvivenza nell' Infarto Miocardico (GISSI): Six- month effects of early treatment with lisinopril and transdermal glyceryl trinitrate singly and together withdrawn six weeks after acute myocardial infarction: the GISSI-3 trial. *J Am Coll Cardiol* 1996, 27:337–344.

Herman AG: Differences in structure of angiotensin-converting enzyme inhibitors might predict differences in action. *Am J Cardiol* 1992, 70:102C–108C.

Hirooka Y, Imaizumi T, Masaki H, *et al.*: Captopril improves impaired endothelium-dependent vasodilation in hypertensive patients. *Hypertension* 1992, 20:175–180.

Howes LG: Critical assessment of ACE inhibitors: part I. *Aust Fam Physician* 1995, 24:425–429.

Jaffe IA: Adverse effects profile of sulphydryl compounds in man. *Am J Med* 1986, 30:471–476.

Johnston CI: Angiotensin converting enzyme inhibitors. In *Handbook of Hypertension, Vol. 5: Clinical Pharmacology of Antihypertensive Drugs.* Edited by Doyle AE. Amsterdam: Elsevier; 1984:272–311.

Kaplan HR, Taylor DG, Olson SC, Andrews LK: Quinapril: a preclinical review of the pharmacology, pharmacokinetics, and toxicology. *Angiology* 1989, 40:335–350.

Kober L, Torp-Pedersen C, Carlsen JE, *et al.* for the Trandolapril Cardiac Evaluation (TRACE) study group: A clinical trial of the angiotensin-converting enzyme inhibitor trandolapril in patients with left ventricular dysfunction after myocardial infarction. *N Engl J Med* 1995, 333:1670–1676.

Lancaster SG, Todd PA: Lisinopril: a preliminary review of its pharmacodynamic and pharmacokinetic properties and therapeutic use in hypertension and congestive heart failure. *Drugs* 1988, 35:646–669.

Latini R, Maggioni AP, Flather M, *et al.*: ACE inhibitor use in patients with myocardial infarction: summary of evidence from clinical trials. *Circulation* 1995, 92:3132–3137.

Leonetti G, Cuspidi C: Choosing the right ACE inhibitor: a guide to selection. *Drugs* 1995, 49:516–535.

Lewis EJ, Hunsicker LG, Bain RP, *et al.*: The effect of angiotensin converting enzyme inhibition on diabetic nephropathy. *N Engl J Med* 1993, 329:1456–1462.

Loeb HS, Johnson G, Herrick A, *et al.*: Effect of enalapril, hydralazine plus isosorbide dinitrate, and prazosin, on hospitalization in patients with chronic congestive heart failure: the V-HeFT VA Cooperative Study Group. *Circulation* 1993, 87(suppl 6):V178.

Mathiesen ER, Hommel E, Giese J, Parving HH: Efficacy of captopril in postponing nephropathy in normotensive insulin dependent diabetic patients with microalbuminuria. *Br Med J* 1991, 303:81–87.

The information here is provided as guidance only. Prescribers should always consult the manufacturer's current prescribing information.

43

Nash DT: Comparative properties of angiotensin-converting enzyme inhibitors: relations with inhibition of tissue angiotensin-converting enzyme and potential clinical implications. *Am J Cardiol* 1992, 69:26C–32C.

Nelson KM, Yeager BF: What is the role of angiotensin-converting enzyme inhibitors in congestive heart failure and after myocardial infarction? *Ann Pharmacother* 1996, 30:986–993.

Pellizzer A-M, Krum H: ACE inhibitors in cardiovascular disease: which patient? Which drug? Which dose? *Aust Fam Physician* 1996, 25:1067–1077.

Perindopril: a new ACE inhibitor for hypertension. *The Medical Letter* 1999 in press.

Pfeffer MA, Braunwald E, Moyé LA, *et al.*, on behalf of the SAVE Investigators: Effect of captopril on mortality and morbidity in patients with left ventricular dysfunction after myocardial infarction: results of the Survival and Ventricular Enlargement (SAVE) trial. *N Engl J Med* 1992, 327:669–677.

Pfeffer MA, Lamas GA, Vaughan DE, *et al.*: Effect of captopril on progressive ventricular dilatation after anterior myocardial infarction. *N Engl J Med* 1988, 319:80–86.

PROGRESS Management Committee: PROGRESS-perindopril protection against recurrent stroke study: status in July 1996. *J Hypertension* 1996, 14(suppl 6):S47–S51.

Reid JL, MacFadyen RJ, Squire IB, Lees KR: Blood pressure response to the first dose of angiotensin-converting enzyme inhibitors in congestive heart failure. *Am J Cardiol* 1993, 71:57E–60E.

Ruddy MC, Kostis JB, Frishman WH: Drugs that affect the renin-angiotensin system. In *Cardiovascular Pharmacotherapeutics*. Edited by Frishman WH, Sonnenblick EH. New York: McGraw-Hill; 1997:131–192.

Safar ME, London GM, Asmar RG, *et al.*: An indirect approach for the study of the elastic modules of the brachial artery in patients with essential hypertension. *Cardiovasc Res* 1986, 20:563–567.

Santoro D, Natali A, Palombo C, *et al.*: Effects of chronic angiotensin converting enzyme inhibition on glucose tolerance and insulin sensitivity in essential hypertension. *Hypertension* 1992, 20:181–191.

Sharpe N, Smith H, Murphy J, Hannan S: Treatment of patients with symptomless left ventricular dysfunction after myocardial infarction. *Lancet* 1988, i:255–259.

Swedberg K, Held P, Kjekshus J, *et al.*, on behalf of the CONSENSUS II Study Group: Results of the Cooperative New Scandinavian Enalapril Survival Study II (CONSENSUS II). *N Engl J Med* 1992, 327:678–684.

The Acute Infarction Ramipril Efficacy (AIRE) Study Investigators: Effects of ramipril on mortality and morbidity of survivors of acute myocardial infarction with clinical evidence of heart failure. *Lancet* 1993, 342:821–828.

The American College of Cardiology/American Heart Association Task Force on Practice Guidelines (Committee on Evaluation and Management of Heart Failure): Guidelines for the evaluation and management of heart failure. *Circulation* 1995, 92:2764–2784.

The Fourth Internal Study of Infarct Survival (ISIS-4) Collaborative Group: A randomised factorial trial assessing early oral captopril, oral mononitrate, and intravenous magnesium sulphate in 58,050 patients with suspected acute myocardial infarction. *Lancet* 1995, 345:669–685.

The SOLVD Investigators: Effects of enalapril on survival in patients with reduced left ventricular ejection fractions and congestive heart failure. *N Engl J Med* 1991, 325:293–302.

The SOLVD Investigators: Effects of enalapril on mortality and the development of heart failure in asymptomatic patients with reduced left ventricular ejection fractions. *N Engl J Med* 1992, 327:685–691.

Todd PA, Benfield P: Ramipril: a review of its pharmacological properties and therapeutic efficacy in cardiovascular disorders. *Drugs* 1990, 39:110–135.

Voors AA, Herre Kingma J, van Gilst WH: Drug differences between ACE inhibitors in experimental settings and clinical practice. *J Cardiovasc Risk* 1995, 2:413–422.

Wadworth AN, Brogden RN: Quinapril: a review of its pharmacological properties, and therapeutic efficacy in cardiovascular disorders. *Drugs* 1991, 41:378–399.

Waeber B, Nussberger J, Brunner HR: Angiotensin converting enzyme inhibitors. In *New Strategies in Hypertension*. Edited by Kaplan NM, Brenner BM, Laragh JH. New York: Raven Press; 1989:97–113.

Weinberger MH: Influence of an angiotensin converting enzyme inhibitor on diuretic-induced metabolic effects in hypertension. *Hypertension* 1983, 5(suppl III):III132–III138.

Wiseman LR, McTavish D: Trandolapril: a review of its pharmacodynamic and pharmacokinetic properties, and therapeutic use in essential hypertension. *Drugs* 1994, 48:71–90.

Zannad F: Trandolapril: How does it differ from other angiotensin converting enzyme inhibitors? *Drugs* 1993, 46(suppl 2):172–182.

As described in the previous chapter, the renin-angiotensin system (RAS) plays an important role in the body's regulation of arterial blood pressure. The effector hormone of the RAS is angiotensin II, which maintains the systemic vascular resistance and extracellular fluid volume through its direct and indirect vasoconstrictive and blood volume expansion effects (Fig. 4.1). In particular, angiotensin II constricts vascular smooth muscle and increases central sympathetic outflow. In addition, angiotensin II stimulates the release of norepinephrine and epinephrine from the sympathetic nervous system and the adrenal medulla. It exerts antinatriuretic and antidiuretic effects in the kidneys and promotes the release of vasopressin from the pituitary gland and the release of aldosterone from the adrenal cortex (sona glomerulosa).

In addition to its effects on cardiovascular homeostasis, angiotensin II increases myocardial contractility, contributes to the control of cellular growth and differentiation, and causes ventricular hypertrophy. Its effect on growth may be pathogenic in patients with chronic cardiovascular disease associated with hypertension.

Angiotensin II exerts its effects by binding to plasma membrane receptors. Two distinct angiotensin II receptor subtypes have been characterized by radioligand binding studies, AT_1 and AT_2. Furthermore, isoforms of AT_1 have been cloned and sequenced in mice and subsequently named AT_{1A} and AT_{1B}. The AT_1 receptor mediates the majority, if not all, of the biologic effects of angiotensin II. Stimulation of the AT_1 receptor causes the direct and indirect vasoconstrictive and volume expanding effects of angiotensin II, as well as cell growth and proliferation and angiogenesis (Table 4.1). The AT_1 receptor can be selectively inhibited by a group of drugs, the angiotensin II receptor blockers (ARBs), which include **candesartan, irbesartan, losartan, telmisartan,** and **valsartan.**

EFFICACY AND USE

The ARBs are approved for clinical use in the treatment of systemic hypertension. It is not established whether the ARBs have a greater hypotensive action than the angiotensin-converting enzyme (ACE) inhibitors. They are not associated with cough as a complication, in contrast to the ACE inhibitors.

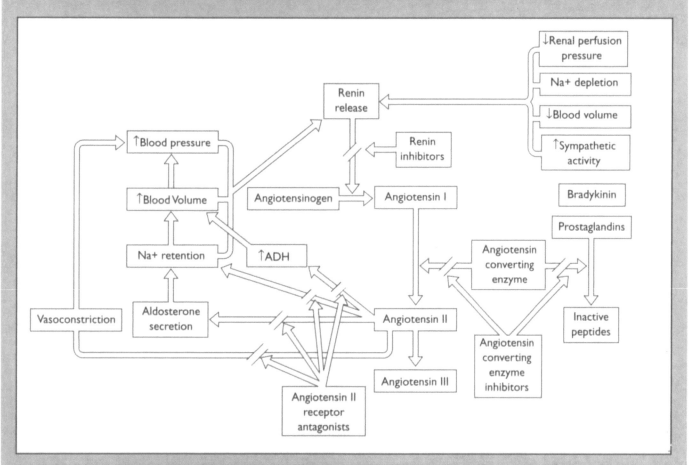

FIGURE 4.1 Schematic representation of renin-angiotensin aldosterone system. (*Adapted from* Foote EF, Halstenson CE: New therapeutic agents in the management of hypertension: angiotensin-II receptor antagonists and renin inhibitors. *Ann Pharmacother* 1993; 27:1495–1503.)

The information here is provided as guidance only. Prescribers should always consult the manufacturer's current prescribing information.

45

The drugs have been used in patients with congestive heart failure (CHF) and appear to be as effective as ACE inhibitors in improving hemodynamics; however, the ARBs are not yet approved for use in CHF. A recent study suggests that the combined use of ACE inhibitors and ARBs may be more efficacious than either class used alone. In diabetic patients, ARBs may also have renal protective actions similar to ACE inhibitors, but this needs to be proven conclusively.

The available ARBs have varied pharmacokinetic effects, as summarized in Table 4.2, and some drugs in the class may be more efficacious than another in control of blood pressure (BP). Multiple morbidity and mortality trials are now in progress that compare individual ARBs to ACE inhibitors and other drugs used to treat hypertension.

MODE OF ACTION

The ARBs bind selectively to the AT_1 receptor and exert their direct pharmacologic effects on BP by this mechanism. An-giotensin II levels are elevated with ARBs, and the unblocked AT_2 receptor will be stimulated. The AT_2 receptor is expressed at high density during *fetal life*, and in lesser amounts in the adult heart, adrenal medulla, and brain. These receptors are upregulated during vascular injury and myocardial infarction (MI). The AT_2 receptor mediates an *antiproliferative and vasodilator effect of angiotensin II* and may potentiate the actions of AT_{1A} blockade, which will have similar effects.

The theoretical benefit of combining ARBs and ACE inhibitors in hypertension and CHF is based on two premises:

1. ACE inhibition does not eliminate angiotensin II production by non-ACE synthetic mechanisms. There may be a gradual loss of pharmacologic action as angiotensin II levels increase.
2. ACE inhibition potentiates the formation of bradykinin, a vasodilator that is not affected by ARBs.

TABLE 4.1 FUNCTIONS OF AT_1 AND AT_2 RECEPTORS

Functions of AT_1 receptor	Functions of AT_2 receptor
Always expressed	Only expressed during stress or injury
Mediates renal reabsorption of sodium through tubules	Decreases renal reabsorption of sodium
Mediates vasoconstriction	Mediates vasodilatation
Mediates cell growth; inhibits endothlial function, smooth muscle proliferation, stimulates connective tissue deposit in media, facilitates LDL transport to media.	Inhibits cell growth (antiproliferation)

	Losartan	Valsartan	Irbesartan	Candesartan	Telmisartan
Trade name	Cozaar	Diovan	Avapro	Atacand	Micardis
Manufacturer	Merck	Novartis	Bristol-Myers Squibb	AstraZeneca	Boehringer Ingelheim
Indication	Hypertension	Hypertension	Hypertension	Hypertension	Hypertension
Duration of action (h)	≈ 24	≈ 24	≈ 24	≥ 24	≥ 24
Onset of action (h)	1	2	2	2–4	1
T_{max} (h)	1	2–4	1–2	3–5	1
Peak effect (h)	≈ 6	≈ 4–6	3–6	6–8	—
Bioavailability	33%	$\approx 25\%$	60%–80%	$\approx 15\%$	42%–58%
Food effect*	AUC ↓ 10%	AUC ↓ 40%; C_{max} ↓ 50%	No effect	No effect	AUC ↓ 6%–20%
Vd (L)	≈ 34 (≈ 12) ‡	17	53–93	≈ 10	≈ 500
Metabolism enzymes, primary	CYP2C9; CYP3A4	Unknown	CYP2C9	—	Acyl-glucuronide
Elimination $T_{1/2}$ (h)	≈ 2 (≈ 6–9)‡	≈ 6	11–15	≈ 9	≈ 24
Elimination (urine/ feces)†	$\approx 35\% / \approx 60\%$	$\approx 13\% / \approx 83\%$	$\approx 20\% / \approx 80\%$	$\approx 33\% / \approx 67\%$	< 1% / > 97%
Plasma bound	> 98% (> 99%)‡	95%	90%	> 99%	> 99%
Dosage range (mg/d)	25–100 (QD or BID dosing)	80–320 (QD dosing)	75–300 (QD dosing)	8–32 (QD dosing)	20–80 (QD dosing)
Dosage adjustment in the elderly	No adjustment required	No adjustment required	No adjustment required	No adjustment required	No adjustment required
Dosage adjustment in hepatic impairment	Reduce intial dose	Use with caution§	No adjustment required	No adjustment required	Use with caution¶
Dosage adjustment in renal impairment	No adjustment required	No adjustment required**	No adjustment required	No adjustment required	No adjustment required**

*All agents listed here can be taken with or without food regardless of food effect.

†% of a dose recovered in urine/ % of a dose recovered in feces.

‡Active metabolite E3174.

§Initial dosage adjustments are not required in patients with mild to moderate hepatic impairment. **Caution is advised when valsartan and telmisartan are administered to patients with severe renal impairment.

¶An alternative treatment should be considered.

AUC—area under the plasma concentration-time curve; BID —twice daily; C_{max}—peak plasma concentration; QD—daily; $T_{1/2}$—half-life; T_{max}—time to peak plasma concentration; V_d—volume of distribution.

CANDESARTAN

(Atacand®)

Candesartan binds to angiotensin II subtype 1 (AT$_1$) receptors selectively and competitively with "insurmountable" binding. Candesartan cilexetil is completely transformed to the active compound candesartan during absorption from the gastrointestinal tract. In contrast to other agents in this class, candesartan has a low bioavailability of about 15%. Candesartan has an elimination half-life of about 9 hours, and tight receptor binding which allows for once daily dosing.

Ambulatory BP monitoring has shown that the benefits of once daily candesartan cilexetil persist for 24 h without affecting normal circadian variations. Candesartan cilexetil 8 mg/d was found to be as effective as usual therapeutic dosages of enalapril, losartan potassium, hydrochlorothiazide, and amlodipine in comparative studies. At 16 mg/d, candesartan cilexetil reduced trough diastolic BP significantly more than losartan potassium 50 mg/d in one study, and candesartan cilexetil 16 mg/d titrated as necessary to 32 mg/d more than losartan potassium 50 mg/d titrated as necessary to 100 mg/d in another study. The combination of candesartan cilexetil with either amlodipine or hydrochlorothiazide resulted in further antihypertensive effects.

Results from a few clinical studies suggest that candesartan may also be beneficial in patients with left ventricular hypertrophy and in diabetic patients with proteinuria; however, in a recent clinical trial (RESOLVD) that studied patients with heart failure, candesartan did not show significant clinical benefits, although combination therapy with enalapril had a favorable effect on ventricular remodeling. Further studies are needed to establish the efficacy of candesartan in the management of heart failure patients.

SPECIAL GROUPS

Race: no effect
Children: safety and effectiveness have not been established
Elderly: no initial dosage adjustment is required
Renal impairment: no initial dosage adjustment is required
Hepatic impairment: no initial dosage adjustment is required
Pregnancy: category C (first trimester); category D (second and third trimester)
Candesartan should be discontinued as soon as pregnancy is detected
Breast-feeding: not recommended; candesartan may be excreted in breast milk

DOSAGE

Usual initial dose is 16 mg once daily. The dosage may be titrated within the range 8–32 mg/d according to response. Hydrochlorothiazide has an additive effect.

IN BRIEF

INDICATIONS
Treatment of hypertension. Candesartan cilexetil can be used alone or in combination with other antihypertensive agents.

CONTRAINDICATIONS
Hypersensitivity
Pregnancy

DRUG INTERACTIONS
Because candesartan is not significantly metabolized by the cytochrome P450 system and has no effects on P450 enzymes, interactions with drugs that inhibit or are metabolized by those enzymes would not be anticipated.

ADVERSE EFFECTS
CNS: headache (>1%), dizziness (4%), fatigue (>1%)
Respiratory: upper respiratory tract infection (6%), cough (1%–2%, less common than with ACE inhibitors)
GI: diarrhea (>1%), abdominal pain (>1%), nausea/vomiting (>1%)
Hematologic: small decreases in hemoglobin and hematocrit, anemia (rare), leukopenia (rare), thrombocytopenia (rare)
Renal: increased blood urea nitrogen (BUN) or serum creatinine (uncommon)

PHARMACOKINETICS AND PHARMACODYNAMICS
Duration of action: ≥24 h
Onset of action: 2–4 h
Time to peak serum concentration: 3–5 h
Peak effect: 6–8 h
Bioavailability: ≈ 15%
Effect of food: no effect
Metabolism: candesartan undergoes minor hepatic metabolism to form an inactive metabolite
Elimination: ≈ 33% recovered in urine, ≈ 67% recovered in feces
Elimination half-life: ≈ 9 h
Protein binding: >99%

MONITORING
BP, electrolytes, serum creatinine, BUN.

OVERDOSE
Treatment should be symptomatic and supportive. Candesartan is not removed by hemodialysis.

PATIENT INFORMATION
Because dizziness may occur in some patients, use caution when driving or doing other things that require alertness. Consult with physician immediately if pregnancy is detected. Notify physician if persistent or unusual side effects occur. Do not discontinue therapy without your physician's advice.

AVAILABILITY
Tablets—4 mg, 8 mg, 16 mg, 32 mg

IRBESARTAN
(Avapro®)

Irbesartan suppresses the activity of angiotensin II via selective and competitive antagonism of the angiotensin II subtype 1 (AT_1) receptor. Compared to other agents in this class, irbesartan has a high bioavailability of about 60%–80%. Irbesartan has a long elimination half-life of 11–15 h, thus allowing for once daily dosing.

Irbesartan was demonstrated to reduce BP to a comparable extent to enalapril and atenolol. When compared to losartan 100 mg/d, irbesartan 300 mg/d was found to reduce BP to a greater extent in one study involving patients with mild to moderate hypertension. Similar to losartan and valsartan, the addition of hydrochlorothiazide to irbesartan resulted in additive antihypertensive effects.

Preliminary studies evaluating the efficacy of irbesartan in patients with heart failure and in diabetic patients with proteinuria have generated encouraging results; however, these findings need to be confirmed in further studies.

SPECIAL GROUPS

Race: the magnitude of BP lowering appeared somewhat less in black patients in some trials

Children: safety and effectiveness have not been established

Elderly: no dosage adjustment is required

Renal impairment: no dosage adjustment is required

Hepatic impairment: no dosage adjustment is required

Pregnancy: category C (first trimester); category D (second and third trimester). Irbesartan should be discontinued as soon as pregnancy is detected

Breast-feeding: not recommended; irbesartan may be excreted in breast milk

DOSAGE

Usual initial dose is 150 mg/d. Patients may be titrated to 300 mg once daily. Hydrochlorothiazide has an additive effect. Patients not adequately managed by the maximum dose of 300 mg once daily are unlikely to derive additional benefit from a higher dose or twice-daily dosing.

IN BRIEF

INDICATIONS
Treatment of hypertension. Irbesartan can be used alone or in combination with other antihypertensive agents.

CONTRAINDICATIONS
Hypersensitivity
Pregnancy

DRUG INTERACTIONS
In vitro studies show appreciable inhibition of the formation of oxidized irbesartan metabolites with the known cytochrome CYP2C9 substrates/inhibitors, tolbutamide, and nifedipine; however, clinical consequences were insignificant

ADVERSE EFFECTS
CNS: headache (≥1%), dizziness (≥1%), fatigue (4%)
Respiratory: upper respiratory tract infection (9%), cough (3%, less than with ACE inhibitors)
GI: diarrhea (3%), dyspepsia (2%), nausea/vomiting (≥1%)
Hematologic: decreased hemoglobin of 0.2 g/dL (0.2%), neutropenia (0.3%)
Renal: increased BUN or serum creatinine (<1%)

PHARMACOKINETICS AND PHARMACODYNAMICS
Duration of action: 24 h
Onset of action: 2 h
Time to peak serum concentration: 1–2 h
Peak effect: 3–6 h
Bioavailability: 60%–80%
Effect of food: no effect
Metabolism: cytochrome P450 2C9 is the primary enzyme involved in the metabolism of irbesartan. No active metabolites have been identified
Elimination: ≈ 20% recovered in urine, ≈ 80% recovered in feces
Elimination half-life: 11–15 h
Protein binding: 90%

MONITORING
BP, electrolytes, serum creatinine, BUN, CBC.

OVERDOSE
Treatment should be symptomatic and supportive. Irbesartan is not removed by hemodialysis.

PATIENT INFORMATION
Because dizziness may occur in some patients, use caution when driving or doing other things that require alertness. Consult with physician immediately if pregnancy is detected. Notify physician if persistent or unusual side effects occur. Do not discontinue therapy without your physician's advice.

AVAILABILITY
Tablets—75 mg, 150 mg, 300 mg
Combination formulation:
Avalide—150 mg irbesartan/12.5 mg hydrochlorothiazide

LOSARTAN (Cozaar®)

Losartan potassium was the first nonpeptide angiotensin II receptor antagonist available for oral treatment of hypertension in the United States. This agent binds competitively and selectively to the angiotensin II subtype 1 (AT$_1$) receptor, thus blocking the physiological effects induced by angiotensin II. Losartan undergoes considerable first-pass metabolism with a bioavailability of about 33%. Approximately 14% of an oral dose of losartan is converted to an active carboxylic acid metabolite E3174. In contrast to losartan potassium, E3174 is a partial "insurmountable" antagonist of the AT1 receptor. This active metabolite has a terminal half-life of 6–9 h and contributes substantially to losartan's antihypertensive effect.

Losartan decreases BP to a similar extent as enalapril, atenolol, and felodipine extended release when administered as monotherapy (50–100 mg once daily) in patients with mild to moderate hypertension. Further BP reduction was observed when hydrochlorothiazide was combined with losartan. Approximately 30% of patients with severe hypertension have responded to the combination product.

Losartan is currently indicated for the treatment of hypertension. Ongoing trials are evaluating the effects of losartan in patients with recent myocardial infarction (OPTIMAL) and in patients with hypertension and left ventricular hypertrophy (LIFE). Preliminary results of the ELITE II heart failure trial found that losartan (50 mg/d) was numerically (but not statistically) less effective than captopril (50 mg tid) in a population age ≥60 years.

SPECIAL GROUPS

Race: BP response is notably less in black patients when compared to white patients
Children: safety and effectiveness have not been established
Elderly: no dosage adjustment is required
Renal impairment: no dosage adjustment is required
Hepatic impairment: reduction of the initial dose is required
Pregnancy: category C (first trimester); category D (second and third trimester). Losartan should be discontinued as soon as pregnancy is detected
Breast-feeding: not recommended; losartan may be excreted in breast milk

DOSAGE

Usual initial dose is 50 mg once daily. Dose can be titrated up to 100 mg/d (in one or two divided doses.) Lower initial dose of 25 mg should be given to patients at high risk for hypotension, volume depletion, and those with hepatic dysfunction.

IN BRIEF

INDICATIONS
Treatment of hypertension. Losartan can be used alone or in combination with other antihypertensive agents.

CONTRAINDICATIONS
Hypersensitivity
Pregnancy

DRUG INTERACTIONS
In vitro studies show notable inhibition of the formation of the active metabolite of losartan by inhibitors of cytochrome P450 3A4 (eg, ketoconazole, troleandomycin) or P450 2C9 (sulfaphenazole). The pharmacodynamic effect of concomitant use of losartan and these inhibitors have not been examined. Interactions also occur with cimetidine and phenobarbital; however, the clinical effects of these interactions are undetermined.

ADVERSE EFFECTS
CNS: headache (>1%), dizziness (4%), fatigue (4%)
Respiratory: upper respiratory tract infection (7%), cough (3%–4%, less than with ACE inhibitors)
GI: diarrhea (2%–3%), dyspepsia (1%–2%)
Hematologic: slight decreases in hemoglobin and hematocrit.
Renal: increased BUN or serum creatinine (<1%)

PHARMACOKINETICS AND PHARMACODYNAMICS
Duration of action: 24 h
Onset of action: 1 h
Time to peak serum
concentration: losartan, 1 h; E3174, 3–4 h
Peak effect: ≈ 6 h
Bioavailability: ≈ 33 %
Effect of food: AUC decrease by 10%
Metabolism: ≈ 14% of losartan is converted to active metabolite E3174
Elimination: ≈ 35% recovered in urine, ≈ 60% recovered in feces
Elimination half-life: losartan, ≈ 2 h; E3174, ≈ 6–9 h
Protein binding: losartan, 98.7%; E3174, 99.8%

MONITORING
BP, electrolytes, serum creatinine, BUN, CBC.

OVERDOSE
Treatment should be symptomatic and supportive. Losartan and E3174 are not removed by hemodialysis.

PATIENT INFORMATION
Because dizziness may occur in some patients, use caution when driving or doing other things that require alertness. Consult with physician immediately if pregnancy is detected. Notify physician if persistent or unusual side effects occur. Do not discontinue therapy without your physician's advice.

AVAILABILITY
Tablets, film coated—25 mg, 50 mg
Combination formulation:
Hyzaar—50 mg losartan potassium/12.5 mg hydrochlorothiazide

TELMISARTAN (Micardis®)

Telmisartan is a nonpeptide angiotensin II receptor antagonist, which inhibits the angiotensin II subtype 1 (AT_1) receptor selectively and competitively. Telmisartan has an extended elimination half-life of about 24 h. This allows the agent to have a longer lasting antihypertensive effect.

In two studies that used ambulatory BP monitoring, telmisartan given once daily was shown to provide better diastolic BP control for the full dosing interval than losartan potassium 50 mg or amlodipine 5 or 10 mg. In patients with mild to moderate hypertension, telmisartan 40–160 mg once daily was found to be at least as effective as atenolol 50 or 100 mg and lisinopril 10–40 mg. Telmisartan 80 mg/d was demonstrated to be more effective than enalapril 20 mg/d in one study. Similar to the other agents in this class, telmisartan is approved by the Food and Drug Administration for the treatment of hypertension.

SPECIAL GROUPS

Race: BP response in black patients (usually in low-renin population) is noticeably less than that in white patients

Children: safety and effectiveness have not been established

Elderly: no initial dosage adjustment is required

Renal impairment: no dosage adjustments are required in patients with mild to moderate renal impairment

Hepatic impairment: use with caution; an alternative treatment can be considered

Pregnancy: category C (first trimester); category D (second and third trimester). Telmisartan should be discontinued as soon as pregnancy is detected

Breast-feeding: not recommended; telmisartan may be excreted in breast milk

DOSAGE

Usual initial dose is 40 mg once daily. The dosage may be titrated within the range of 20–80 mg/d according to response. Initiate treatment under close medical supervision for patients with hepatic impairment or biliary obstructive disorders. Correct the condition of patients with depletion of intravascular volume prior to initiation of therapy and monitor closely.

IN BRIEF

INDICATIONS
Treatment of hypertension. Telmisartan can be used alone or in combination with other antihypertensive agents.

CONTRAINDICATIONS
Hypersensitivity
Pregnancy

DRUG INTERACTIONS
Digoxin—Coadministration led to a variable increase in digoxin serum concentrations
Warfarin—Coadministration led to a decrease in warfarin serum concentrations; however, this decrease did not result in a change in the coagulation parameters

ADVERSE EFFECTS
CNS: headache (1%), dizziness (1%), fatigue (1%)
Respiratory: upper respiratory tract infection (7%), cough (less common than with ACE inhibitors)
GI: diarrhea (3%), abdominal pain (1%), nausea/vomiting (1%)
Hematologic: decreased hemoglobin of > 2g/dL (<1%), anemia (rare)
Renal: increased BUN or serum creatinine (<1%)

PHARMACOKINETICS AND PHARMACODYNAMICS
Duration of action: ≥ 24 h
Onset of action: 1 h
Time to peak serum
  concentration: 1 h
Bioavailability: 42%–58%
Effect of food: AUC decreased by 6%–20%
Metabolism: biotransformation is minimal
Elimination: <1% recovered in urine, >97% recovered in feces
Elimination half-life: ≈ 24 h
Protein binding: >99%

MONITORING
BP, electrolytes, serum creatinine, BUN, CBC, serum digoxin concentration.
Note—Patients on dialysis may develop orthostatic hypotension; monitor BP closely.

OVERDOSE
Treatment should be symptomatic and supportive. Telmisartan is not removed by hemodialysis.

PATIENT INFORMATION
Because dizziness may occur in some patients, use caution when driving or doing other things that require alertness. Consult with physician immediately if pregnancy is detected. Notify physician if persistent or unusual side effects occur. Do not discontinue therapy without your physician's advice.

AVAILABILITY
Tablets—40 mg, 80 mg

VALSARTAN (Diovan®)

Valsartan was the next angiotensin II receptor antagonist that became available for the treatment of hypertension after losartan. Similar to losartan, valsartan binds competitively and selectively to the angiotensin II subtype 1 (AT_1) receptor. Valsartan also undergoes extensive first-pass metabolism with a bioavailability of approximately 25%. Valsartan has an elimination half-life of about 6 h, which allows for once a day dosing.

The antihypertensive efficacy of valsartan was demonstrated to be similar to those of losartan, lisinopril, enalapril, amlodipine, and hydrochlorothiazide in patients with mild to moderate essential hypertension. Addition of hydrochlorothiazide was shown to provide BP control in patients who responded inadequately to valsartan monotherapy. At this time, valsartan is indicated only for the treatment of hypertension. The role of this agent in the treatment of heart failure remains to be determined in an ongoing trial named Val-HeFT.

SPECIAL GROUPS

Race: no information

Children: safety and effectiveness have not been established

Elderly: increased AUC and half-life of valsartan have been observed; however, dosage adjustments are not usually required

Renal impairment: caution is advised when valsartan is administered to patients with severe renal impairment

Hepatic impairment: use with caution; initial dosage adjustments are not required in patients with mild to moderate hepatic insufficiency

Pregnancy: category C (first trimester); category D (second and third trimester). Valsartan should be discontinued as soon as pregnancy is detected

Breast-feeding: not recommended; valsartan may be excreted in breast milk

DOSAGE

Usual initial dose is 80 mg once daily. Dosage may be increased to 160–320 mg/d gradually, if necessary.

IN BRIEF

INDICATIONS
Treatment of hypertension. Valsartan can be used alone or in combination with other antihypertensive agents.

CONTRAINDICATIONS
Hypersensitivity
Pregnancy

DRUG INTERACTIONS
The enzyme(s) responsible for valsartan metabolism has not been identified but do not seem to be CYP 450 isozymes. The inhibitory or induction potential of valsartan on CYP 450 is also unknown.

ADVERSE EFFECTS
CNS: headache (>1%), dizziness (>1%), fatigue (2%)
Respiratory: upper respiratory tract infection (8%), cough (>1%, less than with ACE inhibitors)
GI: diarrhea (2%–3%), dyspepsia (1%–2%), abdominal pain (2%), nausea/vomiting (>1%)
Hematologic: decreased hemoglobin and hematocrit of > 20% (<1%)
Renal: increased BUN or serum creatinine (<1%)
Other: increased serum potassium of > 20% (4%)

PHARMACOKINETICS AND PHARMACODYNAMICS
Duration of action: ≈ 24 h
Onset of action: 2 h
Time to peak serum
concentration: 2–4 h
Peak effect: ≈ 4–6 h
Bioavailability: ≈ 25%
Effect of food: AUC decreased by 40%; C_{max} decreased by 50%
Metabolism: the primary metabolite, valeryl 4-hydroxy valsartan, is inactive
Elimination: ≈ 13% recovered in urine, ≈ 83% recovered in feces
Elimination half-life: ≈ 6 h
Protein binding: 95%

MONITORING
BP, electrolytes, serum creatinine, BUN, CBC, liver function tests.

OVERDOSE
Treatment should be symptomatic and supportive. It is not known if valsartan is removable by hemodialysis.

PATIENT INFORMATION
Because dizziness may occur in some patients, use caution when driving or doing other things that require alertness. Consult with physician immediately if pregnancy is detected. Notify physician if persistent or unusual side effects occur. Do not discontinue therapy without your physician's advice.

AVAILABILITY
Capsule—80 mg, 160 mg
Combination formulation:
Diovan HCT—80 or 160 mg valsartan/12.5 mg hydrochlorothiazide

SUGGESTED BIBLIOGRAPHY

Gheorghiade M, Cody RJ, Francis GS, *et al.*: Current medical therapy for advanced heart failure. *Am Heart J* 1998, 135:S231–S248.

Gillis JC, Markham A: Irbesartan: a review of its pharmacodynamic and pharmacokinetic properties and therapeutic use in the management of hypertension. *Drugs* 1997, 54:885–902.

Goa KL, Wagstaff AJ: Losartan potassium: a review of its pharmacology, clinical efficacy and tolerability in the management of hypertension. *Drugs* 1996, 51:820–845.

Hamroff G, Katz SD, Mancini D, *et al.*: Addition of angiotensin II receptors blockade to maximal angiotensin-converting-enzyme inhibition improves exercise capacity in patients with severe congestive heart failure. *Circulation* 1999; 99:990–992.

Kang PM, Landau AJ, Eberhardt RT, *et al.*: Angiotensin II receptor antagonists: a new approach to blockade of the renin-angiotensin system. *Am Heart J* 1994, 127:1388.

Le Jemtel TH, Sonnenblick EH, Frishman WH: Diagnosis and management of heart failure. In Alexander RW, Schlant RC, Fuster V: *Hurst's the Heart* 9th ed. New York: McGraw-Hill 1998:745–781.

Kostis JB, Frishman WH, Gradman AH: The renin angiotensin system, hypertension, and angiotensin receptor blockers (monograph). Philadelphia: Mosby-Wolfe Med Communications 1999.

Markham A, Goa KL: Valsartan: a review of its pharmacology and therapeutic use in essential hypertension. *Drugs* 1997, 54:299–311.

McClellan KJ, Goa KL: Candesartan cilexetil: a review of its use in essential hypertension. *Drugs* 1998, 56:847–869.

McClellan KJ, Markham A: Telmisartan. *Drugs* 1998, 56:1039–1044.

Pitt B, Segal R, Martinez FA, *et al.* on behalf of the ELITE Study Investigators: Randomised trial of losartan versus captopril in patients over 65 with heart failure (Evaluation of Losartan in the Elderly Study: ELITE). *Lancet* 1997, 349:747–752.

Pohl M, Cooper M, Ulrey J, *et al.*: Safety and efficacy of irbesartan in hypertensive patients with type II diabetes and proteinuria [abstract]. *Am J Hypertens* 1997, 10:105A.

Ruddy MC, Kostis JB, Frishman WH: Drugs that affect the renin-angiotensin system. In *Cardiovascular Pharmacotherapeutics Companion Handbook*. Edited by Frishman WH, Sonnenblick EH. New York: McGraw-Hill; 1998:107–151.

Tonkon M, Awan N, Niazi I, *et al.*: Combination of irbesartan with conventional therapy including angiotensin converting enzyme inhibitors [abstract]. *Heart Failure '97.* May 24–27, 1997, Cologne.

Vijay N, Alhaddad IA, Denny DM, *et al.*: Irebesartan compared with lisinopril in heart failure [abstract]. *Heart Failure '97.* May 24–27, 1997, Cologne.

5

ANTIARRHYTHMIC AGENTS

In recent years there has not been a great influx of new antiarrhythmic agents for clinical use besides the introduction of **ibutilide** and **dofetilide**, drugs that are mainly used to treat supraventricular tachyarrhythmias. Azimilide, with its unique pharmacological profile, may prove to be a beneficial agent in the treatment of ventricular tachyarrhythmias. In addition, the implantable cardioverter defibrillator has become a standard therapy for life-threatening ventricular arrhythmias, limiting the use of antiarrhythmic drugs except as adjunctive therapy.

Despite considerable advances in our understanding of basic and clinical arrhythmia mechanisms and the availability of more than a dozen drugs with antiarrhythmic activity, several factors limit the enthusiasm with which these agents are currently being prescribed. These include

1. The cardiac toxicities of antiarrhythmic drugs, particularly their propensity to cause or exacerbate more severe arrhythmias (ie, proarrhythmia), to depress electrical function, including sinus node activity and cardiac conduction, and to depress myocardial mechanical function including contractility.
2. The disappointing results of several recent trials demonstrating an unfavorable risk/benefit ratio and even mortality in "high risk" patients with premature ventricular beats treated with various conventional and newer antiarrhythmic drugs.
3. Evidence for the beneficial role of beta blockers in post-myocardial infarction (MI) patients and emerging evidence for a beneficial role of low-dose **amiodarone** in various high-risk patients.
4. The noncardiac toxicities of these agents.
5. The advent and evolution of new antiarrhythmic technologies and procedures, including antiarrhythmic devices and ablation procedures.
6. The truism that the treatment of an arrhythmia in an individual patient is still an empiric process even after careful consideration of all clinical factors and armed with full knowledge of all available antiarrhythmic agents.
7. The limitations and potential hazards of empiric therapy.
8. The limitations of noninvasive (eg, ambulatory ECG monitoring, event recorders, exercise ECG, signal-averaged ECG, tilt table testing) and invasive electrophysiologic testing methods for managing patients with arrhythmias.

Consequently, it is now generally accepted that only those arrhythmias that cause hemodynamic compromise, unacceptable symptomatology, or have a high propensity to cause clinical deterioration should be considered for drug therapy. These cautions notwithstanding, cardiac arrhythmias are a major cause of morbidity and mortality, particularly in patients with underlying ischemic, structural, or cardiomyopathic cardiovascular disease, and appropriate therapy can preserve both life and quality of life.

For drug treatment of life-threatening arrhythmias, beta-adrenergic blockers are now playing a more significant role.

Because of these factors, the indications for usage of most antiarrhythmic agents are now more restricted, and the Food and Drug Administration (FDA) recommends that many of these agents be started in a hospital setting, particularly for patients with the most severe arrhythmias or underlying cardiac disease. Thus, therapy for each patient should be individualized, risks and benefits evaluated, and specific therapeutic goals established. Efficacy and toxicity of antiarrhythmics are determined by clinical outcomes. Drug levels are sometimes helpful, particularly to check for patient compliance, as any amount of a drug may be sufficient to produce toxicity or proarrhythmia. This fact sometimes makes it very difficult to determine whether an arrhythmia is aggravated by an antiarrhythmic or is caused by an underlying condition.

In this chapter, the antiarrhythmic agents are presented according to the traditional Vaughn Williams classification with which most physicians are familiar (Table 5.1); however, it is important to realize that this classification is limited and separates the antiarrhythmics on the basis of only one dominant mechanism, whereas many antiarrhythmic agents exert more than one effect. The greatest limitation of this grouping is its inability to facilitate a ready extrapolation for therapeutic efficacy from one drug to the next, even within a particular class. Another limitation is the great variability and individuality among members within a class, which prevents secure substitution of one agent for another. A new classification has been proposed, the Sicilian Gambit, that takes into account the underlying arrhythmia mechanism: abnormal impulse formation (eg, automaticity, triggered arrhythmias, conduction abnormalities, or reentry phenomena). It also classifies antiarrhythmic agents on the basis of their numerous effects on myocardial cell targets that include cell receptors, ion channels, and electrolyte pumps.

GENERAL CONTRAINDICATIONS AND PRECAUTIONS FOR ANTIARRHYTHMIC THERAPY

Considerable caution should be exercised when starting a patient on an antiarrhythmic agent. It is recommended that class I or III antiarrhythmics be started in a hospital setting, particularly for those patients with the most severe arrhythmias or most severe underlying cardiac abnormalities. The following contraindications generally apply to all antiarrhythmic drugs:

Hypersensitivity
Sinus node dysfunction
Long QT interval
Advanced conduction disease (particularly 2° and 3° heart block)
Advanced heart failure or markedly depressed cardiac function

It is important to remember that all antiarrhythmics can potentially cause or exacerbate mechanical or electrical dysfunction, including depression of automaticity and conduction, and all have a potential for proarrhythmia.

TABLE 5.1 CLASSIFICATION OF ANTIARRHYTHMIC AGENTS

Class	Drug	Main electrophysiological/pharmacological effect
Ia	Quinidine Procainamide Disopyramide Moricizine	Depression of V_{max}; increased AP duration; increased Q-T interval; widening of the QRS complex. Moderate effects on phase 0 and ERP
Ib	Lidocaine Mexiletine Tocainide	Depression of V_{max}; decreased AP duration; unchanged Q-T interval or QRS complex. Minimal effects on phase 0 and little effect on ERP
Ic	Flecainide Propafenone	Marked depression of V_{max}; unchanged AP duration; increased QRS complex without primary change in QT interval. Minimal effects on ERP
II	Sympathetic inhibitors eg, beta blockers	Inhibition of sympathetic activity; decreased Q-Tc interval in congenital long QT syndrome
III	Amiodarone Azimilide Bretylium Sotalol (d,l-sotalol) Ibutilide Dofetilide	Increased AP duration; increased Q-T interval
IV	Verapamil Diltiazem	Blocking of slow inward calcium current
Miscellaneous	Digitalis Atropine Adenosine	Inhibition of Na/K pump; vagal effect Antivagal effect. Vagal-like effect

AP—action potential; ERP— effective refractory period; V_{max}—the maximum rate of depolarization of the cell; it equates with the fast inward sodium current.

All class I antiarrhythmics depress automaticity and slow the rate of rise of the action potential. Class I drugs are divided into three subgroups on the basis of their effects on the total action potential duration (Table 5.1): Class Ia drugs (**quinidine, procainamide, disopyramide**) increase the duration of the action potential; class Ib drugs (**lidocaine, mexiletine, tocainide**) shorten it; Class Ic drugs (**flecanide, propafenone**) have little effect. There are other important differences among the three subgroups. For example, the Q-T interval tends to be prolonged by drugs in classes Ia and Ic, and the class Ic drugs have the greatest negative inotropic action. All class I agents are primarily approved for life-threatening arrhythmias as a result of more restrictive labeling, which appeared after the CAST report.

EFFICACY AND USE

The class Ia drugs, a well established group, have retained a role in the treatment of arrhythmias despite the development of new types of antiarrhythmic drugs. All three representatives of this class have several similar effects on clinical electrophysiological parameters (Table 5.1). These drugs have a tendency to increase the Q-T and His-ventricular intervals. **Quinidine** and **disopyramide**, to a lesser extent, can be useful for reverting and controlling supraventricular arrhythmias. This group also offers potential treatment for debilitating ventricular ectopic activity, and some cases of ventricular tachycardia respond well to the drugs. Meta-analysis suggests that they do not improve prognosis by suppressing asymptomatic postinfarction ventricular ectopy or by maintaining sinus rhythm after cardioversion from atrial fibrillation.

The Class Ib drugs are generally the least potent and the least effective of the three subgroups in their suppression of arrhythmias, but they are often better tolerated than class Ia agents. **Lidocaine** is still used in various acute settings because of its intravenous formulation and relative rapid action. Nevertheless, class Ib drugs do not appear to reduce mortality compared with placebo. Their main mode of action is shortening of duration of membrane repolarization.

Class Ic agents are generally very potent in slowing conduction of the cardiac impulse and in suppressing spontaneous ventricular premature complexes. Their noncardiac side effects appear to be relatively minor, but they are highly proarrhythmogenic in a segment of the population. Although seen as an important advance in the control of arrhythmias, the class Ic drugs have recently been shown to have deleterious effects on mortality when used after infarction (Fig. 5.1). This has led to controversy regarding the use of Class Ic drugs in any arrhythmia other than a life-threatening one, and has led some to question the safety of all class I antiarrhythmic drugs in patients with myocardial dysfunction. Patients with poor left ventricular function are also most at risk from any negative inotropic effects of these drugs. It is all the more disturbing that in the CAST study active treatment of patients at high risk with class Ic drugs was associated with a threefold increase in mortality.

MODE OF ACTION

Depression of automaticity in pacemaker fibers is a property common to all class I antiarrhythmic agents (Table 5.1). It is fortunate that most antiarrhythmic agents depress subsidiary pacemaker cells to a greater degree than those of the sinoatrial node, although toxic doses of some can suppress all cardiac pacemaker activity and result in arrest of the heartbeat.

Drugs within this group have a local anesthetic effect on nerve and myocardial cell membranes. They inhibit the fast inward sodium current and thus slow the maximum rate of depolarization. Their dominant effect is to slow the rate of rise in the action potential (V_{max}). A reduction in V_{max} has been found to be associated with (1) an increase in the threshold of excitability; (2) a depression of the conduction velocity; and (3) a prolongation of the effective refractory period. These actions are also consistently associated with inhibition of the spontaneous diastolic depolarization in automatic myocardial cells.

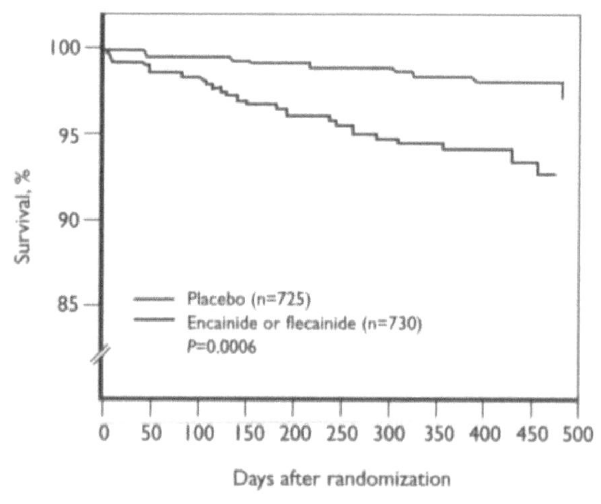

FIGURE 5.1 *The effect of flecainide or encainide on survival of patients after myocardial infarction in the CAST study.*

Placebo (n=725)
Encainide or flecainide (n=730)
P=0.0006

INDICATIONS

	Diso	Flec	Lido	Mexil	Moric	Procain	Propa	Quin	Tocain
Atrial fibrillation	(+)	+	–	–	–	(+)	(+)	+	–
Atrial flutter	(+)	+	–	–	–	(+)	(+)	+	–
Atrial tachycardia	(+)	–	–	–	–	(+)	–	+	–
Atrial extrasystoles	(+)	–	–	–	–	–	–	+	–
Supraventricular tachycardia	(+)	+	–	–	–	(+)	(+)	+	–
Life-threatening VT	+	+	+	+	+	+	+	–	+
Ventricular tachycardia	(+)	–	(+)	(+)	(+)	(+)	(+)	+	(+)
Premature ventricular contractions	(+)	–	(+)	(+)	(+)	(+)	–	+	(+)
Wolfe-Parkinson-White syndrome	–	–	–	–	–	(+)	(+)	–	–
Digitalis arrhythmias	–	–	(+)	–	–	(+)	–	–	–
Arrhythmias caused by surgery/anesthesia	–	–	(+)	–	–	(+)	–	–	–
Post MI arrhythmias	–	–	(+)	–	–	(+)	–	(+)	–
Maintenance of sinus rhythm after cardioversion	(+)	–	–	–	–	(+)	–	+	–

+—FDA approved; – —not FDA approved; (+)—clinical use not FDA approved. Diso—disopyramide; Flec—flecainide; Lido—lidocaine; Mexil—mexiletine; MI—myocardial infarction; Moric—moricizine; Procain—procainamide; Propa—propafenone; Quin—quinidine; Tocain—tocainide.

DISOPYRAMIDE PHOSPHATE

(Disopyramide phosphate, Disopyramide phosphate extended release, Norpace®, Norpace®CR)

Disopyramide depresses myocardial responsiveness and the electro-physiologic conduction rate. Diastolic depolarization is slowed in tissues with augmented automaticity, and the effective refractory period of the atrium and the ventricles is increased, but conduction in accessory pathways is prolonged. Disopyramide has a direct nega-tive inotropic effect on the myocardium, particularly in patients with abnormal heart function. It also exhibits prominent anticholinergic actions, which is a major factor limiting its usage. Disopyramide is a class Ia antiarrhythmic agent available in conventional and sustained-release formulations.

SPECIAL GROUPS

Race: no differences in response
Children: safety and effectiveness have not been established; some experiences have been published—age specific
Elderly: dosage adjustment is required
Renal impairment: dosage adjustment is required
Hepatic impairment: dosage adjustment is required
Pregnancy: category C; should only be used if clearly indicated
Breast-feeding: not recommended; the drug is excreted in breast milk

DOSAGE

Adults: Loading dose—300–400 mg po followed by maintenance regimen—400–800 mg po daily; Maximum dose is 1.6 g/d. Daily doses can be given in four divided doses q 6 h with nonsustained release products, or in two equally divided doses q 12 h with con-trolled or extended release products.

Patients < 50 kg, or with hepatic, renal impairment: Loading dose—150–200 mg po followed by 400 mg/d in two or four divided dos-es, depending on the dosage form used.

The controlled or extended release formulation of disopyramide should not be used initially if rapid plasma concentrations are desired and is not recommended for patients with severe renal impairment.

Maintenance dose with nonsustained release products in patients with severe renal impairment:

CrCl	Maintenance Dose
30–40 mL/min	100 mg q 8 h
15–30 mL/min	100 mg q 12 h
< 15 mL/min	100 mg q 24 h

Children: Use nonsustained release formulation given in divided doses q 6 h

Age	Maintenance Dose
< 1 yr	10–30 mg/kg/d
1–4 yrs	10–20 mg/kg/d
4–12 yrs	10–15 mg/kg/d
12–18 yrs	6–15 mg/kg/d

IN BRIEF

INDICATIONS
Life-threatening ventricular arrhythmias
Supraventricular arrhythmias (unlabeled use)

CONTRAINDICATIONS
History of disopyramide-associated proarrhythmic events or heart blocks
Hypersensitivity
Second or third degree heart block without a pace maker
Long QT syndrome
Severe congestive heart failure (CHF)
Untreated glaucoma
Caution in myasthenia gravis patients
Urinary dysfunction
Cardiogenic shock

DRUG INTERACTIONS
Warfarin
Beta blockers
Hepatic enzyme inducers
Anticholinergics
Antidiabetics
Antiarrhythmics
Alcohol
Macrolides

ADVERSE EFFECTS
Cardiovascular: edema, chest pain, weight gain, syncope, hypotension, CHF exacerbation
CNS: dizziness, headache, fatigue, nervousness
GI: nausea, vomiting, diarrhea, constipation, bloating
Anticholinergic effects: dry mouth, blurred vision, urinary hesitancy or retention

PHARMACOKINETICS AND PHARMACODYNAMICS
Duration of action: 1.5–8.5 h (immediate release)
Onset of action: 30 min–3.5 h
Peak effect: 30 min–3 h
Bioavailability: 87%–95%
Effect of food: not known
Metabolism: hepatic; primary metabolite has antiarrhythmic and anticholinergic actions
Excretion: 80% renal (about 50% unchanged, 30% metabolites); 15% biliary; hemodialyzable
Plasma half-life: 5–7 h (prolonged in renal impairment)
Protein binding: approximately 50% (range, 35%–95% depending on serum concentration)

MONITORING
Electrocardiogram (ECG), BP, baseline left ventricular function, periodic plasma levels, CNS and CHF symptoms. Signs and symptoms of anticholinergic effects on the GI and GU systems.

OVERDOSE
There is no specific antidote; treatment should be supportive and symptomatic. Electrocardiographic monitoring is essential. A mechanical respirator and endocardial pacer may be helpful. Medications such as digitalis, diuretics, dopamine, isoproterenol, and neostigmine may be used when indicated. Hemodialysis or charcoal hemoperfusion may help.

PATIENT INFORMATION
Report confusion, constipation, blurred vision, syncope, palpitations, urination difficulty, edema, shortness of breath to physician. Do not discontinue therapy without your physician's advice.

AVAILABILITY
Capsules (immediate release)—100 mg, 150 mg
Capsules (extended or controlled release)—100 mg, 150 mg

FLECAINIDE ACETATE (Tambocor®)

Flecainide is a class Ic antiarrhythmic agent. It produces a dose-related decrease in intracardiac conduction throughout the heart, with its most marked effect on the His-Purkinje system. It also prolongs refractoriness, especially in the ventricles. Flecainide generally has a minimal effect on sinus node function. Its relatively selective effects on retrograde pathways of atrioventricular (AV) nodal and anomalous AV conduction make it effective in terminating paroxysmal re-entrant supraventricular tachycardia in most patients.

It has also been shown to control atrial fibrillation/flutter. Flecainide, of the antiarrhythmic type Ic agents tested in the CAST I study, has shown the lethal aspects of antiarrhythmic drugs, with a higher mortality rate in the antiarrhythmic treated patients compared to placebo (Fig. 5.1). The study was terminated prematurely (encainide and moricizine were the other two drugs included in the CAST study).

SPECIAL GROUPS

Race: no differences
Children: safety and effectiveness have not been established
Elderly: lower doses recommended due to age-related decline in clearance
CHF: dosage reduction may be needed
Renal impairment: reduction in dosage warranted (renal clearance < 35 mL/min, dose reduced by 25%–50%)
Hepatic impairment: only if benefit outweighs the risk; then dose to be reduced and serum drug levels recommended
Pregnancy: category C; should only be used if clearly indicated
Breast-feeding: drug is excreted in breast milk

DOSAGE

For sustained ventricular tachycardia, initiate at 100 mg every 12 h; increase in increments of 50 mg twice daily every 4 d as needed. Usual maintenance dose is 150 mg every 12 h; limit to 400 mg/d. For patients with paroxysmal supraventricular tachycardia and patients with paroxysmal atrial fibrillation, initiate at 50 mg every 12 h. Increase in increments of 50 mg twice daily every 4 d as needed; limit to 300 mg/d in patients with paroxysmal supraventricular tachycardia. For patients with severe renal impairment (CrCl < 35 mL/min), decrease initial dose to 50 mg every 12 h; increase doses at intervals of > 4 days if needed and monitor plasma levels closely.

IN BRIEF

INDICATIONS
Life-threatening ventricular arrhythmias
Supraventricular tachyarrhythmias

CONTRAINDICATIONS
Hypersensitivity
Right bundle branch block when associated with a left hemiblock without a pacemaker
Recent myocardial infarction
Cardiogenic shock
Second- or third-degree heart block without a pacemaker
Sinus node dysfunction
Probably patients with poor LV function (< 30%–40%)

DRUG INTERACTIONS
Antiarrhythmic agents
Digoxin
Beta blockers
Verapamil
Diltiazem
Alkalinizing and acidifying agents
Cimetidine
Ritonavir

ADVERSE EFFECTS
CV: new or worsened arrhythmias, sudden cardiac death, CHF, sick sinus syndrome, AV blocks, hypotension
CNS: somnolence, headache, coma, dizziness, fatigue
GI: nausea, anorexia, abdominal pain
Other: drug fever, dyspnea, visual disturbances

PHARMACOKINETICS AND PHARMACODYNAMICS
Time to peak plasma
concentration: 3 h (1–6 h)
Bioavailability: 85%–90% well absorbed
Effect of food: no effect
Metabolism: hepatic
Excretion: ≈ 30% is excreted unchanged in the urine
Plasma half-life: 10–20 h, 16–24 h with PVCs, and 19–39 h in renal dysfunction patients
Protein binding: 37%–60%

MONITORING
ECG and vital signs daily during initiation period for PR and QRS prolongation, and every 3–6 months on maintenance dose.

OVERDOSE
Hemodynamic, symptomatic and supportive care. Pressor agents and pacing can be useful. Emesis or lavage can be followed by activated charcoal. Charcoal hemoperfusion may be tried.

PATIENT INFORMATION
Report dizziness, rapid heart rate, shortness of breath, or exercise intolerance to physician. Do not discontinue therapy without physician's advice.

AVAILABILITY
Tablets—50, 100, 150 mg

LIDOCAINE HYDROCHLORIDE

(Lidocaine HCl, Xylocaine®)

Lidocaine is a class Ib agent that has a variable effect on the effective refractory period of the atrioventricular node. It shortens the effective refractory period and action potential of the His-Purkinje system, but it does not seem to affect the excitability of normal cardiac cells.

Unlike quinidine and procainamide, it has little effect on autonomic tone and generally does not produce a substantial drop in blood pressure (BP), decreased myocardial contractility, or diminished cardiac output in the recommended doses; however, as with most anti-arrhythmic agents, it can further depress cardiac function in patients with baseline cardiac dysfunction. In patients with normal sinus nodes, it is the drug of choice for the treatment of ventricular arrhythmias in the acute setting, especially in myocardial infarction (MI), and it is used parenterally for the acute treatment of arrhythmias that arise from cardiac surgery or catheterization. It is useful in preventing a recurrence of ventricular fibrillation and treating ventricular tachycardia fibrillation before and after DC shock. It has been found useful in the correction of digitalis-induced arrhythmias that persist despite the administration of potassium and withdrawal of the glycoside. A meta-analysis of the use of lidocaine after MI showed no evidence of reduction in mortality. The results do not suggest any dramatic benefit from treatment with lidocaine, and the potential for adverse effects in some patients.

SPECIAL GROUPS

Race: no differences in response

Children: safety and effectiveness have not been established; reduce dosage when used in children

Elderly: dosage adjustment required due to reduction in patients' capacity to metabolize the drug

CHF: dosage reduction warranted

Renal impairment: use usual dose with caution

Hepatic impairment: dose reduction warranted

Pregnancy: category B; should only be used if clearly indicated

Breast-feeding: breastfeed with caution; drug is excreted in milk

DOSAGE

Initial IV bolus dose: 1–1.5 mg/kg at 25–50 mg/min, may repeat 0.5–0.75 mg/kg in 5–10 min if initial response is inadequate up to a total dose of 3 mg/kg. Patients with CHF or cardiogenic shock may require a smaller dose.

Maintenance infusion: 1–4 mg/min. Slower rate, 1–2 mg/min, may be sufficient for patients with CHF, liver disease, > 70 years old, or < 90 kg body weight.

IN BRIEF

INDICATIONS
Intravenous (IV) use for acute treatment of ventricular tachyarrhythmias.

CONTRAINDICATIONS
Hypersensitivity to any amide-type local anesthetic
Second or third degree heart block without a pacemaker
Sinus node dysfunction
Stokes-Adams syndrome
Atrial fibrillation and accessory AV pathway (Wolff-Parkinson-White syndrome)

DRUG INTERACTIONS
Antiarrhythmic agents
Succinylcholine
Cimetidine
Beta blockers

ADVERSE EFFECTS
CV: hypotension, bradycardia, cardiovascular collapse, cardiac arrest.
CNS: drowsiness, headache, confusion, disorientation, paresthesia, seizure, coma
Others: nausea, vomiting, respiratory depression

PHARMACOKINETICS AND PHARMACODYNAMICS
Duration of action: 10–20 min (IV bolus), 2 h (IM)
Onset of action: immediate with IV, 10 min with IM.
Bioavailability: nearly complete following IM injection
Effect of food: not applicable
Metabolism: 90% hepatic. The two major metabolites, monoethylglycinexylidide and glycinexylidide, have neurotoxic and antiarrhythmic effects
Excretion: renal; less than 10% as parent drug and the remainder as metabolites
Plasma half-life: 2 h; increased with CHF or liver disease (2–7 h and 5.5–7.7h, respectively), and up to 10 h in MI with CHF
Protein binding: 65%–75%

MONITORING
Continuous ECG, vital signs, serum electrolyte concentrations. Serum drug concentrations during prolonged (> 24 hours) or high-dose infusions (unbound concentration preferred in post-MI patients).

OVERDOSE
Hemodynamic support, discontinue the drug especially for CNS toxicity manifestations.

AVAILABILITY
IM injection—100 mg/mL
For direct IV injection—10, 20 mg/mL
For preparation of IV continuous infusion—40, 100, 200 mg/mL
For IV infusion— 2, 4, 8 mg/mL in 5% dextrose

MEXILETINE HYDROCHLORIDE (Mexiletine HCl, Mexitil®)

Mexiletine has class Ib antiarrhythmic properties. It is structurally similar to lidocaine (except that it is available in oral form for the treatment of arrhythmias), but their antiarrhythmic effects are not identical. Mexiletine reduces the rate of depolarization by blockade of the sodium channel, reduces conduction velocity in the His-Purkinje system, and slightly reduces the effective refractory period and the duration of the action potential; however, it consistently increases the ratio of the effective refractory period-to-action potential duration; this action is thought to correlate with its antiarrhythmic action. Mexiletine is effective in suppressing ventricular arrhythmias associated with acute MI and its efficacy is similar to that of procainamide, quinidine, and disopyramide. Nevertheless, a trend toward an increase in mortality was noted in the IMPACT study, suggesting that a good antiarrhythmic activity may not be sufficient to guarantee a favorable effect in terms of mortality.

SPECIAL GROUPS

Race: no differences in response

Children: safety and effectiveness have not been established

Elderly: dosage adjustment required due to reduction in patients' capacity to metabolize the drug

CHF: dosage reduction warranted

Renal impairment: adjustment recommended for CrCl <10 mL/min

Hepatic impairment: dose reduction warranted

Pregnancy: category C; should only be used if clearly indicated

Breast-feeding: not recommended; drug is excreted in breast milk

DOSAGE

Initiate in capsule form at 200 mg every 8 h, increase or decrease in increments or decrements of 50–100 mg/dose every 2–3 d as needed. For rapid control of ventricular arrhythmias, loading dose of 400 mg may be administered followed by a 200 mg dose 8 h later. Limit to 1200 mg/d when given every 8 h (ie, 400 mg/dose) or 900 mg/d when given every 12 h (ie, 450 mg/dose).

Note: Dosage adjustments should be made no more frequently than every 2–3 d. Some patients may tolerate twice-daily dosing. For patients adequately maintained on a dose of 300 mg or less every 8 h, total daily dose may be given divided every 12 h. Patients not adequately controlled by dosing every 8 h may respond to dosing every 6 h.

IN BRIEF

INDICATIONS
Life-threatening ventricular arrhythmias

CONTRAINDICATIONS
Second or third degree heart block without a pacemaker
Sinus node dysfunction
Cardiogenic shock
Hypersensitivity

DRUG INTERACTIONS
Class I antiarrhythmic agents
Theophylline
Cimetidine
Hepatic enzyme-inducing agents
Urinary alkalinizers/acidifiers
Narcotics
Atropine
Aluminum-magnesium hydroxide
Allopurinol
Caffeine
Metoclopramide

ADVERSE EFFECTS
CV: hypotension, bradycardia, palpitations, chest pain, increased ventricular arrhythmias, cardiovascular collapse, cardiac arrest
CNS: dizziness, lightheadedness, tremor, nervousness, drowsiness, confusion, disorientation, paresthesia
GI: nausea, vomiting, heartburn, constipation, diarrhea
Others: rash, unsteady gait

PHARMACOKINETICS AND PHARMACODYNAMICS
Duration of action: unknown
Onset of action: 1–4 h (average 2 h)
Peak effect: approximately 2–4 hours post administration
Bioavailability: well absorbed (80%)
Effect of food: may delay absorption
Metabolism: hepatic, mostly inactive metabolites
Excretion: 10%–15% excreted unchanged in urine. Urinary acidification accelerates excretion; alkalinization decreases excretion
Plasma half-life: 10–14 h; increased in patients with heart failure, hepatic impairment, or acute myocardial infarction
Protein binding: 60%–66%

MONITORING
ECG daily during initiation period, and every 3–6 mo on maintenance dose. Observe for neurologic abnormalities when initiating therapy.

OVERDOSE
Treatment is mainly supportive and symptomatic. Acidification of urine may be performed to accelerate excretion of mexiletine. Atropine may be indicated if hypotension or bradycardia occurs.

PATIENT INFORMATION
Mexiletine may be taken with food to decrease gastrointestinal upset. This medication may cause abdominal pain, nausea, vomiting, dizziness, and tremor. Report side effects to physician. Do not discontinue therapy without your physician's advice.

AVAILABILITY
Capsules—150, 200, 250 mg

MORICIZINE HYDROCHLORIDE (Ethmozine®)

Moricizine is a class I antiarrhythmic, being classified as either class Ia or Ic, but it is more accurate to classify it as Ic. The drug decreases excitability, conduction velocity and, automaticity as a result of slowed AV nodal and His-Purkinje conduction. It does not markedly affect atrial, AV nodal, or left ventricular refractory periods, and has minimal effect on ventricular repolarization, but it can cause a transient rise in BP and heart rate. Moricizine is approved for the treatment of life-threatening ventricular arrhythmias, including sustained ventricular tachycardia. As with encainide and flecainide, which were used in the CAST study, the moricizine arm of the study was discontinued because no statistically significant benefit of moricizine over placebo occurred, and because an adverse trend appeared after long-term treatment.

SPECIAL GROUPS

Race: no differences in response
Children: safety and effectiveness have not been established
Elderly: dosage adjustment required due to reduction in patients' capacity to metabolize the drug
CHF: dosage reduction may be warranted
Renal impairment: start with low dose and titrate to response
Hepatic impairment: dose reduction is needed
Pregnancy: category B; should only be used if clearly indicated
Breast-feeding: not recommended; drug is excreted in breast milk

DOSAGE

Loading dose: 200 mg po q 8 h; titrate up q 3 d
Maintenance dose: Usual 200–300 mg po q 8 h

IN BRIEF

INDICATIONS
Life-threatening ventricular arrhythmias

CONTRAINDICATIONS
Hypersensitivity
Second or third degree heart block without a pacemaker
Sinus node dysfunction
Right bundle branch block when associated with left hemiblock without a pacemaker
Cardiogenic shock

DRUG INTERACTIONS
Antiarrhythmic agents
Theophylline
Cimetidine
Diltiazem
Digoxin

ADVERSE EFFECTS
CV: proarrhythmia, sustained ventricular tachycardia, CHF, sick sinus syndrome, AV blocks
CNS: dizziness (lessened by administering in smaller doses), headache, fatigue, insomnia
GI: nausea, anorexia, abdominal pain, diarrhea
Other: drug fever, blurred vision, dyspnea

PHARMACOKINETICS AND PHARMACODYNAMICS
Duration of action: 10–24 h
Onset of action: within 2 h
Bioavailability: well absorbed but limited by high first pass metabolism (34%–38%)
Effect of food: may delay absorption
Metabolism: hepatic, extensive with at least 26 metabolites (approximately two are active). It seems to induce its own metabolism
Excretion: biliary/fecal, 56%; renal, 39% (less than 1% of a dose is excreted as parent drug)
Plasma half-life: 2 h with single dose (may be longer with chronic administration)
Protein binding: 92%–95%

MONITORING
ECG daily during initiation period for PR and QRS prolongation, and every 3–6 mo on maintenance dose.

OVERDOSE
Gastric lavage if indicated.
Hemodynamic and respiratory support, ventricular pacing, and defibrillation if needed.

PATIENT INFORMATION
Side effects may include dizziness, palpitations, headache, and nausea. Report side effects to physician. Do not discontinue therapy without your physician's advice.

AVAILABILITY
Tablets—200 mg, 250 mg, 300 mg

PROCAINAMIDE HYDROCHLORIDE

(Procainamide HCl, Procainamide HCl extended-release, Procanbid®, Pronestyl®, Pronestyl® Filmlok®, Pronestyl-SR® Filmlok®)

Procainamide exhibits the electrophysiologic effects of the Class Ia antiarrhythmic drugs. Like lidocaine and quinidine, it suppresses automaticity in the His-Purkinje system. Its anticholinergic action may also increase the conductivity of the AV node. Procainamide decreases the conduction velocity in the atria, ventricles and His-Purkinje system, and may cause no change or a slight direct decrease in the conduction velocity in the AV node. It is used prophylactically for paroxysmal atrial fibrillation, paroxysmal atrial tachycardia, and atrial and ventricular premature beats. Arrhythmias caused by surgery or anesthesia may be responsive to parenteral procainamide. In therapeutic plasma concentrations, the drug causes prolongation of the PR, QRS, and QT intervals. Blood cell dyscrasias, including agranulocytosis, occur occasionally with procainamide, and its prolonged use has been associated with lupus-like reactions, a major reason for its decline in use. N-acetyl procainamide (NAPA), an active metabolite of procainamide, with class III actions, is being investigated as a prototype for newer agents.

SPECIAL GROUPS

Race: no differences in response
Children: safety and effectiveness have not been established. IM injection is not recommended
Elderly: dosage adjustment is required for reduced renal function and other co-morbid conditions (eg, CHF)
Renal impairment: dosage adjustment is required
Hepatic impairment: dosage adjustment may be required
Pregnancy: category C: weigh potential benefits vs risk
Breast-feeding: excreted into breast milk; dosing while nursing is not recommended

DOSAGE

For initial management of arrhythmias in adults, a loading-dose infusion of 12–17 mg/kg (at a rate of 20–30 mg/min) may be given followed by a continuous infusion of 1–4 mg/min. Infusion rate should be lower in patients with renal impairment or hemodynamic instability. Consult procainamide package literature for information on proper dilution of procainamide prior to intravenous administration.

Extended-release and sustained-release tablets are intended for maintenance dosing regimen. Usual maintenance dose for ventricular arrhythmias is 50 mg/kg/day in divided doses q 6 h for extended-release tablets and q 12 h for sustained release tablets (Procanbid). Usual maintenance dose for supraventricular arrhythmias in adults is 1 g q 6 h using extended-release tablets.

For the treatment of arrhythmias that occur during surgery and anesthesia, an IM or IV (preferably IM) dose of 100–500 mg can be given.

IN BRIEF

INDICATIONS
Ventricular arrhythmias
Supraventricular arrhythmias (unlabeled use)
Atrial fibrillation/atrial flutter (unlabeled use)

CONTRAINDICATIONS
History of procainamide-induced systemic lupus erythematosus (SLE)
Second or third degree heart block without a pacemaker
Severe sinus node dysfunction
Long QT syndrome
Torsade de pointes due to other type Ia agents
Hypersensitivity

DRUG INTERACTIONS
H$_2$–receptor antagonists (cimetidine, ranitidine)
Neuromuscular blocking agents
Anticholinesterase and anticholinergic agents
Amiodarone
Antihypertensive agents
Other class I agents
Ofloxacin
Sparfloxacin
Trimethoprim

ADVERSE EFFECTS
CV: Torsade de pointe, hypotension, arrhythmias, tachycardia, QT prolongation
Blood: agranulocytosis, bone marrow depression, neutropenia
GI: anorexia, bitter taste, nausea, vomiting, diarrhea
Skin: pruritus, maculopapular rash
CNS: dizziness, lightheadedness, confusion, psychosis
Other: Sjögren's syndrome, increased LFT with liver failure, systemic lupus erythematosus-like syndrome

PHARMACOKINETICS AND PHARMACODYNAMICS
Duration of action: 4–12 h
Onset of action: 5–10 min (oral); immediate (IV)
Peak effect: 60–90 min (oral), immediate (IV), 15–60 min (IM)
Bioavailability: 75%–95% (oral)
Effect of food: not known
Metabolism: hepatic, 25% converted to active metabolite NAPA, up to 40% in rapid acetylators or renal impairment patients
Excretion: renal 50%–60% unchanged, NAPA is excreted more slowly in renal impairment or heart failure patients
Plasma half-life: procainamide—2.5–4.5 h (normal renal function); 5.3–20.7 h (renal dysfunction); 12.5–14 h (anephric) NAPA—6–8 h (normal renal function), 33–48 h (renal failure)
Protein binding: 15%–20%

MONITORING
BP, ECG, plasma concentrations of procainamide and NAPA, signs and symptoms of toxicity, antinuclear antibody (ANA) titers, CBC, electrolytes (Mg, K).

OVERDOSE
Treatment is primarily symptomatic and supportive. Symptoms of overdose may include hypotension, widening QRS, junctional tachycardia, conduction delay, oliguria, nausea/vomiting, and confusion. Gastric lavage may be performed and emesis may be induced if ingestion is recent. Fluid replacement, vasopressors, and mechanical cardiorespiratory support may be indicated. Hemodialysis may also be useful. Peritoneal dialysis is not effective. To manage torsade de pointes, 2 gm Mg IV over 15 min, then 8–16 g Mg over 24 h via continuous infusion. Replenish K if needed. The proarrhythmia event will also respond to isoproterenol, cardiac pacing, and defibrillation if ventricular fibrillation (VF) occurs.

PATIENT INFORMATION
Report symptoms of nausea/vomiting, sore throat, rash, joint pain, shortness of breath to physician. Do not chew sustained release tablets. Some sustained release tablets contain a wax core that slowly releases the medication; the empty and nonabsorbable wax core is eliminated and may be found in feces. Do not discontinue therapy without physician's advice.

AVAILABILITY
Tablets, extended release (Procainamide hydrochloride Extended-release)—250 mg, 500 mg, 750 mg
Tablets, sustained release (Procanbid)—500 mg, 1000 mg
Tablets, sustained release (Pronestyl-SR Filmlok)—500 mg
Injection—100 mg/mL, 500 mg/mL

PROPAFENONE HYDROCHLORIDE

(Rythmol®)

Propafenone is a class Ic agent with basic local anesthetic and membrane-stabilizing effects. It also has mild beta blocking and calcium blocking properties. It decreases the depolarization velocity and slows conduction in the atria, AV node, and especially in the His-Purkinje system, with resulting lengthening of the PR interval and QRS complex duration. The drug has little or no effect on the atrial functional refractory period, but AV nodal functional and effective refractory periods are prolonged. Propafenone also prolongs the ventricular refractory period and slows conduction in accessory pathways in both directions. The individual maintenance dose should be determined under cardiologic surveillance, including ECG monitoring and BP control. Therapy should be initiated under hospital conditions.

SPECIAL GROUPS

Race: no difference in response
Children: safety and effectiveness have not been established
Elderly: dosage adjustment required due to reduction in patients' capacity to metabolize the drug
CHF: contraindicated in uncontrolled CHF
Renal impairment: reduction in dosage may be warranted
Hepatic impairment: dose reduction is warranted
Pregnancy: category C; should only be used if clearly indicated
Breast-feeding: not recommended; excretion in milk unknown

DOSAGE

Initiate at 150 mg every 8 h; increase after 3–4 d, if needed, to 225 mg every 8 h. Dose may be further increased after an additional 3-4 d, to 300 mg every 8 h if needed and tolerated.

IN BRIEF

INDICATIONS
Life-threatening ventricular arrhythmias
Supraventricular tachyarrhythmias (unlabeled use)

CONTRAINDICATIONS
Second or third degree heart block without a pacemaker
Sinus node dysfunction
Bradycardia
Bronchospastic diseases
Uncontrolled CHF
Marked hypotension
Cardiogenic shock
Manifest electrolyte imbalance
Hypersensitivity

DRUG INTERACTIONS
Antiarrhythmic agents	Anesthetics
Digoxin	Anticoagulants
Beta blockers	Cyclosporine
Calcium channel blockers	Rifampin
Cimetidine	Ritonavir

ADVERSE EFFECTS
CV: proarrhythmia, AV block, hypotension
Lungs: worsening of asthma, chronic obstructive pulmonary disease
CNS: dizziness, headache, anxiety
GI: abnormal taste, nausea, constipation
Other: drug fever, blurred vision, dyspnea

PHARMACOKINETICS AND PHARMACODYNAMICS
Duration of action: 8–12 h
Onset of action: 2–4 h
Peak effect: 2–6 h
Bioavailability: well absorbed, but limited by its high first pass metabolism and its genetically determined metabolism (2%–23%). However, it will increase with chronic dosing as hepatic metabolism is saturable
Effect of food: food does not affect bioavailability significantly during multiple dose administration
Metabolism: in > 90% of patients, it is extensively metabolized into two active metabolites—5-hydroxypropafenone and N-depropylpropafenone; in < 10% of patients, metabolism of propafenone is slowed, and little, if any, of the 5-hydroxy metabolite is formed
Excretion: renal (38% as metabolites, < 1% as unchanged drug); fecal (53% as metabolites)
Plasma half-life: fast metabolizer—2–10 h; poor metabolizer—10–32 h
Protein binding: 85–95%

MONITORING
ECG and vital signs daily during initiation period, and every 3–6 mo on maintenance dose. CNS symptoms.

OVERDOSE
Hemodynamic, symptomatic and supportive care. Pressor agents and pacing may be useful.

PATIENT INFORMATION
Report dizziness, rapid heart rate, shortness of breath, or exercise intolerance to physician. Do not discontinue medication without physician's advice.

AVAILABILITY
Tablets—150, 300 mg

QUINIDINE (Quinidine gluconate, Quinaglute®, Dura-Tabs®, Quinidine polygalacturonate, Cardioquin® Quinidine sulfate, Quinora®, Quinidex®, Extentabs®)

Quinidine, considered to be a class Ia agent, is useful in preventing the recurrence of paroxysmal atrial tachycardia, paroxysmal arrhythmias arising out of the AV junction, ventricular tachycardias, and atrial and ventricular premature beats. It is also useful prophylactically after correction of atrial fibrillation or flutter. Quinidine has both direct and indirect (anticholinergic) effects on cardiac disease. Automaticity, conduction velocity, and membrane responsiveness are decreased, possibly because quinidine inhibits the movement of potassium ions across membranes. The effective refractory period is prolonged, and the anticholinergic action reduces vagal tone. An alpha-adrenergic blocking action often produces increased beta-adrenergic effects, such as peripheral vasodilatation. Use of quinidine alone during atrial flutter can produce a paradoxical acceleration of ventricular response during slowing of atrial rate; this effect is mediated by quinidine's vagolytic effect on the atrioventricular node.

Patients with congenital long QT syndrome or a history of torsades de pointes should not be given quinidine because of the increased risk for arrhythmias. Evidence suggests that although quinidine reduces the recurrence of atrial fibrillation after cardioversion, it may significantly increase the risk of death.

SPECIAL GROUPS

Race: no differences in response

Children: safety and effectiveness have not been established; however, quinidine gluconate used to treat malaria in children has shown an efficacy and safety profile comparable to adults

Elderly: initiate with lowest dose and titrate to response

Renal impairment: use usual dose with caution

Hepatic impairment: dosage adjustment is required

Pregnancy: category C; should only be used if clearly indicated; quinidine has oxytocic property; quinine use during pregnancy has caused fetal blindness and congenital deafness

Breast-feeding: not recommended; drug is excreted in breast milk

IN BRIEF

INDICATIONS
Paroxysmal supraventricualr tachycardia
Paroxysmal ventricular tachycardia
Atrial fibrillation/flutter
Maintenance of sinus rhythm after conversion
Junctional tachycardia
Premature atrial or ventricular contractions
Life-threatening Plasmodium falciparum malaria (IV quinidine gluconate)

CONTRAINDICATIONS
Hypersensitivity
Myasthenia gravis
Second or third degree AV block without a pacemaker
Torsade de pointes
Digitalis toxicity with AV conduction disorder
History of thrombocytopenic purpura associated with quinidine
History of long QT syndrome
Concurrent use of sparfloxacin or ritonavir
Intraventricular conduction defects exhibiting marked QRS widening

DRUG INTERACTIONS
Hepatic enzyme inducers	Amiodarone
Urinary alkalinizers	Antacids
Sodium bicarbonate	Beta blockers
Phenothiazines	Cholinergic drugs
Rauwolfia alkaloids	Cimetidine
Anticholinergics	Succinylcholine
Quinine	Nifedipine
Verapamil	Tricyclic antidepressants
Digoxin	Sucralfate
Bretylium	Disopyramide
Warfarin	Procainamide
Neuromuscular blocking agents	Propafenone

ADVERSE EEFFECTS
CV: torsade de pointes, hypotension, widening of QRS complex
Blood: thrombocytopenia, may cause hemolysis in patients with glucose-6-phosphate dehydrogenase deficiency
GI: diarrhea, bitter taste, anorexia, nausea, vomiting, abdominal pain
Skin: pruritus, urticaria
CNS: dizziness, vertigo, cinchonism, headache
Others: vision disturbances, elevation of serum skeletal muscle creatine phosphokinase, systemic lupus erythematosus, IM injection causes pain and muscle damage

PHARMACOKINETICS AND PHARMACODYNAMICS
Duration of action: 6–8 h; 12 h (extended release)
Onset of action: 1–3 h
Peak effect: 1–2 h (oral quinidine sulfate); 3–5 h (oral quinidine gluconate); 1 h (IM)
Bioavailability: not known
Effect of food: may delay absorption; increased oral quinidine gluconate
Metabolism: hepatic with two active metabolites
Excretion: 10%–50% renal (unchanged)
Plasma half-life: 6 h (4–10 h)
Protein binding: 80%

MONITORING
CBC, renal and hepatic function tests, BP, ECG, electrolytes K, Mg, and quinidine concentration with dosage changes and chronic administration.

DOSAGE

Quinidine is expressed in molar basis: 267 mg of quinidine gluconate or 275 mg of quinidine polygalacturonate is equivalent to 200 mg of quinidine sulfate. The following dosages are expressed in terms of the respective salts.

Quinidine Sulfate: For the conversion of atrial fibrillation— 200 mg po q 2–3 h for 5–8 doses in adults. Usually, clinicians used 300–400 mg po q 6 h. If pharmacological conversion back to sinus rhythm does not occur with plasma concentrations of 9 μg/mL, increase in dose would increase the risk of toxicity. For paroxysmal supraventricular tachycardia and paroxysmal ventricular tachycardia— 400–600 mg po q 2–3 h until paroxysm is terminated. For the maintenance of sinus rhythm after conversion— 200–400 mg po tid or qid or 300–600 mg extended release tablets q 8–12 h.

Quinidine Polygalacturonate: Initial dose—275–825 mg po followed by a second dose in 3–4 h. If no response after three or four equal doses, the dose may be increased by 137.5–275 mg for three or four more doses before further increasing the dosage. Usual maintenance dose—275 mg po bid or tid.

Quinidine Gluconate: For the suppression and prevention of atrial, AV junctional, and PVC—324–648 mg po as extended release tablet q 8–12 h. Maintenance dose for sinus rhythm after conversion, as extended release—324 mg q 8–12 h, increasing to 648 mg q 8–12 h if necessary and if tolerated.

Injections: For atrial fibrillation/flutter (can be used for ventricular arrhythmias)—5–10 mg/kg at an initial rate up to 0.25 mg/kg/min (if no conversion occurs at 10 mg/kg, attempt another mean for conversion). There is a high risk for hypotension. Monitor ECG for widening of QRS and prolongation of QT intervals, disappearance of the P wave, symptomatic bradycardia, or tachycardia. Consult quinidine package literature for proper dilution of intravenous injection.

OVERDOSE

Gastric lavage, emesis, and charcoal administration if recent ingestion. Symptomatic treatment (fluid, norepinephrine), BP and ECG monitoring, and cardiac pacing if necessary. Administration of drugs which delay elimination should be avoided (cimetidine, thiazide diuretics, carbonic anhydrase inhibitors). Artificial ventilation if indicated. Hemodialysis or forced diuresis may be effective, but not peritoneal dialysis. To manage torsade de pointes, 2 gm Mg IV over 15 min, then 8–16 g Mg over 24 h via continuous infusion. Replenish K if needed. The proarrhythmia event will also respond to isoproterenol, cardiac pacing, and defibrillation if ventricular fibrillation (VF) occurs.

PATIENT INFORMATION

Quinidine may be taken with food to reduce gastrointestinal upset. Report any symptoms of blurred vision, dizziness, tinnitus, diarrhea, abnormal bleeding or bruising, rash, or fainting. Do not crush or chew sustained release tablets; scored tablets may be cut in half. May see the core of the tablet in stool. Do not discontinue therapy without your physician's advice.

AVAILABILITY

Tablets (Quinidine sulfate)—200 mg, 300 mg
Tablets, quinidine sulfate sustained release (Quinidex Extentabs)—300 mg
Tablets, quinidine gluconate sustained release (Quinaglute Dura-Tabs)—324 mg
Tablets, quinidine polygalacturonate (Cardioquin)—275 mg
Injection (quinidine gluconate)—80 mg/mL (50 mg/mL quinidine)

TOCAINIDE HYDROCHLORIDE (Tonocard®)

Tocainide, like mexiletine, is a class Ib agent. It is an orally active analogue of lidocaine that has only a minimal effect on PR, QRS, and QT intervals of the ECG. The drug has little impact on atrial rhythm disturbances. It is mainly effective on ventricular arrhythmias and may be effective in suppressing premature ventricular beats. It has been demonstrated to be effective when class Ia drugs have failed, and is effective on those arrhythmias that respond to IV lidocaine. Often, tocainide, quinidine, and procainamide appear to have approximately equal efficacy on ventricular arrhythmias. Tocainide and quinidine can be combined advantageously, which may allow the use of lower doses of each. Tocainide appears to be only marginally effective on the severe, life-threatening arrhythmias.

SPECIAL GROUPS

Race: no differences in response
Children: safety and effectiveness have not been established
Elderly: dosage adjustment required due to reduction in patients' capacity to eliminate the drug
CHF: dosage reduction warranted
Renal impairment: adjustment recommended
Hepatic impairment: dose reduction warranted
Pregnancy: category C; should only be used if clearly indicated
Breast-feeding: not recommended; drug is excreted in breast milk

DOSAGE

Loading dose: 600 mg then 400 mg after 4–6 h
Maintenance dose: 400 mg po q 8 h, usual maintenance dose is 1.2–1.8 g daily, maximum 2.4 g/d in divided doses. Reduce initial maintenance dose by 50% in hepatic dysfunction. With CrCl 10–30 mL/min, reduce dose by 25%; with CrCl < 10 mL/min, reduce dose by 50%

IN BRIEF

INDICATIONS
Life-threatening ventricular arrhythmias

CONTRAINDICATIONS
Second or third degree AV block without a pacemaker
Sinus node dysfunction
Hypersensitivity to tocainide or to amide-type local anesthetics

DRUG INTERACTIONS
Class I antiarrhythmic agents
Rifampin
Cimetidine
Beta blockers
Caffeine
Theophylline

ADVERSE EFFECTS
CV: hypotension, bradycardia, may aggravate ventricular arrhythmias. May worsen CHF
CNS: vertigo, dizziness, drowsiness, confusion, disorientation, ataxia, paresthesia
Lungs: pulmonary fibrosis, interstitial pneumonitis, dyspnea, respiratory arrest
GI: nausea, vomiting, diarrhea, anorexia
Blood: agranulocytosis, bone marrow depression
Others: rash and fever with cross-sensitivity between tocainide and lidocaine, blurred vision, tremor

PHARMACOKINETICS AND PHARMACODYNAMICS
Duration of action: 8–16 h
Onset of action: 1–2 h (delayed by food)
Peak effect: approximately 1 h post-administration
Bioavailability: well absorbed (90%)
Effect of food: absorption is delayed
Metabolism: 30% by the liver, stereo-dependent, negligible first-pass
Excretion: urine (approximately 40% as unchanged drug)
Plasma half-life: 11–16 h in normal persons; 14–19 h in patients with CHF or arrhythmias; 20–25 h in patients with renal dysfunction
Protein binding: 5%–25%

MONITORING
ECG daily during initiation period, and every 3–6 mo on maintenance dose. Observe for neurologic abnormalities when initiating therapy. WBC counts during the first 3 mo of therapy. Baseline chest radiograph, and follow up if signs and symptoms of pulmonary fibrosis or interstitial pneumonitis occur.

OVERDOSE
Hemodynamic support. Discontinue the drug, especially for CNS toxicity manifestations. May worsen CHF.

PATIENT INFORMATION
Report numbness, drowsiness, dizziness, or tremors of extremities. Nausea can be common. Side effects may be minimized by taking tocainide with food. Do not discontinue therapy without your physician's advice.

AVAILABILITY
Tablets—400 mg, 600 mg

For many years it has been known that cardiac arrhythmias could be initiated or worsened by stress or emotion or the cardiac effects of increased catecholamines. Until the development of the beta blockers, however, no drugs were capable of controlling tachycardia, which had its origins in increased adrenergic activity. The individual drugs in this category are listed in the chapter on beta blockers. Sotalol, a beta blocker and class II antiarrhythmic with additional class III properties, is described in the next section (antiarrhythmic agents: class III).

EFFICACY AND USE

The responsiveness of different arrhythmias to beta blockade is shown in Table 5.2. In general, beta$_1$ and nonselective beta blockers are equally effective in treating supraventricular tachycardias and ventricular arrhythmias. Drugs with moderate to high intrinsic sympathomimetic activity (ISA) tend to behave like full antagonists in conditions of high sympathetic drive. In conditions of less stress they may be less effective than drugs with lower or no ISA. Beta$_1$-selective and nonselective drugs appear to be equally effective for ventricular arrhythmias after myocardial infarction. Beta blockers have been demonstrated to be effective at reducing sudden death and reinfarction in this setting. The efficacy of beta blockers in this regard sets them apart from other first-line antiarrhythmic agents. New data are emerging to support the efficacy of amiodarone in reducing sudden cardiac death and mortality in postinfarction patients.

Beta blockers can be effective in the treatment of supraventricular tachycardia (Table 5.3). Under conditions of exercise or stress, the beta blockers may be effective in suppressing premature ventricular beats and may be effective in treating re-current sustained ventricular tachycardia (Table 5.3). A combination of a class II and a class IV agent can be very effective in controlling paroxysmal supraventricular tachycardia, although this is not recommended in atrioventricular nodal disease or heart failure.

The addition of a beta blocker to a digitalis regimen can enhance ventricular function in atrial fibrillation. The combination of beta blockers and class I drugs is associated with a high conversion rate of atrial fibrillation to sinus rhythm; however, beta blockers and digitalis or other classes of antiarrhythmic drugs should be combined with caution because of the risk of complete heart block and asystole.

MODE OF ACTION

(For the use of individual beta blockers in arrhythmias, see individual drug pages).

Increased catecholamines or sympathetic stimulation have insignificant effects on the action potential of ventricular muscle, but their effect on automatic tissue within the heart is different. They increase the diastolic depolarization rate and impulse formation by specialized cardiac fibers that slow pacemaker activity. In the intact heart, sympathetic stimulation leads to increased pacemaker activity, with increased conduction in the atrioventricular node but no increase in the Purkinje fibers. This heterogeneous shortening of the refractoriness of the conduction apparatus lowers the threshold for ventricular fibrillation. Beta blockers can depress the rate of rise of the slow response action potentials, particularly in the presence of high levels of catecholamines and high extracellular potassium concentrations. Beta blockers also inhibit the enhanced spontaneous diastolic

TABLE 5.2 EXPECTED RESPONSE OF SUPRAVENTRICULAR AND VENTRICULAR CARDIAC ARRHYTHMIAS TO TREATMENT WITH BETA BLOCKERS

Arrhythmia	Response
Supraventricular arrhythmia	
Sinus tachycardia	Excellent
Paroxysmal supraventricular tachycardia (including Wolff-Parkinson-White syndrome)	Good: both elective and prophylactic
Chronic ectopic supraventricular tachycardia	Good: sinus rhythm sometimes restored
Atrial fibrillation	Ventricular rate reduced: sinus rhythm rarely restored in chronic setting, and may by restored in acute setting
Atrial flutter	Ventricular rate reduced: sinus rhythm rarely restored in chronic setting, and may be restored in acute setting
Ventricular arrhythmia	
Ventricular premature beats	Fair to good, unless related to digitalis toxicity, exercise or stress, ischemic heart disease, mitral valve prolapse, or the long QT syndrome
Ventricular tachycardia (sustained)	Fair to good, but good when it results from digitalis toxicity, exercise or stress, or the long QT syndrome, chronic infarction or acute ischemia
Paroxysmal ventricular tachycardia	Fair to good, particularly in cases unresponsive to other antiarrhythmic therapy, depending on mechanism
Ventricular fibrillation refractory to initial defibrillation	Good if (1) it results from digitalis toxicity or sympathomimetic amines, or (2) it is refractory to initial defibrillation

Data from Skluth H, Grauer K, Gums J: Ventricular arrhythmias: an assessment of newer therapeutic agents. Postgrad Med 1989, 85:137–153.

depolarizations induced by catecholamines, and therefore diminish automaticity. In the absence of sympathetic tone, propranolol has little effect on heart rate, but pindolol produces rises in resting heart rate regardless of whether the patient is in sinus rhythm. Atrioventricular nodal conduction is generally delayed by beta blockers, leading to prolongation of the PR interval and the effective refractory period. The refractoriness of both antegrade and retrograde accessory pathways in pre-excitation syndromes (such as Wolff-Parkinson-White syndrome) is generally unaffected by beta blockers at rest, but beta blockers can blunt the shortening of refractoriness induced by catecholamines. At rest and during exercise, beta blockers do not significantly affect conduction and refractoriness of His-Purkinje tissue or normal ventricular muscle, but the QT interval may be slightly shortened, suggesting a slight acceleration of ventricular muscle repolarization. In addition, some of the effects of beta blockers may be secondary to decreasing myocardial ischemia or other mechanisms.

TABLE 5.3 AGENTS FOR CONTROLLING VENTRICULAR RATE IN SUPRAVENTRICULAR TACHYCARDIAS

Agent	Loading dose	Usual maintenance dose	Comments
Digoxin* (Lanoxin)	10–15 µg/kg ideal body weight, up to 1–1.5 mg IV or po over 24 h	PO: 0.125–0.5 mg/d	Max response may take several hours and days to achieve steady state; caution in renal dysfunction
Esmolol (Brevibloc)	0.5 mg/kg IV over 1 min	50–300 µg/kg/min continuous infusion with bolus between increases in dosage	Hypotension; short half-life (8 min); additive effects with Dig, CCB
Propranolol (Inderal)	0.5–1 mg IV over ≤ 1 mg/min, repeat after 2 min if needed (max 0.15 mg/kg)	PO: 10–120 mg TID	Caution with CHF and asthma; additive effects with Dig, CCB
Metoprolol (Lopressor)	5 mg at 1 mg/min IV every 5 min × 3 doses	PO: 25–100 mg BID	Caution with CHF and asthma; additive effects with Dig, CCB
Verapamil* (Isoptin, Calan)	5–10 mg (0.075–0.15 mg/kg) IV over ≥ 2 min; may repeat with 10 mg (0.15 mg/kg) 15–30 min after completion of initial dose if needed	CI: 5–10 mg/hr; PO: 40–120 mg TID or 120–480 mg ER daily	Hypotension with IV; additive effects with BB, digoxin; may ↑ dig level
Diltiazem* (Cardizem)	0.25 mg/kg over 2 min; may repeat with 0.35 mg/kg over 2 min if needed	CI: 5–15 mg/hr; PO: 60–90 mg TID or QID or 180–360 mg ER daily	Hypotension; additive effects with Dig, CCB; may ↑ dig and theophylline levels
Adenosine (Adenocard)	6 mg rapid IV push followed with flush; may repeat with 12 mg x 2 at 2 min intervals	Not applicable	Patient may have chest tightness, breathlessness, transient/complete heart block

*Caution not to use calcium channel blockers and digoxin in rapid atrial fibrillation with Wolfe-Parkinson-White Syndrome.

BB—beta blockers; BID—twice daily; CCB—calcium channel blockers; CHF—congestive heart failure; CI—continuous infusion; Dig—digoxin; ER—extended release; IV—intravenous; Max—maximum; po—oral; QID—four times daily; TID—thrice daily.

Class III antiarrhythmic drugs, such as amiodarone, bretylium, and sotalol, are believed to exert their antiarrhythmic effect by causing a homogeneous prolongation of the action potential duration, and thus of the effective refractory period. Drugs belonging to other groups may also have such an action, including disopyramide (class I).

There are ample data from electrophysiologic studies as well as clinical trials defining the therapeutic efficacy of the class III agents, potassium channel blocking, in treating supra- and ventricular cardiac tachyarrhythmia. The concept of treating cardiac arrhythmia by delaying conduction has been replaced by the principle of delaying action potential duration, as well as lengthening the repolarization period.

It has been recognized that there is an efflux of potassium out of myocardial tissues during myocardial cells ischemia or shortly after reoxygenation. This mechanism is regulated through the different types of potassium channels, namely the ATP-dependent potassium channel (K_{ATP}), in which the depletion of ATP, which occurs during hypoxia state, will lead to intracellular acidosis, leakage of potassium out of the myocytes, and influx of sodium and calcium into cardiac cells. The accumulation of potassium outside of the cells will depolarize the myocardial cell membrane. These cumulative events will shorten the action potential duration as well as the effective refractory period, and will predispose the heart to tachyarrhythmias in situations of myocardial damage, electrolyte imbalance, and electrophysiologic instability.

The class III agents, by blocking the efflux of potassium from the cardiac cells, prolong refractoriness and repolarization in both atrial and ventricular tissues. These pharmacologic properties seem to offer a solution to alleviate the proarrhythmic conditions from a damaged myocardium, or to convert atrial fibrillation back to sinus rhythm, and prevent their recurrence.

EFFICACY AND USE

The major effect of amiodarone is to delay repolarization. It is used orally to inhibit and prevent the recurrence of life-threatening ventricular arrhythmias that do not respond to other antiarrhythmic agents. The reason for its restricted use lies in its potentially life-threatening adverse effects. The drug appears to be effective in managing a wide variety of ventricular and supraventricular arrhythmias. Data from most clinical reports indicate that it is effective in patients with life-threatening arrhythmias, including otherwise refractory cases. Amiodarone also appears to be effective in suppressing and preventing paroxysmal re-entrant supraventricular tachycardias, as well as in preventing atrial fibrillation, and can be used in Wolff-Parkinson-White syndrome.

Bretylium is used in treating life-threatening ventricular tachycardia or ventricular fibrillation. It is used in acute situations only; however, if more prolonged treatment is required, an infusion is recommended. One of the main limitations to its use is its hypotensive effect. Sotalol has both beta blocking (class II) and class III actions. It is a relatively well tolerated drug. Despite the apparent additional antiarrhythmic activity, sotalol has not been demonstrated to be superior to other beta blockers in suppressing the gamut of arrhythmias for which beta blockers are currently used, including those post MI patients. On the other hand, sotalol has emerged with a very

positive profile in the Electrophysiologic Study vs. Electrocardiographic Monitoring (ESVEM) trial, where it was compared with other antiarrhythmics. For a complete description of sotalol, see the individual drug page.

All class III antiarrhythmic agents have the potential to induce arrhythmias. They lengthen the Q-T interval, and this can predispose to the evolution of the form of ventricular tachycardia known as torsade de Pointes. Low plasma potassium levels, possibly caused by diuretic use, increase the likelihood of this arrhythmia development.

CLINICAL SIGNIFICANCE

In treating atrial fibrillation, orally administered sotalol was shown to be effective in converting atrial fibrillation back to sinus rhythm in 8%–54% of patients. This drug also had a 40%–52% success rate in preventing the recurrence of atrial fibrillation post-successful cardioversion. Amiodarone demonstrated a success rate of pharmacological cardioversion in the range of 60%–89% while assuring a 61%–79% success rate of patients remaining in sinus rhythm after 1 year with low-dose oral amiodarone (200 mg po daily range). Specifically, in the most recent trials for preventing atrial fibrillation in post-coronary artery bypass graft (CABG) patients, intravenous and orally administered amiodarone have demonstrated efficacy while maintaining a low profile of side effects. Recently, the newer class III agents, ibutilide and dofetilide, have emerged as effective agents for conversion of acute episodes of atrial fibrillation to sinus rhythm.

Sotalol and amiodarone have also been used with good results in reducing ventricular tachyarrhythmia-related death in patients post-MI (BASIS, CAMIAT, EMIAT), in patients with CHF (GESICA), in patients with nonischemic cardiomyopathy (CHF STAT), and also in patients post-cardiac arrest (CASH). It is worth noting that the benefits obtained with amiodarone therapy were associated with the concurrent administration of a beta blocker, and with d,l sotalol, which already had the beta-adrenergic antagonist effect. Even though the implantable cardioverter devices have shown beneficial results in reducing sudden cardiac death, the addition of an antiarrhythmic drug still plays a role in modulating implantable cardioverter device electrical discharges.

MODE OF ACTION

The precise mechanisms underlying the activity of the class III drugs are incompletely understood. Their principal effect on cardiac tissue is to delay repolarization by inhibiting potassium efflux and thereby prolonging the action potential duration and the effective refractory period. The drugs also appear to inhibit the transmembrane influx of extracellular sodium ions via the fast channel. In this respect, they also exhibit minor class I antiarrhythmic activity. Amiodarone noncompetitively inhibits beta-adrenergic activity, which may contribute to its antiarrhythmic effect. Nevertheless, its effects on action potential and refractory period are believed to be the basis of its activity.

Amiodarone has some class Ia and Ic antiarrhythmic actions also. It has complex and varied effects on thyroid function, inhibiting extrathyroidal deiodinases, which result in decreased peripheral conversion of thyroxine to triiodothyronine. After initiation of amiodarone therapy, there is usually a rise in release of thyroid-stimulating hormone, but levels soon fall back to baseline values. Cases of hypo- and hyperthyroidism have been reported.

Bretylium acutely produces an initial increase and then a decrease in norepinephrine release from sympathetic nerve endings. Such an indirect beta blocking effect may contribute to its activity; however, bretylium, like amiodarone, directly prolongs the action potential duration and refractoriness of cardiac tissue.

Sotalol, a beta blocker, also has class III antiarrhythmic effects. Like the other two representatives of this class, it extends the action potential duration and the period of refractoriness.

d-Sotalol, an investigational d-isomer of sotalol, has class III anti-arrhythmic properties as its predominant mode of action. Unlike its parent compound, d-sotalol exhibits much less beta blocking properties. The compound prolongs the action potential duration and the effective refractory period. Trials involving d-sotalol have been terminated prematurely due to an increase in mortality rate in the d-sotalol group compared to the placebo group.

Ibutilide, with class III properties, has been studied in patients with supraventricular and ventricular arrhythmias, and is approved for use as an intravenous agent for converting atrial fibrillation and flutter.

Dofetilide, a newly developed intravenous class III potassium-channel blocking agent, was recently approved by the FDA for treating life-threatening ventricular tachycardia, supraventricular tachyarrhythmias, and atrial fibrillation/flutter.

Azimilide, an orally-active class III potassium-channel blocking agent that blocks multiple potassium ion currents, may soon become available for maintaining normal sinus rhythm in patients with supraventricular tachycardias who have been cardioverted. In addition, azimilide is currently being investigated for its effect on mortality in post MI patients.

INDICATIONS

Indications	Amiodarone	Bretylium	Sotalol	Ibutilide	Dofetilide
Life-threatening ventricular arrhythmias	+	+	+	−	(+)
Ventricular fibrillation	+	+	−	−	(+)
Refractory ventricular arrhythmias	+	+	+	−	(+)
Supraventricular arrhythmias	(+)	−	(+)	+	+

+—FDA approved; − —not FDA approved; (+) clinical uses not FDA approved.

AMIODARONE HYDROCHLORIDE (Pacerone, Cordarone®)

Amiodarone is probably the most potent antiarrhythmic drug available. It prolongs the action potential duration and refractory period in all cardiac tissues by a direct action in the tissues, without significantly affecting membrane potential. It is a very complex drug, considered to be predominantly a class III agent with some class I, class II, and antisympathetic properties. The drug has a mild negative inotropic effect but usually does not depress left ventricular function. It causes coronary and peripheral vasodilatation, and therefore decreases peripheral vascular resistance, but only causes hypotension with large oral and intravenous doses. Amiodarone has significant antianginal properties. It is often an effective antiarrhythmic agent when others have failed. Some data suggest it may reduce mortality by as much as 25%–50% in survivors of acute myocardial infarction. Although another study suggested it has only minor benefits on mortality in severe heart failure, this is an area of active investigation. Other preliminary data have been more promising, resulting in a renewed interest in amiodarone. Investigational trials of intravenous amiodarone are being conducted in the management of patients with cardiac arrest; a higher rate of survival upon arrival to hospital was found in patients who received intravenous amiodarone in addition to standard therapy, compared with patients who received standard therapy alone for cardiac arrest in a study conducted by Kudenchuk *et al.* The general usefulness of amiodarone is limited by its severe adverse reaction profile. Many patients develop photosensitivity (requiring the use of barrier creams) and skin discoloration. All patients should be monitored for signs of pulmonary fibrosis and thyroid (amiodarone has a significant iodine moiety) and liver disorders. It is important to realize that amiodarone loading requires a minimum of 1–3 wks and that its effects persist for weeks and even months after its withdrawal.

SPECIAL GROUPS

Race: no differences in response

Children: safety and effectiveness have not been established; limited data suggest that amiodarone may be useful in the management of refractory supraventricular or ventricular arrhythmias in selected cases

Elderly: dosage adjustment based on comorbid conditions

Renal impairment: no dosage adjustment is required

Hepatic impairment: use usual dose with caution; elevation of hepatic enzymes (AST, ALT, alkaline phosphatase, bilirubin), as well as cases of hepatic injury (resembling alcoholic hepatitis or cirrhosis), have been reported. Therefore, regular monitoring of liver enzymes is recommended

Pregnancy: category D; amiodarone has shown embryotoxicity with fetal resorption, growth retardation. Amidarone and its metabolite cross the placenta. QT prolongation and transient sinus bradycardia have been reported in neonates of limited cases of pregnant women receiving amiodarone in their second or third semester of pregnancy

Breast-feeding: not recommended; amiodarone and its metabolite N-desethylamiodarone are distributed in maternal milk in concentrations higher than concurrent maternal plasma level

IN BRIEF

INDICATIONS
Treatment of refractory life-threatening ventricular arrhythmias
Supraventricular arrhythmias (not FDA approved)

CONTRAINDICATIONS
Hypersensitivity
Sinus node dysfunction
2° and 3° AV block without a pacemaker
Hemodynamic instability
Long QT syndrome
Cardiogenic shock

DRUG INTERACTIONS
Anesthetics (inhalation)	Disopyramide	Cimetidine
Indapamide	Cyclosporine	Hydantoins
Quinidine	Fentanyl	Beta blockers
Photosensitizing medication	Lidocaine	Procainamide
Calcium channel blockers	Ritonavir	Theophylline
Flecainide	Cholestyramine	Digoxin
Warfarin		

ADVERSE EFFECTS
Amiodarone exhibits a high profile of toxicity and side effects. It becomes more prevalent as dosage increases. With a dosage of 400 mg or more daily, adverse reactions occur in 75% of patients taking amiodarone, and 5%–20% require discontinuation of therapy.
Pulmonary: most severe and potentially fatal adverse reaction associated with amiodarone. It could be pulmonary interstitial pneumonitis (or alveolitis), hypersensitivity pneumonitis, or pulmonary fibrosis (10%–17% at dosage up to 400 mg/d). These have been reported fatal in 10% of the cases. Worsening of asthma could occur.
Hepatic: elevation of liver function test (3%–50%), rarely hepatic injury.
CV: pro-arrhythmias, new or worsened heart failure (3%), hypotension mostly associated with IV amiodarone (16%), atropine-resistant sinus bradycardia (1%–5%).
CNS: malaise, fatigue, ataxia, tremor, insomnia, headache, and more rarely, peripheral neuropathy.
Thyroid: hyperthyroidism (2%), hypothyroidism (2%–4%).
GI: nausea/vomiting (10%–33%, usually during the oral loading phase), constipation, abdominal pain.
Ocular: visual disturbances, asymptomatic corneal microdeposits, optic neuropathy, or optic neuritis.
Skin: photosensitivity (10%), pigment deposit resulting in a blue-gray discoloration of the skin (2%–5%) associated with long-term therapy.
Hematology: thrombocytopenia (< 2%).

PHARMACOKINETICS AND PHARMACODYNAMICS
Duration of action: weeks to months
Onset of action: 2–3 d, up to 2–5 mo for oral formulation
Peak concentration: variable, 3–7 h
Bioavailability: 22–86%
Effect of food: not determined
Metabolism: extensive hepatic metabolism, at least one active metabolite (N-desethylamiodarone)
Excretion: biliary, may undergo enterohepatic recirculation; not dialyzable
Plasma half-life: 2–10 d initially, 26–107 d with chronic administration for the parent compound, and 20–118 d for the major metabolite N-DEA
Protein binding: approximately 96%

MONITORING
ECG monitored for HR, PR, QRS, QT, QTc. Baseline and every 3–6 mo tests: LFT, PFT, thyroid, chest radiograph, ophthalmic slit-lamp examination. Electrolytes (K, Mg).

OVERDOSE
For recent ingestion, use emesis or lavage. Beta adrenergic agonists or cardiac pacing for atropine-resistant sinus bradycardia. Vasopressor for hypotension.

DOSAGE

PO loading: 800–1600 mg/d in divided doses x 1–3 wk, then reduce dose to 600–800 mg/d in 1–2 divided doses for 4 weeks.

Maintenance dosage: 200–600 mg/d (usually 400 mg/d for recurrent VT, and 200 mg/d for supraventricular arrhythmia)

IV dosing for ventricular arrhythmias: Load 150 mg over 10 min (15 mg/min). Then 360 mg over the next 6 h (1 mg/min). Maintenance infusion: 540 mg over 18 h (0.5 mg/min) up to 2–3 wks. Supplemental dose of 150 mg over 10 min can be given for breakthrough arrhythmias. Consult amiodarone package literature for proper dilution of drug prior to administration. Intravenous amiodarone concentration should not exceed 2 mg/mL unless a central venous catheter is used.

PATIENT INFORMATION

Take with food. Patients should be warned about skin discoloration and photosensitivity, and to report any shortness of breath, tiredness, abdominal discomfort, or visual abnormality. Follow up with regular visits to physician's office. Do not discontinue therapy without physician's advice.

AVAILABILITY

Tablet—200 mg
Injection for IV infusion—50 mg/mL

BRETYLIUM TOSYLATE

(Bretylium tosylate, Bretylol®)

Bretylium is used for acute life-threatening ventricular tachyarrhythmias and ventricular fibrillation, including part of cardiac resuscitation protocols. The specific mechanism of its antiarrhythmic and antifibrillatory effect has not been determined. A direct effect on the myocardial cell membrane appears to produce a rapid suppression of ventricular fibrillation, and an initial release of norepinephrine at the peripheral adrenergic nerve terminal occurs, followed by an adrenergic blockade of norepinephrine release in response to sympathetic nerve stimulation. The blockade of further norepinephrine release is thought to contribute to the suppression of ventricular tachycardia. Bretylium is considered to be a class III agent that also has sympatholytic antihypertensive activity. Its use can lead to postural decrease in BP.

SPECIAL GROUPS

Race: no differences in response
Children: safety and effectiveness have not been established
Elderly: dosage adjustment may be required based on renal function
Renal impairment: dosage adjustment is required
Hepatic impairment: no dosage adjustment required
Pregnancy: category C; there is a potential risk for reduced uterine blood flow with fetal hypoxia, and bradycardia
Breast-feeding: not recommended; excretion in breast milk unknown

DOSAGE

For ventricular fibrillation, existing and life-threatening, initiate a 5 mg/kg undiluted intravenous injection over 1 min, followed by 10 mg/kg injection over 1 min every 15–30 min if necessary, to a total of 30–35 mg/kg. Maintenance infusion (intermittent) should be diluted and administered in a dose of 5–10 mg/kg over a 8–10 min period or longer, repeated every 6 h. For other ventricular arrhythmias, administer diluted intravenous infusion (intermittent) in a dose of 5–10 mg/kg over a 8–10 min period, repeated every 1–2 h if needed. Maintenance infusion every 6–8 h as above, or administered as a constant infusion (diluted) given at a rate of 1–2 mg/min. With intramuscular administration, give 5–10 mg/kg undiluted and repeated every 1–2 h as needed. Maintenance dose is 5–10 mg/kg every 6–8 h. Do not exceed 5 mL volume in any one site for IM injection.

IN BRIEF

INDICATIONS
Ventricular fibrillation
Refractory ventricular tachycardia
Life-threatening ventricular arrhythmias

CONTRAINDICATIONS
Aortic stenosis
Severe pulmonary hypertension
Suspected digitalis-induced VT (may increase the rate of VT or induce VF)
Hypersensitivity
Coadministration with sparfloxacin

DRUG INTERACTIONS
Digitalis
Sympathomimetics
Sparfloxacin
Dopamine
Norepinephrine
Other antiarrhythmics, such as procainamide, quinidine, lidocaine

ADVERSE EFFECTS
CV: hypotension (usually orthostatic and supine) up to 50% of the patients, transient hypertension, increase in PVC and arrhythmia events, bradycardia, angina
GI: nausea, vomiting
Others: repeated IM injections at the same site lead to muscle damage (atrophy, necrosis, fibrosis, and inflammation changes) nasal stuffiness, diarrhea, renal dysfunction, abdominal pain, hiccup, loss of appetite

PHARMACOKINETICS AND PHARMACODYNAMICS
Duration of action: 6–24 h (6–12 h after a single dose)
Onset of action: 5–10 min (IV injection for ventricular fibrillation); 20–120 min (IV injection for ventricular tachycardia)
Peak effect: 6–9 h (IM)
Bioavailability: not applicable
Effect of food: not applicable
Metabolism: none
Excretion: renal, unchanged. Removed by dialysis
Plasma half-life: 6–17 h, 16–32 h in renal impairment
Protein binding: 1%–6%

MONITORING
BP and constant ECG monitoring.

OVERDOSE
Hypotension usually responds to Trendelenburg positioning and volume expansion with IV fluid or plasma. Dopamine or norepinephrine may also be indicated.

PATIENT INFORMATION
Not applicable.

AVAILABILITY
Injection—50 mg/mL (10 mL, 20 mL)
IV infusion—
  1 mg/mL in 5% dextrose (500 mL)
  2 mg/mL in 5% dextrose (250 mL)
  4 mg/mL in 5% dextrose (250 mL, 500 mL)

DOFETILIDE

(Tikosyn®)

Dofetilide has recently been approved for the conversion and maintenance of atrial fibrillation and atrial flutter. In addition, this agent has been investigated for life-threatening ventricular tachyarrhythmias, as well as for usage in conjunction with the implantable cardioverter defibrillator.

Dofetilide is a class III antiarrhythmic agent devoid of properties related to other classes I, II, or IV. In vitro and in vivo studies have shown that dofetilide selectively blocks the rapid component of cardiac delayed rectifier potassium current (Ikr), does not have effects on the time-independent inward rectifier (Iki), the transient outward current (Ito), or the inward calcium current.

Dofetilide does not affect the inotropic properties of the heart. This agent may possess the reverse use dependent characteristic, which may predispose patients to torsade de pointes. Several investigators have reported a dose-dependent negative chronotropic effect. When used with the implantable cardioverter defibrillator, dofetilide (epicardial patches) reduces the defibrillation threshold. It also increases the ventricular fibrillation threshold.

SPECIAL GROUPS

Race:	no differences in response
Children:	safety and effectiveness have not been established
Elderly:	dosage adjustment based on co-morbid conditions
Renal impairment:	dosage adjustment is required
Hepatic impairment:	dosage adjustment is expected as 50% of the drug is metabolized through the liver
Pregnancy:	no information available yet
Breast-feeding:	not recommended; excretion of drug in breast milk unknown

DOSAGE

(based on clinical trials as the official insert is still under approval process by the FDA)

Oral: Ventricular tachyarrhythmias— 0.25–1 mg bid, reduced to once daily if QT increases > 15% compared to baseline, and discontinue if QT increases > 25% compared to baseline or > 500 ms (> 600 ms for bundle branch block).

Maintenance of sinus rhythm after atrial fibrillation/atrial flutter conversion—0.125–0.5 mg po bid (maximum effect at 0.5 mg bid)

Intravenous: Ventricular tachyarrhythmias—1.5–15 mcg/kg

Conversion of atrial fibrillation/atrial flutter—4–8 mcg/kg over 15 min, can be repeated after 15 min if no response.

Supraventricular tachycardia—Loading dose is 1–10 mcg/kg over 15 min

Maintenance dose is 0.12–0.5 mcg/kg continuous infusion

IN BRIEF

INDICATIONS
Conversion and maintenance of atrial fibrillation/flutter

CONTRAINDICATIONS
Hypersensitivity
Baseline QTc > 420 msec

DRUG INTERACTIONS
Nothing specific available; however, drugs known to induce torsade de pointes (eg, tricyclic antidepressants, selective serotonic reuptake inhibitors, antiarrhythmics, cisapride, astemizole, seldane, erythromycin, haloperidol, protease inhibitors) should be avoided.

ADVERSE EFFECTS
CV: proarrhythmias torsade de pointes (4%–8%)
CNS: headache, fatigue
Other: muscle cramp

PHARMACOKINETICS AND PHARMACODYNAMICS
Duration of action:	4 h after oral dose, 3 h after IV dosing
Onset of action:	2 h with po, immediate with IV
Peak concentration:	1–2.5 hr, immediate with IV
Bioavailability:	96%–100%
Effect of food:	delay absorption but not the extent
Metabolism:	hepatic metabolism (50%)
Excretion:	renal (50% unchanged in the urine)
Plasma half-life:	7.5 hr with po, 7.5–9.7 hr with IV, prolonged in renal impairment patients
Protein binding:	not applicable

MONITORING
ECG monitoring for HR, PR, QRS, QT, QTc. Electrolytes (K, Mg).

OVERDOSE
For recent ingestion, use emesis or lavage.
Magnesium, pacing, isoproterenol may be indicated for torsade de pointes. Replenish potassium.

PATIENT INFORMATION
Patients should be warned about fatigue, headache, muscle cramps, and rapid heart rate.

AVAILABILITY
No information from the manufacturer yet.

The information here is provided as guidance only. Prescribers should always consult the manufacturer's current prescribing information.

75

IBUTILIDE FUMARATE (Corvert®)

Ibutilide is similar to the other class III agents by its action in increasing the refractory period and the action potential duration; however, it is unique because its antiarrhythmic effect solely relies on the prolongation of the action potential duration. Animal studies demonstrated that ibutilide prolongs the action potential duration through the activation of a slow inward sodium current, whereas the other class III agents prolong the refractory period and the action potential duration by blocking the cardiac delayed rectifier potassium current. Interestingly, ibutilide increases the action potential duration at low dose but shortens it at high dose (100 fold concentration).

Ibutilide prolongs the conduction time from the atria to the bundle of His, the AV Wenkebach cycle, atrial and ventricular refractoriness, right ventricular monophasic APD, and the QTc interval. There is no significant increase in the PR interval or QRS complex. In a study of healthy volunteers, the (+) enantiomer prolonged the QT interval more than the (-) enantiomer; however, no correlation could be made between the drug's effectiveness and the QT prolongation. In addition, ibutilide does not possess the reverse use dependent effect such as with sotalol. It has been suggested that ibutilide terminates re-entry supraventricular tachyarrhythmias by prolonging the atrial refractoriness without significantly affecting the conduction velocity. Ibutilide has negligible effects on heart rate, cardiac contractility, and BP.

SPECIAL GROUPS

Race: no differences in response
Children: safety and effectiveness have not been established
Elderly: no dosage adjustment is required
Renal impairment: use usual dose with caution
Hepatic impairment: no data; dosage adjustment is probably not required
Pregnancy: category C; should only be used if clearly indicated
Breast-feeding: not recommended; not known if the drug is excreted in human milk

DOSAGE

≥ 60 kg–1 mg IV push over 10 min
< 60 kg–0.01 mg/kg IV push over 10 min
Can repeat x 1, 10 min after completion of the first infusion if no response.

IN BRIEF

INDICATIONS
IV use for rapid termination of recent onset of atrial fibrillation/atrial flutter

CONTRAINDICATIONS
History of polymorphic VT
Hypersensitivity
Concurrent use of other class III antiarrhythmic agents and other drugs with the risk of causing ventricular arrhythmias

DRUG INTERACTIONS
Class I and III antiarrhythmic agents
Ketoconazole
Cisapride
Selected serotonin reuptake inhibitor (SSRI)
Phenothiazines
TCA
Macrolides

ADVERSE EFFECTS
CV: hypotension, sustained polymorphic ventricular tachycardia (ie, torsade de pointes), nonsustained polymorphic ventricular tachycardia, nonsustained monomorphic ventricular extrasystoles, nonsustained monomorphic ventricular tachycardia, bundle branch block
CNS: headache
GI: nausea

PHARMACOKINETICS AND PHARMACODYNAMICS
Onset of action: 20–30 minutes of the start of infusion
Peak effect: approximately ≥ 40 min post-injection
Effect of food: not applicable
Metabolism: extensively metabolized in liver
Excretion: both parent drug and metabolites are excreted primarily in the urine; 5%–7% as unchanged drug
Plasma half-life: 6 hr (range 2–12 hr)
Protein binding: 40%

MONITORING
Continuous ECG monitoring up to 4 hr after the injection(s) or until the QTc has returned to baseline. ECG monitoring for more than 4 h post injection is required in patients with hepatic dysfunction.

OVERDOSE
Treatment is symptomatic and supportive. To manage torsade de pointes, 2 gm Mg IV over 15 min, then 8– 16 gm Mg over 24 hr via continuous infusion. Replenish K. The proarrhythmia event will also respond to isoproterenol, cardiac pacing, and defibrillation if ventricular fibrillation (VF) occurs.

PATIENT INFORMATION
Inform about the risks of arrhythmias.

AVAILABILITY
Injection—0.1 mg/mL

SOTALOL HYDROCHLORIDE
(Betapace®)

Sotalol is a racemic mixture of two optical isomers d and l. Both isomers have class III antiarrhythmic effects; however, only the d,l-sotalol exhibits both class II antiadrenergic activities (without the membrane stabilizing property) as well as the class III activities, such as prolongation of the refractory period without affecting conduction, whereas d-sotalol only exhibits class III characteristics. Sotalol nonselectively blocks the $beta_1$ receptors within the myocardium and the $beta_2$ receptors within the bronchial and vascular smooth muscle. Sotalol does not have intrinsic sympathomimetic property. Studies have confirmed sotalol's ability to increase the action potential duration, its inverse correlation with heart rate, its lack of effect on the resting membrane potential, and maximum rate of depolarization. Sotalol selectively inhibits the rapidly activated inward component of the delayed rectifier potassium current I_{kr}. Sotalol increases the atria and ventricular refractory periods and the AV nodal conduction without affecting the atrial, His-Purkinje, or ventricular conduction velocity. Thus, sotalol prolongs QT and QTc intervals and does not affect PR and QRS intervals. Sotalol expresses its class III effects at a higher serum drug concentration than required for the class II properties.

SPECIAL GROUPS

Race: no differences in response

Children: safety and efficacy have not been established in children < 18 years of age. Fatigue and sinus bradycardia have occurred necessitating discontinuation of the drug

Elderly: dosage adjustment is required

Renal impairment: dosage adjustment is required

Hepatic impairment: no dosage adjustment required

Pregnancy: category B; crosses placenta, therefore usage of sotalol in pregnant women requires that the benefit clearly outweighs the risk

Breast-feeding: not recommended; excretion in breast milk is 2.5–5.5 times the maternal serum drug concentration

DOSAGE

Start with low doses and titrate up slowly. Usual starting dose is 80 mg po bid. Can titrate up every 2–3 d up to 240 mg and 320 mg daily in divided dosages 2 or 3 times daily. Usual maintenance dose is 160–320 mg/d, but some patients with life-threatening refractory ventricular arrhythmias may require doses as high as 480 mg or 640 mg daily.

IN BRIEF

INDICATIONS
Treatment and prevention of supraventricular tachycardia (not FDA approved)
Documented life-threatening ventricular arrhythmias

CONTRAINDICATIONS
Hypersensitivity
History of polymorphic VT
Concurrent use of other class III antiarrhythmic agents and other drugs with the risk of developing ventricular arrhythmias
Asthma
Severe CHF
Sinus bradycardia
Second and third degree AV block without a pacemaker
Long QT syndrome, cardiogenic shock

DRUG INTERACTIONS
Class I and III antiarrhythmic agents
Ketoconazole
Astemizole
Terfenadine
Cisapride
SSRI
Phenothiazines
TCA
Macrolides
Beta-blockers
Sparfloxacin

ADVERSE EFFECTS
CNS: fatigue, dizziness (20%)
CV: torsade de pointes (1%–4%), new or worsened CHF, sinus bradycardia
Respiratory: dypsnea (21%)
Blood: bleeding (2%), and rarely thrombocytopenia, leukopenia, and eosinophilia
GI: nausea, vomiting are the most frequent (10%), diarrhea (7%), dyspepsia (6%), abdominal pain, colon problems (3%), flatulence (2%)
Other: rash (5%), fever, infection, hyperglycemia, hyperlipidemia

PHARMACOKINETICS AND PHARMACODYNAMICS
Duration of action: approximately 24 h
Onset of action: 30 min–1 h
Peak effect: 1–3 h after oral dose
Bioavailability: 90%–100%
Effect of food: up to 20 % reduction in bioavailability
Metabolism: minor hepatic metabolism; no active metabolites have been identified
Excretion: 80%–90% as unchanged drug in the urine
Plasma half-life: 15.5 ± 1.2 h; 24.2 ± 7.5 h in moderate renal insufficiency; 34 ± 27 h in endstage renal disease; sotalol is cleared during dialysis
Protein binding: none

MONITORING
Heart rate, QT, QTc, and electrolytes K, Mg.

OVERDOSE
Gastric lavage if recent ingestion. Supportive therapy. To manage torsade de pointes, 2 gm Mg IV over 15 min, then 8–16 gm Mg over 24 h via continuous infusion. Replenish K if needed. The proarrhythmia event will also respond to isoproterenol, cardiac pacing, and defibrillation if VF occurs.

PATIENT INFORMATION
To be initiated in the hospital. Side effects may include bradycardia, palpitations, fatigue, dizziness, and shortness of breath. Do not discontinue therapy without your physician's advice.

AVAILABILITY
Tablets (scored)—80 mg, 120 mg, 160 mg, 240 mg

ANTIARRHYTHMIC AGENTS: CLASS IV

Class IV antiarrhythmic drugs interfere with entry of calcium ions through the slow channel. Only two agents of this type have any important effects on arrhythmias: verapamil and diltiazem. The dihydropyridine calcium antagonist (eg, nifedipine) has no useful antiarrhythmic activity. Verapamil and diltiazem are profiled in the chapter on calcium antagonists.

EFFICACY AND USE

Calcium antagonists are primarily useful for the treatment of supraventricular arrhythmias (Table 5.3). Because of their effect on conduction through the AV node, they can effectively blunt the ventricular response during atrial fibrillation and are useful in the chronic prevention of paroxysmal supraventricular re-entrant tachycardia; however, they do not convert atrial fibrillation to normal sinus rhythm, and their chronic use as oral agents for the prevention of re-entrant supraventricular tachycardias is becoming less prominent as catheter ablative procedures are advancing in frequency.

Digitalis may control the ventricular response to atrial fibrillation at rest, but marked increases in ventricular responsiveness may be seen during exercise, which can limit the exercise capacity of such patients. Exercise-induced tachycardia in patients with atrial fibrillation can be markedly attenuated by the addition of verapamil in patients receiving digitalis. Verapamil has also been used in the management of ventricular responsiveness in patients with atrial fibrillation complicating MI. Diltiazem and beta blockers can also be used for these purposes.

Paroxysmal supraventricular tachyarrhythmias, which have a re-entrant mechanism involving the AV node, can usually be terminated within 1–2 minutes after sufficient dose of intravenous verapamil. Verapamil alters the conduction and refractoriness of the AV node and can terminate these re-entrant rhythms by interrupting the circuit. The efficacy of verapamil and diltiazem in this type of arrhythmia is extremely high: over 80% of such episodes convert to sinus rhythm within minutes. Verapamil and diltiazem are generally considered second-line alternatives to adenosine for this indication. In humans, verapamil shows no ability to suppress chronic ventricular premature contractions or sustained ventricular tachycardia; however, because of its negative inotropic effect, caution must be used in giving intravenous verapamil to any patient who has compromised left ventricular function. Hypotension and bradycardia are also important concerns

with these agents, and extreme caution should be exercised when attempting to combine them with other negative inotropic agents, such as beta blockers or disopyramide, especially when there is a combination of a low ejection fraction (< 30%) and a high pulmonary wedge pressure (> 20 mmHg).

In patients with sick sinus syndrome, great caution must be exercised because of a possibility of prolonged asystole. Calcium-channel blockers are contraindicated in patients with Wolff-Parkinson-White Syndrome because of a potential preferential enhancement of the bypass tract conduction. Also, calcium-channel blockers are not indicated in wide-complex tachycardia unless the clinician is certain that a supraventricular tachycardia without anterograde accessory pathway conduction is present. One exception to this rule is a rare form of ventricular tachycardia that is usually seen in young healthy individuals and is typically sensitive to verapamil.

With verapamil, BP is reduced to 90/60 mmHg in approximately 5%–10% of patients. One percent to 2% may become symptomatic. Significant sinus bradycardia or the development of 2°–3° heart block may occur in 0.5%–2% of patients with verapamil or diltiazem. As with all other antiarrhythmic agents, arrhythmogenesis may be promoted. Constipation is a side effect that limits the use of verapamil in some individuals, especially in the elderly population. For information on the use of individual calcium antagonists in the treatment of arrhythmias, see the chapter on calcium antagonists.

MODE OF ACTION

Unlike class I antiarrhythmic drugs, whose predominant actions are on the fast sodium channel, the calcium antagonists depress sinoatrial automaticity and AV nodal depolarization predominantly by their effect on the slow inward current that is carried by calcium. Blockade of this calcium channel slows the conduction and prolongs the refractoriness within the sinus and atrioventricular nodes. These pharmacological effects result in slowing of the sinus discharge rate, an extension of the PR interval of the ECG, and a reduction of ventricular responsiveness to atrial arrhythmias. Calcium antagonists may also block arrhythmias that involve the AV node. They have little effect on normal Purkinje fibers on cardiac myocytes; however, abnormal Purkinje fibers in which sodium channels have been activated may be blocked by calcium antagonists such as verapamil. These drugs may therefore also be effective in ventricular arrhythmias.

ADENOSINE

Adenosine is used for the parenteral therapy of supraventricular arrhythmias as a cardioverting agent.

ATROPINE

Atropine is used for the parenteral management of symptomatic sinus bradycardia.

CARDIAC GLYCOSIDES (DIGITALIS, DIGOXIN)

Cardiac glycosides have been in clinical use for more than 200 years. Their value in the control of CHF has been questioned and re-established, and they continue to have a role in the treatment of various cardiac arrhythmias.

EFFICACY AND USE

Digoxin is a drug of choice for controlling rapid ventricular rates when associated with atrial fibrillation or flutter (Table 5.3). It is often useful to combine digoxin with a beta blocker or with a calcium-channel blocker such as propranolol or verapamil, which give added control of the ventricular rhythm.

Glycosides usually are not indicated in the treatment of supraventricular tachycardia associated with Wolff-Parkinson-White syndrome because digitalis may enhance the conduction of the accessory pathway and, in atrial fibrillation, produce rapid ventricular rates and even ventricular fibrillation.

Cardiac glycosides slow heart rate when sinus tachycardia is caused by heart failure, but they are usually ineffective in the absence of failure.

Atrial flutter may be converted to atrial fibrillation, and this, in turn, may convert to sinus rhythm during continued therapy. In some instances the propensity to atrial fibrillation may be exacerbated by the use of digoxin. Paroxysmal atrial flutter may sometimes convert to sinus rhythm when digitalis is withdrawn.

Cardiac glycosides are used in the prevention and treatment of recurrent episodes of paroxysmal re-entrant tachycardia involving the AV mode.

For information on the use of digitalis preparations in the treatment of arrhythmias, see the chapter on inotropic and vasopressor agents.

MODE OF ACTION

Cardiac glycosides decrease conduction velocity through the AV node and prolong its effective refractory period by increasing vagal activity through a direct action on the AV node and by a sympatholytic effect. With normal doses, conduction velocity and refractoriness of the His-Purkinje system are not directly affected. Cardiac glycosides shorten the effective refractory period of the atria and decrease conduction velocity by a reflex increase in vagal tone and a direct effect on the atria. With therapeutic doses, prolongation of the PR interval, shortening of the QT interval, and ST segment depression occur but are not quantitatively related to the degree of digitalization. Therapeutic doses have little effect on the ventricles; however, digitalis may induce nitrate-reversible vasoconstriction of both normal and atherosclerotic epicardial coronary arteries.

The therapeutic/toxic window with regard to digoxin's antiarrhythmic actions/electrophysiologic effects is relatively narrow, and digoxin can cause a large variety of atrial, junctional, or ventricular tachyarrhythmias and sinoatrial and AV nodal conduction abnormalities, some of which may be life threatening (Table 5.1). The tachyarrhythmias are apparently related to a mechanism of so-called triggered arrhythmias caused by after-depolarizations. Arrhythmias are more common in the setting of hypokalemia, although severe digoxin toxicity may cause hyperkalemia. Digoxin antibodies can be used to reverse the effects of severe digoxin toxicity.

ADENOSINE (Adenocard®)

Adenosine is an endogenous nucleoside found in all cells of the body. When administered as an IV bolus, it slows conduction through the AV node. Adenosine can interrupt a re-entrant pathway involving the AV node and restore normal sinus rhythm in patients with paroxysmal supraventricular tachycardia, including that associated with the Wolff-Parkinson-White syndrome. Because of its extremely short half-life (< 10 s), it can be given safely to patients with broad-complex tachycardia, poor left ventricular function, or severe hypotension, and those receiving concomitant beta blockade. It may also be used as an aid in the diagnosis of broad- or narrow-complex supraventricular tachycardia; however, adenosine can cause AV block and is not beneficial in atrial fibrillation or flutter or in most ventricular arrhythmias. A very small percentage of patients may develop atrial fibrillation after an adenosine bolus. A rare form of catecholamine-sensitive idiopathic ventricular tachycardia is adenosine-sensitive and will terminate after administration of adenosine, beta blockers, or occasionally, calcium channel blockers. Its short half-life means that most side effects are transient. A comparative study of patients with narrow-complex tachycardia found that the efficacy of adenosine was 100%, whereas that of verapamil was 73%.

SPECIAL GROUPS

Race: no difference in response
Children: safety and effectiveness have not been established; however, studies performed to date on adenosine use as an anti-arrhythmic have not demonstrated pediatric-specific problems
Elderly: no dosage adjustment required
CHF: no dosage reduction warranted
Renal impairment: no reduction in dosage warranted
Hepatic impairment: no dose reduction needed
Pregnancy: category C; should only be used if clearly indicated
Breast-feeding: drug unlikely excreted in milk due to its short half-life

DOSAGE

Rapid administration: IV followed with saline flush of the line.
Initial dose: 6 mg IV push (over a 1–2 second period)
   If no response, 12 mg can be given 2 min later and repeated again if necessary.
Patients receiving dipyridamole concurrently: 1 mg IV push has been reported as effective.

IN BRIEF

INDICATIONS
Paroxysmal supraventricular tachyarrhythmias, including that associated with Wolff-Parkinson-White syndrome
AV reciprocating tachycardia
Wide complex QRS tachycardia suspected to be of supraventricular origin

CONTRAINDICATIONS
Second or third degree heart block without a pacemaker
Sinus node dysfunction
Hypersensitivity

DRUG INTERACTIONS
Dipyridamole
Theophylline
Drugs affecting cardiac conduction
Carbamazepine

ADVERSE EFFECTS
CV: transient post-conversion arrhythmias (AV block, PVC, sinus bradycardia, atrial fibrillation) or asystole, chest pain, palpitation
Lungs: dyspnea, bronchospasm with asthmatic patients
CNS: headache, dizziness, apprehension
Other: facial flushing, nausea

PHARMACOKINETICS AND PHARMACODYNAMICS
Duration of action: 10–20 s
Onset of action: approximately 8–10 s
Bioavailability: not measured
Effect of food: not applicable
Metabolism: rapidly metabolized into two clinically inactive metabolites: inosine and adenosine mono-phosphate
Excretion: renally, as inactive metabolites
Plasma half-life: 1–10 s
Protein binding: not applicable

MONITORING
ECG and vital signs post-administration for signs of AV blocks, asystole, and bronchospasm.

OVERDOSE
No case report. Not likely to be clinically relevant due to its short half-life.

PATIENT INFORMATION
Not applicable.

AVAILABILITY
Injection—3 mg/mL (2 and 5 mL vials)

ATROPINE SULFATE   (Atropine)

Atropine blocks the cholinergic impulse to the sinoatrial (SA) node. The pharmacologic activity of atropine results almost completely from l-hyoscyamine. As a racemic mixture, it possesses about 50% of the antimuscarinic potency of l-hyoscyamine. In general, it is more potent than scopalamine in its antimuscarinic action in the heart and on bronchial and intestinal smooth muscle. Larger doses progressively block normal vagal inhibition of the SA node. Atropine has a positive chronotropic effect, accelerating sinus rate by direct parasympathetic blockade. It is effective in reversing sinus bradycardia secondary to extracardiac causes. It shortens SA conduction time and stimulates AV functional pacemaker activity, but shortens AV nodal conduction time.

SPECIAL GROUPS

Race:	no difference in response
Children:	use with caution, as cases of respiratory distress, seizures, muscular hypotonia, and coma have been reported
Elderly:	use with caution
CHF:	use with caution
Renal impairment:	use with caution
Hepatic impairment:	use with caution
Pregnancy:	category C; should only be used if clearly indicated
Breast-feeding:	should not be used if breast feeding

DOSAGE

Administration: IV, IM, SQ, or via endotracheal tube (then dose should be 2–2.5 times the IV dose, diluted in 10 mL sodium chloride solution in adult and in 1–2 mL in children). Rapid administration and dose not less than 0.5 mg is recommended as paradoxical bradycardia has been reported with slow administration

Children: 0.01 mg/kg max 0.4 mg, may repeat every 4–6 h if needed.

For bradycardia during CPR: usual adult dose is 0.5–1 mg IV, can repeat every 3–5 min

For asystole: 1 mg IV every 3–5 min to a max of 0.04 mg/kg, as 2.5 mg usually produces full vagal blockade

IN BRIEF

INDICATIONS
(Intravenous formulation only)
Type I second degree AV block
Symptomatic sinus bradycardia
Use in bradycardia associated with MI is controversial
Chronic sinus node dysfunction

CONTRAINDICATIONS
Narrow angle glaucoma
Obstructive disease of the GI tract
Intestinal atony or megacolon
Hiatal hernia with reflux esophagitis
Tachycardia
Acute hemorrhage
Myasthenia gravis
Obstructive uropathy
Hypersensitivity

DRUG INTERACTIONS
Anticholinesterase inhibitors
Drugs with anticholinergic effects (phenothiazines, antiparkinsonians, amantadine, TCA, meperidine, type Ia antiarrhythmics)
Ketoconazole
Wax matrix potassium chloride preparations

ADVERSE EFFECTS
CV: tachycardia, palpitation, chest pain, MI
Lungs: dyspnea, bronchospasm with asthmatic patients
CNS: headache, disorientation, delirium, excitement, slurred speech
GI: dry mouth, thirst, impaired GI motility, constipation
Skin: flush, dry skin
Other: blurred vision, mydriasis, dry nose, anaphylaxis reaction due to sulfite ingredient in the drug (in particular, for asthmatic patients)

PHARMACOKINETICS AND PHARMACODYNAMICS

Duration of action:	4 h
Onset of action:	approximately 15 min
Bioavailability:	rapid, complete absorption from all dosage forms
Effect of food:	unknown
Metabolism:	metabolized into several metabolites in liver
Excretion:	30%–50% excreted as unchanged drug in urine
Plasma half-life:	biphasic—2–3 h initially, then 12 h or longer in the terminal phase
Protein binding:	18%

MONITORING
ECG, BP, mental status, and respiratory status.

OVERDOSE
May produce narcosis with respiratory depression and/or atropine poisoning, particularly in children. Symptoms include dry skin and mucous membranes, flushing, hyperthermia, tachycardia. Onset of symptoms may be considerably delayed. They may recur in spite of initial response to narcotic antagonists. Naloxone is a specific antidote for respiratory depression. Repeated injections may be needed. Establishment of airway and artificial ventilation may be needed. If patient is not comatose, consider gastric lavage and administration of a slurry of activated charcoal.

PATIENT INFORMATION
Report shortness of breath, chest pain, difficulty in urination, flushing, dry skin, nervousness, thirst, and other CNS effects to physician.

AVAILABILITY
Injection—0.05, 0.1, 0.3, 0.4, 0.5, 0.8, 1 mg/mL

SUGGESTED BIBLIOGRAPHY

Anderson JL, Jolivette DM, Fredell PA: Summary of efficacy and safety of flecainide for supraventricular arrhythmias. *Am J Cardiol* 1988, 62:62D–66D.

Antman EM, Beamer AD, Cantillon C, *et al.*: Long-term oral propafenone therapy for suppression of refractory symptomatic atrial fibrillation and atrial flutter. *J Am Coll Cardiol* 1988,12:1005–1011.

Burkart F, Pfisterer M, Kiowski W, *et al.*: Effect of antiarrhythmic therapy on mortality in survivors of myocardial infarction with asymptomatic complex ventricular arrhythmias: Basel Antiarrhythmic Study of Infarct Survival (BASIS). *J Am Coll Cardiol* 1990, 16:1711–1718.

Cairns JA, Connolly SJ, Gent M, Roberts R: Post-myocardial infarction mortality in patients with ventricular premature depolarizations: Canadian Amiodarone Myocardial Infarction Arrhythmia Trial Pilot Study. *Circulation* 1991, 84:550–557.

Cairns JA, Connolly SJ, Roberts R, *et al.*, for the Canadian Amiodarone Myocardial Infarction (CAMIAT) Investigators: Randomized trial of outcome after myocardial infarction in patients with frequent or repetitive ventricular premature depolarizations: CAMIAT. *Lancet* 1997, 349:675–682.

Campbell TJ: Clinical use of class Ia antiarrhythmic drugs. In *Handbook of Experimental Pharmacology: Antiarrhythmic Drugs.* Edited by Vaughan Williams EM. Heidelberg: Springer Verlag; 1989:175–200.

Capucci A, Lenzi T, Boriani G, *et al*: Effectiveness of loading oral flecainide for converting recent-onset atrial fibrillation to sinus rhythm in patients without organic heart disease or with only systemic hypertension. *Am J Cardiol* 1992, 70:69–72.

Cavusoglu E, Frishman WH: Sotalol: a new β-adrenergic blocker for ventricular arrhythmias. *Prog Cardiovasc Dis* 1995, 37:423–440.

Coplen SE, Antman EH, Berlin JE, *et al.*: Efficacy and safety of quinidine therapy for maintenance of sinus rhythm after cardioversion: a meta-analysis of randomized control trials. *Circulation* 1990, 82: 1106–1116.

Cruickshank JM, Prichard BNC: Arrhythmias. In *Beta Blockers in Clinical Practice.* London: Churchill; 1987:577–636.

Daoud E, Strickberger S, Man K, *et al.*: Preoperative amiodarone as prophylaxis against atrial fibrillation after heart surgery. *N Engl J Med* 1997, 337:1785–1791.

DeCara JM, Pollak A, Dubrey S, *et al.*: Positive atrial inotropic effects of dofetilide following cardioversion of atrial fibrillation [abstract]. *J Am Coll Cardiol* 1998, 31(2 Suppl A):432A.

Dolak GL for the CASCADE Investigators: Clinical predictors of implantable cardioverter-defibrillator shocks (results of the CASCADE trial). *Am J Cardiol* 1994, 73:237–241.

Donovan KD, Power BM, Hockings BE, *et al.*: Intravenous flecainide versus amiodarone for recent onset atrial fibrillation. *Am J Cardiol* 1995, 75:693–697.

Doval HC, Nul DR, Grancelli HO, *et al.*, for Grupo de Estudio de la Sobrevida en la Insuficiencia Cardiaca en Argentina (GESICA): Randomized trial of low-dose amiodarone in severe congestive heart failure. *Lancet* 1994, 344:493–498.

Ellenbogen KA, Stambler BS, Wood MA, *et al.*: Efficacy of intravenous inutilide for rapid termination of atrial fibrillation and atrial flutter: a dose-response study. *J Am Coll Cardiol* 1996, 28:130–136.

Ferreira E, Sunderji R, Gin K: Is oral sotalol effective in converting atrial fibrillation to sinus rhythm? *Pharmacotherapy* 1997, 17:1233–1237.

Frishman WH, Vahdat S, Bhatta S: Innovative pharmacologic approaches to cardiopulmonary resuscitation. *J Clin Pharmacol* 1998, 38:765–772.

Gottlieb CD, Horowitz LN: Potential interactions between antiarrhythmic medication and the automatic implantable cardioverter defibrillator. *Pacing Clin Electrophysiol* 1991, 14:898–904.

Gottlieb SS: The use of antiarrhythmic agents in heart failure: implications of CAST. *Am Heart J* 1989, 118:1074–1077.

Greene HL: The efficacy of amiodarone in the treatment of ventricular tachycardia or ventricular fibrillation. *Prog Cardiovasc Dis* 1989, 31:439–446.

Guarnieri T, Nolan S, Gottlieb SO, *et al.*: Intravenous amiodarone for the prevention of atrial fibrillation after open heart surgery: The Amiodarone Reduction in Coronary Heart (ARCH) Trial. *J Am Coll Cardiol* 1999; 34:343–347.

Hagemeijer F: Verapamil in the management of supraventricular tachyarrhythmias occurring after a recent myocardial infarction. *Circulation* 1978, 57:751–755.

Halinen MO, Huttunen M, Paakkinen S, *et al.*: Comparison of sotalol with digoxin-quinidine for conversion of acute atrial fibrillation to sinus rhythm (the Sotalol-Digoxin-Quinidine Trial). *Am J Cardiol* 1995, 76:495–498.

Harron DWG, Shanks RG: Clinical use of class Ib antiarrhythmic drugs. In *Handbook of Experimental Pharmacology: Antiarrhythmic Drugs.* Edited by Vaughan Williams EM. Heidelberg: Springer Verlag; 1989:201–234.

Hessen SE, Michelson EL: Antiarrhythmic drugs. In *Cardiovascular Pharmacotherapeutics.* Edited by Frishman WH, Sonnenblick EH. New York:McGraw Hill; 1997:281–322.

Hine LK, Laird N, Hewitt P, *et al.*: Meta-analytic evidence against prophylactic use of lidocaine in acute myocardial infarction. *Arch Intern Med* 1989, 149:2694–2698.

Hombach V, Braun V, Hopp HW, *et al.*: Electrophysiological effects of cardioselective and non-selective beta-adrenoceptor blockers with and without ISA at rest and during exercise. *Br J Clin Pharmacol* 1982, 13:285S–293S.

Hood MA, Smith WM: Adenosine versus verapamil in the treatment of supraventricular tachycardia: a randomized double-crossover trial. *Am Heart J* 1992, 123:1543–1549.

IMPACT Research Group: International Mexiletine and Placebo Antiarrhythmic Coronary Trial (IMPACT). II: results from 24 hour electrocardiogram. *Eur Heart J* 1986, 7:749–759.

Indolfi C, Piscione F, Russolillo E, *et al.*: Digoxin-induced vasoconstriction of normal and atherosclerotic epicardial coronary arteries. *Am J Cardiol* 1991, 68:1274–1278.

Julian DG, Camm AJ, Frangin G, *et al.*, for the European Myocardial Infarct Amiodarone Trial (EMIAT) Investigators: Randomized trial of effect of amiodarone on mortality in patients with left ventricular dysfunction after recent myocardial infarction: EMIAT. *Lancet* 1997, 349:667–674.

Juul-Moller S, Edvardsson N, Rehnqvist-Ahlberg N: Sotalol versus quinidine for the maintenance of sinus rhythm after direct current conversion of atrial fibrillation. *Circulation* 1990, 82:1932–1939.

Kaber L, The Danish Investigations of Arrhythmia and Mortality on Dofetilide (DIAMOND) Study Group: Dofetilide, a new class III antiarrhythmic drug reduces hospital admissions for congestive heart failure: secondary endpoints of the DIAMOND-CHF study [abstract]. *J Am Coll Cardiol* 1998, 31(2 Suppl A):33A.

Kerin NZ, Faitel K, Naini M: The efficacy of intravenous amiodarone for the conversion of chronic atrial fibrillation: amiodarone vs quinidine for conversion of atrial fibrillation. *Arch Intern Med* 1996, 156:49–53.

Kober L, The DIAMOND Study Group: Dofetilide improves heart failure in patients with atrial fibrillation and left ventricular dysfunction: a Diamond subanalysis [abstract]. *J Am Coll Cardiol* 1999, 33(2 Suppl A):186A.

Kochiadakis GE, Igoumenidis NE, Marketou ME *et al.*: Low-dose amiodarone versus sotalol for suppression of recurrent symptomatic atrial fibrillation. *Am J Cardiol* 1998, 81:995–998.

Kudenchuk PJ, Cobb LA, Copass MK, *et al.*: Amiodarone for resuscitation after out-of-hospital cardiac arrest due to ventricular fibrillation. *N Engl J Med* 1999, 341:871–878.

Kumar A: Intravenous amiodarone for therapy of atrial fibrillation and flutter in critically ill patients with severe depressed left ventricular function. *South Med J* 1996, 89:779–785.

Larbuisson R, Venneman I, Stiels B: The efficacy and safety of intravenous propafenone versus intravenous amiodarone in the conversion of atrial fibrillation or flutter after cardiac surgery. *J Cardiothorac Vasc Anesth* 1996, 10:229–234.

Lee JT, Kroemer HK, Silberstein DJ, *et al.*: The role of genetically determined polymorphic drug metabolism in the beta blockade produced by propafenone. *N Engl J Med* 1990, 322:1764–1768.

Lehman R, Greenbaum RA, Campbell TJ, *et al.*: Patients with longer QT (QTc) interval are more likely to remain in sinus rhythm after one year treatment on dofetilide: The EMERALD (European and Australian Multicenter Evaluation Research on Atrial Fibrillation Dofetilide) study [abstract]. *J Am Coll Cardiol* 1999, 33 (2 Suppl A):132A.

Morganroth J, Chen CC, Sturm S, Dreifus LS: Oral verapamil in the treatment of atrial fibrillation/flutter. *Am J Cardiol* 1982, 49:981–985.

Moss AJ, Hall WJ, Cannon DS, *et al.*: Improved survival with an implanted defibrillator in patients with coronary disease at high risk for ventricular arrhythmia: Multicenter Automatic Defibrillator Implantation Trial Investigators. *N Engl J Med* 1996, 335:1933–1940.

Nicklas JM, McKenna WJ, Stewart RA, *et al.*: Prospective, double-blind, placebo-controlled trial of low-dose amiodarone in patients with severe heart failure and asymptomatic frequent ventricular ectopy. *Am Heart J* 1991, 122:1016–1021.

Parker RB, McCollum PL, Bauman JL: Propafenone: a novel type Ic antiarrhythmic agent. *Drug Intel Clin Pharm* 1989, 23:196–203.

Petersen TR for the Norwegian Multicenter Study Group: Six year follow up of the Norwegian Multicenter Study on timolol after acute myocardial infarction. *N Engl J Med* 1985, 313:1055–1058.

Pfisterer ME, Kiowski W, Brunner H, *et al.*: Long-term benefit of 1 year amiodarone treatment for persistent complex ventricular arrhythmias after myocardial infarction. *Circulation* 1993, 87:309–311.

Schofield PM, Reid F, Bennett DH: A comparison of atenolol and sotalol in the treatment of patients with paroxysmal supraventricular tachycardia. *Br Heart J* 1987, 57:105–106.

Siebel J, Cappato R, Rüppel R, *et al.* and the CASH Investigators: ICD versus drugs in cardiac arrest survivors: preliminary results of the Cardiac Arrest Study, Hamburg. *PACE* 1993, 16:552–558.

Singh BN, Ellrodt G, Peters T: Verapamil: a review of its pharmacological properties and therapeutic use. *Drugs* 1978, 15:169–197.

Singh SN, Berk MR, Yellen LG, *et al.*: Oral dofetilide for conversion of patients with chronic atrial fibrillation or atrial flutter to normal sinus rhythm: a multicenter study [abstract]. *J Am Coll Cardiol* 1998, 31(2 Suppl A):369A.

Singh SN, Berk MR, Yellen LG, *et al.*: Efficacy and safety of dofetilide in maintaining normal sinus in patients with atrial fibrillation/flutter: a multicenter study [abstract]. *Circulation* 1997, 96:383.

Singh SN, Galk R, Farahi J, *et al.*: Restoration of sinus rhythm in subjects with atrial fibrillation improves exercise capacity: a SAFIRE-D (Symptomatic Atrial Fibrillation Investigative Research on Dofetilide) Substudy [abstract]. *Circulation* 1998, 98(Suppl 1):432.

Singh SN, Fletcher RD, Fisher SG, *et al.* for the Survival Trial of Antiarrhythmic Therapy in Congestive Heart Failure: Amiodarone in patients with congestive heart failure and asymptomatic ventricular arrhythmias. *N Engl J Med* 1995, 333:77–82.

Skluth H, Grauer K, Gums J: Ventricular arrhythmias: an assessment of newer therapeutic agents. *Postgrad Med* 1989, 85:137–153.

Stambler BS, Wood MA, Ellenboken KA: Comparative efficacy of intravenous ibutilide versus procainamide for enhancing termination of atrial flutter by atrial overdrive pacing. *Am J Cardiol* 1996, 77:960–966.

Steinbeck G, Andersen D, Bach P, *et al.*: A comparison of electrophysiologically and guided antiarrhythmic drug therapy with beta blocker therapy in patients with symptomatic sustained ventricular tachyarrhythmias. *N Engl J Med* 1992, 327:987–992.

Strasberg B, Arditti A, Sclarovsky S, *et al.*: Efficacy of intravenous amiodarone in the management of paroxysmal or new atrial fibrillation with fast ventricular response. *Int J Cardiol* 1985, 7:47–58.

Task Force of the Working Group on Arrhythmias of the European Society of Cardiology: The Sicilian Gambit: a new approach to the classification of antiarrhythmic drugs and their actions on arrhythmogenic mechanisms. *Circulation* 1991, 84:1831–1851.

Teo KT, Yusuf S, Furberg CD: Effects of prophylactic antiarrhythmic drug therapy in acute myocardial infarction: an overview of results from randomized controlled trials. *JAMA* 1993, 270: 1589–1595.

The AVID Investigators: A comparison of antiarrhythmic drug therapy with implantable defibrillators in patients resuscitated from near fatal ventricular arrhythmias. *N Engl J Med* 1997, 337:1576–1583.

The Cardiac Arrhythmia Suppression Trial (CAST) Investigators: Preliminary report: effect of encainide and flecanide on mortality in a randomized trial of arrhythmia suppression after myocardial infarction. *N Engl J Med* 1989, 321:406–412.

The Cardiac Arrhythmia Suppression Trial II Investigators: Effect of the antiarrhythmic agent moricizine on survival after myocardial infarction. *N Engl J Med* 1992, 327:227–233.

The ESVEM Investigators: Determinants of predicted efficacy of antiarrhythmic drugs in the Electrophysiologic Study Versus Electrocardiographic Monitoring trial. *Circulation* 1993, 87: 323–329.

Torp-Pedersen C, Møller M, Bloch-Thomsen PE, *et al.* for the Danish Investigations on Arrhythmia and Mortality on Dofetilide (DIAMOND) Study Group: Dofetilide in patients with congestive heart failure and left ventricular dysfunction. *N Engl J Med* 1999; 341: 857–865.

Vaughan Williams EM: Classification of antiarrhythmic action. In *Handbook of Experimental Pharmacology: Antiarrhythmic Drugs.* Edited by Vaughan Williams EM. Heidelberg: Springer Verlag; 1989:45–67.

Waldo AL, Camm AJ, De Ruyter H, *et al.*: Effects of d-sotalol on mortality in patients with left ventricular dysfunction after recent and remote myocardial infarction. *Lancet* 1996, 348:7–12.

Wit AL, Hoffman BF, Rosen MR: Electrophysiology and pharmacology of cardiac arrhythmias. IX: cardiac electrophysiological effects of beta-adrenergic receptor stimulation and blockade. *Am Heart J* 1975, 90:795–803.

Wit AL, Rosen MR, Hoffman BF. Relationship of normal and abnormal electrical activity of cardiac fibers to the genesis of arrhythmias. II: Re-entry. *Am Heart J* 1974, 88:798–807.

Woosley RL, Tang T, Stone W: Pharmacology, electrophysiology, and pharmacokinetics of mexiletine. *Am Heart J* 1984, 107:1058–1065.

Wyse DG, Morganroth J, Leidengham R, *et al.*: New insights into the definition and meaning of proarrhythmia during initiation of antiarrhythmic drug therapy from the Cardiac Arrhythmia Suppression Trial and its pilot study. *J Am Coll Cardiol* 1994, 23:1130–1140.

Zaremski DG, Nolan PE Jr, Slack MK, *et al.*: Treatment of resistant atrial fibrillation: A meta-analysis comparing amiodarone and flecanide. *Arch Intern Med* 1995, 155:1885–1891.

Zehender M, Hohnloser S, Mueller B, *et al.*: Effects of amiodarone versus quinidine and verapamil in patients with chronic atrial fibrillation: results of a comparative study and a 2-year follow-up. *J Am Coll Cardiol* 1992, 19:1054–1059.

6

ANTITHROMBOTIC THERAPY

Antiplatelet agents prevent platelets from adhering to damaged vessel wall or to one another, a vital step in the initiation of clot formation, particularly in arteries. Anticoagulant therapy is used to prevent clots from forming or extending by inhibiting the formation of the fibrin framework of the blood clot. Thrombolytic therapy activates the enzyme pathways that lyse the fibrin meshwork of the blood clot to restore blood flow after a clot has blocked a vessel. Figure 6.1 shows the clotting process cascade.

Antithrombotic therapy may use more than one type of drug in sequence (eg, a thrombolytic agent to dissolve a clot and an antiplatelet with or without an anticoagulant drug to prevent the clot from reforming on the injured artery wall). All antithrombotic drugs increase the risk of bleeding. Combinations of these drugs, particularly thrombolytics and anticoagulants, may increase this risk. These risks must be balanced against the desired therapeutic goals.

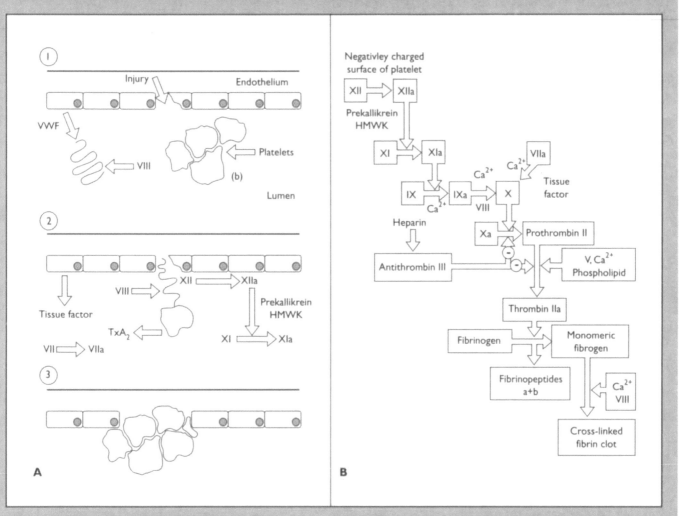

FIGURE 6.1 Stages of hemostasis. **A**, 1) Injury of vascular endothelium; 2) adherence of platelets and initiation of extrinsic and intrinsic coagulation pathways; 3) aggregated platelets provide a negatively charged surface on which the clotting cascade produces thrombin IIa. **B**, Antithrombin III inactivates factors Xa and thrombin IIa. This effect is much enhanced by heparin. The other anticoagulants work in a similar way by inhibiting the formation of active factors II, VII, IX, and X. a—activated clotting factors; HMWK—high molecular weight kininogen; VWF—Von Willebrand factor.

ANTITHROMBOTIC THERAPY: ANTICOAGULANTS

Anticoagulants are available as rapid acting parenteral agents (such as **heparin**, low molecular weight **heparins** (LMWH), **danaparoid**, and **lepirudin**) and oral agents (such as **warfarin**). Anticoagulant therapy is usually initiated with a parenteral agent, followed by long-term oral **warfarin** therapy. Heparin and LMWH, are the preferred anticoagulants of choice in pregnancy. **Lepirudin** and **danaparoid** may be used safely in patients with heparin-induced thrombocytopenia.

EFFICACY AND USE

In patients with recently diagnosed deep vein thrombosis (DVT) or thrombophlebitis, anticoagulant therapy can prevent extension and embolization of the thrombus and reduce the risk of pulmonary embolism (PE) or recurrent thromboembolic events. In patients with acute PE, anticoagulation reduces the risk of extension of the thrombus, recurrence, and death.

Anticoagulant therapy is also useful in DVT and PE prophylaxis after major abdominal, gynecologic, orthopedic, or thoracic surgery, especially in high-risk patients. In patients with acute myocardial infarction (MI), anticoagulant therapy can reduce the risk of systemic thromboembolic complications. **Heparin** and LMWHs are indicated as an adjunct therapy together with thrombolytic and/or antiplatelet therapy in patients with acute MI or unstable angina to lyse the clot and prevent reocclusion of the artery. In addition, **heparin** is used during heart surgery and angioplasty with and without stent placement.

In patients with recent cerebral embolism, especially if the heart is the suspected origin of thrombi, anticoagulation may reduce the risk of recurrence. Cerebral hemorrhage should be ruled out, and the risk of cerebral hemorrhage should be weighed against the risk of recurrent embolic event in a patient before initiating anticoagulant therapy. The treatment is of less value in patients with transient ischemic attacks (TIA).

Some other common indications for anticoagulation include patients with shock, congestive heart failure (CHF), chronic atrial fibrillation or flutter, previous MI, and history of thromboembolism.

MODE OF ACTION

Heparin potentiates the inhibition of antithrombin III on activated clotting factors, including IIa (thrombin), IXa, Xa, XIa, and XIIa (Fig. 6.1B). **Heparin** is not absorbed through the gastrointestinal (GI) tract and should be given either intravenously or subcutaneously. Because of the short half-life, **heparin** has a rapid onset of action with a short duration of action.

LMWHs act primarily through the inhibition of factor Xa (Table 6.1). Different from regular **heparin**, these agents provide more predictable dose response with less interpatient variability. Compared to **heparin**, LMWHs have longer half-lives and lower risk of bleeding for equivalent antithrombotic effect.

Danaparoid is a low molecular weight heparinoid approved for DVT prophylaxis. Similar to LMWHs, its antithrombotic effect is primarily related to its potent anti-factor Xa activity. It has the lowest cross-reactivity with **heparin** (10%–20%) and has been used safely in patients with type 2 **heparin**-induced thrombocytopenia.

Different from **heparin**, **lepirudin** (**hirudin**) is a direct antithrombin. It exerts its anticoagulant activity independent of a cofactor and binds to both free and clot-bound thrombin. This may have the advantage of preventing clot-bound thrombin to stimulate further thrombogenesis. **Lepirudin** also inhibits thrombin-induced platelet activation. **Lepirudin** is only approved for use in patients with **heparin**-induced thrombocytopenia, although it is probably also effective in the management of other acute thromboembolic problems.

Warfarin inhibits the synthesis of clotting factors II, VII, IX, and X by competitively inhibiting vitamin K–dependent gamma carboxylation of the precursor proteins. Following the initiation of **warfarin** therapy, factor VII (plasma half-life of 4–6 h) is depleted first, followed by factors IX, X, and II (plasma half-lives of 20–24 h, 48–72 h, and ≥ 60 h, respectively). Although prothrombin time (PT) and International Normalized Ratio (INR) are prolonged after factor VII depletion, peak antithrombotic effect is not achieved until all four factors are depleted from the circulation, which usually takes several days. Therefore, for more rapid anticoagulation in acute thromboembolic events, therapy with a direct-acting agent, such as **heparin** or a LMWH, is used. Oral **warfarin** therapy is initiated for long-term maintenance with concurrent heparin or LMWH therapy for the first 5–10 d.

Generic (brand) name	Mean molecular weight (daltons)	Bioavailability	Anti-Xa:Anti IIa	Half-life (hours)	Approved dosing for DVT prophylaxis
Ardeparin (Normiflo)	6000	90%–92%	1.9:1	3	50 U/kg twice daily
Dalteparin (Fragmin)	5000	87%	2.7:1	2–4	2500 or 5000 U* once daily
Enoxaparin (Lovenox)	4500	92%	3.8:1	3–6	30 mg twice daily or 40 mg once daily
Danaparoid† (Orgaran)	5500	100%	22:1	18—28	750 U twice daily

TABLE 6.1 LOW MOLECULAR WEIGHT HEPARINS AND HEPARINOIDS APPROVED BY THE FOOD AND DRUG ADMINISTRATION

*High dose is recommended for high-risk patients.

†A heparinoid.

INDICATIONS

	Heparin	Ardeparin	Dalteparin	Enoxaparin	Danaparoid	Lepirudin	Warfarin
Venous thrombosis (T/P)	+	+ (P)*	+ (P)*	+	+ (P)*	+*	+
Pulmonary embolism (T/P)	+	+ (P)*	+ (P)*	+	+ (P)*	+*	+
Atrial fibrillation (T/P)	+	–	–	–	–	–	+
Disseminated intravascular coagulation	+	–	–	–	–	–	–
Peripheral arterial embolism (T/P)	+	–	–	–	–	+*	–
Extracorporeal circulation	+	–	–	–	–	–	–
Adjunctive management of coronary occlusion	(+)	–	+*	+*	–	–	–

*Limited indications only (see discussions of each drug).

+—FDA approved; – —not FDA approved; (+)—not FDA approved but commonly used; T/P—treatment/prophylaxis.

HEPARIN SODIUM, OR CALCIUM

(Heparin Sodium, Calciparine®)

Heparin acts indirectly at multiple sites in the intrinsic and extrinsic clotting systems by potentiating the inhibitory action of antithrombin III. Inhibition of activated factor Xa by heparin interferes with thrombin generation and thereby inhibits the various actions by thrombin in coagulation. It also prevents formation of a fibrin clot by inhibiting the thrombin-activated formation of fibrin-stabilized factor. Because heparin does not cross the placenta, therefore it does not affect blood clotting in the fetus. Heparin is the anticoagulant of choice during pregnancy. Although complications in pregnancy have been reported, the incidence seems to be somewhat lower than with coumarin-related oral anticoagulants.

Heparin is used when rapid anticoagulation is desired. It is effective in unstable angina. It can reduce mortality in patients with acute MI (when used alone or as an adjunctive to thrombolytic therapy) (Table 6.2). Although heparin can improve patency of the occluded vessel, it is associated with an increase in bleeding complications, including intracerebral hemorrhage. It has been shown to reduce mortality as an adjunctive therapy to thrombolysis plus aspirin (Table 6.3). It is also useful in venous thrombosis, pulmonary thromboembolism, maintaining extracorporeal circulation, and after vascular surgery grafts. Low dose heparin is widely used for patients at high risk of venous thrombosis, such as bedridden patients with severe heart failure, and before surgical arthroplasty of the hip joint.

SPECIAL GROUPS

Race: no differences in response

Children: dosage adjustment based on weight, age, and coagulation test results

Elderly: no dosage adjustment is required

Renal impairment: dosage adjustment based on weight and coagulation test results

Hepatic impairment: dosage adjustment based on weight and coagulation test results

Pregnancy: category C; the preferred anticoagulant during pregnancy but should only be used if clearly indicated

Breast-feeding: not excreted in human milk; dosage adjustment based on weight and coagulation test results

IN BRIEF

INDICATIONS
Prophylaxis and treatment:
  Venous thrombosis
  Pulmonary embolism
  Atrial fibrillation with thromboembolism
  Peripheral arterial embolism
  *Unstable angina
  *Evolving stroke
  *Acute MI
Prevention of clotting in:
  Cardiac/ arterial surgery
  Blood transfusion
  Dialysis and other extracorporeal interventions
  Disseminated intravascular coagulation (DIC)
*Not approved by the Food and Drug Administration (FDA)

CONTRAINDICATIONS
Known hypersensitivity
Active major bleeding
Thrombocytopenia or other blood dyscrasias

DRUG INTERACTIONS
Other anticoagulants
Thrombolytics
Antiplatelets
NSAIDs
Antibiotics (cefotetan, cefoperazole, cefmetazole, ticarcillin, piperacillin, etc.)

ADVERSE EFFECTS
Blood: bleeding/clotting problems, thrombocytopenia, hyperkalemia, hyperlipidemia
GI: liver function abnormalities
Endocrine: hypoaldosteronism
Skin: local skin reactions, hematoma, cutaneous necrosis, alopecia
Other: allergic vasospastic reaction, fever, chills, urticaria, anaphylactoid reaction, osteoporosis

PHARMACOKINETICS AND PHARMACODYNAMICS
Duration of action: 1.5 h (intravenous); >12 h (subcutaneous)
Onset of action: immediate (intravenous); 20–30 min (subcutaneous)
Peak effect: 2 min (intravenous); 2–4 h (subcutaneous)
Bioavailability: 100% (intravenous); variable (subcutaneous)
Effect of food: not applicable
Clearance/Excretion: mainly metabolized by liver and eliminated in urine; up to 50% of unchanged heparin may be eliminated with high doses of heparin
Plasma half-life: 30–180 min
Protein binding: extensively bind to plasma proteins and endothelium

MONITORING
Lab: CBC, liver function, serum potassium and aPTT (1.5–2.5 times control; not required for low-dose heparin). Clinical evidence of active or occult bleeding.

OVERDOSE
Supportive; blood transfusion is indicated for acute, significant blood loss and protamine may be used to neutralize heparin (1 mg protamine/100 μ heparin).

PATIENT INFORMATION
Consult physician in the event of bleeding or bruising, hair loss, change in condition of skin, coldness, pain, or color changes in the legs, tingling or sensation loss, or local reactions at the injection site. Elderly patients are at greater risk for hemorrhage. Do not take other drugs without consulting your physician. Aspirin, ibuprofen, or other platelet-active medications should not be taken while on heparin unless prescribed by your physician. Inform all physicians and dentists that heparin is being used. Carry identification stating heparin is being used.

DOSAGE

Prophylaxis for DVT: 5000 U subcutaneously (SQ) every 8–12 h until the patient is fully ambulatory

Treatment guidelines for thromboembolic events: IV 60–100 µ/kg bolus, followed by 15–25 µ/kg/h and adjusted based on coagulation test results

SQ 10,000–20,000 U loading dose, followed by 8000–10,000 U every 8 h or 15,000–20,000 U every 12 h; dose should be adjusted based on coagulation test results

Open heart and vascular surgery: minimum initial dose is 150 µ/kg; usually for procedures <60 min, 300 µ/kg is used, and for procedures >60 min, 400 µ/ kg is used

Heparin lock: 10–100 U in the hub and replace after each use

TABLE 6.2 THE INFLUENCE OF HEPARIN ON PATENCY OF THE INFARCT-RELATED ARTERY IN PATIENTS WHO RECEIVED RT-PA*

	Comparatice regimen	Timing of angiography	Heparin
TAMI-III	None	90 min	
HART	Heparin	18 h	
Bleich	None	Day 2	
ECSG-6	None	Day 4	
Australian Heart Failure	24 h intravenous heparin	Day 7	

*Odds ratio and 95% confidence limits.

Adapted from Prins MH, Hirsh J: Heparin as an adjunctive treatment after thrombolytic therapy for acute myocardial infarction. Am J Cardiol 1991, 67: A3–A11.

TABLE 6.3 COMBINED RESULTS FROM THE GISSI-2 AND ISIS-3 STUDIES OF THE EFFECT OF HEPARIN ADMINISTRATION ON ALL-CAUSE MORTALITY

	Heparin	No heparin	P value
Mortality	6.8%	7.3%	< 0.005

The information here is provided as guidance only. Prescribers should always consult the manufacturer's current prescribing information.

89

ARDEPARIN SODIUM (Normiflo®)

Ardeparin, a LMWH, is produced by perioxidative cleavage of porcine source heparin. Ardeparin has an average molecular weight of 6000 Daltons with an anti-Xa/IIa ratio of 1.9:1. Similar to other LMWHs, ardeparin offers potential advantages over heparin with its longer duration of action and predictable antithrombotic properties. It is effective in preventing DVT in patients undergoing orthopedic surgery. The role of ardeparin in the prevention and treatment of other thromboembolic complications awaits further clinical evaluations. Bleeding and thrombocytopenia are the major concerns of ardeparin therapy. Ardeparin use is contraindicated in patients with a history of heparin-induced thrombocytopenia due to the possible cross-reactivity problem (>90%).

SPECIAL GROUPS

Race: no data
Children: safety and effectiveness have not been established
Elderly: no dosage adjustment is required
Renal impairment: no dosage adjustment is required, use with caution in severe renal dysfunction
Hepatic impairment: no data, use with caution
Pregnancy: category C; should only be used if clearly indicated
Breast-feeding: unknown if the drug is excreted in human milk; use with caution

DOSAGE

50 anti-Factor Xa U/kg twice a day subcutaneously, starting the night prior to the surgery and continuing for up to 14 d or until the patient is fully ambulatory, whichever is shorter.

IN BRIEF

INDICATIONS
Prophylaxis against DVT that may lead to PE in patients undergoing total knee replacement surgery

CONTRAINDICATIONS
Known hypersensitivity to ardeparin, heparin, sulfite, or pork
Known heparin-induced thrombocytopenia
Active major bleeding

DRUG INTERACTIONS
Anticoagulants
Thrombolytics
Antiplatelets
NSAIDs

ADVERSE EFFECTS
Blood: hemorrhage, thrombocytopenia
GI: liver function abnormalities
CNS: epidural or spinal hematoma (especially with spinal or epidural anesthesia and spinal puncture)
Skin: local irritation, pruritus, rash, pain, bullous eruption, necrosis
Rare: hypersensitivity reaction (ardeparin contains metabisulfite), fever, anaphylactoid reaction

PHARMACOKINETICS AND PHARMACODYNAMICS
(based on plasma anti-Factor Xa activity)
Duration of action: 12 h
Onset of action: <2 h
Peak effect: 2–3 h
Bioavailability: 90%–92%
Clearance: mainly via renal excretion as unchanged drug
Plasma half-life: 3 h
Protein binding: no data

MONITORING
Lab: CBC, anti-factor Xa level (?), liver function test. Clinical evidence of active or occult bleeding.

OVERDOSE
Supportive; the antithrombotic effect may be partially neutralized with protamine.

PATIENT INFORMATION
Ardeparin can cause excessive bleeding and low platelet problems.

AVAILABILITY
Syringes—
  5000 anti-Factor Xa U/0.5 mL
  10,000 anti-Factor Xa U/0.5 mL

DALTEPARIN SODIUM (Fragmin®)

Dalteparin, an LMWH, is derived through nitrous acid depolymerization of porcine source heparin. It has an average molecular weight of 5000 Daltons. Similar to other LMWHs, the antithrombotic effect of dalteparin results primarily from its anti-Factor Xa activity (anti-Xa/IIa ratio = 2.7:1). Dalteparin, administered once daily subcutaneously, starting prior to hip replacement or abdominal surgery and continuing for 5–10 d after surgery, is effective in preventing thromboembolic complications in high-risk patients. While 5000 IU dalteparin is more effective than the 2500 IU dose in patients undergoing abdominal surgery, a higher dose increases the risk of bleeding. Thus, high dose should only be used in patients with a high risk of thromboembolic complications, such as in those with underlying malignancy. Dalteparin 2500 IU regimen is at least as effective as heparin 5000 IU given twice daily subcutaneously in patients undergoing abdominal surgery. It is not clear if dalteparin therapy is more efficacious, especially when compared to heparin 5000 IU every 8 h or adjusted-dose regimen. In two large clinical studies, dalteparin, 120 IU/kg every 12 h administered subcutaneously with concurrent oral aspirin, was effective in reducing death, MI, or recurrent angina in patients with a recent onset of unstable angina or non–Q-wave MI. Dalteparin therapy may be more effective than heparin therapy in patients suffering from acute coronary syndrome with more predictable therapeutic effect and less monitoring requirement. Because of the potential for cross-reactivity (> 90%), dalteparin is also contraindicated in patients with a history of heparin-induced thrombocytopenia.

SPECIAL GROUPS

Race: no data
Children: safety and effectiveness have not been established
Elderly: no data, dosage adjustment is probably not required
Renal impairment: slower clearance, use with caution
Hepatic impairment: no data, use with caution
Pregnancy: category B; should only be used if clearly indicated
Breast-feeding: unknown if the drug is excreted in human milk, used with caution

DOSAGE

1) Abdominal surgery:
Patients with low to moderate risk: 2500 IU subcutaneously once daily for 5–10 d starting 1–2 h prior to surgery
Patients with high risk: 5000 IU subcutaneously once daily for 5–10 d starting the evening before surgery; or 2500 IU subcutaneously starting 1–2 h prior to surgery with a second 2500 IU giving 12 h later and followed by 5000 IU subcutaneously once daily for 5–10 d
2) Hip replacement surgery:
Administer first dose, 2500 IU, subcutaneously within 2 h before surgery and second dose of 2500 IU in the evening after the surgery (at least 6 h after the first dose; otherwise, the second dose should be omitted); dalteparin 5000 IU is then administered subcutaneously once daily from first postoperative day and continued for 5–10 d. Alternatively, dalteparin 5000 IU can be administered the evening before the surgery, followed by 5000 IU once daily, starting in the evening of the surgery and continued for 5–10 d.
3) Unstable angina/non–Q-wave MI:
120 IU/kg (max. 10,000 IU) subcutaneously every 12 h with concurrent aspirin therapy for 5–8 d or until the patient is clinically stable.

IN BRIEF

INDICATIONS
Prophylaxis against DVT that may lead to PE in high risk patients undergoing hip replacement surgery, and also patients undergoing abdominal surgery who are at risk for thromboembolic complications. Patients at risk include those who are over 40 years of age, obese, undergoing surgery under general anesthesia lasting longer than 30 minutes, or who have additional risk factors, such as malignancy or a history of DVT or PE.
Prevention of ischemic complications in patients with unstable angina or non–Q-wave MI (use with concurrent aspirin)

CONTRAINDICATIONS
Known hypersensitivity to dalteparin, heparin, or pork
Known heparin-induced thrombocytopenia
Active major bleeding
Patients undergoing regional anesthesia should not receive dalteparin for unstable angina on non–Q-wave MI

DRUG INTERACTIONS
Anticoagulants
Thrombolytics
Antiplatelets
NSAIDs

ADVERSE EFFECTS
Blood: hemorrhage, thrombocytopenia
GI: liver function abnormalities
CNS: epidural or spinal hematoma (especially with spinal or epidural anesthesia and spinal puncture)
Skin: local irritation, pruritus, rash, pain, bullous eruption, necrosis
Rare: hypersensitivity reaction, fever, anaphylactoid reaction

PHARMACOKINETICS AND PHARMACODYNAMICS
(based on plasma anti-Factor Xa activity)
Duration of action: 10–24 h
Onset of action: < 2 h
Peak effect: 2–4 h
Bioavailability: 87%
Clearance: mainly via kidney as unchanged drug
Plasma half-life: 2–4 h
Protein binding: no data

MONITORING
Lab: CBC, anti-factor Xa level (?), liver function test. Clinical evidence of active or occult bleeding.

OVERDOSE
Supportive; the antithrombotic effect may be partially neutralized with protamine.

PATIENT INFORMATION
Dalteparin can cause excessive bleeding and low platelet problems.

AVAILABILITY
Syringes—
2500 anti-Factor Xa IU/ 0.2 mL
5000 anti-Factor Xa IU/ 0.2 mL
Multiple-dose Vials:
10,000 anti-Factor Xa IU/mL, 9.5 mL

DANAPAROID SODIUM (Orgaran®)

Danaparoid is the only low molecular weight heparinoid available in the United States. Danaparoid, derived from porcine source, has a mean molecular weight of 5500 Daltons. The antithrombotic effect is related to its anti-A and anti-IIa effect with an antiXa/IIa ratio greater than 22.

Bleeding and thrombocytopenia are still the major concerns of danaparoid therapy. Among all currently available LMWH/ heparinoids, danaparoid is the least likely agent to cause cross-reactivity with heparin (10%–20%). Its use is still contraindicated in patients with a history of type 2 heparin-induced thrombocytopenia (HIT) without the results of in vitro antiplatelet antibody test. Although clinical data are limited for patients with positive HIT and negative test results, danaparoid may be used safely to treat and prevent thromboembolic complications associated with HIT.

SPECIAL GROUPS

Race: no data; dosage adjustment is probably not required
Children: safety and effectiveness have not been established
Elderly: dosage adjustment is not required
Renal impairment: no dosage adjustment is required; used with caution in patients with serum creatinine ≥2 mg/dL
Hepatic impairment: no data; dosage adjustment is probably not required
Pregnancy: category B; should only be used if clearly indicated
Breast-feeding: unknown if the drug is excreted in human milk; use with caution

DOSAGE

750 anti-Xa U (0.6 mL) twice daily administered SQ beginning 1–4 h before surgery and not sooner than 2 h after surgery. Treatment should be continued until the patient is fully ambulatory (up to 14 d).

IN BRIEF

INDICATIONS
Prophylaxis against DVT that may lead to PE in patients undergoing elective hip replacement surgery.

CONTRAINDICATIONS
Known hypersensitivity to danaparoid, heparin, sulfite, or pork
Known heparin-induced thrombocytopenia associated with a positive in vitro test for antiplatelet antibody in the presence of danaparoid
Active major bleeding
Severe hemorrhagic diathesis

DRUG INTERACTIONS
Anticoagulants
Thrombolytics
Antiplatelets
NSAIDs

ADVERSE EFFECTS
Blood: hemorrhage, thrombocytopenia
GI: nausea, constipation
CNS: epidural or spinal hematoma (especially with spinal or epidural anesthesia and spinal puncture), fever
Skin: local irritation, pruritus, rash, pain
Rare: hypersensitivity (danaparoid contains sulfite)

PHARMACOKINETICS AND PHARMACODYNAMICS
(based on plasma anti-Factor Xa activity)
Duration of action: 24 h
Onset of action: <2 h
Peak effect: 2–5 h
Bioavailability: 100%
Clearance: not metabolized, up to 50% cleared renally
Plasma half-life: 18–28 h
Protein binding: no data

MONITORING
Lab: CBC, anti-factor Xa level (?). Clinical evidence of active or occult bleeding.

OVERDOSE
Supportive; the antithrombotic effect may be partially neutralized with protamine.

PATIENT INFORMATION
Danaparoid can cause excessive bleeding and low platelet problems.

AVAILABILITY
Ampules—750 anti-Factor Xa U/0.6 mL
Syringes—750 anti-Factor Xa U/0.6 mL

ENOXAPARIN SODIUM (Lovenox®)

Enoxaparin is the first LMWH available in the United States. Enoxaparin is produced by alkaline degradation of heparin benzyl ester derived from porcine intestinal mucosa. The average molecular weight is about 4500 Daltons. The antithrombotic effect of enoxaparin is primarily due to its anti-Factor Xa activity (anti-Xa/IIa ratio = 3.8:1). The approximate anti-Factor Xa activity is 1000 IU per 10 mg of enoxaparin.

Enoxaparin therapy, 30 mg twice daily or 40 mg once daily given subcutaneously (SQ), is effective in reducing the risk for DVT and PE in high-risk surgical patients. It may be more effective than the conventional heparin therapy, 5000 U SQ every 8 h. Clinical data also support that enoxaparin administered 1 mg/kg SQ every 12 h or 1.5 mg/kg SQ once daily is as effective as heparin in the management of patients with DVT or PE. In addition, clinical data demonstrate that in combination with aspirin, enoxaparin administered 1 mg/kg SQ every 12 h is more effective than intravenous (IV) heparin therapy in the reduction of ischemic complications, such as death, MI, or recurrent angina in patients with unstable angina or non–Q-wave MI.

SQ enoxaparin, producing more rapid and predictable antithrombotic effect with less monitoring requirements, is also more convenient than IV heparin therapy. With these advantages and convenient route of administration, selected patients with noncomplicated DVT may be discharged early and be managed at home. It is important to remember that, similar to heparin, bleeding and thrombocytopenia are problems seen with enoxaparin therapy. Enoxaparin should not be administered in patients with a history of heparin-induced thrombocytopenia (cross-reactivity >90%).

SPECIAL GROUPS

Race: no data
Children: safety and effectiveness have not been established
Elderly: no dosage adjustment is required
Renal impairment: dosage adjustment should be considered in patients with a creatinine clearance <30 mL/min
Hepatic impairment: no data
Pregnancy: category B; should only be used if clearly indicated
Breast-feeding: unknown if the drug is excreted in human milk; use with caution

DOSAGE

Knee replacement surgery: 30 mg every 12 h SQ for 7–10 d; start 12–24 h after the surgery
Hip replacement surgery: 30 mg every 12 h or 40 mg daily SQ; may be started 12 h prior to the surgery. After initial phase, continuing prophylaxis with 40 mg daily for 21 d is recommended
Abdominal surgery: 40 mg daily SQ for 7–10 d; start 2 h prior to surgery
DVT/PE: 1mg/kg every 12 h or 1.5 mg/kg daily SQ; warfarin therapy should be initiated and enoxaparin should be continued for 5 d or until the INR is therapeutic for two consecutive days
Unstable angina/non–Q-wave MI: 1 mg/kg every 12 h SQ for ≥ 2 d until the patient is clinically stable (with aspirin)

IN BRIEF

INDICATIONS
Prophylaxis against DVT that may lead to PE in patients undergoing hip or knee replacement surgery and in high risk patients undergoing abdominal surgery
Treat DVT with or without PE when used in conjunction with warfarin
Prevention of ischemic complications in patients with unstable angina or non–Q-wave MI with concurrent aspirin

CONTRAINDICATIONS
Known hypersensitivity to enoxaparin, heparin, or pork
Known heparin-induced thrombocytopenia
Active major bleeding

DRUG INTERACTIONS
Anticoagulants
Thrombolytics
Antiplatelets
NSAIDs

ADVERSE EFFECTS
Blood: hemorrhage, thrombocytopenia
GI: liver function abnormalities
CNS: epidural or spinal hematoma (seen with spinal or epidural anesthesia and spinal puncture)
Skin: local irritation, pain, pruritus, urticaria, hematoma, ecchymosis
Rare: anaphylactoid reaction

PHARMACOKINETICS AND PHARMACODYNAMICS
(based on plasma anti-Factor Xa activity)
Duration of action: 12 h or longer
Onset of action: <30 min
Peak effect: 3–5 h
Bioavailability: 92%
Clearance: mainly via kidney, 40% of radioactivity and 8%–20% anti-Factor Xa were recovered in urine in 24 h
Elimination half-life: 4.5 h (range: 3–6 h)
Protein binding: less protein binding, compared with heparin

MONITORING
Lab: CBC, liver function test.
Clinical evidence of active or occult bleeding.

OVERDOSE
Supportive; the antithrombotic effect may be partially neutralized with protamine.

PATIENT INFORMATION
Enoxaparin can cause excessive bleeding and low platelet problems; report any unusual bleeding or easy bruising to your physicians.

AVAILABILITY
Ampules—30 mg/0.3 mL
Syringes—30 mg/0.3 mL; 40 mg/0.4 mL; 60 mg/0.6 mL; 80 mg/0.8 mL; 100 mg/1 mL

LEPIRUDIN

(Refludan®)

Lepirudin is a recombinant hirudin derived from yeast cells. Hirudin is a thrombin inhibitor produced by the medicinal leech, Hirudo medicinalis. Lepirudin inhibits both free and clot-bound thrombin and causes a dose-dependent elevation of activated partial thromboplastin time (aPTT). Its antithrombotic effect is not dependent on cofactors such as antithrombin. Lepirudin is not inhibited by activated platelets or other proteins known to neutralize heparin in vivo. As a result, lepirudin provides a more stable and predictable level of anticoagulation than heparin and can be used to manage patients with documented type II heparin-induced thrombocytopenia.

SPECIAL GROUPS

Race: no data
Children: safety and effectiveness have not been established
Elderly: dose should be adjusted based on creatinine clearance
Renal impairment: dose reduction with more frequent monitoring if creatinine clearance is below 60 mL/min or serum creatinine is above 1.5 mg/dL
Hepatic impairment: no specific dosage adjustments; more frequent monitoring is recommended
Pregnancy: category B; should only be used if clearly indicated
Breast-feeding: not recommended; not known if the drug is excreted in human milk

DOSAGE

Bolus dose: 0.4 mg/kg (up to 44 mg) over 15–20 sec IV
Maintenance: 0.15 mg/kg/h (up to 16.5 mg/h) IV; adjusted based on aPTT measured (4 h after bolus and at least once daily). Treatment should be continued for 2–14 d or longer if indicated. Dose should be adjusted in patients with concurrent thrombolytic therapy or renal insufficiency.
Concurrent warfarin therapy: Reducing lepirudin dose to reach an aPTT ratio just above 1.5 before first dose of warfarin. Once an international normalized ratio (INR) of 2 is achieved, lepirudin therapy should be discontinued.

IN BRIEF

INDICATIONS
Prevent further thromboembolic complications in patients with heparin-induced thrombocytopenia and associated thromboembolic disease.

CONTRAINDICATIONS
Known hypersensitivity to hirudins
End-stage renal disease
Active major bleeding
Severe hemorrhagic diathesis
Recent major surgery/bleeding
Bacterial endocarditis
Severe uncontrolled hypertension
Recent cerebral vascular accident
Anomaly of vessels or organs
Baseline aPTT ratio ≥ 2.5

DRUG INTERACTIONS
Anticoagulants
Thrombolytics
Antiplatelets
NSAIDs

ADVERSE EFFECTS
Blood: bleeding and clotting disorders
GI: liver function abnormalities
Skin: rash, pruritus, urticaria, flushes, chills
Severe/rare: anaphylaxis, anaphylactoid reaction

PHARMACOKINETICS AND PHARMACODYNAMICS
Duration of action: no data
Onset of action: rapid
Peak effect: 4 h
Clearance: partially metabolized by catabolic hydrolysis. 48% renal clearance with 35% as unchanged drug
Plasma half-life: 1.3 h
Protein binding: no data

MONITORING
Lab: CBC, aPTT ratio (1.5–2.5). Clinical evidence of active or occult bleeding.

OVERDOSE
Supportive—no specific antidote is available.

PATIENT INFORMATION
Lepirudin can cause excessive bleeding.

AVAILABILITY
Vials—50 mg

WARFARIN SODIUM
(Warfarin, Coumadin®)

Warfarin is the most widely used oral anticoagulant. It has a relatively narrow therapeutic index. As with the other drugs in this class, the status of the coagulant system should be constantly monitored. Because warfarin is almost entirely metabolized in the liver, impaired hepatic function might be expected to increase sensitivity to the drug. Hepatic impairment also reduces the synthesis of endogenous clotting factors, further enhancing the therapeutic response to warfarin. In a trial involving 1214 patients, warfarin or placebo was given randomly at a mean of 27 d after MI. Treatment continued for an average of 37 mo. In the warfarin group, there was a 24% reduction in deaths ($P < 0.03$) and a 34% reduction in reinfarctions ($P < 0.001$). Cerebrovascular accidents were reduced by 55%. Incidence of serious bleeding was 0.6% per year. This study underlines the value of prophylaxis with anticoagulant therapies after infarction. Drug interactions with warfarin may be associated with synergism (impaired hemostasis, reduced clotting factor synthesis), antagonism (vitamin K), and altered physiologic control loop for vitamin K (hereditary resistance to warfarin).

The most serious risks associated with warfarin are hemorrhage in any tissue or organ, and less frequently, necrosis or gangrene of the skin and other tissues. The risk of hemorrhage is related to the intensity and the duration of anticoagulation. Hemorrhage and tissue necrosis have, in some cases, been reported to result in death or permanent disability. Skin necrosis appears to be associated with local thrombosis and usually appears within a few days of the start of anticoagulant therapy.

Anticoagulant therapy with warfarin may enhance the release of atheromatous plaque emboli. This may increase the risk of systemic cholesterol microembolization, including the purple toe syndrome. Some cases have progressed to extensive tissue necrosis or death. One of the more recently approved indications for warfarin is for the prophylaxis of thromboembolism associated with atrial fibrillation.

Special Note: The Fifth American College of Chest Physicians Consensus Conference on Antithrombotic Therapy (1998) provided recommendations for therapeutic ranges for oral anticoagulant therapy. An internationalized normalized ratio (INR) of 2.5 is recommended for all indications, including recurrent systemic embolism, with the exception of mechanical prosthetic heart valve. An INR of 3.0 is recommended for this indication. The recommendations for therapeutic ranges are provided as INR values instead of prothrombin time (PT) ratios because the variations in responsiveness of commercial thromboplastins is so wide that the term *typical North American thromboplastin* is no longer valid. The INR is calculated as the observed Patient PT/Normal PT (ISI), where ISI is the International Sensitivity Index for the relevant thromboplastin used in the test. All laboratories today should report the INR value of each measured PT (Table 6.4).

IN BRIEF

INDICATIONS
Prophylaxis and treatment:
  Venous thrombosis
  PE
  Atrial fibrillation with embolization
  Thromboembolism associated with prosthetic heart valves

CONTRAINDICATIONS
Known hypersensitivity
Pregnancy
Recent surgery or trauma involving brain, eye, or spinal cord
Active major bleeding
Blood dyscrasias
Arterial aneurysm
Severe hypertension
Endocarditis, pericarditis, or pericardial effusions

DRUG INTERACTIONS
Because of narrow therapeutic index, many drugs may affect the response to warfarin. It is important to monitor the patient closely when any alterations in a patient medication profile occur.

Phenytoin—may increase/decrease response

Agents that may increase response:	Agents that may decrease response:
Acetaminophen	Alcohol (chronic use)
Alcohol (acute)	Aminoglutethimide
Allopurinol	Barbiturates
Amiodarone	Carbamazepine
Anabolic steroids	Cholestyramine
Antiplatelets	Corticosteroids
Cimetidine	Corticotropin
Clofibrate	Estrogen-containing products
Co-trimoxazole	Glutethimide
Disulfiram	Mercaptopurine
Erythromycin	Methaqualone
Ethacrynic acid	Nafcillin
Fluoroquinolones	Rifampin
Glucagon	Spironolactone
Influenza virus vaccine	Sucralfate
Isoniazid	Trazodone
Lovastatin	Vitamin K
Methylthiouracil	
Metronidazole	
Miconazole	
Nalidixic acid	
Neomycin, oral	
NSAIDs	
Other anticoagulants	
Pentoxifylline	
Propafenone	
Propoxyphene	
Propylthiouracil	
Quinidine	
Quinine	
Sulfonamides	
Tamoxifen	
Tetracycline	
Thyroid drugs	
Thrombolytics	
Tricyclic antidepressants	
Thiazides	
Vitamin E	

SPECIAL GROUPS

Race: no differences in response

Children: safety and effectiveness have not been established

Elderly: dosing based on coagulation test results; use smaller initial doses

Renal impairment: use with caution; dosing based on coagulation test results

Hepatic impairment: use with caution; dosing based on coagulation test results

Pregnancy: category X; should not be used

Breast-feeding: excreted in human milk as inactive metabolites; infants nursed by warfarin-treated mothers had no change in PT/INR

DOSAGE

Adults—initiate with 2–5 mg/d for 2–4 d; adjust dose to maintain desired therapeutic INRs as per recommendation by the American College of Chest Physicians (ACCP) and the National Heart, Lung and Blood Institute (NHLBI) (Table 6.4).

The dose of warfarin injection is the same as the oral dose and should only be administered intravenously. The dose should be given as a slow bolus over 1–2 min.

ADVERSE EFFECTS

Blood: bleeding, leukopenia, agranulocytosis, cholesterol microembolization, purple toe syndrome
GI: nausea, vomiting, anorexia, diarrhea, abnormal liver function test
Skin: dermatitis, urticaria, alopecia, skin necrosis or gangrene, subcutaneous infarction, vasculitis, and local thrombosis
Other: fever, hypersensitivity

PHARMACOKINETICS AND PHARMACODYNAMICS

Duration of action: 4–5 d
Onset of action: 1–3 d
Peak effect: 3–6 d
Bioavailability: 78%–100%
Effect of food: no effect on absorption; variations in food vitamin K content can affect therapeutic response
Clearance/Excretion: metabolized by hepatic microsomal enzymes and excreted in the urine mainly as inactive metabolites
Plasma half-life: 1.5–2.5 d
Protein binding: 97%–99%

MONITORING

Lab: CBC, liver function, PT, and INR. Clinical evidence of active or occult bleeding.

OVERDOSE

Supportive—For significant blood loss, whole blood transfusion, fresh frozen plasma, or clotting factor concentrates may be administered. Vitamin K should be reserved as the last alternative to reverse the effect of warfarin (Table 6.5).

PATIENT INFORMATION

Contact physician if excessive bleeding, unusual bruising, skin changes, hair loss, or fever occurs. Inform your physician and dentist that warfarin is being used. Do not take other drugs, change diet pattern, or take food/vitamin supplements before discussing with your physician or pharmacist.
Carry an identification indicating that warfarin is used.

AVAILABILITY

Tablets—1, 2, 2.5, 3, 4, 5, 6, 7.5, 10 mg
Vials—2 mg

TABLE 6.4 THERAPEUTICS RANGE FOR WARFARIN THERAPY RECOMMENDED BY ACCP AND NHLBI

Target INR*	Indications
2.5 (range: 2–3)	Acute myocardial infarction[†]
	Atrial fibrillation[†]
	PE—treatment
	System embolism—prevention
	Tissue heart valves[†]
	Valvular heart diseases[†]
	Venous thromboembolism—both prevention and treatment
3.0 (range: 2.5–3.5)	Mechanical prosthetic valves[‡]
	Systemic embolism, recurrent[‡]

*INR = (observed PT ratio)^{ISI}; INR:International Normalized Ratio; ISI: International Sensitivity Index.

†Prevention for systemic embolism.

‡ With aspirin 81 mg/d.

TABLE 6.5 VITAMIN K DOSE RECOMMENDED FOR RAPID REVERSAL IN WARFARIN OVERDOSE

INR	Vitamin K regimen*	Comments[†]
<6	Not recommended if the patient is not bleeding	Hold warfarin for a few days
6–10	1–2 mg	Reduce INR in 8 h, repeat dose of 0.5 mg at 24 hr if INR remains high
10–20	3–5 mg	Reduce INR in 6 h, repeat the dose every 12 h if needed
>20	5–10 mg	Repeat the dose every 12 h if needed

*Vitamin K may be administered orally, subcutaneously, or intravenously. For intravenous administration, the dose should be diluted and administered over 10–20 minutes to minimize the risk of anaphylactoid reactions.

†INR should be checked every 6–8 h. Resume warfarin therapy at a lower dose when INR is in therapeutic range in patients who are clinically stable. After high dose of vitamin K, concurrent heparin therapy may be required until patients become responsive to warfarin.

ANTITHROMBOTIC THERAPY: ANTIPLATELET AGENTS

With the increased awareness that blood platelets play an important role in the pathogenesis of arterial vaso-occlusive conditions (Fig. 6.1), interest in antiplatelet therapy has increased markedly. The chief function of the platelets is to interact with vascular endothelium and soluble plasma factors in the hemostatic process. Under normal physiologic conditions, platelets are mostly inert. Their adhesion to the subendothelial matrix is prevented by an intact vascular wall. In response to vessel trauma, platelets adhere to newly exposed adhesive proteins, forming a protective monolayer of cells. Within seconds, these platelets are activated by agonists such as thrombin, collagen, and adenosine diphosphate (ADP), causing them to change shape and release stored vesicles. The constituents of the vesicles are mostly involved in the further activation of platelets and the propagation of the hemostatic process. Ultimately these activated platelets aggregate to form a hemostatic plug—closing the lesion in the endothelium and preventing further loss of blood from the site. Under certain pathologic conditions (ie, rupture of an atherosclerotic plaque), these platelet aggregates can form thrombi leading to cardiovascular ischemic events, including unstable angina and myocardial infarction.

Aspirin, dipyridamole, the ADP receptor blockers (ticlopidine, clopidogrel), and the glycoprotein IIb/IIIa integrin receptor antagonists (abciximab, eptifibatide, tirofiban), are the major antiplatelet agents used clinically.

EFFICACY AND USE

The value of antiplatelet therapy on cardiovascular morbidity and mortality has been established largely through the clinical use of aspirin. The long-acting antiplatelet effect of aspirin can be achieved with doses that avoid many of the problems associated with its use in inflammatory disorders. Aspirin is recommended in patients with transient ischemic attack, ischemic stroke, angina pectoris, acute MI, and recurrent MI, as well as in patients undergoing revascularization procedures.

The antithrombotic activity of dipyridamole is more evident when artificial surfaces (prosthetic heart valves, grafts, cannulae) are involved. Dipyridamole's effects are more obvious on synthetic surfaces than on biologic ones, and so, despite a beneficial trend in decreasing vascular events after MI and in reducing occlusion rates in coronary artery grafts, it has no proven benefit in unstable angina or stroke. Dipyridamole may work synergistically with warfarin. Based on clinical observations, there is no additional benefit of adding dipyridamole to other antiplatelet therapy.

Ticlopidine and clopidogrel are effective in many situations where altered platelet function plays a pathologic role. The drugs

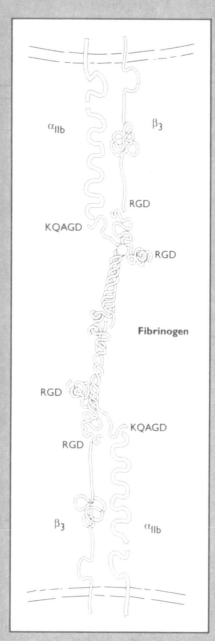

FIGURE 6.2
GPIIb/IIIa structure and interactions binding platelets by divalent fibrinogen. (*Adapted from* Colman RW *et al*: *Hemostasis and Thrombosis: Basic Principles and Clinical Practice.* Philadelphia: Lippincott; 1994:1638–1660.)

The information here is provided as guidance only. Prescribers should always consult the manufacturer's current prescribing information.

97

have little proven benefit in the treatment of angina pectoris. They are used with aspirin in preventing thrombotic events after coronary artery angioplasty and stenting. Ticlopidine has been studied extensively in the prevention of cerebrovascular disease. When compared with placebo in 1000 patients, as part of a study in the secondary prevention of stroke, ticlopidine treatment resulted in a 30% reduction in the relative risk of strokes, MI, or vascular death. When compared with aspirin in the Ticlopidine Aspirin Stroke Study (TASS) study, ticlopidine was found to be superior in terms of all-cause mortality as well as nonfatal stroke. Clopidogrel has also been found to be more efficacious than aspirin in patients with a recent ischemic stroke or MI, or in those with symptomatic peripheral vascular disease.

The binding of fibrinogen to activated platelets (Fig. 6.2) has been identified as the final step in platelet aggregation. This binding can be inhibited by the glycoprotein IIb/IIIa integrin receptor antagonists. A drug with this mechanism could prevent thrombosis resulting from vessel damage or atherosclerotic plaque rupture regardless of the extent of platelet activation.

Abciximab is a parenteral IIb/IIIa receptor antagonist used in high-risk percutaneous coronary intervention or in patients with unstable angina refractory to conventional therapy. Eptifibatide (Integrelin) is approved for use in patients with unstable angina or non–Q-wave MI and in patients undergoing elective percutaneous cardiovascular interventions. Tirofiban is also approved for use in acute coronary syndromes. Xem-lofiban, sibrafiban, orbofiban, and lefradifiban are being evaluated in clinical trials.

MODES OF ACTION

Aspirin affects platelet function by acetylating the enzyme cyclooxygenase. It inactivates the enzymes permanently and prevents formation of thromboxane A2. The effect of aspirin lasts the lifetime of the affected platelets. Its effect on endothelial cell-derived prostacyclin is dose-dependent and less prolonged.

Dipyridamole increases platelet cyclic adenosine monophosphate (AMP). Cyclic AMP inhibits the release of calcium from the dense tubular reticulum, reduces the secretion of serotonin and ADP, and thereby increases the resistance of the platelet to activation.

Ticlopidine and clopidogrel, thienopyridine compounds, are prodrugs that are active antiplatelets in vivo but not in vitro. These drugs act by blocking ADP receptors within the platelet membrane (Fig. 6.3) and act independently of arachidonic acid pathways. The drugs produce a thromboasthenia-like state, resulting in a reduction in platelet aggregation, a prolongation of the bleeding time, a decrease in platelet degranulation, and a reduction in platelet and fibrin deposition on artificial surfaces.

The glycoprotein IIb/IIIa receptor antagonists bind to the receptors of activated platelets and inhibit platelet aggregation.

INDICATIONS

	Aspirin	Dipyridamole	Ticlopidine	Clopidogrel	GP IIb/IIIa
Primary and secondary prophylaxis of MI	+	–	(+)	+	+*
Prophylaxis of stroke	(+)	–	+	+	–
Prophylaxis for transient ischemic attack	+	(+)	+	+	–
Peripheral vascular disease	–	(+)	–	+	–

*Only approved for limited indications.

+—FDA approved; – —not FDA approved; (+)—clinical uses, not FDA approved.

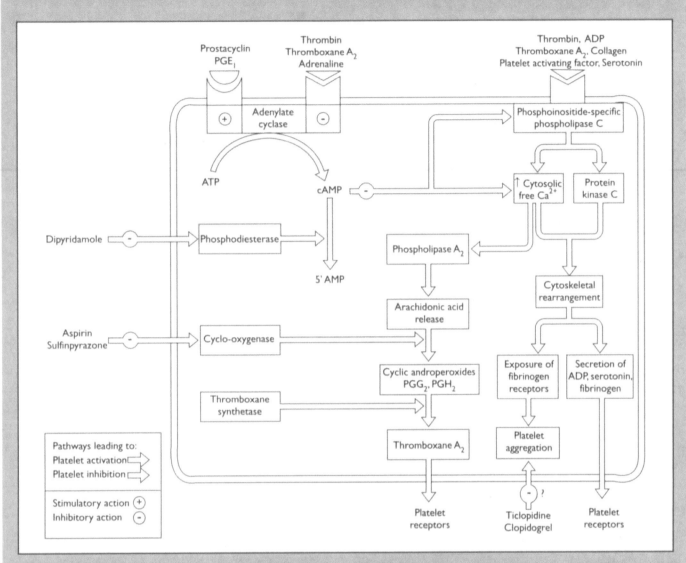

FIGURE 6.3 Sites of action of some of the antiplatelet drugs and the associated mechanisms of platelet activation. Platelet activation results from mobilization of calcium, which in turn results from agonist binding to the platelet receptor. (*Adapted from* Saltiel E, Ward A: Ticlopidine: a review of its pharmacodynamic and pharmacokinetic properties, and therapeutic efficacy in platelet-dependent disease states. *Drugs* 1987, 34:222–262.)

ASPIRIN

Aspirin inhibits cyclooxygenase-dependent platelet aggregation permanently, and doses as low as 80 mg daily can be effective. Secondary prevention trials using 300–1200 mg daily have consistently demonstrated a decreased incidence of transient ischemic attacks (TIAs), strokes, and death. Adding another antiplatelet drug does not appear to improve outcome. Aspirin also reduces progression of unstable angina to MI or death.

The ISIS-2 study examined the short-term (5 week) outcome in patients with suspected acute MI randomized to intravenous streptokinase, 160 mg enteric-coated aspirin daily, both, or neither. Therapy was initiated within 24 h of initial symptoms and continuing the aspirin for 1 mo. The study showed that aspirin decreased nonfatal reinfarction, stroke, and vascular mortality. Streptokinase alone increased nonfatal reinfarction, but the combination of aspirin with streptokinase decreased nonfatal reinfarction and vascular mortality (Fig. 6.4).

The Physicians' Health Study, a primary prevention study of 22,071 healthy male physicians, demonstrated a 39% lower incidence of nonfatal MI, but a 19% higher (although not statistically significant) incidence of strokes (Fig. 6.5).

Aspirin is effective in decreasing early vascular graft occlusion. In combination with dipyridamole, aspirin has been shown to be as effective as, and safer than, anticoagulants in maintaining vessel patency after angioplasty. Treatment with aspirin for 5 years reduced the incidence of MI from 12% to 5% and reduced the incidence of new angiographic lesions from 35% to 23%. Antithrombotic treatment with either aspirin or warfarin has been shown to reduce the risk of stroke and systemic embolism in patients with atrial fibrillation.

IN BRIEF

INDICATIONS
Cardiovascular use only (not all indications are FDA approved)
Prevention of arterial and venous thrombosis in:

Transient ischemic attacks

MI (primary/secondary prophylaxis)

Unstable angina

Acute pericarditis

Prosthetic heart valves (with an oral anticoagulant or dipyridamole)

Arteriovenous shunt for hemodialysis

Microcirculatory thrombosis seen in thrombocytosis

Transluminal angioplasty of coronary, iliac, femoral, popliteal, or tibial artery (+/– dipyridamole)

Aortocoronary-artery bypass

Other uses: Kawasaki syndrome; diabetic retinopathy

CONTRAINDICATIONS
Known hypersensitivity to salicylate or NSAIDs

Active internal bleeding or bleeding diathesis

History of asthma, nasal polyps, chronic urticaria

Hemophilia

DRUG INTERACTIONS (less problematic with low dose)
Urine acidifiers such as ascorbic acid (vitamin C)

Urine alkalinizers such as antacids

Alcohol

ACE inhibitors

Beta-blockers

Diuretics

Corticosteroids

Methotrexate

Probenecid

Carbonic anhydrase inhibitors

Anticoagulants

Other antiplatelets

NSAIDs

Thrombolytics

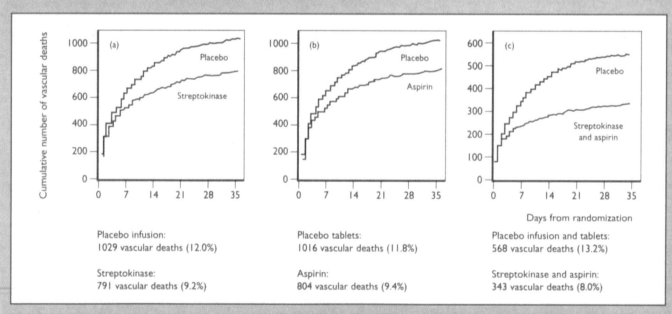

Placebo infusion:
1029 vascular deaths (12.0%)

Streptokinase:
791 vascular deaths (9.2%)

Placebo tablets:
1016 vascular deaths (11.8%)

Aspirin:
804 vascular deaths (9.4%)

Placebo infusion and tablets:
568 vascular deaths (13.2%)

Streptokinase and aspirin:
343 vascular deaths (8.0%)

FIGURE 6.4 Cumulative vascular mortality on days 0-35 of ISIS-2 study. **A,** All patients allocated to receive streptokinase compared with all patients allocated to placebo infusion. **B,** All patients allocated to receive aspirin compared with all patients allocated to placebo tablets. **C,** All patients allocated to both streptokinase and aspirin regimens compared with all patients allocated to placebo infusion and tablets. (Adapted from ISIS 2 Collaborative Group: Randomised trial of intravenous streptokinase, oral aspirin, both or neither among 17,187 cases of suspected acute myocardial infarction. Lancet 1988, 2:349–360.)

ASPIRIN (CONTINUED)

SPECIAL GROUPS

Race: no differences in response

Children: not recommended in children with acute febrile illness due to the risk for Reye's syndrome

Elderly: no dosage adjustment is required

Renal impairment: use with caution in patients with chronic renal insufficiency, especially avoid high dose

Hepatic impairment: use with caution

Pregnancy: category D; avoid use in the third trimester of pregnancy and only use if clearly indicated in the first and second trimesters

Breast-feeding: excreted in human milk; used with caution

DOSAGE

Transient ischemic attack in males: 1300 mg/d in 2–4 divided doses; dose as low as 300 mg/d may be effective if tolerance is a problem with higher doses

MI/unstable angina: 80–325 mg once daily; the first dose should be the plain aspirin and the dose should be chewed or crushed or dispersed in solution and administered as soon as possible for more rapid antiplatelet effect

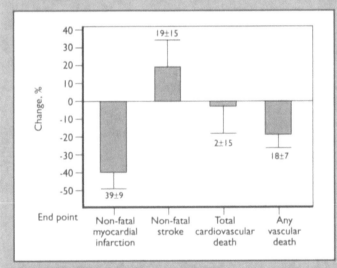

FIGURE 6.5 Effect of aspirin on primary prevention of myocardial infarction in the USPHS trial. (*Adapted from* The Steering Committee of the Physicians' Health Study Research Group: final report on the aspirin component of the ongoing Physicians' Health Study. *N Engl J Med* 1989, 321:129–135.)

ADVERSE EFFECTS

Blood: prolonged bleeding time, blood dyscrasias

GI: nausea, dyspepsia, discomfort, ulceration, bleeding, occult blood loss, liver dysfunction

CNS: tinnitus

Kidney: progressed renal dysfunction, especially in patients with chronic renal insufficiency

Other: anaphylaxis, bronchospasm, angioedema, hives, rashes, Reye's syndrome,

PHARMACOKINETICS AND PHARMACODYNAMICS

Duration of action: 7–10 d for antiplatelet effect; 4–6 h for analgesic, antipyretic effect

Onset of action: rapid if the first dose is chewed or crushed or dispersed in solution before the administration

Peak effect: no data

Bioavailability: 50%–100% (depends on formulations)

Effect of food: decrease the rate/extent of absorption

Clearance: hydrolyzed to salicylic acid in liver, plasma, and erythrocytes, and further metabolized by liver

Excretion: mainly as metabolites and some as unchanged aspirin in urine

Plasma half-life: (salicylic acid) 2–3 h with low dose; over 20 h with the higher anti-inflammatory dose

Protein binding: 50%–90%; concentration dependent

MONITORING

Clinical evidence of active or occult bleeding (especially if used with other agents that may affect hemostasis); gastrointestinal intolerance.

OVERDOSE

Manifests first as tinnitus and hearing loss, vomiting, oliguria, acute renal failure, behavioral changes, central stimulation followed by central depression, acid base and electrolyte disturbances, dehydration, hyperpyrexia and hyperglycemia or hypoglycemia. Treatment may include emptying stomach via induction of emesis or gastric lavage, administering activated charcoal, monitoring and supporting vital function, correcting hypothermia, fluid, electrolyte and acid-base imbalances, correcting ketosis, and adjusting plasma glucose concentrations as needed.

Monitor serum salicylate concentration until it is apparent that concentration is decreasing to nontoxic range. Induce forced alkaline diuresis to increase salicylate excretion; however, bicarbonate should not be administered orally for this purpose because salicylate absorption may be increased. Also, if acetazolamide is used, the increased risk for severe metabolic acidosis and salicylate toxicity must be considered.

Institute exchange transfusion, hemodialysis, peritoneal dialysis, or hemoperfusion as needed in severe overdose. Monitor for pulmonary edema and convulsions and institute appropriate therapy if required. Administer blood or vitamin K, if necessary, to treat hemorrhage.

PATIENT INFORMATION

May cause gastrointestinal irritation (take with food or after meals). Tablet forms always administered with full glass of water, with patient remaining upright for 15–30 min after administration. Tablets should not be placed directly on tooth or gum surface because of possible injury to tissues. No chewing before swallowing for at least 7 d following tonsillectomy or oral surgery. Use caution when taking other medications. Do not take within 3 h of ketoconazole, within 3–4 h of oral tetracycline, within 1–2 h of any other oral medication, or within 2 h of cellulose-containing laxative. Use caution with other medications containing aspirin or other salicylates (including diflunisal) or when significant quantities of sodium are used. If breathing difficulties (rare), changes in hearing function, or rashes, dizziness, or other untoward effects (black, tarry stools or blood in urine) occur, contact physician immediately.

Do not take aspirin 5 d prior to any surgery, unless otherwise directed by physician.

AVAILABILITY

Available in various strengths and formulations.

DIPYRIDAMOLE (Dipyridamole, Persantine®)

Dipyridamole, a vasodilator as well as an inhibitor of platelet activity, decreases platelet aggregation in a number of thromboembolic disorders. When combined with anticoagulant drugs, there is evidence of added benefit, especially in patients undergoing vascular grafts or those with prosthetic heart valves. When used in combination with other antiplatelet drugs, there is no convincing evidence that dipyridamole has contributed significantly to the benefit derived, except possibly when artificial grafts may have contributed to the risk of thrombosis. When used as monotherapy, dipyridamole does not improve the survival of patients with acute MI, reduce the incidence of postoperative deep vein thrombosis, or produce beneficial effects in patients suffering transient ischemic attacks. Recently the FDA approved a combination formulation of extended release dipyridamole and aspirin for prevention of secondary stroke in patients who have had transient ischemic attack or stroke.

SPECIAL GROUPS

Race: no differences in response
Children: safety and effectiveness have not been established in children under 12 y of age
Elderly: no dose adjustment necessary
Renal impairment: renal elimination is relatively minor; no need to reduce dose
Hepatic impairment: no data; dosage adjustment is probably not required
Pregnancy: category B; should only be used if clearly indicated
Breast-feeding: use with caution; excreted in breast milk

DOSAGE

75–100 mg four times daily (as an adjunct to warfarin therapy)

IN BRIEF

INDICATIONS
Prophylaxis of thromboembolism after cardiac valve replacement (as an adjunct to warfarin therapy).

CONTRAINDICATIONS
Known hypersensitivity
History of problematic hypotension

DRUG INTERACTIONS
Any agents that may affect BP
Anticoagulants
Other antiplatelets
NSAIDs
Thrombolytics

ADVERSE EFFECTS
CV: hypotension, flushing, angina
CNS: headache, dizziness, syncope
GI: intolerance, nausea, vomiting, diarrhea
Skin: rash, pruritus

PHARMACOKINETICS AND PHARMACODYNAMICS
Duration of action: no data
Onset of action: no data
Peak effect: no data
Bioavailability: 37%–66%
Effect of food: no data
Clearance/Excretion: metabolized in the liver, excreted in the bile, and eliminated in feces; small amount is eliminated in urine
Plasma half-life: 40–80 min (initial phase); 10–12 h (terminal phase)
Protein binding: 91%–99%

MONITORING
BP, heart rate, and clinical evidence of active or occult bleeding (especially if used with warfarin).

OVERDOSE
Supportive—hypotension is the main concern; fluid and pressor may be used if necessary; not dialyzable.

PATIENT INFORMATION
Can produce gastrointestinal discomfort (take with food, preferably before meals). May also cause dizziness, headache, weakness, or flushing. If chest pain increases, contact physician immediately. Use caution when taking other medications.

AVAILABILITY
Tablets—25, 50 ,75 mg
Combination formulation:
Aggrenox®—extended release dipyridamole 200 mg/aspirin 25 mg

CLOPIDOGREL BISULFATE (Plavix®)

Clopidogrel, a thienopyridine derivative, inhibits ADP-induced platelet aggregation. Clopidogrel is a prodrug with no direct antiplatelet activity in vitro. After biotransformation, an unknown metabolite is responsible for its pharmacologic effect. Although chemically similar to ticlopidine, clopidogrel causes less neutropenia (<450 neutrophils/µL) or agranulocytosis.

Clinical data support prophylactic use of clopidogrel in patients at risk of ischemic events, especially in those with recent history of myocardial infarction or ischemic stroke, and in those with peripheral arterial disease. The CAPRIE trial demonstrated that clopidogrel was more effective than aspirin in 19,185 patients. Clopidogrel was demonstrated to provide 7%–8% benefit over aspirin in patients with MI, stroke, and peripheral arterial disease. Aspirin remains the least expensive agent for primary and secondary prevention in patients at risk of ischemic events. Clopidogrel may be the preferred antiplatelet alternative in patients who have known histories of aspirin allergy or intolerance, and in those who experience recurrent ischemic events while maintaining on aspirin therapy. Clopidogrel may also be useful in patients undergoing percutaneous transluminal coronary angioplasty (PTCA), stent, coronary artery bypass graft (CABG), and in patients presenting with unstable angina. Because clopidogrel does not affect the cyclooxygenase pathway, it may act synergistically with aspirin to inhibit platelet aggregation. The contribution of clopidogrel plus aspirin has been found to be effective in preventing stent thrombosis. The combination is also being investigated in patients with unstable angina and acute MI.

SPECIAL GROUPS

Race: no differences in response
Children: safety and effectiveness have not been established
Elderly: no dosage adjustment is required
Renal impairment: no dosage adjustment is required
Hepatic impairment: no data; dosage adjustment is probably not required
Pregnancy: category B; should only be used if clearly indicated
Breast-feeding: not recommended; not known if the drug is excreted in human milk

DOSAGE
75 mg once daily

IN BRIEF

INDICATIONS
Prevention of ischemic events, MI, stroke, and vascular death in patients with recent MI, recent stroke, and peripheral arterial disease.

CONTRAINDICATIONS
Hypersensitivity
Active pathologic bleeding

DRUG INTERACTIONS
Anticoagulants
Other antiplatelets
NSAIDs
Thrombolytics

ADVERSE EFFECTS
Side effects that were more common vs. aspirin include rash, diarrhea, purpura, and pruritus.

PHARMACOKINETICS AND PHARMACODYNAMICS
Duration of action: 5 d after treatment is discontinued
Onset of action: 2 h after a single dose
Peak effect: between day 3 and day 7 after repeated doses
Bioavailability: 50%
Effect of food: none
Clearance: mainly hepatic; by hydrolysis and glucuronidation
Excretion: mainly as metabolites; urine—50%; feces—46%
Plasma half-life: up to 11 d for platelet-bound clopidogrel and 8 h for a major metabolite; neither one has direct antiplatelet effect
Protein binding: 98%

MONITORING
For prolonged use, monitor well being and observe for side effects.

OVERDOSE
Supportive—platelet transfusion may be administered to rapidly reverse prolonged bleeding time.

PATIENT INFORMATION
Clopidogrel may cause prolonged bleeding; report any unusual bleeding and inform physicians prior to any surgical procedures or starting any new drugs.

AVAILABILITY
Tablets—75 mg

TICLOPIDINE HYDROCHLORIDE (Ticlid®)

Ticlopidine, a thienopyridine derivative, inhibits ADP-induced platelet aggregation. Ticlopidine has no direct antiplatelet activity in vitro. Its metabolites are responsible for the pharmacologic effect observed in vivo. Ticlopidine may also interfere with the binding of von Willebrand factor to platelet receptors. With the therapeutic dose of ticlopidine, 20%–30% platelet inhibition can be achieved. This effect is irreversible for the life of the platelets. Clinical studies have supported the effectiveness of ticlopidine in stroke prevention; however, the side effect profile of ticlopidine, especially the bone marrow toxicity, precludes its use as the first line agent. Aspirin remains the preferred agent of choice in patients with a history of transient ischemic attack or stroke.

Because ticlopidine has no effect on the cyclooxygenase pathway, it may act synergistically with aspirin. The combination of ticlopidine and aspirin has been studied in high-risk patients undergoing coronary stenting. Lower rates of stent thrombosis and cardiovascular complications were observed with the combination. Ticlopidine may also be useful in peripheral arterial obliterative disease, CABG, postsaphenous vein bypass grafting, diabetic retinopathy, and in patients with MI or unstable angina.

SPECIAL GROUPS

Race: no differences in response
Children: safety and effectiveness have not been established
Elderly: no dosage adjustment is required
Renal impairment: use with caution; dosage reduction may be required
Hepatic impairment: contraindicated in severe liver dysfunction; use with caution in mild/moderate liver dysfunction
Pregnancy: category B; should only be used if clearly indicated
Breast-feeding: not recommended; not known if the drug is excreted in human milk

DOSAGE

250 mg twice daily with food

IN BRIEF

INDICATIONS
Prevention of thrombotic stroke in patients with transient ischemic attack or with a history of completed thrombotic stroke.

CONTRAINDICATIONS
Hypersensitivity
Active pathologic bleeding
Neutropenia
Thrombocytopenia
Severe hepatic dysfunction

DRUG INTERACTIONS
Antacids
Cimetidine
Digoxin
Theophylline
Phenytoin
Anticoagulants
Other antiplatelets
NSAIDs
Thrombolytics

ADVERSE EFFECTS
Hematological: bone marrow suppression, neutropenia, thrombocytopenia, agranulocytosis, pancytopenia, bleeding
GI: nausea, vomiting, diarrhea, dyspepsia, liver function abnormalities
Skin: rash, pruritus
Severe/Rare: neutropenia, agranulocytosis, hypersensitivity such as Stevens-Johnson syndrome, erythema multiforme, and exfoliative dermatitis

PHARMACOKINETICS AND PHARMACODYNAMICS
Duration of action: 7–10 d
Onset of action: within 2–3 d
Peak effect: 8–11 d
Bioavailability: >80%
Effect of food: increase absorption by 20% when taken after a meal
Clearance: metabolized by liver
Excretion: urine—60%, mainly as metabolites
feces—23%, 1/3 as unchanged drug
Plasma half-life: 10–12 h
Protein binding: 98%

MONITORING
Lab: white blood cell count with differential; clinical evidence of active or occult bleeding.

OVERDOSE
Supportive—platelet transfusion may be administered to rapidly reverse prolonged bleeding time.

PATIENT INFORMATION
Ticlopidine may cause prolonged bleeding or affect white blood cells; report any unusual bleeding, fever, chills, and sore throat; inform physicians prior to any surgical procedures or starting any new drugs.

AVAILABILITY
Tablets—250 mg

ABCIXIMAB (ReoPro®)

Abciximab is the Fab fragment of the chimeric human-murine monoclonal antibody 7E. Abciximab binds to glycoprotein (GP) IIb/IIIa receptor of human platelets and inhibits platelet aggregation by preventing the binding of fibrinogen, von Willebrand factor, and other adhesive molecules to activated platelets. Maximal inhibition of platelet aggregation can be achieved when more than 80% of GP IIb/IIIa receptors are blocked by abciximab. This can be achieved after the bolus dose of 0.25 mg/kg of abciximab and maintained by continuous intravenous infusion. Platelet function gradually returns to normal after discontinuation of abciximab infusion.

Clinical efficacy of abciximab in patients undergoing percutaneous coronary intervention and in patients with unstable angina not responding to conventional medical therapy has been evaluated and supported by four studies: EPIC, EPILOG, CAPTURE, and EPISTENT. Abciximab therapy was associated with a significant reduction in death, MI, and need for urgent cardiac intervention. All patients received concurrent heparin and aspirin unless contraindicated. These benefits were observed early and sustained beyond 6 mo after the therapy.

SPECIAL GROUPS

Race: no differences in response
Children: safety and effectiveness have not been established
Elderly: no dosage adjustment is required
Renal impairment: no dosage adjustment is required
Hepatic impairment: no data; dosage adjustment is probably not required
Pregnancy: category C; should only be used if clearly indicated
Breast-feeding: use with caution; not known if the drug is excreted in human milk

DOSAGE*

Percutaneous coronary intervention (PCI): 0.25mg/kg intravenous bolus over 10–60 min before PTCA, followed by a continuous infusion of 0.125 µg/kg/min (up to 10 µg/min) for 12 h
Unstable angina with PCI planned in 24 h: 0.25mg/kg intravenous bolus over 10–60 min followed by a continuous infusion of 10 µg/min for 18–24 h, concluding 1 h after the PCI
*Recommended with concurrent heparin and aspirin therapy

IN BRIEF

INDICATIONS
Prevention of cardiac ischemic complications in patients undergoing PCI or in patients with unstable angina failing conventional therapy with planned PCI within 24 h.

CONTRAINDICATIONS
Hypersensitivity
Intracranial pathology
Active internal bleeding or bleeding diathesis
Severe GI or GU bleeding within 6 wks
History of stroke within 2 yrs or with a significant residual neurologic deficit
Severe uncontrolled hypertension
Thrombocytopenia
Major surgery or severe trauma within 6 wks
Vasculitis
Dextran use
Warfarin use with a PT > 1.2 times control

DRUG INTERACTIONS
Any agents that can affect hemostasis:
Anticoagulants
Thrombolytics
Other antiplatelets
NSAIDs
Dextran

ADVERSE EFFECTS
Major: bleeding and clotting disorders, thrombocytopenia
CV: hypotension, bradycardia, chest pain
CNS: headache, intracranial hemorrhage, stroke
GI: bleeding, abdominal discomfort, nausea, vomiting
Severe/Rare: hypersensitivity

PHARMACOKINETICS AND PHARMACODYNAMICS
Duration of action: ≥ 48 hrs
Onset of action: rapid
Clearance: unknown
Excretion: unknown
Plasma half-life: initial phase: <10 min; second phase: 30 min
Protein binding: unknown

MONITORING
Lab: CBC, PT, APTT, ACT. Clinical evidence of active or occult bleeding.

OVERDOSE
Supportive—avoid prolonged infusion; platelet transfusion may restore platelet function.

PATIENT INFORMATION
Administration of abciximab has been associated with an increased risk of bleeding, including intracranial, retroperitoneal, gastrointestinal, and genitourinary bleeding.

AVAILABILITY
Vials—10 mg/5 mL (2 mg/mL)

EPTIFIBATIDE

(Integrilin®)

Eptifibatide, a reversible peptide antagonist of the platelet GP IIb/IIIa receptor, inhibits platelet aggregation in a dose- or concentration-dependent way. More than 90% and 40%–50% of inhibition can be achieved and maintained, respectively, at steady state with the high-dose and low-dose regimens used clinically.

In patients with acute coronary syndrome (unstable angina or non–Q-wave MI) who were managed medically or underwent early percutaneous cardiovascular intervention (PCI), adjunct epitifibatide therapy reduced the risk of death and MI. This benefit was observed at 72 h; however, the benefit diminished over time and was not statistically significant at the end of the 6-mo period. In patients undergoing elective PCI, eptifibatide reduced the rate of death, MI, or urgent intervention. Again, the benefit was diminished over time and did not reach statistical significance at the end of the 6-mo period. Similar to other GP IIb/IIIa receptor antagonists, concurrent aspirin and heparin therapy is recommended unless otherwise contraindicated.

SPECIAL GROUPS

Race: no data

Children: safety and effectiveness have not been established

Elderly: no dosage adjustment is required; limited data in patients more than 75 years of age and less than 50 kg of weight

Renal impairment: not recommended

Hepatic impairment: no data; dosage adjustment is probably not required

Pregnancy: category B; should only be used if clearly indicated

Breast-feeding: use with caution; not known if the drug is excreted in human milk

DOSAGE*

Acute Coronary Syndrome (ACS): 180 µg/kg intravenous bolus over 1–2 min, followed by 2 µg/kg/min continuous infusion for 72 h, until hospital discharge, or until the time of CABG, whichever occurs first. If PCI is performed, the infusion may be reduced to 0.5 µg/kg/min during the procedure and resumed 2 µg/kg/min for 20–24 h after the procedure (maximum duration of infusion up to 96 h).

Percutaneous Cardiovascular Intervention (PCI): 135 µg/kg intravenous bolus over 1–2 min, immediately before the procedure, followed by 0.5 µg/kg/min for 20–24 h.

*Recommended with concurrent heparin and aspirin therapy.

IN BRIEF

INDICATIONS
Prevention of cardiac ischemic complications in patients with ACS (unstable angina or non–Q-wave MI) and in patients undergoing elective PCI.

CONTRAINDICATIONS
Known hypersensitivity

Bleeding diathesis or active bleeding within 30 d

Severe hypertension—SBP > 200 mmHg; DBP > 110 mmHg

Major surgery within 6 wks

History of stroke within 30 d or hemorrhagic stroke

Platelet count < 100,000/mm³

Renal insufficiency; serum creatinine > 2 mg/dL for 180 µg/kg bolus and 2 µg/kg/min infusion; serum creatinine > 4 mg/dL for 135 µg/kg bolus and 0.5 µg/kg/min infusion

DRUG INTERACTIONS
Anticoagulants

Thrombolytics

Other antiplatelets

NSAIDs

ADVERSE EFFECTS
Blood: bleeding and clotting disorders, thrombocytopenia

CNS: intracranial hemorrhage, stroke

Severe/Rare: hypersensitivity

PHARMACOKINETICS AND PHARMACODYNAMICS
Duration of action: 4–6 h (dose dependent)

Onset of action: within 15 min

Clearance: renal and plasma

Excretion: urine—50%, mainly unchanged

Plasma half-life: 2.5 h

Protein binding: 25%

MONITORING
Lab: CBC, PT, APTT, ACT. Clinical evidence of active or occult bleeding.

OVERDOSE
Supportive—avoid prolonged infusion and platelet transfusion may restore platelet function.

PATIENT INFORMATION
Administration of eptifibatide has been associated with an increased risk of bleeding including intracranial, retroperitoneal, gastrointestinal, and genitourinary bleeding.

AVAILABILITY
Vials—20 mg/10 mL (2 mg/mL); 75 mg/100 mL (0.75 mg/mL)

TIROFIBAN HYDROCHLORIDE (Aggrastat®)

Tirofiban, a reversible nonpeptide antagonist of the platelet GP IIb/IIIa receptor, inhibits platelet aggregation. With the recommended dosing regimen, more than 90% of inhibition is achieved by the end of the 30-min bolus infusion and maintained by the continuous infusion.

Compared to conventional heparin therapy, tirofiban used alone or in combination with heparin, reduced the risk of refractory ischemia, MI, or death in patients with acute coronary syndrome (ACS), unstable angina, or non–Q-wave MI. The benefit was observed early in the course and sustained beyond 6 mo after the therapy. Concurrent heparin therapy is more efficacious in risk reduction than using tirofiban alone. Tirofiban therapy may be used as an adjunct in patients solely managed medically or in those undergoing PTCA or subsequent CABG. All patients should also receive aspirin unless contraindicated.

SPECIAL GROUPS

Race: no difference in plasma clearance
Children: safety and effectiveness have not been established
Elderly: slower clearance, no dosage adjustment is required
Renal impairment: reduce dose by 50% in patients with a creatinine clearance < 30 mL/min
Hepatic impairment: no dosage adjustment is required in mild/moderate liver dysfunction
Pregnancy: category B; should only be used if clearly indicated
Breast-feeding: not recommended; not known if the drug is excreted in human milk

DOSAGE*

0.4 µg/kg/min for 30 min, followed by 0.1 µg/kg/min for 48–108 h. The infusion should be continued through angiography and for 12–24 h after angioplasty or atherectomy.
*Recommended with concurrent heparin and aspirin therapy.

IN BRIEF

INDICATIONS
Prevention of cardiac ischemic complications in patients with ACS (unstable angina or non–Q-wave MI).

CONTRAINDICATIONS
Hypersensitivity
Active internal bleeding
Intracranial pathology
Acute pericarditis
History of stroke within 30 d or hemorrhagic stroke
Severe hypertension (SBP > 180 mmHg; DBP > 110 mmHg)
Major surgery or severe trauma within 30 d
Dissecting aortic aneurysm

DRUG INTERACTIONS
Anticoagulants
Thrombolytics
Other antiplatelets
NSAIDs

ADVERSE EFFECTS
Major: bleeding and clotting disorders, thrombocytopenia
CV: bradycardia, coronary artery dissection
CNS: headache, dizziness
GI: nausea
Severe/Rare: hypersensitivity

PHARMACOKINETICS AND PHARMACODYNAMICS
Duration of action: 4–8 h
Onset of action: achieved 90% platelet inhibition within 30 min
Clearance: renal and plasma, minimally metabolized
Excretion: mainly unchanged; urine—65%; feces— 25%
Plasma half-life: 2 h
Protein binding: 65%

MONITORING
Lab: CBC, PT, APTT, ACT. Clinical evidence of active or occult bleeding.

OVERDOSE
Supportive—can be removed by dialysis; platelet transfusion may restore platelet function.

PATIENT INFORMATION
Administration of tirofiban has been associated with an increased risk of bleeding including intracranial, retroperitoneal, gastrointestinal, and genitourinary bleeding.

AVAILABILITY
Vials—12.5 mg/50 mL (250 µg/mL)
Premixed bags—25 mg/500 mL (50 µg/mL)

ANTITHROMBOTIC THERAPY: THROMBOLYTIC AGENTS

Thrombolytic therapy has played a critical part in cardiovascular medicine as a result of the appreciation that infarction is caused by a blood clot. A localized vascular occlusion is initiated by changes at the endothelial surface, possibly involving a plaque fissure or ulceration. The activation, adherence, and aggregation of platelets, along with the release of coagulation proteins, initiate the clotting cascade. This allows the development of a critical concentration of thrombin sufficient to convert fibrinogen into fibrin. After cross-linkage, fibrin forms a clot anchored to the original site of endothelial surface derangement.

A dynamic situation occurs with the fibrinolytic mechanism being activated on the fibrin network as fibrin continues to be formed. The eventual outcome of the vessel depends on the net balance between the clotting and lysing systems. Clinically, this process is manifest as unstable angina (subtotal occlusion), subendocardial infarction (transient occlusion), and transmural infarction (sustained occlusion) (Fig. 6.1A).

Thrombolytic therapy increases plasmin release locally to break down the clot, while minimizing the risk of adverse events, such as bleeding. Five thrombolytic agents are available: alteplase (tissue-type plasminogen activator, or tPA), an enzyme naturally secreted by endothelial cells; streptokinase (SK) derived from ß hemolytic streptococci; urokinase (UK), a trypsin-like enzyme produced in the kidney; anistreplase (anisoylated streptokinase plasminogen activator complex [APSAC]), streptokinase bound to plasminogen and acylated to "time release" its activity; and reteplase, an unglycosylated recombinant plasminogen activator consisting of the Kringle 2 and protease domains of tPA, with a 3–4 times longer half-life than tPA (Table 6.6).

EFFICACY AND USE

Thrombolytic treatment decreases mortality after coronary thrombosis (Table 6.7). Although streptokinase was first ad-ministered to patients with acute MI more than 30 years ago, thrombolysis has only recently become widely used because of the development of recombinant DNA technology, which allows large-scale production of tPA.

Anistreplase has the advantage of its simple single intravenous regimen that gives possibility for early out-of-hospital use. The survival benefits from thrombolytic therapy are beginning to be fully appreciated, especially when used with aspirin (Fig. 6.4). Aspirin reduces the rate of reinfarction after thrombolysis and lowers the incidence of stroke following MI.

Thrombolytic therapy should be instituted as soon as possible following the onset of clinical symptoms of acute MI. Current recommendations are to initiate thrombolytic therapy when indicated within 30 min of hospital arrival. Aspirin may be administered to inhibit platelet aggregation and reduce the thrombogenic tendency during or following post-thrombolytic anticoagulant therapy. Angioplasty, coronary bypass surgery, or repeat revascularization procedure may be necessary to provide long-lasting protection against reocclusion.

Cardiac rupture may be a risk with the late administration of thrombolytics. The observation that early atenolol treatment in acute MI may reduce deaths from cardiac rupture suggests that thrombolytic therapy should be combined with beta blockade. Allergic reactions, including the rare anaphylactic reactions, have been associated almost exclusively with streptokinase and anistreplase because of foreign protein components. Transient hypotension associated with streptokinase infusion is a frequent finding. Hypotension may also occur at the time of reperfusion with successful thrombolysis and recanalization. Arrhythmias occurring during thrombolytic therapy have been used as a

TABLE 6.6 THROMBOLYTIC AGENTS CURRENTLY AVAILABLE					
Characteristic	Streptokinase	Anistreplase	Urokinase	Alteplase	Reteplase
Molecular weight (daltons)	47,000	131,000	31,000–55,000	70,000	39,571
Plasma clearance time (min)	15–25	50–90	15–20	4–8	11–19
Fibrin specificity	Minimal	Minimal	Moderate	Moderate	Moderate
Plasminogen binding	Indirect	Indirect	Direct	Direct	Direct
Potential allergic reaction	Yes	Yes	No	No	No
Typical dose	1.5 million U	30 U	2 million U	100 mg (max)	10 U + 10 U
Administration	1-hr IV infusion	5 min IV infusion	1 million U IV bolus, then 1 million U IV over 1 h	15 mg bolus, then 0.75 mg/kg (max 50 mg) over 30 min, then 0.5 mg/kg (max 35 mg) over 60 min	Two 10 U IV boluses, each over 2 min, and 30 min apart
Approximate cost	$300	$2000	$2750	$2200	$2200

Adapted from Forman R, Frishman WH: Thrombolytic agents. In Cardiovascular Pharmacotherapeutics Companion Handbook. Edited by Frishman WH, Sonnenblick EH. New York: McGraw Hill; 1998:327.

nonangiographic marker of reperfusion. Ventricular fibrillation has also been reported. The most common complication of thrombolytic therapy is hemorrhage, and the most devastating complication is intracerebral bleedings, which occurs more often in the elderly. Intracerebral hemorrhage is less frequent with streptokinase than alteplase. Streptokinase is the most cost effective thrombolytic, especially in the elderly.

MODE OF ACTION

Fibrin and fibrinogen are degraded by the enzyme plasmin that is converted from its inactive proenzyme plasminogen (Fig. 6.6). Fibrinolytic therapy aims at increasing plasmin formation by means of additional plasminogen activation. The PT may be prolonged up to 24 h after discontinuing therapy, a result of relative depletion of fibrinogen or other clotting factors.

TABLE 6.7 MAJOR CLINICAL TRIALS OF INTRAVENOUS THROMBOLYTIC THERAPY IN ACUTE MYOCARDIAL INFARCTION

STUDY	Patients receiving active treatment, n	Dose	Intracranial bleeding, %	Mortality
Streptokinase (SK)				
GISSI-1	5860	1.5 MU over 1 h	0.2	21 d mortality, 10.7% vs control, 13% ($P = 0.0002$)
ISIS-2	8592	1.5 MU over 24 h	Not available	5 wk mortality, 9.2% vs control, 12.0% ($P = 0.000005$)
Alteplase (tPA)				
ASSET	2516	100 mg over 3 h	1.4	1 mo mortality, 7.2% anistreplase vs 9.8% control ($P = 0.0011$)
Anistreplase (APSAC)				
AIMS	624	30 units bolus injection	Not available	30 d mortality, 6% vs control, 12% ($P = 0.0006$)
Comparative				
GISSI-2	20,749	SK 1.5-MU/1 h	0.29	8.5%
		tPA 100 mg/3 h	0.42	8.9%
ISIS-3	46,000	SK 1.5 MU/1 h	0.30	10.5%
		AAPSAC 30 units/3–5 min	0.58	10.6%
		tPA 0.6 mg/kg/4 h	0.73	10.3%
GUSTO	41,021	SK 1.5 mL units/1 h	0.50	7.3%
		tPA 15 mg and 1.25 mg/kg/90 min (not to exceed 100 mg)	0.72	6.3%

AIMS—APSAC Intervention Mortality Study; APSAC—Anisoylated Plasminogen Streptokinase Activator Complex; GISSI—Gruppo Italiano per lo Studio della Sopravivenza nell'Infarcto Miocardio 1,2; ISIS—International Study of Infarct Survival 2,3; GUSTO—Global Utilization of Streptokinase and tPA for Occluded Coronary Arteries; SK—Streptokinase; tPA—tissue-type plasminogen activator.

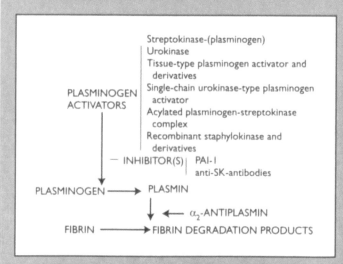

FIGURE 6.6 Schematic representation of the fibrinolytic system. Plasminogen is a proenzyme and is activated by plasminogen activators into the active enzyme plasmin. Plasmin degrades fibrin into degradation products. Fibrinolysis may be inhibited at the level of plasminogen activators by PAI-1 (plasminogen activator inhibitor) and anti-SK (streptokinase) antibodies or the level of plasmin by α_2-antiplasmin. (*From Forman R, Frishman WH: Thrombolytic agents. In Cardiovascular Pharmacotherapeutics. Edited by Frishman WH, Sonnenblick EH. New York: McGraw Hill; 1997:382; with permission.*)

The information here is provided as guidance only. Prescribers should always consult the manufacturer's current prescribing information.

109

ALTEPLASE, RECOMBINANT

(Activase®)

Alteplase is a recombinant tissue plasminogen activator (t-PA) derived from genetically engineered Chinese Hamster ovary cells. At therapeutic concentration, fibrinolysis is initiated by binding of t-PA to fibrin in the thrombus and converting the entrapped plasminogen to plasmin. This localized thrombolytic activity theoretically may reduce the systemic proteolysis and the risk of bleeding. The experience from GISSI-2, ISIS-3, and GUSTO-1 trials has shown an increased risk of stroke and cerebral hemorrhage in the t-PA groups.

When alteplase therapy was initiated promptly in patients with acute MI, infarct artery patency was documented in 71% of patients by coronary angiogram at 90 min. Alteplase, administered either as an accelerated or 3-h infusion, has been compared to streptokinase in patients with acute MI. Although patients treated with alteplase had similar or slightly better mortality, an increase in stroke and intracerebral hemorrhage was observed.

In patients with acute ischemic stroke, early thrombolysis with alteplase has been shown to improve neurological recovery and reduce the incidence of disability. These benefits were observed when the treatment was initiated within 3 h of symptom onset. The potential benefits of administering alteplase to stroke patients should always be assessed against the risk of intracranial hemorrhage. The risk is increased especially in patients presenting with severe neurological deficit or of advanced age.

In patients with pulmonary embolism who are hemodynamically unstable, thrombolytic therapy may be beneficial. Improvement in pulmonary perfusion scan and embolism-induced pulmonary hypertension has been observed with alteplase therapy when used appropriately.

SPECIAL GROUPS

Race: no differences in response
Children: safety and effectiveness have not been established
Elderly: adjust the dose based on weight
Renal impairment: no data; use with caution
Hepatic impairment: no data; use with caution
Pregnancy: category C; should only be used if clearly indicated
Breast-feeding: not clear if the drug is excreted in human milk; use with caution

IN BRIEF

INDICATIONS
Acute MI
Acute ischemic stroke
PE

CONTRAINDICATIONS
Active internal bleeding
Known bleeding diathesis
History of cerebrovascular accident
Recent intracranial or intraspinal surgery or trauma
Intracranial neoplasm, arteriovenous malformation or aneurysm
Severe uncontrolled hypertension
Evidence of intracranial or subarachnoid hemorrhage
History of recent stroke or intracranial hemorrhage

DRUG INTERACTIONS
Anticoagulants
Thrombolytics
Antiplatelets
NSAIDs

ADVERSE EFFECTS
Bleeding: intracranial, retroperitoneal, gastrointestinal, genitourinary or respiratory, venous/arterial catheter sites, ecchymosis
CV: cholesterol embolization, cardiogenic shock, arrhythmias, hypotension
GI: nausea, vomiting
Rare: allergic or anaphylactoid reaction, laryngeal edema, rash, and urticaria

PHARMACOKINETICS AND PHARMACODYNAMICS
Duration of action: no data
Onset of action: rapid
Peak effect: thrombolysis occurs within 40–50 min
Bioavailability: 100%
Clearance: mainly metabolized by liver and excreted in urine
Plasma half-life: < 5 min
Protein binding: no data

DOSAGE

Acute MI: The following two regimens should be used with concurrent administration of heparin and aspirin. Treatment should be initiated as soon as possible, preferably within 12 h after the onset of chest pain:

1. Accelerated Infusion—15 mg intravenous bolus, followed by 0.75 mg/kg (up to 50 mg) infused over 30 min, and then 0.5 mg/kg (up to 35 mg) infused over 60 min. A maximum total dose is 100 mg for patients weighing more than 67 kg.

2. Three-hour Infusion—60 mg infused over 60 min (with 6–10 mg administered as a bolus first), followed by 20 mg/h infusion for 2 h to deliver a total dose of 100 mg. For patients weighing less than 65 kg, a total dose of 1.25 mg/kg is recommended.

Acute ischemic stroke: 0.9 mg/kg (up to 90 mg) administered intravenously over 60 min with 10% of the total dose administered as a bolus over the first minute. Treatment should be initiated within 3 h after the onset of stroke symptoms. Avoid aspirin and heparin use during the first 24 h.

PE: 100 mg intravenously over 2 h. Heparin therapy should be initiated near the end or following the alteplase infusion when partial thromboplastin time or thrombin time returns to twice of normal or less.

MONITORING
Lab: CBC, PT, aPTT, fibrinolytic activity. Clinical evidence of active or occult bleeding.

OVERDOSE
Supportive—no data.

PATIENT INFORMATION
Alteplase can cause excessive bleeding.

AVAILABILITY
Vials—50 mg and 100 mg (potency: 580,000 IU/mg)

ANISTREPLASE (Eminase®)

Anistreplase (anisoylated plasminogen streptokinase activator complex [APSAC]) is a complex of streptokinase with human plasminogen. In vitro studies show APSAC to have thrombolytic potency 10 times that of streptokinase. This indicates that its thrombolytic action is dependent on fibrin binding. The streptokinase-plasminogen complex of anistreplase dissociates at a slower rate than does the deacylation rate, ensuring that the fibrinolytic activity of the drug is controlled by the latter. The deacylation half-life is about 105 minutes in human plasma or whole blood in vitro, and the plasma clearance half-life of fibrinolytic activity has been reported to be 90–112 min in patients with acute MI. These pharmacologic differences, however, may be irrelevant in clinical practice.

Data suggest that the patency rate (70%–80%) achieved with AP-SAC may be less than that with tPA, but the reocclusion rate may be smaller. However, the ISIS-3 study showed that mortality reduction was similar with streptokinase, tPA, and APSAC. Streptokinase was associated with less life-threatening bleeding (Table 6.7). Of particular merit is the single bolus dose of anistreplase, which may make it particularly useful for out-of-hospital use.

SPECIAL GROUPS

Race: no differences in response
Children: safety and effectiveness have not been established
Elderly: no dosage adjustment is required
Renal impairment: no dosage adjustment is required; use with caution
Hepatic impairment: use with caution; dosage reduction may be required
Pregnancy: category C; should only be used if clearly indicated
Breast-feeding: not recommended; not known if the drug is excreted in human milk

DOSAGE

Acute MI: Thrombolytic therapy should be initiated as soon as possible after the onset of symptoms. The dose of anistreplase is 30 units administered intravenously over 2–5 min.

IN BRIEF

INDICATIONS
Acute MI

CONTRAINDICATIONS
Active internal bleeding
Known bleeding diathesis
Known hypersensitivity reaction to anistreplase or streptokinase
History of cerebrovascular accident
Recent (< 2 mo) intracranial or intraspinal surgery or trauma
Intracranial neoplasm, arteriovenous malformation or aneurysm
Severe uncontrolled hypertension
Recent trauma, including cardiopulmonary resuscitation

DRUG INTERACTIONS
Anticoagulants
Thrombolytics
Antiplatelets
NSAIDs

ADVERSE EFFECTS
Bleeding: intracranial, retroperitoneal, gastrointestinal, genitourinary or respiratory, venous/arterial catheter sites, ecchymosis
CV: arrhythmias, hypotension
GI: nausea, vomiting
Other: fever, chills, urticaria, pruritus, anaphylactic or anaphylactoid reactions, angioedema, bronchospasm, Guillain-Barre syndrome, vasculitis, eosinophilia, arthralgia

PHARMACOKINETICS AND PHARMACODYNAMICS
(based on thrombolytic activity measured)
Duration of action: 4–6 h
Onset of action: immediate
Peak effect: no data, but reperfusion occurs in 45 min
Bioavailability: 100%
Clearance: unclear; activated by deacylation in vivo
Plasma half-life: 70–120 min
Protein binding: no data

MONITORING
Lab: CBC, PT, TT, aPTT, fibrinolytic activity. Clinical evidence of active or occult bleeding.

OVERDOSE
Supportive—no data.

PATIENT INFORMATION
Anistreplase can cause excessive bleeding.

AVAILABILITY
Vials—30 units

RETEPLASE, RECOMBINANT

(Retavase®)

Reteplase is a recombinant plasminogen activator derived from *Escherichia coli*. It catalyzes the cleavage of endogenous plasminogen to generate plasmin, which in turn degrades the fibrin matrix of the thrombus producing thrombolysis.

Three clinical studies, INJECT, RAPID 1, and RAPID 2 have supported the efficacy of reteplase in restoring coronary artery flow when administered within 6 or 12 h after the onset of acute MI. With few exceptions, patients were also treated with aspirin and heparin. In the INJECT study, the double-bolus reteplase (10 U and 10 U) was compared to streptokinase therapy (1.5 MU over 60 min). Although reteplase was associated with better early coronary patency, both treatments showed similar 35 d and 6 mo mortality rates. While fewer patients developed CHF and cardiogenic shock, more patients had hemorrhagic strokes in the reteplase group. In RAPID 1 and RAPID 2, reteplase was compared to two different alteplase regimens in patients after acute MI. More patients achieved complete restoration of coronary blood flow with reteplase at 60 and 90 min after the initiation of therapy. The reocclusion rates and the incidence of bleeding complications were similar for reteplase and alteplase therapy.

With its efficacy in restoring coronary artery blood flow, convenient dosing, and administration, reteplase may be useful in treating patients with acute MI before they reach the hospital. This implies earlier thrombolysis, which may further improve the outcome of these patients.

SPECIAL GROUPS

Race: no data

Children: safety and effectiveness have not been established

Elderly: no dosage adjustment is recommended

Renal impairment: no data; use with caution

Hepatic impairment: no data; use with caution

Pregnancy: category C; should only be used if clearly indicated

Breast-feeding: not clear if the drug is excreted in human milk; use with caution

DOSAGE

Two 10 U bolus injections; each bolus is given intravenously over 2 min with the second bolus given 30 min after initiation of the first bolus. Treatment should be initiated as soon as possible, preferably within 12 h after the onset of chest pain. Patients should also receive adjunctive therapy with heparin and aspirin.

IN BRIEF

INDICATIONS
Thrombolysis in patients with acute MI to improve ventricular function.

CONTRAINDICATIONS
Active internal bleeding
History of cerebrovascular accident
Recent intracranial or intraspinal surgery or trauma
Intracranial neoplasm, arteriovenous malformation or aneurysm
Known bleeding diathesis
Severe uncontrolled hypertension
Known hypersensitivity

DRUG INTERACTIONS
Anticoagulants
Thrombolytics
Antiplatelets
NSAIDs

ADVERSE EFFECTS
Bleeding: intracranial, retroperitoneal, gastrointestinal, genitourinary or respiratory, venous/arterial catheter sites
CV: cholesterol embolization, arrhythmias, hypotension
GI: nausea, vomiting
Rare: allergic or anaphylactoid reaction

PHARMACOKINETICS AND PHARMACODYNAMICS
(based on thrombolytic activity measured)
Duration of action: up to 48 h
Onset of action: rapid
Peak effect: lysis occurs within 60–90 min
Clearance: mainly metabolized by liver and excreted in urine
Plasma half-life: 13–16 min
Protein binding: no data

MONITORING
Lab: CBC, PT, aPTT, fibrinolytic activity. Clinical evidence of active or occult bleeding.

OVERDOSE
Supportive—no data.

PATIENT INFORMATION
Reteplase can cause excessive bleeding.

AVAILABILITY
Kit—reteplase 18.8 mg (10.8 U)/vial, 2 vials; 10 mL sterile water/vial; 2 vials syringes, dispensing pins, needles, alcohol swabs (two of each)

STREPTOKINASE (Kabikinase®, Streptase®)

Streptokinase, obtained from beta-hemolytic streptococci, activates plasminogen indirectly after forming a complex with it. The formed plasmin formed acts on fibrinogen and fibrin to yield degradation products. The resistance attributable to antibodies varies, but systemic doses of 250,000 units induce a systemic fibrinolytic state in more than 90% of patients. Generally, doses of 750,000 to 1.5×10^6 units are used for patients with evolving MI. Major trials have demonstrated its efficacy and the value of early thrombolysis (Fig. 6.4). Reductions in mortality and the reinfarction rate have been demonstrated for the combination of streptokinase with heparin or aspirin and atenolol (Fig. 6.4 and Table 6.7). Rapid infusion of large doses (> 500 units/min) can induce hypotension, but the relative reduction in BP can reduce myocardial work and have an oxygen-sparing effect. The production of systemic fibrinolysis also can result in decreased blood viscosity. Both effects may be beneficial.

SPECIAL GROUPS

Race: no differences in response
Children: safety and effectiveness have not been established
Elderly: no dosage adjustment is required
Renal impairment: no dosage adjustment is required; use with caution
Hepatic impairment: use with caution; dosage adjustment may be required
Pregnancy: category C; avoid use during first 18 wks of pregnancy; otherwise, use with caution
Breast-feeding: not recommended; not known if the drug is excreted in human milk

DOSAGE

Acute MI: Although therapeutic benefits have been reported in patients up to 24 h after the onset of symptoms, treatment should be initiated as soon as possible for maximum benefit.
Intravenous—1.5×10^6 IU infused over 60 min
Intracoronary—20,000 IU bolus, followed by 2,000 IU/min infusion for 60 min (a total of 140,000 IU).
Pulmonary embolism, deep vein thrombosis, arterial thrombosis, or embolism: 250,000 IU bolus infused over 30 min, followed by 100,000 IU/hr continuous infusion for up to 24 h for pulmonary embolism, 72 h for deep vein thrombosis, and 24–72 h for arterial thromboembolism. Treatment should be initiated as soon as possible, preferably within 7 d after onset of the symptoms.
Arteriovenous cannulae occlusion: Instill 250,000 IU streptokinase in 2 mL solution into occluded cannula, clamped the cannula for 2 h, then aspirate the contents and flush with saline.

IN BRIEF

INDICATIONS
Acute MI
PE
DVT
Arterial thrombosis or embolism
Occlusion of arteriovenous cannulae

CONTRAINDICATIONS
Active internal bleeding
Known bleeding diathesis
Known hypersensitivity reaction to streptokinase
Recent cerebrovascular accident (< 2 mo)
Recent intracranial or intraspinal surgery (< 2 mo)
Intracranial neoplasm, arteriovenous malformation or aneurysm
Severe uncontrolled hypertension
Recent trauma, including cardiopulmonary resuscitation

DRUG INTERACTIONS
Anticoagulants
Thrombolytics
Antiplatelets
NSAIDs

ADVERSE EEFFECTS
Bleeding: intracranial, retroperitoneal, gastrointestinal, genitourinary or respiratory, venous/arterial catheter sites, ecchymosis
CV: arrhythmias, hypotension, cholesterol embolization, cardiogenic shock
GI: nausea, vomiting
Other: fever, chills, urticaria, pruritus, anaphylactic or anaphylactoid reactions, angioedema, polyneuropathy, noncardiogenic pulmonary edema

PHARMACOKINETICS AND PHARMACODYNAMICS
Duration of action: 12–24 h; fibrinolytic activity only lasts for a few hours
Onset of action: rapid
Peak effect: rapid
Bioavailability: 100%
Clearance: cleared by circulating antibodies and the reticuloendothelial system
Plasma half-life: 18–83 min
Protein binding: no data

MONITORING
Lab: CBC, PT, TT, aPTT, fibrinolytic activity. Clinical evidence of active or occult bleeding.

OVERDOSE
Supportive—no data.

PATIENT INFORMATION
Streptokinase can cause excessive bleeding.

AVAILABILITY
Vials—250,000, 750,000, 1.5 million IU

UROKINASE (Abbokinase®)

Urokinase (UK), an enzyme produced by the kidney and found in the urine, is a direct plasminogen activator. There are two forms of UK with different molecular weights but similar activity. Abbokinase, the commercially available product of UK, contains primarily the low molecular weight form. UK is structurally different from t-PA with low antigenicity and low binding affinity for fibrin.

Intracoronary UK administration at a rate of 6000 IU/min up to a maximum dose of 750,000 IU resulted in recanalization in more than 60% of patients suffering from MI. In the TIMI-5 study, intravenous (IV) administration of UK, t-PA, or a combination of both, achieved 62%, 71%, and 76% coronary patency rate, respectively. The difference was not statistically significant.

In the NIH-sponsored Urokinase Streptokinase Pulmonary Embolism Trial, patients with massive PE receiving UK (4400 IU/kg/h IV for 24 h) had significantly greater pulmonary reperfusion on lung scanning and greater reduction of pulmonary hypertension than those receiving streptokinase therapy (100,000 IU/h IV for 24 h). In another study, IV UK (3 million IU over 2 h) was compared to t-PA (100 mg over 2 h) in patients with PE. Although earlier resolution of emboli was observed in the t-PA group, no significant difference was observed at 24 h when assessed by lung scanning.

In patients who have received streptokinase within the prior 12 months and have high antibody titers to streptokinase, UK can be used safely and effectively.

SPECIAL GROUPS

Race: no differences in response
Children: safety and effectiveness have not been established
Elderly: no dosage adjustment is required
Renal impairment: no dosage adjustment is required; use with caution
Hepatic impairment: use with caution; dosage adjustment is probably required
Pregnancy: category B; should only be used if clearly indicated
Breast-feeding: not known if the drug is excreted in human milk; use with caution

IN BRIEF

INDICATIONS
PE
Coronary artery thrombosis
Intravenous catheter clearance

CONTRAINDICATIONS
Active internal bleeding
Known bleeding diathesis
History of cerebrovascular accident
Recent intracranial or intraspinal surgery (< 2 mo)
Intracranial neoplasm, arteriovenous malformation, or aneurysm
Severe uncontrolled hypertension
Recent trauma, including cardiopulmonary resuscitation

DRUG INTERACTIONS
Anticoagulants
Thrombolytics
Antiplatelets
NSAIDs

ADVERSE EFFECTS
Bleeding: intracranial, retroperitoneal, gastrointestinal, genitourinary or respiratory, venous/arterial catheter sites, ecchymosis
CV: hypotension, hypertension, tachycardia
GI: nausea, vomiting
Rare: allergic reaction, bronchospasm, skin rash, fever, chills, rigors

PHARMACOKINETICS AND PHARMACODYNAMICS
Duration of action: 12–24 h; fibrinolytic activity only lasts for a few hours
Onset of action: immediate
Peak effect: rapid
Bioavailability: 100%
Clearance/Excretion: metabolized by liver; only small amounts are eliminated in urine and bile
Plasma half-life: < 20 min
Protein binding: no data

DOSAGE

PE: Urokinase 4400 IU/kg administered intravenously over 10 min, followed by continuous infusion of 4400 IU/kg/hr for 12 h; thrombin time (TT) should be determined 3–4 h after initiation of therapy and maintained greater than twice the normal control. Appropriate anticoagulant therapy should be initiated after urokinase therapy.

Coronary artery thrombosis (within 6 h of the onset of the symptoms): A bolus dose of heparin 2000–10,000 U should be administered by rapid intravenous injection, followed by intracoronary administration of urokinase at a rate of 6000 IU/min (1500 IU/mL) for up to 2 h. The duration of treatment is guided by angiography performed every 15 min. The average urokinase dose used was 500,000 IU with a 60% response rate. Heparin should be continued after clot lysis.

Occluded catheter: Urokinase 5000 IU/mL is used and only the amount that equals to the internal volume of the catheter should be injected slowly into the catheter. Specific instructions provided by the manufacturer should be followed to ensure aseptic application and proper urokinase indwelling time before each aspiration attempt, and to avoid the risk for air emboli.

MONITORING

Lab: CBC, TT, PT, aPTT, fibrinolytic activity. Clinical evidence of active or occult bleeding.

OVERDOSE

Supportive—no data.

PATIENT INFORMATION

Urokinase can cause excessive bleeding.

AVAILABILITY

Vials—5,000 IU, 9,000 IU, 250,000 IU

SELECTED BIBLIOGRAPHY

ACC-AHA Guidelines for the Management of Patients with Acute Myocardial Infarction: A report from the American College of Cardiology/American Heart Association: Task Force on Practice Guidelines (Committee on Management of Acute Myocardial Infarction). *J Am Coll Cardiol* 1996, 28:1328–1428.

AIMS Trial Study Group: Long-term effects of intravenous anistreplase in acute myocardial infarction: final report of the AIMS study. *Lancet* 1990, 335:427–431.

Albers GW, Sherman DG, Gress DR, *et al.*: Stroke prevention in nonvalvular atrial fibrillation: a review of prospective randomized trials. *Ann Neurol* 1991, 30:511–518.

Amiral J, Bridey F, Wolf M, *et al.*: Antibodies to marcomolecular platelet factor 4-heparin complexes in heparin-induced thrombocytopenia: a study of 44 cases. *Thromb Haemost* 1995, 73:21–28.

Anderson JL: Development and evaluation of anisoylated plasminogen streptokinase activator complex (APSAC) as a second generation thrombolytic agent. *J Am Coll Cardiol* 1987, 10:22B–27B.

Antiplatelet Trialists Collaboration: Collaborative overview of randomized trials of antiplatelet therapy. I: prevention of death, myocardial infarction, and stroke by prolonged antiplatelet therapy in various categories of patients. *Br J Med* 1994, 308:81–106.

Antman EM, Guigliano RP, Gibson CM, *et al.* for the TIMI 14 Investigators: Abciximab facilitates the rate and extent of thrombolysis: results from the Thrombolysis in Myocardial Infarction (TIMI) 14 Trial. *Circulation* 1999, 99:2720–2732.

Armstrong PW: Heparin in acute coronary disease: requiem for a heavyweight [editorial]. *N Engl J Med* 1997, 337:492.

Bode C, Smalling R, Gunther B, *et al.*: Randomized comparison of coronary thrombolysis achieved with double bolus reteplase (recombinant plasminogen activator) and front-loaded, accelerated alteplase (recombinant tissue plasminogen activator) in patients with acute myocardial infarction. *Circulation* 1996, 94:891–898.

Cannon CP: Aggrastat in the treatment of unstable angina. *Curr Pract Med* 1998, 1:55–58.

CAPRIE Steering Committee: A randomised, blinded trial of clopidogrel versus aspirin in patients at risk of ischaemic events (CAPRIE). *Lancet* 1996, 348:1329–1339.

CAPTURE Investigators: Randomised, placebo-controlled trial of abciximab before, during and after coronary intervention in refractory unstable angina: the CAPTURE study. *Lancet* 1997, 349:1429–1435.

Challapalli R, Lefkovits J, Topol EJ: Clinical trials of recombinant hirudin in acute coronary syndromes. *Coronary Artery Disease* 1996, 7:429–437.

Cohen M, Demers C, Gurfinkel E, *et al.* for the Efficacy and Safety of Subcutaneous Enoxaparin vs Non–Q-Wave Coronary Events Study Group: A comparison of low molecular weight heparin with unfractionated heparin for unstable coronary artery disease. *N Engl J Med* 1997, 337:447–452.

Collen D: Fibrin-selective thrombolytic therapy for acute myocardial infarction. *Circulation* 1996, 93:857–865.

Danhof M, de Boer A, Magnani HN, *et al.*: Pharmacokinetic considerations of orgaran (org 10172) therapy. *Haemostasis* 1992, 22:73–84.

EPIC Investigators: Use of a monoclonal antibody directed against the platelet glycoprotein IIb/IIIa receptorin high-risk coronary angioplasty. *N Engl J Med* 1994, 330:956–961.

EPILOG Investigators: Platelet glycoprotein IIb/IIIa receptor blockade and low dose heparin during percutaneous coronary revascularization. *N Engl J Med* 1997, 336:1689–1696.

EPISTENT Investigators: Randomised, placebo-controlled and balloon-angioplasty-controlled trial to assess safety of coronary stenting with use of platelet glycoprotein IIb/IIIa blockade. *Lancet* 1998, 352:87–92.

ESSENCE trial results: Breaking new ground: efficacy and safety of subcutaneous enoxaparin in non–Q-wave coronary events. *Can J Cardiol* 1998, 14(suppl E):15E–19E.

Fifth ACCP Consensus Conference on Antithrombotic Therapy. *Chest* 1998, 114(suppl):439S–769S.

Forman R, Frishman WH: Thrombolytic agents. In *Cardiovascular Pharmacotherapeutics*. Edited by Frishman WH, Sonnenblick EH. New York: McGraw Hill;1997:381–398.

Foster RH, Wiseman LR: Abciximab: an updated review of its use in ischaemic heart disease. *Drugs* 1998, 56:629–665.

Frishman WH, Klein MD, Blaufarb I, *et al.*: Antiplatelet and other antithrombotic drugs. In *Cardiovascular Pharmacotherapeutics*. Edited by Frishman WH, Sonnenblick EH. New York: McGraw Hill; 1997:323–379.

Gent M, Easton JD, Hachinski VC, *et al.*: The Canadian American Ticlopidine Study (CATS) in thromboembolic stroke. *Lancet* 1989, 1:1215–1220.

GISSI (Gruppo Italiano per lo Studio della Streptochinasi nell'Infarcto Miocardico): Effectiveness of intravenous thrombolytic treatment in acute myocardial infarction. *Lancet* 1986, 1:397–401.

GISSI Group, GISSI 2: A factorial randomised trial of alteplase versus streptokinase and heparin versus no heparin among 12,490 patient with acute myocardial infarction. *Lancet* 1990, 336:65–71.

Glycoprotein (GP) IIb/IIIa Inhibitors in Acute Coronary Syndromes: Applying Evidence from Clinical Trials to Medical Practice. Data presented concurrently with the 48th Annual Scientific Session of the American College of Cardiology, March 6, 1999: New Orleans, Louisiana. Presentations in Focus™, supported by an education grant from COR Therapeutics Inc. and Key Pharmaceuticals Inc., 1999.

Granger CB, Califf RM, Topol EJ: Thrombolytic therapy for acute myocardial infarction. *Drugs* 1992, 44:293–325.

Greinacher A, Alban S: Heparinoids as alternative for parenteral anticoagulation therapy in patients with heparin-induced thrombocytopenia. *Hamostaseologie* 1996, 16:41–49.

Greinacher A, Amiral J, Dummel V, *et al.*: Laboratory diagnosis of heparin-associated thrombo-cytopenia and comparison of platelet aggregation test, heparin-induced platelet activation test, and platelet factor 4-heparin enzyme linked immunosorbent assay. *Transfusion* 1994, 34:381–385.

Greinacher A, Volpel H, Janssens U, *et al.*: Recombinent hirudin provides safe and effective anti-coagulation in patients with heparin-induced thrombocytopenia: a prospective study. *Circulation* 1999, 99:73–80.

Grotta JC, Norris JW, Kamm B: Prevention of stroke with ticlopidine: who benefits the most? TASS baseline and angiographic subgroup. *Neurology* 1992, 42:111–115.

GUSTO Investigators: An international randomized trial comparing four thrombolytic strategies for acute myocardial infarction. *N Engl J Med* 1993, 329:673–682.

Hass WK, Easton JD, Adams HP, *et al.*: A randomized trial comparing ticlopidine hydrochloride with aspirin for the prevention of stroke in high risk patients. *N Engl J Med* 1989, 321:501.

Hennekens CH, O'Donnell CJ, Ridker PM, *et al.*: Current issues concerning thrombolytic therapy for acute myocardial infarction. *J Am Coll Cardiol* 1995, 25(suppl):18s–22s.

Hirsh J, Fuster V: Guide to anticoagulant therapy. Part 1: heparin. *Circulation* 1994, 89:1449–1468.

Hirsh J, Fuster V: Guide to anticoagulant therapy. Part 2: Oral anticoagulants. *Circulation* 1994, 89:1469–1493.

Hirsh J, Raschke R, Warkentin TE, *et al.*: Heparin: mechanism of action, pharmacokinetics dosing considerations, monitoring, efficacy and safety. *Chest* 1995, 108:258S–275S.

Hirsh J, Warkentin TE, Raschke R, *et al.*: Heparin and low-molecular-weight heparin: mechanisms of actions, pharmacokinetics, dosing consideration, monitoring, efficacy and safety. *Chest* 1998, 114(suppl):489s–510s.

Hirsh J: Low-molecular-weight heparin: a review of the results of recent studies of the treatment of venous thromboembolism and unstable angina. *Circulation* 1998, 98:1575–1582.

IMPACT II Investigators: Randomised placebo-controlled trial of effect of eptifibatide on complications of percutaneous coronary intervention: IMPACT-II. *Lancet* 1997, 349:1422–1428.

INJECT Study Group: Randomised, double-blind comparison of reteplase double-bolus administration with streptokinase in acute myocardial infarction (INJECT): trial to investigate equivalence. *Lancet* 1995, 346:329–336.

ISIS 2 Collaborative Group: Randomised trial of intravenous streptokinase, oral aspirin, both or neither among 17,187 cases of suspected acute myocardial infarction. *Lancet* 1988, 2:349–360.

ISIS-3: A randomized comparison of streptokinase vs tissue plasminogen activator vs anistreplase and of aspirin plus heparin vs aspirin alone among 41,299 cases of suspected acute myocardial infarction. *Lancet* 1992, 339:753–770.

Jang I-K, Brown DFM, Giugliano RP, *et al* and the MINT Investigators: A multicenter, randomized study of argatroban versus heparin as adjunct to tissue plasminogen activator (TPA) in acute myocardial infarction: Myocardial Infarction with Novastatin and TPA (MINT) Study. *J Am Coll Cardiol* 1999, 33:1879–1885.

Krumholz HM, Pasternak RC, Weinstein MC, *et al.*: Cost effectiveness of thrombolytic therapy with streptokinase in elderly patients with suspected acute myocardial infarction. *N Engl J Med* 1992, 327:7–13.

Levine M, Gent M, Hirsh J, *et al.*: A comparison of low-molecular-weight heparin administered primarily at home with unfractionated heparin administered in the hospital for proximal deep vein thrombosis. *N Engl J Med* 1996, 334:677–681.

McEwen J, Strauch G, Perles P, *et al.*: Clopidogrel bioavailability is unaffected by food or antacids. *J Clin Pharmacol* 1996, 36:856.

Monealescot G, Phillippe F, Ankri A, *et al.*: Early increase in von Willebrand factor predicts adverse outcome in unstable coronary artery disease: beneficial effects of enoxaparin. *Circulation* 1998, 98:294–299.

Monreal M, Costa J, Salva P: Pharmacological properties of hirudin and its derivatives: potential clinical advantages over heparin. *Drugs Aging* 1996, 8:171–182.

Noble S, Spencer CM: Enoxaparin: a review of its clinical potential in the management of coronary artery disease. *Drugs* 1998, 56:259–272.

Organisation to Assess Strategies for Ischemic Syndromes (OASIS-2) Investigators: Effects of recombinant hirudin (lepirudin) compared with heparin on death, myocardial infarction, refractory angina, and revascularisation procedures in patients with acute myocardial ischaemia without ST elevation: a randomised trial. *Lancet* 1999, 353:429–438.

Patrono C: Aspirin as an antiplatelet agent. *N Engl J Med* 1994, 329:1287–1294.

Phillips DR, Scarborough RM: Clinical pharmacology of eptifibatide. *Am J Cardiol* 1997, 80:11B–20B.

Pineo GF, Hull RD: Unfractionated and low-molecular-weight heparin: comparison and current recommendations. *Med Clin North Am* 1998, 82:587–599.

PRISM Study Investigators: A comparison of aspirin plus tirofiban with aspirin plus heparin for unstable angina. *N Engl J Med* 1998, 338:1498–1505.

PRISM-PLUS Study Investigators: Inhibition of platelet glycoprotein IIb/IIIa receptor with tirofiban in unstable angina and non–Q-wave myocardial infarction. *N Engl J Med* 1998, 338:1488–1497.

PURSUIT Trial Investigators: Inhibition of platelet glycoprotein IIb/IIIa with eptifibatide in patients with acute coronary syndromes. *N Engl J Med* 1998, 339:436–443.

RESTORE Investigators: Effects of platelet glycoprotein IIb/IIIa blockade with tirofiban on adverse cardiac events in patients with unstable angina or acute myocardial infarction undergoing coronary angioplasty. *Circulation* 1997, 96:1445–1453.

Saltiel E, Ward A: Ticlopidine: a review of its pharmacodynamic and pharmacokinetic properties, and therapeutic efficacy in platelet-dependent disease states. *Drugs* 1987, 34:222–262.

SCATI (Studio sulla Calciparina nell' Angina e nella Trombosi Ventricolare nell 'Infarcto) Group: Randomized controlled trial of subcutaneous calcium-heparin in acute myocardial infarction. *Lancet* 1989, 2:182–186.

Sharis PJ, Cannon CP, Loscalzo J: The antiplatelet effects of ticlopidine and clopidogrel. *Ann Intern Med* 1998, 129:394–405.

Smalling R, Bode C, Kalbfleisch J, *et al.*: More rapid, complete, and stable coronary thrombolysis with bolus administration of reteplase compared with alteplase infusion in acute myocardial infarction. *Circulation* 1995, 91:2725–2732.

Smith P, Amesen H, Holme I: The effect of warfarin on mortality and reinfarction after myocardial infarction. *N Engl J Med* 1990, 323:147–152.

Stein B, Fuster V, Israel DH, *et al.*: Platelet inhibitor agents in cardiovascular disease: an update. *J Am Coll Cardiol* 1989, 14:813–836.

The Dutch TIA Trial Study Group: A comparison of two doses of aspirin (30 mg vs 283 mg a day) in patients after a transient ischemic attack or minor ischemic stroke. *N Engl J Med* 1991, 325:1261–1266.

The ECASS Study Group: Intravenous thrombolysis with recombinant tissue plasminogen activator for acute hemispheric stroke: The European Cooperative Acute Stroke Study (ECASS). *JAMA* 1995, 274:1017–1025.

The European Myocardial Infarction Project Group: Prehospital thrombolytic therapy in patients with suspected acute myocardial infarction. *N Engl J Med* 1993, 329:383–389.

The Global Use of Strategies to Open Occluded Coronary Arteries (GUSTO III) Investigators: A comparison of reteplase with alteplase for acute myocardial infarction. *N Engl J Med* 1997, 337:1118–1123.

The National Institute of Neurological Disorders and Stroke t-PA Stroke Study Group: Tissue plasminogen activator for acute ischemic stroke. *N Engl J Med* 1995, 333:1581–1587.

The Steering Committee of the Physicians' Health Study Research Group: final report on the aspirin component of the ongoing Physicians' Health Study. *N Engl J Med* 1989, 321:129–135.

Theroux P, Ouimet H, McCars J, *et al.*: Aspirin, heparin or both to treat acute unstable angina. *N Engl J Med* 1988, 319:1105–1111.

TIMI Study Group: Comparison of invasive and conservative strategies after treatment with intravenous tissue plasminogen activator in acute myocardial infarction: result of the thrombolysis in myocardial infarction (TIMI) phase II trial. *N Engl J Med* 1989, 320:618–627.

Verstraete M, Fuster V: Thrombogenesis and antithrombotic therapy. In *Hurst's The Heart*, edn 9. Edited by Alexander RW, Schlant RC, Fuster V. New York: McGraw Hill; 1998:1501–1551.

Warkentin TE, Chong BH, Greinacher A: Heparin-induced thrombocytopenia: towards consensus. *Thromb Haemostas* 1998, 79:1–7.

Warkentin TE, Elavathil LJ, Hayward CPM, *et al.*: The pathogenesis of venous limb gangrene associated with heparin-induced thrombocytopenia. *Ann Intern Med* 1997, 127:804–812.

Wilcox RG, Von der Lippe G, Olsson CG, *et al.*: Trial of tissue plasminogen activator for mortality reduction in acute myocardial infarction (ASSET). *Lancet* 1988, ii: 525–530.

Wilde MI, Markham A: Danaparoid: a review of its pharmacology and clinical use in the management of heparin-induced thrombocytopenia. *Drugs* 1997, 54:903–924.

7

BETA-ADRENERGIC BLOCKERS

Beta-adrenergic blocking agents exert their major effects through the beta adrenoceptors in the heart and peripheral vasculature. Both heart rate and myocardial contractility are reduced with beta blockade. Beta receptors are also found in a wide range of other tissues. These agents are generally well tolerated, and are widely used for various cardiovascular and other clinical conditions.

The two main types of beta receptors, $beta_1$ and $beta_2$, frequently coexist in the same tissue. Evidence now also indicates a $beta_3$ receptor in brown fat, which is associated with thermogenesis. Table 7.1 shows the distribution of beta receptors in the body.

During the 1950s, J.W. Black conceived the idea that patients with coronary heart disease might benefit if the work of the heart

TABLE 7.1 DISTRIBUTION AND RESPONSES MEDIATED BY ADRENOCEPTORS

System	Adrenoceptor type	Response to stimulation
Heart	$beta_1$, $beta_2$	Increase in heart rate
	$beta_1$	Increase in conduction velocity
	$beta_1$	Increase in excitability
	$beta_1$	Increase in force of contraction
Blood vessels	alpha	Constriction of arteries and veins
	$beta_1$	Dilation of coronary arteries
	$beta_2$	Dilation of most arteries
Lung	alpha	Bronchoconstriction
	$beta_2$, $beta_1$	Bronchodilatation
Skeletal muscles	$beta_2$	Tremor
	$beta_2$	Stimulation of Na/K pump, resulting in increased contractility and hypokalemia
Bladder detrusor	beta	Relaxatory urgency
Smooth muscles		
Uterine	$beta_2$	Relaxation
Eye	alpha	Mydriasis
Intestinal	$beta_1$	Relaxation
Mast cells	alpha	Augmented releases of mediators of anaphylaxis
	beta	Inhibition of release of mediators of anaphylaxis
Platelets	$alpha_2$, beta	Aggregation promoted
Eye		
Intraocular pressure	$beta_1$	Increase in intraocular pressure
Tear secretion	$beta_2$	Increase in basic secretion
Central nervous system	$beta_1$	Not known
	$alpha_2$	Fall in blood pressure
Metabolism		
Gluconeogenesis	alpha	Promoted
Glycogenolysis	alpha (liver)	Promoted
	$beta_1$ (heart)	Promoted
	$beta_2$ (skeletal muscle; ? liver)	Promoted
Lipolysis (white adipocytes)	$beta_1$, $beta_2$	Promoted
Thermogenesis (brown adipocytes)	$beta_1$, $beta_3$	Promoted
Hormone secretion		
Glucagon	$beta_2$	Promoted
Insulin	alpha	Inhibited
	$beta_2$	Promoted
Parathyroid hormone	$beta_1$	Promoted
Renin	$beta_1$, $beta_2$	Promoted
Neurotransmitter release		Facilitated: skeletal neuromuscular junction
Acetylcholine	alpha	Inhibited: sympathetic ganglia and intestine, with inhibition/relaxation
Noradrenaline	alpha	Inhibited
	beta (? $beta_2$)	Facilitated

Adapted from *Cruickshank JM, Prichard BNC: Beta Blockers in Clinical Practice. Edinburgh: Churchill Livingstone; 1987.*

could be reduced through inhibition of the cardiac beta receptors. Beta blockade results in a reduction in heart rate, myocardial contractility, and myocardial oxygen consumption. His work led to the synthesis of **propranolol**, a nonselective beta blocker that proved effective in treating ischemic heart disease. Its antihypertensive activity came as a surprise. Today, beta blockers are indicated for the treatment of hypertension, angina pectoris, myocardial infarction (MI), arrhythmias, pheochromocytoma, Fallot's tetralogy, congestive cardiomyopathy, portal hypertension, thyrotoxicosis, anxiety, tremor, migraine, and glaucoma.

The manufacture of **propranolol** was followed by a number of other beta blockers with different pharmacology. Examples include those with partial agonist activity (PAA), such as **pindolol and penbutolol**, and beta$_1$-selective (cardioselective) agents, such as **atenolol** and **metoprolol**. The term *partial agonist activity*, also referred to as intrinsic sympathomimetic activity (ISA), implies the capacity of beta blockers to stimulate as well as to inhibit adrenergic receptors (Fig. 7.1).

The numerous available beta blockers can be subdivided on the basis of their pharmacological properties: nonselective drugs without ISA; beta$_1$-selective (or cardioselective) drugs without ISA; drugs with ISA (nonselective, beta$_1$-selective, and beta$_2$-selective); and agents with additional alpha-blocking activity, direct vasodilatory activity, or the "dual-acting" beta blockers (Table 7.2).

Beta blockers can also be classified on the basis of their water solubility (hydrophilicity). The hydrophilic agents are minimally metabolized. These agents tend to have a longer duration of action, which makes them suitable for once-daily administration. Moreover, hydrophilic agents penetrate brain tissue less; thus, they are less likely to produce central nervous system side effects.

MODE OF ACTION

The mode of action of a beta blocker is best described by considering the actions of the sympathetic nervous system. The sympathetic nervous system prepares the body for "fight or flight" by accelerating heart rate, raising blood pressure (BP), and shifting blood from the skin and splanchnic bed to the skeletal muscles. Many of these effects result from stimulation of the beta receptors by the catecholamines, epinephrine and norepinephrine. The former is released by the adrenal medulla and the latter by

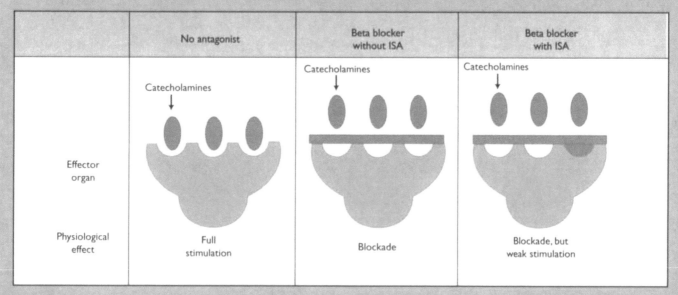

FIGURE 7.1 Nature of beta-adrenoceptor inhibition: effects of intrinsic sympathomimetic activity (partial agonist activity) in the presence of high levels of catecholamines. (*Adapted from* Frishman WH, Charlap S, Kostis JB: Clinical significance of ISA in beta-adrenoceptor blocker drugs. In Kostis, JB et al. (eds): *Beta Blockers in the Treatment of Cardiovascular Disease.* New York: Raven Press; 1984:253–274.)

TABLE 7.2. CLASSIFICATION OF BETA-ADRENERGIC BLOCKERS

Without ISA		With ISA		Dual-acting
Nonselective	**β₁-Selective**	**Nonselective**	**β₁-Selective**	
Nadolol	Atenolol	Carteolol	Acebutolol	Carvedilol
Propranolol	Betaxolol	Penbutolol		Labetalol
Sotalol	Bisoprolol	Pindolol		
Timolol	Esmolol			
	Metoprolol			
ISA—intrinsic sympathomimetic activity.				

sympathetic nerve endings. An exogenously-administered beta blocker binds preferentially and reversibly to the beta receptor, thus competitively inhibiting endogenous catecholamines (Fig. 7.1). Some beta blockers, besides inhibiting sympathetic nerve activity when they occupy the receptor, also possess some sympathomimetic activity (ie, PAA or ISA) (Fig. 7.1).

The BP-lowering mechanism of the beta blockers is not entirely understood. The initial fall in cardiac output is counterbalanced by increased peripheral sympathetic nerve activity, leading to vasoconstriction and increased total peripheral resistance. Peripheral sympathetic nerve activity subsides eventually, which is accompanied by falls in total peripheral resistance and BP. The fall in blood pressure is a result of decreased cardiac output. The acute and chronic hemodynamic effects of beta blockers in hypertensive patients are illustrated in Figure 7.2. Some beta blockers have a direct effect on peripheral resistance via their beta$_2$ ISA, which causes vasodilatation via alpha blockade, which prevents vasoconstriction, or via nonspecific vasodilatory effect. Several other mechanisms have been proposed to explain the above phenomenon: (1) a central action, (2) in-

hibition of sympathetic nervous action by prejunctional beta$_2$ receptor blockade, (3) renin blocking activity, (4) reduction in plasma volume, (5) stimulation of vasodilatory prostaglandins and atrial natriuretic factor, and (6) baroreceptor resetting. These mechanisms are discussed in detail by Cruickshank and Prichard, and Frishman and Sonnenblick.

In patients with acute or chronic myocardial ischemia, beta blockers offset the effects of endogenous catecholamines. This results in reduced heart rate, systolic BP, and myocardial contractility, which in turn reduces myocardial oxygen demand. Beta blockade has been shown to prevent cardiac rupture in patients with MI.

The class II antiarrhythmic properties of beta blockers arise directly through the following: (1) reversal of the catecholamine-induced increase of diastolic depolarization of automatic pacemaker cells; (2) increase in the conduction through the atrioventricular node; (3) shortening of the refractory period of ventricular cells; and (4) indirectly, through modification of factors that predispose a patient to arrhythmias, such as myocardial ischemia or hypokalemia.

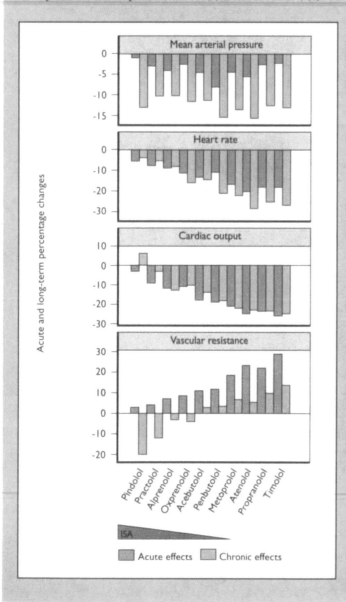

FIGURE 7.2 Acute and chronic hemodynamic effects of 10 beta-adrenoceptor antagonists in hypertensive patients at rest. The degree of ISA decreases from strong (pindolol) to almost none (penbutolol). Metoprolol, atenolol, propranolol, and timolol lack intrinsic sympathomimetic activity. (*Adapted from* Man In't Veld AJ, van der Meiracker AH: Effects of antihypertensive drugs on cardiovascular haemodynamics. In Laragh JH, Brenner BM (eds): *Hypertension.* New York: Raven Press; 1990:2117–2130.)

NONSELECTIVE BETA-ADRENERGIC BLOCKERS WITHOUT ISA

Nonselective beta blockers competitively inhibit the effects of catecholamines at beta$_1$ and beta$_2$ adrenergic sites. To reverse the effect of beta blockade, a higher concentration of the agonist is required.

EFFICACY AND USE

Nonselective beta blockers without ISA are effective in lowering diastolic BP to < 95 mmHg in 40%–50% of patients with mild to moderate hypertension. The BP is lowered in the supine and standing positions and also during exercise. The Medical Research Council trial of mild hypertension showed that in nonsmoking men, **propranolol** decreased the frequency of strokes by 47% and coronary events by 33%. Smoking negated these benefits. Furthermore, **propranolol** significantly reduced the incidence of Q-wave MI (silent and overt); risk for sudden death remained unchanged.

Comparisons between nonselective beta blockers without ISA (**propranolol, timolol, nadolol**) have found no differences in antihypertensive efficacy. Studies comparing nonselective beta blockers without ISA (usually **propranolol**) and agents with mild to modest ISA (**carteolol** and **penbutolol**) indicate similar BP lowering effect. Comparisons of **propranolol** with **pindolol** (which has moderate to high ISA) have shown that they have similar efficacy in lowering daytime BP, but **pindolol** does not significantly lower nocturnal BP. Under conditions of low sympathetic drive, such as sleep, **pindolol** acts as a stimulant to increase the heart rate. Comparisons of nonselective beta blockers without ISA and beta$_1$ selective blockers without ISA (**atenolol, metoprolol**) indicate similar antihypertensive effects. During strenuous exercise, when catecholamine levels are high, systolic BP is probably better controlled by a beta$_1$ selective than by a nonselective beta blocker agent.

Diuretics combine well with **propranolol, nadolol, sotalol,** or **timolol**, producing additive antihypertensive effects. The presence of a beta blocker mitigates, to some extent, the diuretic-induced hypokalemia. Vasodilators combine well with nonselective beta blockers, resulting in additive antihypertensive effects. The reflex increase in heart rate associated with vasodilators is diminished by beta blockade. Calcium antago-nists of the **nifedipine** type combine well with beta blockers, adding additional antihypertensive effect. Central-acting antihypertensive agents, such as **methyldopa**, combine well with beta blockers, such as **propranolol**; they are well tolerated and produce additive antihypertensive effects.

In treating stable angina, **propranolol** is significantly superior to long-acting nitrates. This class of beta blockers is generally more effective than **nifedipine** in reducing angina symptoms and ischemia. In unstable angina, beta blockers without ISA are probably more effective than **nifedipine** in rapid pain relief. Some patients do not respond to these drugs, and some (perhaps 15%) experience a worsening of anginal symptoms. Late intervention trials with oral nonselective beta blockers without ISA (given between days 2 and 28 after MI and continued for up to 3 years) showed a decrease in mortality of about 25%. The incidence of nonfatal reinfarction was also reduced by about 25%. Life-saving benefit has also been achieved in post-infarction patients with coexisting diabetes or congestive heart failure (CHF).

Patients with various arrhythmias may benefit from nonselective beta blockade. In patients with supraventricular tachycardia, ventricular premature beats, sustained ventricular tachycardia, and ventricular fibrillation associated with ischemia, exercise, or emotion, beta blockers are often the drugs of choice. **Sotalol**, which is approved for arrhythmias only, is discussed in the antiarrhythmic drug section.

In Fallot's tetralogy, intravenous **propranolol** improves pulmonary artery flow and arterial oxygen saturation. Long-term treatment with oral **propranolol** is highly effective in abolishing syncopal episodes and improving exercise tolerance. Likewise, beta blockers can benefit patients with congestive cardiomyopathy, hypertrophic obstructive cardiomyopathy, dissecting aneurysms, mitral valve prolapse, mitral stenosis, idiopathic or orthostatic hypotension, and stress-induced cardiac necrosis associated with subarachnoid hemorrhage. Nonselective beta blockers are also prescribed for a number of noncardiovascular conditions, including portal hypertension, thyrotoxicosis, pheochromocytoma, anxiety, migraine, tremor, and raised intraocular pressure.

MODE OF ACTION

Oral beta blockers reduce heart rate, systolic BP, and myocardial contractility, thus reducing myocardial oxygen demand. This reduction in myocardial workload is the main mechanism of action in the ischemic patient. Additionally, in acute MI, beta blockade has been shown to prevent cardiac rupture and life-threatening arrhythmias.

In treating hypertension, both intravenous and oral beta blockade leads to a reduction in cardiac output by 20%–25%. This decrease is maintained on chronic oral therapy. Stroke volume is usually unchanged or possibly slightly increased. A fall in heart rate is the main cause of the fall in cardiac output, but left ventricular contractility is also reduced. The fall in cardiac output is counterbalanced by a reflex increase in peripheral resistance magnified by vasoconstriction caused by peripheral beta$_2$ blockade. A nonselective agent may thus produce a lesser fall in diastolic BP than a beta$_1$ selective agent (which preserves beta$_2$ vasodilatation) (Fig. 7.2).

Except in the presence of high sympathetic tone or poor left ventricular function, BP does not fall immediately after intravenous beta blockade. In responders, the reduction in BP occurs during the first few hours, but maximum reduction may not be achieved after a few months. The fall in coronary blood flow is largely an autoregulatory effect of decreased myocardial oxygen requirement. Autoregulatory processes maintain flow to the brain, whereas less vital tissues, such as skin, muscle, and splanchnic areas, may experience a marked decrease in blood flow.

All the normal hemodynamic responses associated with dynamic exercise or mental stress remain unchanged on nonselective beta blockade except that heart rate, BP, and cardiac output are 15%–25% lower. Factors associated with excessive sympathetic activity, such as hypoglycemia and smoking, may be linked to an increase in BP and a reflex decrease in heart rate when nonselective beta blockers are given.

INDICATIONS

	Nadolol	Propranolol	Sotalol	Timolol
Hypertension	+	+	–	+
Angina	+	+	–	–
Post-myocardial infarction	–	+	–	+
Arrhythmias	–	+	+	–
Hypertrophic obstructive cardiomyopathy	–	+	–	–
Essential tremor	–	+	–	–
Migraine headache	–	+	–	+

+–approved by the FDA; – –not approved by the FDA.

NADOLOL
(Nadolol, Corgard®)

Nadolol, structually similar to propranolol, is a nonselective beta adrenergic antagonist. It has no intrinsic sympathomimetic activity (ISA) or membrane stabilizing activity. Nadolol is water soluble and is not metabolized with a long duration of action, which offers the advantage of once a day dosing. It has been observed that nadolol increased renal blood flow in humans without significant changes in glomerular filtration rate. Its effect on renal hemodynamics remains unclear. Nadolol has also been used as an antiarrhythmic agent in a dose range of 60–160 mg/d.

SPECIAL GROUPS

Race: black hypertensive patients may be less responsive than white patients
Children: safety and effectiveness have not been established
Elderly: starting with low dose and titrate the dose based on clinical response
Renal impairment: dosing interval should be increased and adjusted based on clinical response
Hepatic impairment: use with caution; dosage adjustment is probably not required
Pregnancy: category C; should only be used if clearly indicated
Breast-feeding: not recommended; excreted in human milk

DOSAGE*

Hypertension: Usual dose—40–80 mg daily.
Maximum dose—240–320 mg daily
The dose is 20–40 mg once daily initially, and increased by 40–80 mg/d every 1–2 wk until desired BP control is achieved.
Angina Pectoris: Usual dose—40–80 mg daily.
Maximum dose—> 240 mg daily
The initial dose is 40 mg once daily and increased by 40–80 mg/d every 3–7 d until adequate control of angina is achieved.
*Guidelines for dosing intervals in patients with renal impairment (including elderly patients)

Creatinine Clearance (mL/min/1.73 m²)	Interval
> 50	q 24 h
30–50	q 24–36 h
10–30	q 24–48 h
< 10	q 48 h or longer

IN BRIEF

INDICATIONS
Hypertension
Angina pectoris

CONTRAINDICATIONS
Severe heart failure
Bronchial asthma or related bronchospastic problems
Severe bradycardia with second- or third-degree AV block
Sick sinus syndrome without a permanent pacemaker in place
Cardiogenic shock
Known hypersensitivity

DRUG INTERACTIONS
Beta-agonists
Calcium-channel blockers: verapamil or diltiazem
Diuretics
Other antihypertensive agents
Insulin
Oral hypoglycemic agents
NSAIDs

ADVERSE EFFECTS
CV: bradycardia, peripheral vascular insufficiency/ Raynaud's type, postural hypotension, syncope, hypotension, heart failure, AV block, ventricular arrhythmia, angina
CNS: fatigue, dizziness, drowsiness, paresthesia
Respiratory: dyspnea, bronchospasm, nasal congestion
GI: nausea, vomiting, dyspepsia, constipation
GU: male impotence, ejaculatory failure
Metabolic: dyslipidemia
Other: edema, weight gain, allergic reaction

PHARMACOKINETICS AND PHARMACODYNAMICS
Duration of action: >24 h
Onset of action: <2 h
Peak effect: 2–4 h
Bioavailability: 30%–40%
Effect of food: no effect
Metabolism: not metabolized
Clearance: urine—24.6%; feces—76.9%
Plasma half-life: 10–24 h (↑ in renal impairment)
Protein binding: 30%

MONITORING
BP, heart rate, respiratory status.

OVERDOSE
Supportive: For severe bradycardia, atropine 2 mg IV may be administered or a pacemaker should be placed. For cardiovascular support, glucagon 5–10 mg IV bolus administered over 30 s, followed by 5 mg/h continuous infusion. Fluid therapy with vasopressors/inotropic therapy added if necessary may also be appropriate.

PATIENT INFORMATION
Nadolol therapy should not be discontinued abruptly without consulting a physician. The physician should also be consulted for persistent or unusual problems, such as dizziness/faintness, weight gain, worsening edema, or increasing shortness of breath. Sit or lie down if dizziness occurs and rise slowly from a sitting or lying position.

AVAILABILITY
Tablets—20, 40, 80, 120, 160 mg
Combination Formulations with a diuretic:
Corizide® 40/5 tablets—40 mg nadolol and 5 mg bendroflumethiazide
Corizide® 80/5 tablets—80 mg nadolol and 5 mg bendroflumethiazide

PROPRANOLOL

(Propranolol, Inderal®, Inderal LA®)

Propranolol has been available for over 30 years. It is a lipophilic molecule, is extensively metabolized by the liver, and has a short half-life. It is administered 2–3 times daily except for slow-release formulations, which may be administered once daily. Its use may have contributed to considerable saving of lives in several indications, including hypertension and post-MI. In particular, in the large MRC mild hypertension study, propranolol significantly reduced the incidence of fatal and nonfatal stroke (although the benefits were offset by smoking), silent and overt infarctions, and sudden death. In the BHAT postinfarction study, propranolol reduced mortality and the reinfarction rate by about 25%. This benefit was particularly noticeable in diabetic patients and those with heart failure. In patients with subarachnoid hemorrhage, propranolol reduced stress-induced myocardial necrosis. In humans, chronic propranolol use may reverse left ventricular hypertrophy.

SPECIAL GROUPS

Race: black hypertensive patients may be less responsive than white patients

Children: less extensive data on efficacy and safety in children as in adults, increased bioavailability in patients with Down's syndrome

Elderly: starting with low dose and titrate the dose based on clinical response

Renal impairment: use with caution; titrate the dose based on clinical response

Hepatic impairment: use with caution; titrate the dose based on clinical response

Pregnancy: category C; should only be used if clearly indicated

Breast-feeding: excreted in human milk; used with caution

IN BRIEF

INDICATIONS

Angina	Hypertrophic subaortic stenosis
Cardiac arrhythmias	MI
Essential tremor	Migraine prophylaxis
Hypertension	Pheochromocytoma

CONTRAINDICATIONS

Bronchial asthma or related bronchospastic problems
Cardiogenic shock
Known hypersensitivity
Second- or third-degree AV block
Severe heart failure
Sick sinus syndrome without a permanent pacemaker in place
Severe bradycardia

DRUG INTERACTIONS

Beta agonists
Calcium-channel blockers: verapamil or diltiazem
Cimetidine
Diuretics
Other antihypertensive agents
Insulin
Oral hypoglycemic agents
NSAIDs
Phenytoin
Phenobarbital
Rifampin

ADVERSE EFFECTS

CV: bradycardia, peripheral vascular insufficiency/Raynaud's type, postural hypotension, syncope, hypotension, heart failure, AV block, ventricular arrhythmia, angina
CNS: fatigue, dizziness, drowsiness, depression, hallucinations, disorientation, vivid dream, short-term memory loss, paresthesia
Respiratory: dyspnea, bronchospasm
GI: nausea, vomiting, dyspepsia, constipation
GU: male impotence, ejaculatory failure
Metabolic: dyslipidemia
Other: edema, weight gain, allergic reaction, systemic lupus erythematosus, blood dyscrasias

PHARMACOKINETICS AND PHARMACODYNAMICS

Duration of action: 10–15 min (IV); 6–24 h (po)
Onset of action: immediate (IV); 1–2 h (po)
Peak effect: IV—1 min; regular tablets— 60–90 min; sustained release—6 h
Bioavailability: 100% (IV); 30%–70% (po; sustained release—40%)
Effect of food: delayed absorption
Metabolism: mainly metabolized in liver with at least one active metabolite
Clearance: mainly excreted in urine as metabolites
Plasma half-life: 3.4–6 h
Protein binding: >90%

MONITORING

BP, heart rate, ECG, respiratory status, and appropriate clinical response as per indication.

OVERDOSE

Supportive: For severe bradycardia, atropine 2 mg IV may be administered or a pacemaker should be placed. For cardiovascular support, glucagon 5–10 mg IV bolus administered over 30 s, followed by 5 mg/h continuous infusion. Fluid therapy with vasopressors/inotropic therapy added if necessary may also be appropriate.

PATIENT INFORMATION

Propranolol therapy should not be discontinued abruptly without consulting a physician. The physician should also be consulted for persistent or unusual problems, such as dizziness/faintness, weight gain, worsening edema, or increasing shortness of breath. Sit or lie down if dizziness occurs and rise slowly from a sitting or lying position.

DOSAGE (LA—sustained release form)

Hypertension:* Initial dose—40 mg twice daily; (LA) 80 mg once daily
   Maintenance—120–240 mg/d in 2–3 divided doses; (LA) 120–160
   mg once daily
   Maximum—640 mg/d in 2–3 divided doses

Angina pectoris:* 80–320 mg/d in 2–4 divided doses; (LA) 80–320 mg
   once daily

Arrhythmias: 10–30 mg 3 or 4 times daily before meals and at bedtime

Myocardial infarction: 180–240 mg/d in 2–4 divided doses

Migraine prophylaxis:* Dose range: 160–240 mg/d in divided doses
   starting from 80 mg/d in divided doses and increased gradually to
   achieve optimal control; (LA) 80–240 mg once daily

Essential tremor: Usual dose is 120 mg/d in divided doses, starting from
   40 mg twice daily and titrate the dose based on the response (maximum dose: 240–320 mg/d)

Hypertrophic subaortic stenosis:* 20–40 mg 3 or 4 times daily
   before meals and at bedtime; (LA) 80–160 mg once daily

Pheochromocytoma: 30–60 mg/d in divided doses

Intravenous administration for life-threatening arrhythmias:
   1–3 mg, rate ≤ 1 mg/min; a second dose may be administered
   after 2 min if indicated

* Patients may also be switched from the regular to sustained release formulation for once daily regimen; however, it is not an exact milligram-
   for-milligram switch. To assure the desired therapeutic effect is maintained, dose should be adjusted based on clinical response.

AVAILABILITY

Tablets—10, 20, 40, 60, 80, 90 mg
Solutions—40 mg/5 mL, 80 mg/mL (concentrate)
Capsules (sustained release)—60, 80, 120, 160 mg
Injectable ampules—1 mg/ml, 1 ml
Combination Formulations with a diuretic, HCTZ (hydrochlorothiazide):
  Capsules (sustained release):
    Inderide LA 80/50: propranolol 80 mg/HCTZ 50 mg
    Inderide LA 120/50: propranolol 120 mg/HCTZ 50 mg
    Inderide LA 160/50: propranolol 160 mg/HCTZ 50 mg
  Tablets:
    Inderide 80/25: propranolol 80 mg/HCTZ 25 mg
    Inderide 40/25: propranolol 40 mg/HCTZ 25 mg
    Propranolol/HCTZ 80/25 mg
    Propranolol/HCTZ 40/25 mg

Sotalol, a nonselective beta-adrenergic blocking agent without ISA or membrane stabilizing activity, is water soluble and long acting. Similar to amiodarone, it has class II and III antiarrhythmic actions. The action potential of the myocardial cell is prolonged, resulting in a long QT interval. This proarrhythmia property can occasionally predispose a patient to life-threatening arrhythmias, including ventricular fibrillation. Sotalol is indicated for the treatment of documented ventricular arrhythmias, such as sustained ventricular tachycardia, that, in the judgment of the physician, are life-threatening. A recent study showed greater antiarrhythmic efficacy than other conventional antiarrhythmic agents used for the treatment of ventricular arrhythmias.

For additional information on sotalol, please refer to the chapter on antiarrhythmic agents.

TIMOLOL
(Timolol, Blocadren®)

Timolol is a nonselective beta blocker. It is lipophilic and metabolized by the liver. It does not have intrinsic sympathomimetic, direct myocardial depressant, or membrane stabilizing activities. The mortality curves from the classic Norwegian Multicentre Study Group in postinfarction patients treated with timolol for 7–28 d after the event demonstrated that late intervention caused a significant decrease in mortality and reinfarction over 3 years. This benefit was still present at a 6-year follow-up. Patients receiving timolol who stopped smoking gained the most benefit.

SPECIAL GROUPS

Race: black hypertensive patients may be less responsive than white patients
Children: safety and effectiveness have not been established
Elderly: start with low dose and titrate the dose based on clinical response
Renal impairment: use with caution; titrate the dose based on clinical response
Hepatic impairment: use with caution; titrate the dose based on clinical response
Pregnancy: category C; should only be used if clearly indicated
Breast-feeding: not recommended; excreted in human milk

DOSAGE

Hypertension: 10–30 mg twice daily
Myocardial infarction: 10 mg twice daily
Migraine prophylaxis: initial dose is 10 mg twice daily. The dose should be adjusted based on clinical response to a maximum of 30 mg per day in divided doses. If no effect after 6–8 wk of the maximum dose, therapy should be tapered and discontinued.

IN BRIEF

INDICATIONS
Hypertension
MI
Migraine prophylaxis
Open-angle glaucoma

CONTRAINDICATIONS
Bronchial asthma or related bronchospastic problems
Cardiogenic shock
Known hypersensitivity
Second- or third-degree AV block
Sick sinus syndrome without a permanent pacemaker in place
Severe bradycardia
Severe heart failure

DRUG INTERACTIONS
Beta agonists
Calcium-channel blockers: verapamil or diltiazem
Cimetidine
Diuretics
Other antihypertensive agents
Insulin
Oral hypoglycemic agents
NSAIDs
Phenytoin
Phenobarbital
Rifampin

ADVERSE EFFECTS
CV: bradycardia, peripheral vascular insufficiency/Raynaud's type, postural hypotension, syncope, hypotension, heart failure, AV block, ventricular arrhythmia, angina
CNS: fatigue, dizziness, drowsiness, depression, hallucinations, disorientation, short-term memory loss, paresthesia
Respiratory: dyspnea, bronchospasm
GI: nausea, vomiting, dyspepsia, constipation
GU: male impotence, ejaculatory failure
Metabolic: dyslipidemia
Other: edema, weight gain, pruritus, rash, fever, allergic reaction, blood dyscrasias

PHARMACOKINETICS AND PHARMACODYNAMICS
Duration of action: 12–24 h
Onset of action: 30 min
Peak effect: 1–2 h
Bioavailability: 50%
Effect of food: no effect
Metabolism: 80% metabolized in the liver
Clearance: excreted in the urine as metabolites
Plasma half-life: 4 h
Protein binding: 10%–60%

MONITORING
BP, heart rate, respiratory status, and appropriate clinical response as per indication.

OVERDOSE
Supportive: For severe bradycardia, atropine 2 mg IV may be administered or a pacemaker should be placed. For cardiovascular support, glucagon 5–10 mg IV bolus administered over 30 seconds, followed by 5 mg/h continuous infusion. Fluid therapy with vasopressors/inotropic therapy added if necessary may also be appropriate.

PATIENT INFORMATION
Timolol therapy should not be discontinued abruptly without consulting a physician. The physician should also be consulted for persistent or unusual problems such as dizziness/faintness, weight gain, worsening edema, or increasing shortness of breath. Sit or lie down if dizziness occurs and rise slowly from a sitting or lying position.

AVAILABILITY
Tablets—5, 10, 20 mg
Ophthalmic solutions—0.25%, 0.5 %
Ophthalmic gel-forming solutions— 0.25%, 0.5%
Combination Formulations:
Timolide® 10–25 tablets—10 mg timolol/25 mg hydrochlorothiazide

Since selective beta₁ antagonism was first described in 1968 with **practolol**, other structures with this property have subsequently been developed. The term *cardioselectivity* was used, indicating that beta₂ receptors in the airway would remain unblocked. The implied safety factor, free from drug-induced bronchospasm in the asthmatic patient, is only relative, as selectivity tends to diminish at higher doses. Beta₁ selectivity is a more accurate term than cardioselectivity because both beta₁ and beta₂ receptors coexist in human myocardium in a 3:1 ratio.

EFFICACY AND USE

Beta₁ selective blockers may lower diastolic BP more than non-selective drugs, a result of their beta₂ vasodilatory-sparing action. The beta₁ selective drugs appear more effective than a thiazide diuretic in lowering BP of young, white hypertensive patients, especially in the presence of sympathetic hyperactivity. They have about the same antihypertensive actions as calcium antagonists and angiotensin-converting enzyme (ACE) inhibitors.

The Heart Attack Primary Prevention in Hypertension (HAPPHY) trial, involving more than 6000 moderately hypertensive middle-aged men, showed that total mortality rates were similar in both diuretic and beta blocker groups, although death rate from stroke was significantly lower in the beta blocker group. In the follow-up subgroup analysis, the Metoprolol Atherosclerosis Prevention in Hypertension (MAPH) trial, selective beta₁ blockade with metoprolol significantly reduced MI and sudden death compared with the diuretic in smokers and nonsmokers. Similar to nonselective beta blockers, beta₁ selective agents are cardioprotective and reverse left ventricular hypertrophy by reducing wall thickness. However, in elderly hypertensives, atenolol has been shown to reduce the frequency of stroke but not MI.

Similar to nonselective beta blockers, beta₁ selective agents have greater antihypertensive effect in patients with baseline high or normal plasma renin activity (PRA), such as in Asian and white patients. Black patients and the elderly (usually with low PRA) do not respond as well.

Atenolol is more effective than placebo in the management of hypertension in the third trimester of pregnancy. Atenolol reduced both maternal hospital admissions and neonatal respiratory distress. Birth weights, however, tend to be lower in the atenolol group.

Similar to other beta blockers, beta₁ selective agents work synergistically with antihypertensive agents from other classes. Diuretic-induced hypokalemia may be partially mitigated by the beta₁ blockers, but probably less than by a nonselective agent. Atenolol works synergistically with nifedipine in lowering BP, especially in patients with eclampsia. The combination of a beta₁ selective blocker and an ACE inhibitor is less satisfactory because the effects are less than additive.

Beta₁ selective agents are also effective anti-ischemic agents. Patients with mixed angina who experience frequent silent ischemic episodes may benefit more from beta₁ blockade than from nitrates or nifedipine. Patients with angina and mild to moderate aortic stenosis also respond well to beta blockade.

In unstable angina, beta₁ selective agents were superior to nifedipine in preventing cardiac events in the Holland Interuniversity Nifedipine/Metoprolol (HINT) study. Beta₁ selective beta blockers can be used effectively in combination with nitrates and dihydropyridines. Left ventricular function and atrioventricular conduction are not usually suppressed, though hypotension is seen occasionally.

Early intervention studies of post-MI, such as the First International Study of Infarct Survival (ISIS-1), indicate a 15% reduction in vascular mortality with beta blockers at one week (Fig. 7.3). Most of the life savings appear to occur in the first 24–36 h, and prevention of cardiac rupture is the main benefit. Bradycardia, hypotension, and heart failure can occur but rarely require active intervention. Pooled data from 28 randomized trials suggest that the incidence of reinfarction and cardiac arrest is significantly decreased (15%–18%) by early IV beta blockade. All beta blockers without ISA, including beta₁ selective drugs, decrease mortality by about 25%–30% in late intervention postinfarction patients.

Beta₁ selective drugs also have a role in treating cardiac arrhythmias. Their selectivity for the beta₁ receptor means that they are relatively safe and well tolerated in patients with potential airway problems (although they are not recommended if alternative drugs can be given), in insulin-dependent diabetics and in hypertensives who undergo physical exercise.

Beta₁ adrenergic blockers have also been used as an adjunctive therapy, such as metoprolol, bisoprolols, in patients with symptomatic CHF who are already receiving conventional therapy with diuretics, ACE inhibitors, and digoxin. The results of placebo-controlled clinical trials demonstrate a morbidity and mortality benefit with beta blocker treatment; however, the beta₁ selective agents are not yet approved for use in heart failure patients.

MODE OF ACTION

Beta₁ selective blockade leads to a fall in cardiac output of 20%–25%. This decrease is maintained on chronic oral therapy. This fall is counterbalanced by a small reflex increase in peripheral resistance. The lack of beta₂ blocking effects, however, permits beta₂ vasodilatation; thus, peripheral resistance does not increase to the same degree as with nonselective agents (Fig. 7.2). As a consequence, beta₁ selective agents produce a slightly greater fall in diastolic BP (3–4 mmHg). Beta₁ selective beta blockers suppress resting heart rate, cardiac output, and exercise-induced increase in heart rate to the same extent as nonselective beta blockers; however, when the increase in heart rate involves stimulation of beta₂ as well as beta₁ receptors (for instance, via isoproterenol or epinephrine), nonselective beta blockers cause a greater decrease in stimulated heart rate.

Beta₁ selective agents decrease coronary flow (mainly a reflection of decreased oxygen requirements) to the same degree as nonselective beta blockers; however, blood flow to other organs, such as skin, kidney, and liver, is possibly less affected by the beta₁ selective agents. A beta₁ selective agent may show advantages in terms of lesser impairment of exercise tolerance, probably a result of sparing beta$_2$ blocking effects on muscle gly-colytic processes and possibly on blood glucose and potassium levels during exercise. Beta$_1$ selective agents possibly attenuate the hemodynamic changes of isometric exercise to a greater degree than nonselective agents. The hypertensive reaction to nonselective beta blockers in the presence of excessive sympathetic activity, hypoglycemia, or smoking, is less likely to occur with beta$_1$ selective agents.

INDICATIONS

	Atenolol	Betaxolol	Bisoprolol	Esmolol	Metoprolol
Hypertension	+	+	+	+	+
Angina	+	–	–	–	+
Post MI	+	–	–	–	+
Arrhythmias	–	–	–	+	–

+—approved by the FDA; – —not approved by the FDA.

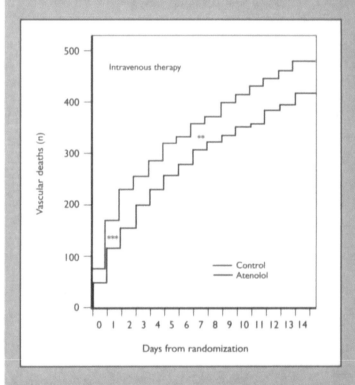

FIGURE 7.3 Mortality reduction in ISIS: comparison of atenolol and placebo. **–2P < 0.4; ***–2P < 0.002. (Adapted from ISIS-1 Collaborative Group: Randomized trial of intravenous atenolol among 16,027 cases of suspected acute myocardial infarction: ISIS-1. Lancet 1986, ii:57–66.)

ATENOLOL
(Atenolol, Tenormin®)

Atenolol, a beta₁ selective blocker without membrane stabilizing activity or ISA, is water soluble and long acting. It was the first once-daily beta blocker in use, and various studies have demonstrated its short- and long-term efficacy and tolerability. Atenolol was shown to decrease the risk of MI and stroke (fatal and nonfatal) in hypertensive patients when compared with a control population. Its effect on stroke prevention was confirmed in elderly hypertensive patients with isolated systolic hypertension. Its secondary cardioprotective property was demonstrated in patients with acute MI. Early intervention reduced mortality significantly. It is more effective than nifedipine and nitrates in abolishing ischemic episodes in mixed angina, and is beneficial in the treatment of angina with aortic stenosis. It crosses the blood-brain barrier marginally, with fewer CNS side effects than lipid-soluble beta blockers. It is not recommended in patients with asthma, but its beta₁ selectivity makes it safer than nonselective agents in patients with reactive airways disease, and it does not prolong insulin-induced hypoglycemia in diabetes. It reduces stress-induced cardiac necrosis in patients with head injuries and reverses left ventricular hypertrophy.

The results of four randomized clinical trials demonstrated the use of oral atenolol in relieving ischemia and improving outcomes in patients with documented silent myocardial ischemia. These studies compared atenolol monotherapy with placebo, calcium-channel blocker monotherapy, calcium-channel blockers and nitrates combination, and the combination of atenolol with calcium-channel blockers (*ie*, nifedipine, amlodipine).

SPECIAL GROUPS

Race: black hypertensive patients may be less responsive than white patients

Children: safety and effectiveness have not been established

Elderly: start with a low dose and titrate the dose based on clinical response

Renal impairment: dosage should be adjusted based on renal function and clinical response

Hepatic impairment: use with caution; dosage adjustment is probably not required

Pregnancy: category D; should not be used

Breast-feeding: not recommended; excreted in human milk

DOSAGE

Hypertension:* 50–100 mg once daily
Angina pectoris: 50–200 mg once daily
Myocardial infarction: Treatment should be initiated with intravenous (IV) atenolol 5 mg administered over 5 min, followed by a second IV dose of 5 mg 10 min later. If the patient tolerates the full IV therapy, 50 mg of atenolol should be administered orally 10 min after the last IV dose, followed by a second 50 mg 12 h later. Then, the patient can receive atenolol orally either 100 mg once daily or 50 mg twice daily for 6–9 d or until discharge from the hospital.
*Guidelines for dosing adjustments in patients with renal impairment (including elderly patients)

Creatinine Clearance (mL/min/1.73 m²)	Maximum dose
15–35	50 mg/d
<15	25 mg/d
on hemodialysis (HD)	25 or 50 mg after HD

IN BRIEF

INDICATIONS
Angina pectoris
Hypertension
MI

CONTRAINDICATIONS
Bronchial asthma or related bronchospastic problems
Cardiogenic shock
Known hypersensitivity
Second- or third-degree AV block
Severe bradycardia
Severe heart failure
Sick sinus syndrome without a permanent pacemaker in place

DRUG INTERACTIONS
Beta agonists
Calcium-channel blockers: verapamil or diltiazem
Diuretics
Other antihypertensive agents
Insulin
Oral hypoglycemic agents
NSAIDs

ADVERSE EFFECTS
CV: bradycardia, peripheral vascular insufficiency/Raynaud's type, postural hypotension, syncope, hypotension, heart failure, AV block, ventricular arrhythmia, angina
CNS: fatigue, dizziness, drowsiness, depression, vertigo, sleep disturbances
Respiratory: dyspnea, bronchospasm, nasal congestion
GI: nausea, diarrhea
GU: male impotence, ejaculatory failure
Metabolic: dyslipidemia
Other: edema, weight gain, allergic reaction, rash, agranulocytosis, lupus syndrome

PHARMACOKINETICS AND PHARMACODYNAMICS
Duration of action:	up to 12 h (IV); >24 h (po)
Onset of action:	immediate (IV); <1 h (po)
Peak effect:	<5 min (IV); 2–4 h (po)
Bioavailability:	100% (IV); about 50% (po)
Effect of food:	↓ bioavailability
Metabolism:	little or no metabolism
Clearance:	mainly renal as unchanged drug
Plasma half-life:	6–7 h (normal renal function)
Protein binding:	6%–16%

MONITORING
BP, heart rate, ECG, and respiratory status.

OVERDOSE
Supportive: For severe bradycardia, atropine 2 mg IV may be administered or a pacemaker should be placed. For cardiovascular support, glucagon 5–10 mg IV bolus administered over 30 s, followed by 5 mg/h continuous infusion. Fluid therapy with vasopressors /inotropic therapy added if necessary may also be appropriate.

PATIENT INFORMATION
Atenolol therapy should not be discontinued abruptly without consulting a physician. The physician should also be consulted for persistent or unusual problems such as dizziness/faintness, weight gain, worsening edema, or increasing shortness of breath. Sit or lie down if dizziness occurs and rise slowly from a sitting or lying position.

AVAILABILITY
Tablets—25, 50, 100 mg
Ampules—5 mg/10 mL
Combination Formulations with a diuretic:
Tenoretic® Tablets—
  50 mg atenolol/25 mg chlorthalidone
  100 mg atenolol/25 mg chlorthalidone

BETAXOLOL (Kerlone®)

Betaxolol, a beta₁ selective blocker devoid of ISA and membrane stabilizing activity, is moderately lipid-soluble and is extensively metabolized by the liver. It is prescribed once daily for hypertension and is also available in topical form for management of elevated intraocular pressure.

SPECIAL GROUPS

Race: black hypertensive patients may be less responsive than white patients

Children: safety and effectiveness have not been established

Elderly: start with a low dose and titrate the dose based on clinical response

Renal impairment: use with caution; starting with lower dose

Hepatic impairment: use with caution; starting with lower dose

Pregnancy: category C; should only be used if clearly indicated

Breast-feeding: not recommended; excreted in human milk

DOSAGE

Hypertension: The initial dose is 10 mg once daily (5 mg for elderly patients or patients with impaired renal function). If the desired effect is not achieved, increase the dose by 5 mg/d increments every 2 wk to maximum doses of 20–40 mg/d.

IN BRIEF

INDICATIONS
Hypertension
Ocular hypertension
Open-angle glaucoma

CONTRAINDICATIONS
Bronchial asthma or related bronchospastic problems
Cardiogenic shock
Known hypersentivity
Second- or third-degree AV block
Severe bradycardia
Severe heart failure
Sick sinus syndrome without a permanent pacemaker in place

DRUG INTERACTIONS
Beta agonists
Calcium-channel blockers: verapamil or diltiazem
Diuretics
Other antihypertensive agents
Insulin
Oral hypoglycemic agents
NSAIDs

ADVERSE EFFECTS
CV: bradycardia, peripheral vascular insufficiency/Raynaud's type, postural hypotension, syncope, hypotension, heart failure, AV block, ventricular arrhythmia, angina
CNS: fatigue, dizziness, drowsiness, depression, headache, sleep disturbances
Respiratory: dyspnea, bronchospasm, nasal congestion
GI: dyspepsia, nausea, diarrhea
GU: male impotence, ejaculatory failure
Metabolic: dyslipidemia
Other: edema, weight gain, allergic reaction, rash, blood dyscrasias

PHARMACOKINETICS AND PHARMACODYNAMICS
Duration of action: >24 h
Onset of action: 2–3 h
Peak effect: 3–4 h
Bioavailability: 89%
Effect of food: no effect
Metabolism: mainly metabolized in the liver
Clearance: 80% via renal excretion (15% as unchanged)
Plasma half-life: 14–22 h
Protein binding: 50%

MONITORING
BP, heart rate, respiratory status, and other appropriate clinical response.

OVERDOSE
Supportive: For severe bradycardia, atropine 2 mg IV may be administered or a pacemaker should be placed. For cardiovascular support, glucagon 5–10 mg IV bolus administered over 30 s, followed by 5 mg/h continuous infusion. Fluid therapy with vasopressors/inotropic therapy added if necessary may also be appropriate.

PATIENT INFORMATION
Betaxolol therapy should not be discontinued abruptly without consulting a physician. The physician should also be consulted for persistent or unusual problems, such as dizziness/faintness, weight gain, worsening edema, or increasing shortness of breath. Sit or lie down if dizziness occurs and rise slowly from a sitting or lying position.

AVAILABILITY
Tablets—10, 20 mg

BISOPROLOL
(Zebata®)

Bisoprolol, a beta₁ selective adrenergic blocking agent, is structurally similar to acebuterol, atenolol, and metoprolol. Bisoprolol does not exhibit intrinsic sympathomimetic activity or membrane-stabilizing activity. At high doses (20 mg or higher), bisoprolol loses its cardioselectivity and inhibits both beta₁ and beta₂ adrenergic receptors. In controlled clinical trials, bisoprolol monotherapy has been shown to produce significant dose-related BP reduction with a 47% to 70% clinical response rate observed in patients with hypertension.

SPECIAL GROUPS

Race: black hypertensive patients may be less responsive than white patients

Children: safety and effectiveness have not been established

Elderly: start with low dose and titrate the dose based on clinical response

Renal impairment: use with caution; starting with lower dose

Hepatic impairment: use with caution; titrate the dose based on clinical response

Pregnancy: category C; should only be used if clearly indicated

Breast-feeding: use with caution; not known if the drug is excreted in human milk

DOSAGE

Hypertension: 2.5–20 mg once daily

The initial dose should be 2.5–5 mg once daily and increase gradually based on BP response

IN BRIEF

INDICATIONS
Hypertension
Ocular hypertension
Open-angle glaucoma

CONTRAINDICATIONS
Bronchial asthma or related bronchospastic problems
Cardiogenic shock
Known hypersensitivity
Second- or third-degree AV block
Severe bradycardia
Severe heart failure
Sick sinus syndrome without a permanent pacemaker in place

DRUG INTERACTIONS
Beta agonists
Calcium-channel blockers: verapamil or diltiazem
Diuretics
Other antihypertensive agents
Insulin
Oral hypoglycemic agents
NSAIDs

ADVERSE EFFECTS
CV: bradycardia, peripheral vascular insufficiency/Raynaud's type, postural hypotension, syncope, hypotension, heart failure, AV block, ventricular arrhythmia, angina
CNS: fatigue, dizziness, drowsiness, depression, vertigo, sleep disturbances
Respiratory: dyspnea, bronchospasm, nasal congestion
GI: nausea, diarrhea
GU: male impotence, ejaculatory failure
Metabolic: dyslipidemia, hyperuricemia
Other: edema, weight gain, allergic reaction, rash, purpura

PHARMACOKINETICS AND PHARMACODYNAMICS
Duration of action: >24 h
Onset of action: 1–2 h
Peak effect: 2–4 h
Bioavailability: 80%
Effect of food: no effect
Metabolism: 50% metabolized by the liver
Clearance: mainly renal (50% as unchanged); <2% in feces
Plasma half-life: 9–12 h
Protein binding: 30%

MONITORING
BP, heart rate, respiratory status, and other appropriate clinical response.

OVERDOSE
Supportive: For severe bradycardia, atropine 2 mg IV may be administered or a pacemaker should be placed. For cardiovascular support, glucagon 5–10 mg IV bolus administered over 30 s, followed by 5 mg/h continuous infusion. Fluid therapy with vasopressors/inotropic therapy added if necessary may also be appropriate.

PATIENT INFORMATION
Bisoprolol therapy should not be discontinued abruptly without consulting a physician. The physician should also be consulted for persistent or unusual problems, such as dizziness/faintness, weight gain, worsening edema, or increasing shortness of breath. Sit or lie down if dizziness occurs or rise slowly from a sitting or lying position.

AVAILABILITY
Tablets—5, 10 mg
Combination Formulations with a diuretic:
Ziac® Tablets—
 2.5 mg bisoprolol/6.25 mg hydrochlorothiazide
 5 mg bisoprolol/6.25 mg hydrochlorothiazide
 10 mg bisoprolol/6.25 mg hydrochlorothiazide

ESMOLOL
(Brevibloc®)

Esmolol, a beta₁ selective blocker with no significant ISA or membrane stabilizing activity, is available only in the IV form. It has an elimination half-life of about 9 min because of rapid and extensive metabolism. Esmolol has a very rapid onset and a very short duration of action. After termination of infusion, substantial recovery from beta blockade is observed in 10–20 min. Esmolol is indicated for the rapid control of ventricular rate in patients with atrial fibrillation or atrial flutter in perioperative, postoperative, or other emergencies when short-term control of ventricular rate with a short-acting beta-adrenergic agent is desirable. Esmolol is also used in patients with noncompensatory sinus tachycardia when rapid heart rate control is indicated. In addition to its antiarrhythmic activity, esmolol is indicated for the treatment of tachycardia and hypertension that occurs intraoperatively or postoperatively. Esmolol may also be useful in managing patients with unstable angina or dissecting aorta.

SPECIAL GROUPS

Race: black hypertensive patients may be less responsive than white patients

Children: safety and effectiveness have not been established

Elderly: start with a low dose and titrate the dose based on clinical response

Renal impairment: titrate the dose based on clinical response

Hepatic impairment: titrate the dose based on clinical response

Pregnancy: category C; should only be used if clearly indicated

Breast-feeding: use with caution; not known if the drug is excreted in human milk

DOSAGE

Supraventricular tachycardia: Treatment should be initiated with a loading infusion of 0.5 mg/kg over 1 min, followed by 50 µg/kg/min infusion. If an adequate response is not achieved after 5–10 min, repeat the same loading dose over 1 min and increase the rate of infusion to 100 µg/kg/min. This titration process should be repeated with a bolus followed by a 50 µg/kg/min increment in infusion rate until a desired response is achieved. Then, the maintenance infusion can be decreased or increased based on the desired endpoint. Most patients respond within the range of 25–200 µg/kg/min. Alternative antiarrhythmic agents, such as a longer acting beta-blocker, verapamil, or digoxin, should also be considered for long-term patient management if indicated.

Intraoperative and postoperative tachycardia and hypertension:
Rapid intraoperative control—Administer an 80 mg (1 mg/kg) IV bolus dose over 30 s, followed by a 150 µg/kg/min infusion and titrate the dose to maintained desired heart rate or BP (up to 300 µg/kg/min)
Gradual postoperative control—Dose titration schedule is the same as the treatment in supraventricular tachycardia; however, higher dosages, up to 250–300 µg/kg/min, may be required for adequate BP control.

IN BRIEF

INDICATIONS
Supraventricular tachycardia
Intraoperative and postoperative hypertension

CONTRAINDICATIONS
Bronchial asthma or related bronchospastic problems
Cardiogenic shock
Known hypersensitivity
Second- or third-degree AV block
Severe bradycardia
Severe decompensated heart failure
Sick sinus syndrome without a permanent pacemaker in place

DRUG INTERACTIONS
Beta-agonists
Calcium-channel blockers: verapamil or diltiazem
Diuretics
Other antihypertensive agents
Digoxin
Insulin
Oral hypoglycemic agents

ADVERSE EFFECTS
CV: bradycardia, hypotension, peripheral vascular insufficiency/Raynaud's type, syncope, heart failure, AV block, ventricular arrhythmia, angina
CNS: fatigue, dizziness, drowsiness, confusion, headache, depression, paresthesia
Respiratory: dyspnea, bronchospasm, nasal congestion
GI: nausea, vomiting
GU: urinary retention
Other: infusion site reactions, edema, weight gain, allergic reaction, rash, purpura

PHARMACOKINETICS AND PHARMACODYNAMICS
Duration of action: 10–20 min
Onset of action: within minutes
Peak effect: <5 min (with bolus); 30 minutes (without bolus)
Bioavailability: 100%
Effect of food: not applicable
Metabolism: metabolized by esterases in the blood
Clearance: (renal) 73%–88%; mainly as metabolites
Plasma half-life: 2 min (distribution); 9 min (elimination)
Protein binding: 55%

MONITORING
BP, heart rate, ECG, respiratory status.

OVERDOSE
Supportive—Esmolol is a short-acting agent. For severe bradycardia, atropine 2 mg IV may be administered or a pacemaker should be placed. For cardiovascular support, glucagon 5–10 mg IV bolus administered over 30 s, followed by 5 mg/hr continuous infusion. Fluid therapy with vasopressors /inotropic therapy added if necessary may also be appropriate.

PATIENT INFORMATION
Esmolol is used for adequate BP or heart rate control.

AVAILABILITY
Ampules—2500 mg/10 mL (250 mg/mL), not for direct IV injection
Vials—100 mg/10 mL (10 mg/mL)

The information here is provided as guidance only. Prescribers should always consult the manufacturer's current prescribing information.

135

METOPROLOL SUCCINATE
METOPROLOL TARTRATE

(Metoprolol Tartrate, Lopressor®)
(Toprol XL®)

Metoprolol is a beta₁ antagonist without the intrinsic sympathomimetic activity. Its beta₁ selectivity is less potent than atenolol. Metoprolol also lacks membrane-stabilizing activity within the usual therapeutic range. In addition to its antihypertensive and anti-ischemic effects, metoprolol has been shown to reduce both morbidity and mortality in patients with acute MI. Clinical data also support chronic metoprolol therapy, which reduces recurrent cardiovascular events in these patients. Metoprolol therapy also provided long-term benefits in reducing mortality and morbidity in patients with mild to moderate congestive cardiomyopathy in the MERIT-HF trial. Other potential uses of this agent include left ventricular hypertrophy and dilated cardiomyopathy with diastolic dysfunction. An equivalent maximal beta-blockade of metoprolol is achieved with oral and intravenous doses in the ratio of approximately 2.5:1.

SPECIAL GROUPS

Race: black hypertensive patients may be less responsive than white patients

Children: safety and effectiveness have not been established

Elderly: start with a low dose and titrate the dose based on clinical response

Renal impairment: no dose reduction is required; titrate the dose based on clinical response

Hepatic impairment: titrate the dose based on clinical response

Pregnancy: category C; should only be used if clearly indicated

Breast-feeding: not recommended; excreted in human milk

DOSAGE

Hypertension: 100–450 mg/d. The initial dose is 100 mg/d in single or divided doses. The dose should be adjusted at weekly intervals (or longer) until the desired BP control is achieved.

Angina pectoris: 100–400 mg/d in two divided doses. Same dose titration as recommended in the management of hypertension

MI: Treatment should be initiated as soon as the patient's hemodynamic status has stabilized; three 5 mg IV bolus injections of metoprolol should be administered at 2 min intervals. If the full 15 mg dose is tolerated by the patients, 50 mg of metoprolol (or 25 mg for those who cannot tolerate the full dose) every 6 h should be initiated 15 min after the last IV dose and continued for 48 h. Then, the dose may be adjusted to 100 mg twice daily.

IN BRIEF

INDICATIONS
Angina pectoris
Hypertension
MI

CONTRAINDICATIONS
Bronchial asthma or related bronchospastic problems
Cardiogenic shock
Known hypersensitivity
Second- or third-degree AV block
Severe bradycardia
Severe decompensated heart failure
Sick sinus syndrome without a permanent pacemaker in place

DRUG INTERACTIONS
Beta agonists
Calcium-channel blockers: verapamil or diltiazem
Diuretics
Other antihypertensive agents
Insulin
Oral hypoglycemic agents
NSAIDs

ADVERSE EFFECTS
CV: bradycardia, hypotension, peripheral vascular insufficiency/Raynaud's type, syncope, cold extremities, heart failure, AV block, ventricular arrhythmia, angina
CNS: fatigue, dizziness, drowsiness, confusion, headache, depression, sleep disturbance
Respiratory: dyspnea, bronchospasm, nasal congestion
GI: nausea, vomiting
GU: male impotence, ejaculatory failure
Metabolic: dyslipidemia
Other: edema, weight gain, allergic reaction, rash

PHARMACOKINETICS AND PHARMACODYNAMICS
Duration of action
(dose-dependent): (IV) 5–8 h; (po) 12–24 h; > 24 h for slow release
Onset of action: (IV) within minutes; (po) 15 min
Peak effect: (IV) 20 min; (po) 1–2 h; >7 h for slow-released
Bioavailability: (IV) 100%; (po) 50%; 40% for slow release
Effect of food: (tartrate salt) increased absorption; (succinate salt) no effect
Metabolism: metabolized in the liver
Excretion: renal (5%–10% as unchanged)
Plasma half-life: 3–7 h
Protein binding: 12%

MONITORING
BP, heart rate, ECG, respiratory status, and clinical improvement.

OVERDOSE
Supportive: For severe bradycardia, atropine 2 mg IV may be administered or a pacemaker should be placed. For cardiovascular support, glucagon 5–10 mg IV bolus administered over 30 s, followed by 5 mg/h continuous infusion. Fluid therapy with vasopressors/inotropic therapy added if necessary may also be appropriate.

PATIENT INFORMATION
Metoprolol therapy should not be discontinued abruptly without consulting a physician. The physician should also be consulted for persistent or unusual problems, such as dizziness/faintness, weight gain, worsening edema, or increasing shortness of breath. Sit or lie down if dizziness occurs and rise slowly from a sitting or lying position.

AVAILABILITY
Tablets—50, 100 mg (Lopressor); 50, 100, 200 mg (Toprol XL)
Ampules—5 mg/5 mL
Combination Formulations with a diuretic:
Lopressor® HCT tablets:
  50/25 50 mg metoprolol/25 mg hydrochlorothiazide
  100/25 100 mg metoprolol/25 mg hydrochlorothiazide
  100/50 100 mg metoprolol/50 mg hydrochlorothiazide

Some beta blockers, in addition to inhibiting the effects of sympathetic activity, possess some stimulant activity of their own, termed PAA or ISA. The partial agonist, however, differs from that of epinephrine or isoproterenol in that the maximal response of the tissue is lower (Fig. 7.4). ISA may be competitively inhibited by a beta blocker with no such property, such as propranolol. The degree of ISA in some of the available beta blockers has been quantified (Fig. 7.5).

EFFICACY AND USE

Beta blockers with ISA cause a decrease in resting heart rate to a lesser degree than beta blockers without ISA. Indeed, a beta blocker with moderate to high ISA can increase resting heart rate if sympathetic tone is low. During exercise or stress, when sympathetic drive is high, beta blockers with ISA act more like full antagonists although the maximum heart rate reduction is usually less than that achieved with beta blockers without ISA. Under resting conditions, cardiac output is minimally depressed by beta blockers with high ISA. Under conditions of high sympathetic drive, the fall in cardiac output approximates that observed with beta blockers without ISA. In patients with chronically impaired left ventricular function (dependent on increased sympathetic drive) given beta blockers with a moderate degree of ISA, such as pindolol, the reduction in cardiac output may cause heart failure. Newer agents with a high degree of ISA (45%–50%) may benefit patients with milder forms of heart failure.

The IPPPSH study, involving more than 6000 moderately hypertensive patients, suggested that a beta blocker with ISA could reduce coronary events in nonsmoking men.

Beta blockers with ISA possess antianginal properties similar to their counterparts without ISA but tend to be less effective (particularly at night when an increase in heart rate can prolong ischemic episodes).

Beta blockers with ISA are shown to be less effective after infarction, achieving only about a 10% decrease in mortality compared to 25%–30% achieved with beta blockers without ISA. However, acebutolol (with only 10% $beta_1$ ISA) was found to be effective in high-risk post-infarction patients. Beta blockers with ISA are probably as effective as non-ISA beta blockers in reducing the rate of reinfarction.

Under experimental conditions, beta blockers with moderate ISA tend to affect the cardiac conduction system to a lesser extent than agents without ISA, except under conditions of high sympathetic tone. Pindolol has antiarrhythmic activity, but may also increase ventricular ectopic beats.

Nonselective agents with ISA, such as pindolol, can still cause marked bronchoconstriction in patients with asthma and hyperreactive airway problems. They also competitively inhibit the bronchodilatory action of $beta_2$ agonists. While adverse reactions, such as cold peripheries and fatigue, tend to be less common with beta blockers with ISA, increased incidence of tremor and muscle cramps have been reported.

MODE OF ACTION

ISA is best expressed in humans when baseline sympathetic activity is minimal. For example, at night, pindolol acts as a stimulant to increase resting heart rate. During exercise, however, the beta antagonism of pindolol predominates and inhibits maximum heart rate acceleration.

Although data are limited, it is probable that the ISA contained within a $beta_1$-selective beta blocker will express itself only through the $beta_1$ receptor, and the ISA of a nonselective beta blocker acts on both $beta_1$ and $beta_2$ receptors. A nonselective agent, however, can possess predominantly $beta_2$-selective ISA. Beta Blockers with significant $beta_2$-ISA lower BP mainly by reducing peripheral resistance (beta$_2$ vasodilatation, Figure 7.2). Possession of significant $beta_1$ ISA results in little peripheral action and minimal effect on cardiac output so that resting BP is lowered to a lesser degree or even increased. Resting BP is lowered by a nonselective beta blocker with moderate nonselective ISA or $beta_2$-selective ISA more by a reduction in peripheral resistance than a fall in cardiac output. Beta$_1$ selective ISA is associated with a diminution or abolition of antihypertensive efficacy.

INDICATIONS

	Nonselective Agents			Beta₁ Selective Agent
	Carteolol	Penbutolol	Pindolol	Acebutolol
Hypertension	+	+	+	+
Arrhythmias	–	–	–	+
Angina	–	–	–	–
Mild Congestive Heart Failure	–	–	–	–

+—approved by the FDA; – —not approved by the FDA.

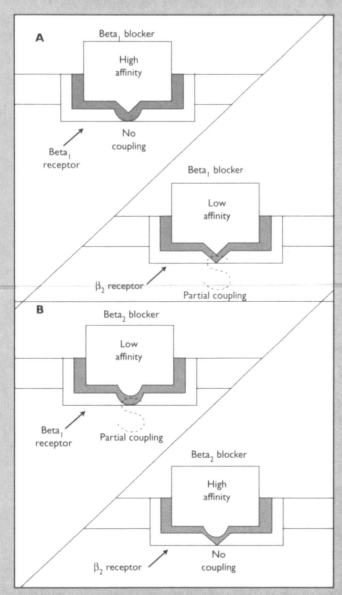

FIGURE 7.4 Examples of receptor affinity/coupling characteristics of a beta₁-selective blocker with beta₂-selective ISA and a beta₂-selective blocker with beta₁-selective ISA. (*Adapted from* Cruickshank JM: Measurement and cardiovascular relevance of partial agonist activity (PAA) involving beta₁- and beta₂- adrenoceptors. *Pharmacol Ther* 1990, 46:199–242.)

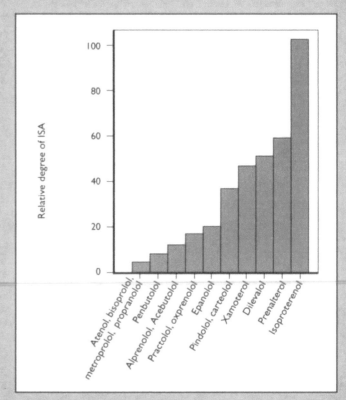

FIGURE 7.5 Relative degree of intrinsic sympathomimetic activity of various beta blockers.

ACEBUTOLOL
(Acebutolol, Sectral®)

Acebutolol is a selective beta₁-adrenergic antagonist with mild ISA within the usual therapeutic range. Its relative potency on beta₁-blockade is only 10%–30% of that of propranolol. At high doses (> 800 mg daily), the beta₁-selectivity of acebutolol diminishes and it inhibits both beta₁-and beta₂-receptors competitively. Both acebutolol and its active metabolite, diacetolol, are responsible for the therapeutic effect observed clinically. It has been shown that serum diacetolol levels have been consistently higher than acebutolol secondary to its long half-life. Diacetolol has similar beta-blockade activity to acebutolol and also possesses weak ISA activity. Diacetolol may contribute substantially to the therapeutic effect of acebutolol. Since diacetolol is primarily cleared by the kidney and can accumulate in patients with renal dysfunction, lower maintenance doses are recommended.

SPECIAL GROUPS

Race: black hypertensive patients may be less responsive than white patients

Children: safety and effectiveness have not been established

Elderly: two-fold increase in bioavailability; start with low dose and titrate the dose based on clinical response

Renal impairment: use with caution; dose reduction is required because diacetolol will accumulate

Hepatic impairment: use with caution; dosage adjustment is probably not required

Pregnancy: category B; should only be used if clearly indicated

Breast-feeding: not recommended; excreted in human milk

DOSAGE

Hypertension: 200–1200 mg/d. The initial dose is 200–400 mg administered as a single dose or twice daily. The dose may be gradually increased based on clinical response up to 600 mg twice daily. Most patients require 400–800 mg/d.

Ventricular arrhythmia: 400–1200 mg/d in 2 divided doses

IN BRIEF

INDICATIONS
Hypertension
Ventricular arrhythmia

CONTRAINDICATIONS
Bronchial asthma or related bronchospastic problems
Cardiogenic shock
Known hypersensitivity
Second- or third-degree AV block
Sick sinus syndrome without a permanent pacemaker in place
Severe bradycardia
Severe decompensated heart failure

DRUG INTERACTIONS
Beta agonists
Calcium-channel blockers: verapamil or diltiazem
Diuretics
Other antihypertensive agents
Insulin
Oral hypoglycemic agents
NSAIDs

ADVERSE EFFECTS
CV: bradycardia, peripheral vascular insufficiency/Raynaud's type, postural hypotension, syncope, hypotension, heart failure, AV block, ventricular arrhythmia, angina
CNS: fatigue, dizziness, drowsiness, depression, headache, sleep disturbances
Respiratory: dyspnea, bronchospasm, nasal congestion
GI: constipation, dyspepsia, nausea, diarrhea, liver function abnormality
GU: male impotence, ejaculatory failure, urinary frequency
Metabolic: dyslipidemia
Other: edema, weight gain, allergic reaction, rash, pruritus, lupus-like syndrome, positive ANA

PHARMACOKINETICS AND PHARMACODYNAMICS
Duration of action: >24 h
Onset of action: 1–2 h
Peak effect: 3–8 h
Bioavailability: 40%
Effect of food: slower absorption and lower peak concentration, but similar extent of absorption
Metabolism: mainly metabolized in the liver, diacetolol is the active metabolite
Excretion: 30%–40% in urine; 50%–60% in stools
Plasma half-life: 3–4 h; 8–13 h (diacetolol)
Protein binding: 26%

MONITORING
BP, heart rate, ECG, respiratory status, and other appropriate clinical response.

OVERDOSE
Supportive: For severe bradycardia, atropine 2 mg IV may be administered or a pacemaker should be placed. For cardiovascular support, glucagon 5–10 mg IV bolus administered over 30 s, followed by 5 mg/h continuous infusion. Fluid therapy with vasopressors /inotropic therapy added if necessary may also be appropriate.

PATIENT INFORMATION
Acebutolol therapy should not be discontinued abruptly without consulting a physician. The physician should also be consulted for persistent or unusual problems such as dizziness/faintness, weight gain, worsening edema, or increasing shortness of breath. Sit or lie down if dizziness occurs and rise slowly from a sitting or lying position.

AVAILABILITY
Capsules—200, 400 mg

CARTEOLOL

(Cartrol®)

Carteolol is a long-acting, nonselective beta-adrenergic receptor antagonist with ISA and without significant membrane stabilizing activity. Because of its partial beta-agonist activity, carteolol does not reduce resting heart rate as much as other beta blockers without ISA. It does not have clinically significant antiarrhythmic activity. Carteolol is either used alone or in combination with other agents for the management of hypertension. It is also available as an ophthalmic solution for open-angle glaucoma.

SPECIAL GROUPS

Race: black hypertensive patients may be less responsive than white patients

Children: safety and effectiveness have not been established

Elderly: start with low dose and adjust dosing intervals based on renal function

Renal impairment: use with caution; adjust dosing intervals based on renal function

Hepatic impairment: use with caution; dosage adjustment is probably not required

Pregnancy: category C; should only be used if clearly indicated

Breast-feeding: use with caution; not known if the drug is excreted in human milk

DOSAGE

2.5–10 mg once daily (usual maintenance dose is 2.5 or 5 mg once daily)
Guidelines for dosing intervals in patients with renal impairment (including elderly patients):

Creatinine Clearance (mL/min/1.73 m^2)	Dosing Interval (hours)
> 60	24
20–60	48
< 20	72

IN BRIEF

INDICATIONS
Hypertension
Open-angle glaucoma

CONTRAINDICATIONS
Bronchial asthma or related bronchospastic problems
Cardiogenic shock
Known hypersensitivity
Second- or third-degree AV block
Severe bradycardia
Severe decompensated heart failure
Sick sinus syndrome without a permanent pacemaker in place

DRUG INTERACTIONS
Beta agonists
Calcium-channel blockers: verapamil or diltiazem
Diuretics
Other antihypertensive agents
Insulin
Oral hypoglycemic agents
NSAIDs

ADVERSE EFFECTS
CV: bradycardia, peripheral vascular insufficiency/Raynaud's type, postural hypotension, syncope, hypotension, heart failure, AV block, ventricular arrhythmia, angina
CNS: fatigue, dizziness, drowsiness, depression, headache, sleep disturbances, paresthesia
Respiratory: dyspnea, bronchospasm, nasal congestion
GI: nausea, diarrhea
GU: male impotence, ejaculatory failure, urinary frequency
Other: edema, weight gain, allergic reaction, rash

PHARMACOKINETICS AND PHARMACODYNAMICS
Duration of action: >24 h
Onset of action: 1–3 h
Peak effect: 6 h
Bioavailability: 85%
Effect of food: slower absorption but no effect on the extent of absorption
Metabolism: partially metabolized with an active metabolite, 8-hydroxycarteolol
Excretion: mainly in urine (50%–70% unchanged; 5% as 8-hydroxycarteolol)
Plasma half-life: 6 h in normal renal function; 8–12 h (8-hydroxycarteolol, active)
Protein binding: 23%–30%

MONITORING
BP, heart rate, respiratory status and other appropriate clinical response.

OVERDOSE
Supportive: For severe bradycardia, atropine 2 mg IV may be administered or a pacemaker should be placed. For cardiovascular support, glucagon 5–10 mg IV bolus administered over 30 s, followed by 5 mg/h continuous infusion. Fluid therapy with vasopressors/inotropic therapy added if necessary may also be appropriate.

PATIENT INFORMATION
Carteolol therapy should not be discontinued abruptly without consulting a physician. The physician should also be consulted for persistent or unusual problems, such as dizziness/faintness, weight gain, worsening edema, or increasing shortness of breath. Sit or lie down if dizziness occurs and rise slowly from a sitting or lying position.

AVAILABILITY
Tablets —2.5, 5 mg
Ophthalmic Solutions—1%, 5 mL and 10 mL

PENBUTOLOL

(Levatol®)

Penbutolol is a long-acting, nonselective beta-adrenergic receptor antagonist with mild ISA. It is not clear if the ISA activity offers additional advantages in a clinical setting. The beta blocking potency of penbutolol is approximately 4 times that of propranolol. Maximum beta antagonism occurs with doses of 10–20 mg. Penbutolol may be used alone or in combination with other agents in the management of hypertension.

SPECIAL GROUPS

Race: black hypertensive patients may be less responsive than white patients

Children: safety and effectiveness have not been established

Elderly: start with low dose and adjust the dose based on clinical response

Renal impairment: use with caution; dosage adjustment is probably not required

Hepatic impairment: use with caution; adjust the dose based on clinical response

Pregnancy: category C; should only be used if clearly indicated

Breast-feeding: use with caution; not known if the drug is excreted in human milk

DOSAGE

20–80 mg once daily (usual maintenance dose is 20 mg once daily)

IN BRIEF

INDICATIONS
Hypertension

CONTRAINDICATIONS
Bronchial asthma or related bronchospastic problems
Cardiogenic shock
Known hypersensitivity
Second- or third-degree AV block
Severe bradycardia
Severe decompensated heart failure
Sick sinus syndrome without a permanent pacemaker in place

DRUG INTERACTIONS
Beta agonists
Calcium-channel blockers: verapamil or diltiazem
Diuretics
Other antihypertensive agents
Insulin
Oral hypoglycemic agents
NSAIDs

ADVERSE EFFECTS
CV: bradycardia, peripheral vascular insufficiency/Raynaud's type, postural hypotension, syncope, hypotension, heart failure, AV block, ventricular arrhythmia, angina
CNS: fatigue, dizziness, drowsiness, depression, headache, sleep disturbances
Respiratory: dyspnea, bronchospasm, nasal congestion
GI: dyspepsia, nausea, diarrhea
GU: male impotence, ejaculatory failure
Metabolic: dyslipidemia
Other: edema, weight gain, allergic reaction

PHARMACOKINETICS AND PHARMACODYNAMICS
Duration of action: > 20 h
Onset of action: <1 h
Peak effect: 2–3 h
Bioavailability: 100%
Effect of food: little effect
Metabolism: extensively metabolized
Excretion: 90% in urine, mainly as metabolites
Plasma half-life: 5 h
Protein binding: 80%–98%

MONITORING
BP, heart rate, respiratory status.

OVERDOSE
Supportive: For severe bradycardia, atropine 2 mg IV may be administered or a pacemaker should be placed. For cardiovascular support, glucagon 5–10 mg IV bolus administered over 30 s, followed by 5 mg/h continuous infusion. Fluid therapy with vasopressors/inotropic therapy added if necessary may also be appropriate.

PATIENT INFORMATION
Penbutolol therapy should not be discontinued abruptly without consulting a physician. The physician should also be consulted for persistent or unusual problems, such as dizziness/faintness, weight gain, worsening edema, or increasing shortness of breath. Sit or lie down if dizziness occurs and rise slowly from a sitting or lying position.

AVAILABILITY
Tablets—20 mg

The information here is provided as guidance only. Prescribers should always consult the manufacturer's current prescribing information.

141

PINDOLOL

(Pindolol, Visken®)

Pindolol is a nonselective beta-adrenergic receptor antagonist with ISA. It is not clear if the ISA activity offers additional advantages in a clinical setting. It also exhibits membrane-stabilizing activity (quinidine-like). Pindolol has less effect on reducing the heart rate and cardiac output at rest, although its effect on blocking stress- or exercise-induced tachycardia is similar to other beta blockers without ISA. Pindolol may be used alone or in combination with other agents in the management of hypertension. It may also be useful in the management of stress- or exercise-induced angina (not an indication approved by the FDA), especially in those patients with resting bradycardia and CHF.

SPECIAL GROUPS

Race: black hypertensive patients may be less responsive than white patients

Children: safety and effectiveness have not been established

Elderly: start with low dose and adjust the dose based on clinical response

Renal impairment: use with caution and adjust the dose based on clinical response

Hepatic impairment: use with caution and adjust the dose based on clinical response

Pregnancy: category B; should only be used if clearly indicated

Breast-feeding: not recommended; excreted in human milk

DOSAGE

10–60 mg/d in 2–3 divided doses (usual maintenance dose is 10–30 mg/d in 2–3 divided doses)

IN BRIEF

INDICATIONS
Hypertension

CONTRAINDICATIONS
Bronchial asthma or related bronchospastic problems
Cardiogenic shock
Known hypersensitivity
Second- or third-degree AV block
Severe bradycardia
Severe decompensated heart failure
Sick sinus syndrome without a permanent pacemaker in place

DRUG INTERACTIONS
Beta agonists
Calcium-channel blockers: verapamil or diltiazem
Diuretics
Other antihypertensive agents
Insulin
Oral hypoglycemic agents
NSAIDs

ADVERSE EFFECTS
CV: bradycardia, peripheral vascular insufficiency/Raynaud's type, postural hypotension, syncope, hypotension, heart failure, AV block, ventricular arrhythmia, angina
CNS: fatigue, dizziness, drowsiness, depression, headache, sleep disturbances
Respiratory: dyspnea, bronchospasm, nasal congestion
GI: nausea, abdominal discomfort, diarrhea, elevated liver enzymes
GU: male impotence, ejaculatory failure
Metabolic: dyslipidemia
Other: edema, weight gain, allergic reaction

PHARMACOKINETICS AND PHARMACODYNAMICS
Duration of action: 24 h
Onset of action: < 3 h
Peak effect: 1–2 h
Bioavailability: 50%–95%
Effect of food: only increase the rate of absorption
Metabolism: 60%–65% metabolized in liver
Excretion: 30%–50% excreted in urine unchanged
Plasma half-life: 3–4 h (↑ in elderly and renal dysfunction)
Protein binding: 40%–60%

MONITORING
BP, heart rate, respiratory status.

OVERDOSE
Supportive: For severe bradycardia, atropine 2 mg IV may be administered or a pacemaker should be placed. For cardiovascular support, glucagon 5–10 mg IV bolus administered over 30 s, followed by 5 mg/h continuous infusion. Fluid therapy with vasopressors/inotropic therapy added if necessary may also be appropriate.

PATIENT INFORMATION
Pindolol therapy should not be discontinued abruptly without consulting a physician. The physician should also be consulted for persistent or unusual problems such as dizziness/faintness, weight gain, worsening edema, or increasing shortness of breath. Sit or lie down if dizziness occurs and rise slowly from a sitting or lying position.

AVAILABILITY
Tablets—5, 10 mg

DUAL-ACTING BETA BLOCKERS

Some beta blockers, such as labetalol and carvedilol, have dual beta- and alpha-blocking properties. These agents improve arterial compliance through alpha blockade, and therefore may be particularly effective in reversing left ventricular hypertrophy. Carvedilol was the first beta blocker approved for use in CHF.

EFFICACY AND USE

Dual-acting agents are effective in lowering BP in patients with hypertension. Labetalol produces a fall in supine BP of the same order as pure beta blockers but is more effective in reducing BP in the upright position. The BP is lowered maximally within I–2 h, and once controlled, it remains low on chronic therapy. Severe hypertension often requires higher dosage. IV labetalol has been used effectively in hypertension associated with pregnancy.

Labetalol appears to be as effective as a thiazide diuretic in lowering supine and standing BP. It is more effective than hydralazine, although probably less effective than minoxidil. It has similar efficacy to methyldopa and clonidine, and is more effective than the sympatholytic agents, like guanethidine, bethanidine, and debrisoquine.

The combination of labetalol with a diuretic is an effective treatment for hypertension, with the fall in BP on the combination being greater than either agent alone. Labetalol has been combined with vasodilators, such as minoxidil, and calcium antagonists, to manage resistant hypertension.

Carvedilol is approved for use in hypertension, but it is also used as an adjunctive therapy in patients with CHF and systolic dysfunction. The drug has been shown to reduce morbidity and mortality in patients with heart failure secondary to either coronary artery disease or idiopathic cardiomyopathy.

Vasodilatory side effects relating to alpha blockade are seen, particularly at higher doses. Postural hypotension, scalp tingling, and genitourinary problems can be a problem in some patients. Classic adverse reactions to beta blockers, such as fatigue and cold peripheries associated to reduced cardiac output, are less common with this class of agents. Coronary risk factors, such as low plasma high-density lipoprotein (HDL) concentrations and high fibrinogen concentrations, are improved. The clinical relevance of these changes has yet to be established. These drugs tend to be lipid neutral, although the clinical significance of this is not yet clear.

MODE OF ACTION

Dual-acting beta blockers have only a moderate effect on resting cardiac output and, therefore, they lower BP primarily through a reduction in total peripheral resistance via alpha blockade or direct nonspecific vasodilatory properties. The afterload reduction may be beneficial when left ventricular function is impaired.

The exact mechanism for carvedilol's benefit in patients with heart failure is not clear. Various mechanisms have been postulated (Table 7.3). There is no clinical experience using labetalol in patients with heart failure.

INDICATIONS

	Labetalol	Carvedilol
Hypertension	+	+
Hypertensive Emergencies	+	–
CHF	–	+

+— approved by the FDA; – —not approved by the FDA.

TABLE 7.3 POSSIBLE MECHANISMS BY WHICH BETA-ADRENERGIC BLOCKERS IMPROVE VENTRICULAR FUNCTION IN CHRONIC CONGESTIVE HEART FAILURE

Upregulation of beta receptors	Increase in coronary blood flow by reducing heart rate and improving diastolic perfusion time; possible coronary dilatation with vasodilator beta blocker
Direct myocardial protective action against catecholamine toxicity	
Improved ability of noradrenergic sympathetic nerves to synthesize norepinephrine	Restoration of abnormal baroreflex function
Decreased release of norepinephrine from sympathetic nerve endings	Prevention of ventricular muscle hypertrophy and vascular remodeling
Decreased stimulation of other vasoconstrictive systems including renin-angiotensin-aldosterone, vasopressin, and endothelin	Antioxidant effects (carvedilol?)
	Shift from free fatty acid to carbohydrate metabolism (improved metabolic efficiency)
Potentiation of kallikrein-kinin system and natural vasodilatation (increase in bradykinin)	Vasodilatation (eg, bucindolol, carvedilol)
Antiarrhythmic effects raising ventricular fibrillation threshold	Antiapoptosis effect
Protection against catecholamine-induced hypokalemia	Modulation of post-receptor inhibitory G-proteins
Interference with anti-β receptor antibodies	Improved left atrial contribution to left ventricular filling

Adapted from Frishman WH: Alpha- and beta-adrenergic blocking drugs. In Frishman WH, Sonnenblick EH (eds): Cardiovascular Pharmacotherapeutics. McGraw Hill: New York; 1997: 80.

The information here is provided as guidance only. Prescribers should always consult the manufacturer's current prescribing information.

143

CARVEDILOL (Coreg®)

Similar to labetalol, carvedilol is a nonselective beta-adrenergic blocking agent with selective alpha$_1$ blocking activity. It has moderate membrane stabilizing activity but no ISA. In general, beta blockers, in addition to their antihypertensive and cardiac protective effects, may provide long-term clinical benefits in patients with heart failure by blocking the deleterious effects of the overacting sympathetic nervous system. Clinical studies have shown that bisoprolol, carvedilol, and metoprolol, when added to conventional therapy, may slow disease progression and reduce mortality and the frequency of hospitalization in patients with mild to moderate heart failure (NYHA class II and III). Although carvedilol is the first beta blocker approved in the United States as an add-on therapy in patients with heart failure, it is not clear if its dual alpha- and beta-adrenergic blocking activity offers additional advantage over other beta blockers. Because beta blockers may exacerbate heart failure, carvedilol therapy should be initiated with low doses (3.125 mg twice daily). Close patient monitoring for hypotension, bradycardia, and worsening of heart failure is recommended, especially during the first 2–4 wks of therapy and after each dose increase. Doses should be increased gradually or reduced based on patient tolerance and clinical response. A 1–3 mo trial period is required to determine the full benefits of carvedilol therapy.

SPECIAL GROUPS

Race: black hypertensive patients may be less responsive than white patients

Children: safety and effectiveness have not been established

Elderly: no differences in response

Renal impairment: titrate the dose based on response

Hepatic impairment: slower clearance; titrate the dose based on response

Pregnancy: category C; should only be used if clearly indicated

Breast-feeding: not recommended; not known if the drug is excreted in human milk

DOSAGE

CHF (NYHA class II or III): If the patient is taking ACE inhibitors, diuretics, or digoxin, the dosing of these agents should be stabilized prior to initiation of carvedilol.
3.125–50 mg twice daily.* The initial dose is 3.125 mg twice daily for 2 wk. If the dose is tolerated, then it may be doubled every 2–4 wk to the highest dose tolerated by the patient (up to 25 mg twice daily in patients weighing less than 85 kg and 50 mg twice daily in patients weighing more than 85 kg).

Hypertension: 6.25–25 mg twice daily.* The initial dose is 6.25 mg twice daily. The dose should be doubled every 1–2 wk based on BP response up to a maximum dose of 25 mg twice daily.

* The dose should be taken with food to slow down the rate of absorption and reduce the incidence of orthostatic effect. In patients with heart failure, slower titration with temporary dose reduction or withdrawal may be required based on clinical assessment; however, this should not preclude later attempts to reintroduce or increase the dose of carvedilol.

IN BRIEF

INDICATIONS
CHF (NYHA class II or III)
Hypertension

CONTRAINDICATIONS
Bronchial asthma or related bronchospastic problems
Cardiogenic shock
Known hypersensitivity
NYHA class IV decompensated heart failure requiring intravenous inotropic therapy
Second- or third-degree AV block
Severe bradycardia
Sick sinus syndrome without a permanent pacemaker in place

DRUG INTERACTIONS
Other antihypertensive agents
Rifampin
Cimetidine
Digoxin
Diltiazem
Verapamil
Certain antiarrhythmics
Catecholamine-depleting agents (such as reserpine, MAO inhibitors)
Insulin
Oral hypoglycemic agents

ADVERSE EFFECTS
CV: bradycardia, syncope, hypotension, postural hypotension, heart failure exacerbation, AV block, angina
CNS: fatigue, drowsiness
Respiratory: dyspnea, bronchospasm, nasal congestion
GI: hepatic injury, nausea, vomiting, diarrhea
GU: male impotence, ejaculatory failure
Metabolic: hyperglycemia, hypoglycemia, dyslipidemia
Other: edema, weight gain, thrombocytopenia, allergic reaction

PHARMACOKINETICS AND PHARMACODYNAMICS
Duration of action: 12–24 h
Onset of action: < 30 min
Peak effect: 1–7 h
Bioavailability: 25%–35%
Effect of food: slower absorption but has no effect on the extent of absorption
Clearance: mainly metabolized in the liver with three active metabolites identified; excreted mainly via the bile into feces and < 2% excreted unchanged in urine
Plasma half-life: 7–10 h
Protein binding: 95%–98%

MONITORING
BP, heart rate, weight, respiratory status, CBC, liver function, blood glucose.

OVERDOSE
Supportive: For severe bradycardia, atropine 2 mg IV may be administered or a pacemaker should be placed. For cardiovascular support, glucagon 5–10 mg IV bolus administered over 30 s, followed by 5 mg/h continuous infusion. Fluid therapy with vasopressors/inotropic therapy added if necessary may also be appropriate.

PATIENT INFORMATION
Carvedilol therapy should not be discontinued abruptly without consulting a physician. The physician should also be consulted if the patient experiences dizziness/faintness or signs and symptoms of worsening heart failure, such as unusual weight gain, worsening of edema, or increasing shortness of breath. Sit or lie down if dizziness occurs and rise slowly from a sitting or lying position.

AVAILABILITY
Tablets—3.125, 6.25, 12.5, 25 mg

LABETALOL (Normodyne®, Trandate®)

Labetalol is an adrenergic receptor blocking agent that has both selective alpha$_1$ and nonselective beta adrenergic receptor blocking actions. In humans, the ratios of alpha to beta blockade have been estimated to be approximately 1:2 and 1:7 after oral and IV administration, respectively. Beta$_2$ agonist activity has also been demonstrated, but labetalol does not possess membrane stabilizing activity. It is effective in increased BP and angina. Vasodilating side effects, such as scalp tingling and postural hypotension, can be a problem for some patients, particularly at higher doses. Several cases of hepatic failure, including deaths, have been reported with labetalol. Patients with severe hypertension often respond to IV labetalol.

SPECIAL GROUPS

Race: black hypertensive patients may be less responsive than white patients
Children: safety and effectiveness have not been established
Elderly: no differences in response
Renal impairment: titrate the dose based on response
Hepatic impairment: increased bioavailability and slower clearance; titrate the dose based on response
Pregnancy: category C; should only be used if clearly indicated
Breast-feeding: excreted in human milk; used with caution

DOSAGE

PO: Initial dose is 100 mg twice daily; dose may be titrated in increments of 100 mg every 2–3 d based on BP response
Usual maintenance dose: 200– 400 mg bid; maximum dose: 1200–2400 mg/d in 2–3 divided dose
Intermittent IV administration: 20 mg (0.25 mg/kg) slow IV over 2 min; additional doses of 20, 40, or 80 mg may be administered every 10 min until a desired supine BP is achieved or a total dose of 300 mg has been injected.
Continuous IV administration: 0.5–2 mg/min
Dose should be titrated based on BP response. The infusion should be continued until an adequate response is achieved or a total dose of 300 mg is infused. The infusion is then discontinued and oral therapy is initiated when supine BP begins to increase. Initial dose is 200 mg, followed in 6–12 h by an additional oral dose of 200 or 400 mg, depending on BP response

IN BRIEF

INDICATIONS
Hypertension

CONTRAINDICATIONS
Bronchial asthma or related bronchospastic problems
Cardiogenic shock
Severe bradycardia with second- or third-degree AV block
Severe heart failure
Sick sinus syndrome without a permanent pacemaker in place

DRUG INTERACTIONS
Beta agonists
Calcium-channel blockers: verapamil or diltiazem
Cimetidine
Diuretics
Other antihypertensive agents
Halothane
Tricyclic antidepressants
Insulin
Oral hypoglycemic agents

ADVERSE EFFECTS
CV: postural hypotension, syncope, hypotension, heart failure exacerbation, bradycardia, AV block, ventricular arrhythmia, angina
CNS: fatigue, drowsiness, headache, paresthesia
Respiratory: dyspnea, bronchospasm, nasal congestion
GI: hepatic injury, jaundice, nausea, vomiting, dyspepsia
GU: male impotence, ejaculatory failure
Metabolic: dyslipidemia
Other: edema, weight gain, allergic reaction

PHARMACOKINETICS AND PHARMACODYNAMICS
Duration of action: 8–24 h (po); 2–4 h (IV)
Onset of action: 20 min (po); 2–5 min (IV)
Peak effect: 1–4 h (po); 5–15 minutes (IV)
Bioavailability: 26%–36% (po); 100% (IV)
Effect of food: delay but increase the extent of absorption
Metabolism: mainly metabolized in the liver and GI mucosa
Excretion: biliary—30%; urine—55%–60% (< 5% unchanged)
Plasma half-life: 6–8 h (po), 5.5 h (IV)
Protein binding: 50%

MONITORING
BP, heart rate, respiratory status.

OVERDOSE
Supportive: For severe bradycardia, atropine 2 mg IV may be administered or a pacemaker should be placed. For cardiovascular support, glucagon 5–10 mg IV bolus administered over 30 s, followed by 5 mg/h continuous infusion. Fluid therapy with vasopressors/inotropic therapy added if necessary may also be appropriate.

PATIENT INFORMATION
Labetalol therapy should not be discontinued abruptly without consulting a physician. The physician should also be consulted for persistent or unusual problems, such as dizziness/faintness, weight gain, worsening edema, increasing shortness of breath, anorexia, jaundice, pruritus, dark urine, flu-like syndrome, and right upper quadrant tenderness. Sit or lie down if dizziness occurs and rise slowly from a sitting or lying position.

AVAILABILITY
Tablets—100, 200, 300 mg
Vials—5 mg/mL, 20 mL, and 40 mL
Syringes—5 mg/mL, 4 mL, and 8 mL

Australia/New Zealand Heart Failure Research Collaborative Group: Randomised, placebo-controlled trial of carvedilol in patients with congestive heart failure due to ischaemic heart disease. *Lancet* 1997, 349:375–380.

Beta-Blocker Heart Attack Trial Research Group: A randomized trial of propranolol in patients with acute myocardial infarction. *JAMA* 1982, 247:1707–1713.

Black JW: Ahlquist and the development of beta-adrenoceptor antagonists. *Postgrad Med J* 1976, 52 (suppl 4):11–13.

Boissel JP, Leizorovicz A, Picolet H, *et al.*: Secondary prevention after high-risk acute myocardial infarction with low-dose acebutolol. *Am J Cardiol* 1990, 66:251–260.

Carson PE: β-blocker therapy in heart failure: pathophysiology and clinical results. *Curr Prob Card* 1999, 24: 421–460.

Cavusoglu E, Frishman WH: Sotalol: a new β-adrenergic blockers for ventricular arrhythmias. *Prog Cardiovasc Dis* 1995, 37:423–440.

Chadda K, Goldstein S, Byington R, Curb JD: Effects of propranolol after acute myocardial infarction in patients with congestive heart failure. *Circulation* 1986, 73:503–510.

CIBIS Investigators and Committees: A randomized trial of β blockade in heart failure: The Cardiac Insufficiency Bisoprolol Study (CIBIS). *Circulation* 1994, 90:1765–1773.

CIBIS II Investigators and Committees: The Cardiac Insufficiency Bisoprolol Study II (CIBIS II): a randomized trial. *Lancet* 1999, 353:9–13.

Coope J, Warrender TS: Randomised trial of treatment of hypertension in elderly patients in primary care. *Br Med J* 1986, 293:1145–1148.

Cruickshank JM: Measurement and cardiovascular relevance of partial agonist activity (PAA) involving beta1- and beta2-adrenoceptors. *Pharmacol Ther* 1990, 46:199–242.

Cruickshank JM, Pennert K, Sorman A, *et al.*: Low mortality from all causes, including myocardial infarction, in well-controlled hypertensives treated with a beta blocker plus other antihyper-tensives. *J Hypertens* 1987, 5:489–498.

DiBona GF, Sawin LL: Effect of metoprolol administration on renal sodium handling in experimental heart failure. *Circulation* 1999, 100:82–86.

Dwyer N, Walter P, Cruickshank JM, *et al.*: Effect of propranolol and phentolamine on myocardial necrosis after subarachnoid haemorrhage. *Br Med J* 1978, 2:990–992.

Engelmeier RS, O'Connell JB, Walsh R, *et al.*: Improvements in symptoms and exercise tolerance by metoprolol in patients with dilated cardiomyopathy. *Circulation* 1985, 72:536–546.

Frishman WH: Secondary prevention of myocardial infarction: the roles of beta-adrenergic blockers, calcium-channel blockers, angiotensin converting enzyme inhibitors and aspirin. In *Triggering of Acute Coronary Syndromes: Implications for Prevention*. Edited by Willich SN, Muller JE. Dordrecht: Kluwer Academic Publishers; 1995:367–394.

Frishman WH: Alpha- and beta-adrenergic blocking drugs. In *Cardiovascular Pharmacotherapeutics*. Edited by Frishman WH, Sonnenblick EH. New York: McGraw Hill; 1997:59–94.

Frishman WH: Alpha- and beta-adrenergic blocking drugs. In *Cardiovascular Pharmacotherapeutics Companion Handbook*. Edited by Frishman WH, Sonnenblick EH. New York: McGraw Hill; 1998:23–64.

Frishman WH: Carvedilol. *N Engl J Med* 1998, 339:1759–1765.

Frishman WH: β-Adrenergic blockers. In *Hypertension Primer*, edn 2. Edited by Izzo JL Jr, Black HR. Dallas: American Heart Association; 1998:362–365.

Frishman WH, Burris FJ, Mroczek WJ, *et al.*: First-line therapy option with low-dose bisoprolol fumarate and low-dose hydrocholorothiazide in patients with stage I and stage II systemic hypertension. *J Clin Pharacol* 1995, 35:182–188.

Frishman WH, Bryzinski BS, Coulson LR, *et al.*: A multifactorial trial design to assess combination therapy in hypertension: treatment with bisoprolol and hydrochlorothiazide. *Arch Intern Med* 1994, 154:1461–1468.

Frishman WH, Cheng A: Secondary prevention of myocardial infarction: the role of β-adrenergic blockers and angiotensin converting enzyme inhibitors: based on symposium *Agents to Prevent Acute Coronary Disease*. *Am Heart J* 1999, 137:S25–S34.

Frishman WH, Christiana J: The current use of beta blockers in cardiovascular disease. In *Cardiology Clinics Annual of Drug Therapy*, vol 2. Edited by Crawford MH. Philadelphia: W.B. Saunders; 1998:37–59.

Frishman WH, Murthy VS, Strom JA, Hershman D: Ultra-short-acting β-adrenergic blocking drugs. In *Cardiovascular Drug Therapy*, edn 2. Edited by Messerli FH. Philadelphia: W.B. Saunders; 1996:507–516.

Frishman WH, Skolnick AE: Secondary prevention post infarction: the role of β-adrenergic blockers, calcium-channel blockers and aspirin. In *Acute Myocardial Infarction*, edn 2. Edited by Gersh BJ, Rahimtoola SH. New York: Chapman and Hall; 1996:766–796.

Frishman WH, Sonnenblick EH: β-Adrenergic blocking drugs and calcium channel blockers. In *Hurst'sThe Heart*, edn 9. Edited by Alexander RW, Schlant RC, Fuster V. New York: McGraw Hill; 1998:1583–1618.

Goldstein S, Hjalmarson A: Metoprolol CR/XL randomized intervention trial in congestive heart failure (MERIT-HF): an update after completed randomization: The International Steering Committee on behalf of the MERIT-HF Study Group [abstract]. *Circulation* 1998, 98 (Suppl):I–364.

Hjalmarson A, Herlitz J, Holmbert S, *et al.*: The Goteborg Metoprolol Trial: effects on mortality and morbidity in acute myocardial infarction. *Circulation* 1983, 67 (Suppl I):I36–I32.

Hohnloser SH, Meinertz T, Klingenheben T, *et al.*: Usefulness of esmolol in unstable angina pectoris. *Am J Cardiol* 1991, 67:1319–1323.

ISIS-1 Collaborative Group: Randomised trial of intravenous atenolol among 16,027 cases of suspected acute myocardial infarction: ISIS-1. *Lancet* 1986, ii:57–66.

Kjekshus J: Comments: beta blockers and heart rate reduction: a mechanism of benefit. *Eur Heart J* 1985, 6 (Suppl A):29–30.

Kjekshus J, Gilpin E, Cali G, *et al.*: Diabetic patients and beta blockers after acute myocardial infarction. *Eur Heart J* 1990, 11:43–50.

Lubsen J, Tijssen JGP, Study Group: Efficacy of nifedipine and metoprolol in the early treatment of unstable angina in the coronary care unit: findings from the Holland Interuniversity Nifedipine/Metoprolol Trial (HINT). *Am J Cardiol* 1987, 60:18A–25A.

Man In't Veld AJ, van den Meiracker AH: Effects of antihypertensive drugs on cardiovascular haemodynamics. In *Hypertension*. Edited by Laragh JH, Brenner BM. New York: Raven Press; 1990, 2117–2130.

Mason JW for the Electrophysiologic Study Versus Electrocardiographic Monitoring Investigators (ESVEM): A comparison of seven antiarrhythmic drugs in patients with ventricular tachyarrhythmias. *N Engl J Med* 1993, 329:452–458.

McAinsh H, Cruickshank JM: Beta blockers and the central nervous system side effects. *Pharmacol Ther* 1990, 46:163–197.

MERIT-HF Study Group: Effect of metoprolol CR/XL in chronic heart failure: Metoprolol CR/XL Randomised Intervention Trial in Congestive Heart Failure (MERIT-HF). *Lancet* 1999, 353: 2001–2007.

Miall WE, Greenberg D: The Medical Working Party on mild to moderate hypertension: the influence of thiazide and beta-blocker treatment on ECG findings. In *Mild Hypertension: Is There Pressure to Treat? An Account of the MRC Trial*. Cambridge: Cambridge University Press; 1987:78–94; 181–185.

MIAMI Trial Research Group: Metoprolol in Acute Myocardial Infarction (MIAMI): a randomised placebo-controlled international trial. *Eur Heart J* 1985, 6:199–226.

Mohindra SK, Udeani GO: Intravenous esmolol in acute aortic dissection. *Ann Pharmacother* 1991, 25:735–738.

MRC Working Party: MRC Trial of Treatment of Mild Hypertension: principal results. *Br Med J* 1985, 291:97–104.

Norwegian Multicentre Study Group: Timolol-induced reduction in mortality and reinfarction in patients surviving acute myocardial infarction. *N Engl J Med* 1981, 304:801–807.

Opie LH, Sonnenblick EH, Frishman WH, Thadani U: Beta-blocking agents. In *Drugs for the Heart*, edn 4. Edited by Opie LH. Philadelphia: W.B. Saunders; 1995:1–30.

Packer M, Bristow MR, Cohn JN, *et al.*: The effect of carvedilol on morbidity and mortality in patient with chronic heart failure. *N Engl J Med* 1996, 334:1349–1355.

Pepine CJ, Cohn PF, Deedwania PC, *et al.*: Effects of treatment on outcome in asymptomatic and mildly symptomatic patients with ischemia during daily life: The Atenolol Silent Ischemia Study (ASIST). *Circulation* 1994, 90:762–768.

Quyyumi AA, Crake T, Wright CM, *et al.*: Medical treatment of patients with severe exertional and rest angina in a double-bind comparison of beta blocker, calcium antagonist and nitrate. *Br Heart J* 1987, 57:505–511.

Rapaport E: Should beta blockers be given immediately and concomitantly with thrombolytic therapy in acute myocardial infarction? *Circulation* 1991, 83:695–697.

Sandberg A, Blomqvist I, Jonsson UE, Lundborg P: Pharmacokinetic and pharmacodynamic properties of a new controlled-release formulation of metoprolol: a comparison with conventional tablets. *Eur J Clin Pharmacol* 1988, 33 (Suppl):S9–S14.

Sharma S, Mitra S, Grover VK, *et al.*: Esmolol blunt the haemodynamic responses to tracheal intubation in treated hypertensive patients. *Can J Anaesth* 1996, 43:778–782.

The SHEP Cooperative Research Group: Prevention of stroke by antihypertensive drug treatment in older persons with isolated systolic hypertension: final results of Systolic Hypertension in the Elderly Program (SHEP). *JAMA* 1991, 265:3255–3264.

Smerling A, Gersony WM: Esmolol for severe hypertension following repair of aortic coarctation. *Crit Care Med* 1990, 18:1288–1290.

Wikstrand J, Warnold I, Olsson G, *et al.*: Primary prevention with metoprolol in patients with hypertension. *JAMA* 1988, 159:1976–1982.

Wilhelmsen L, Berglund G, Elmfeldt D, *et al.*: Beta blockers versus diuretics in hypertensive men: main results from the HAPPHY trial. *J Hypertens* 1987, 5:561–572.

Verapamil, a coronary vasodilator, was reported in 1962 to possess negative inotropic and chronotropic effects that were not seen with other apparently similar vasodilator agents, such as nitroglycerin. The mechanism of action of verapamil was initially thought to be a result of coronary vasodilatation and blockade of myocardial beta adrenergic receptors. Later, however, it was shown that the mechanism of action was not related to beta receptor blockade but to inhibition of the movement of calcium ions into cells, with resulting inhibition of excitation-contraction coupling. **Verapamil** and the later drugs, **nifedipine** and **diltiazem**, became known as calcium antagonists because they inhibit the flux of calcium through the voltage-dependent "L" channel.

Unlike the beta blockers, not all calcium antagonists are chemically related (Table 8.1). The prototype calcium antagonist, **verapamil**, is a benzeneacetronitrile; **nifedipine** is a dihydropyridine derivative; and **diltiazem** is structurally related to the benzothiazepines. The second generation calcium antagonists are mainly nifedipine-like dihydropyridines. These agents differ in potency, tissue specificity, and possibly even in their exact mode of action. Nevertheless, they all have one action in common— that of altering calcium ion homeostasis. **Bepridil**, however, is not chemically related to the other calcium antagonists.

EFFICACY AND USE

In broad terms, the calcium antagonists have found therapeutic use in the treatment of hypertension and angina pectoris. In stable angina pectoris, numerous studies have shown that **nifedipine, verapamil, diltiazem, nicardipine,** and **bepridil** are effective antianginal agents. **Verapamil's** antianginal efficacy is similar to that of **diltiazem**, and both are more potent than the dihydropyridines, particularly **nifedipine**. Aggravation of anginal symptoms has, however, been noted with calcium antagonists. This may occur in up to 10% of patients taking **nifedipine** and may be caused by coronary steal or increased sympathetic tone secondary to peripheral vasodilatation. This effect is less apparent with **verapamil** and **diltiazem**, possibly because of the absence of reflex tachycardia.

In comparable studies, beta blockers and **diltiazem** have similar efficacy. Although early data suggested that calcium antagonists were beneficial in the treatment of the total ischemic burden (silent and painful episodes), more recent results have suggested otherwise, at least with **nifedipine** and **diltiazem**. By comparison, beta blockers have been shown to be beneficial in treating the total ischemic burden.

Combined therapy of a dihydropyridine calcium antagonist and a beta blocker has been found to be effective in the treatment of stable angina, but may be best used when left ventricular function is good. Combination therapy, particularly with **verapamil** or **diltiazem**, should not be used in patients with conduction system disease or with moderate-to-severe left ventricular dysfunction.

TABLE 8.1 CURRENTLY AVAILABLE CALCIUM ANTAGONISTS	
Diphenylalkylamine	Verapamil
Dihydropyridines	Amlodipine
	Felodipine
	Isradipine
	Nicardipine
	Nifedipine
	Nisoldipine
	Nimodipine
Benzothiazepines	Diltiazem
Miscellaneous	Bepridil

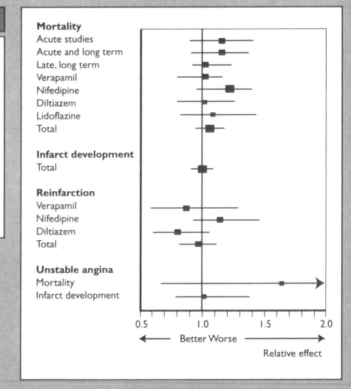

FIGURE 8.1 Meta analysis of trials involving calcium antagonists in acute myocardial infarction and angina, showing relative effects of drugs. (*Adapted from* Held PH, Yusuf S, Furberg CD: Calcium channel blockers in acute myocardial infarction and unstable angina: an overview. *Br Med J* 1989; 299:1187–1192.)

The three types of calcium antagonists have been shown to be effective in the treatment of a rare variant (Prinzmetal's) angina; the benefit being due to coronary dilatation. In theory, calcium antagonists offer a unique approach to the treatment of unstable angina, but in reality, their use as monotherapy in unstable or preinfarction angina has been disappointing (Figure 8.1). The large HINT study was stopped because of an excess of cardiovascular events in the **nifedipine** group. Indeed, in patients with chronic stable angina, a significant excess of cardiovascular events has been noted.

In post-myocardial infarction (MI) (not an official indication for calcium antagonists), the dihydropyridines have been associated with an excess of cardiovascular events. However, **verapamil** and **diltiazem** may be useful in non–Q-wave infarction and prevention of reinfarction, provided left ventricular function is good.

Nifedipine and the other dihydropyridine calcium antagonists have been shown to be relatively well tolerated and effective drugs for the treatment of systemic hypertension. They are about as effective as other commonly used antihypertensive agents, and combine well with angiotensin converting enzyme (ACE) inhibitors and beta blockers. Their combination with diuretics produces a less than additive effect.

The most common side effects of calcium antagonists are secondary to their vasodilating properties, for example, headache, flushing, sweating, dizziness, edema, and ankle swelling. In combination with beta blockers, some of their vasodilatory side effects are reduced. However, the calcium antagonists have few contraindications, unlike the beta blockers. With **diltiazem**, hypotension and depression of atrioventricular nodal conduction can occur, and constipation has also been noted (the most common side effect of **verapamil**).

Calcium antagonists tend to be lipid and biochemically neutral, although the dihydropyridines tend to lower potassium concentrations. They usually have a beneficial effect on left ventricular hypertrophy, insulin resistance, and atheroma. However, the clinical significance of the last finding is unclear, as cardiovascular mortality with the dihydropyridines was increased in the INTACT study.

Verapamil and **diltiazem** have become the drugs of first choice for abolishing acute episodes of paroxysmal supraventricular tachycardia caused by atrioventricular nodal re-entry or by anomalous atrioventricular connections of either the Wolff-Parkinson-White type or concealed bypass tracts. **Verapamil** and **diltiazem** are also very useful for immediate reduction of the ventricular response to atrial fibrillation or atrial flutter. **Verapamil** is used to treat ventricular tachycardia and ventricular fibrillation caused by coronary artery spasm.

Nifedipine has produced subjective improvement in Raynaud's disease in more than 60% of patients. **Verapamil** has had beneficial effects in hypertrophic obstructive cardiomyopathy, but the role of calcium antagonists in congestive heart failure (CHF) is still being examined. Studies have shown that amlodipidine and other agents can be given along with standard heart failure therapies. High doses of **nifedipine** (and **diltiazem**) appear to improve survival of patients with primary pulmonary hypertension.

Bepridil hydrochloride is unique among the calcium antagonists. It is a calcium channel blocker and antianginal agent with type I antiarrhythmic and minimal antihypertensive properties. **Bepridil** has inhibitory effects on both the slow calcium and fast sodium inward currents in both myocardial and vascular smooth muscle.

MODE OF ACTION

Definitive evidence shows that depolarization in atrial tissue is mediated by two inwardly directed ionic currents. When a cardiac cell potential reaches threshold, the membrane permeability for sodium increases (Figure 8.2). The *fast channel* is responsible for this influx of sodium. The time required for the second inward current to reach maximal values is much longer. This current is largely caused by the movement of calcium ions into the cell

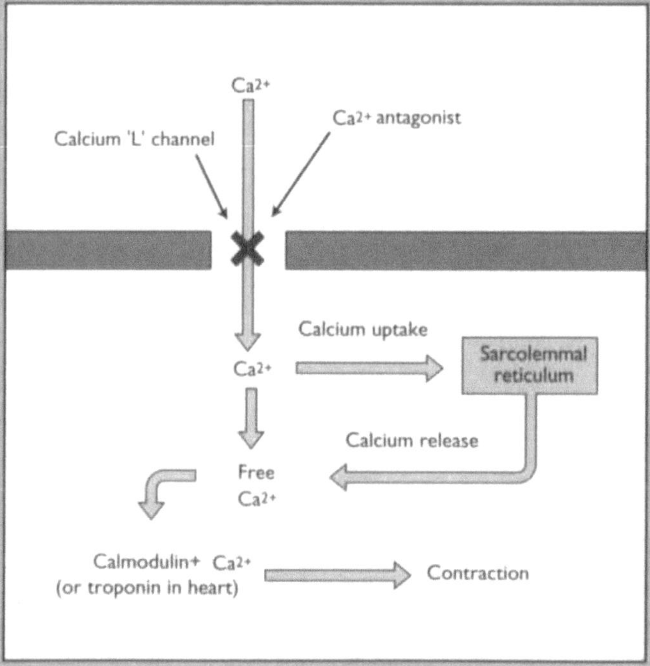

FIGURE 8.2 Mode of action of calcium antagonists.

TABLE 8.2 COMPARATIVE HEMODYNAMICS OF THREE CALCIUM ANTAGONISTS

Property	Verapamil	Nifedipine	Diltiazem
Heart rate	↓	↑	↓
Cardiac output	↓/←→	↑	↓/←→
Inotropic effect	↓	↓/←→	↓
Coronary artery tone	↓	↓	↓
Peripheral vascular resistance	↓	↓↓	↓
Reflex sympathetic activity	↑	↑↑	↑
Atrioventricular conduction	↓	←→	↓
Atrioventricular node refractory period	↑	←→	↑
Blood pressure	↓	↓	↓

↓—decrease; ↑—increase; ←→—no change.

	Amlodipine	Bepridil	Diltiazem	Felodipine	Isradipine	Nicardipine	Nifedipine	Nimodipine	Nisoldipine	Verapamil
Hypertension	+	—	+	+	+	+	+	—	+	+
Angina	+	+	+	—	—	+	+	—	—	+
Hypertrophic cardiomyopathy	—	—	—	—	—	—	—	—	—	(+)
Raynaud's phenomenon	—	—	—	—	—	—	(+)	—	—	—
Arrhythmias	—	—	+	—	—	—	—	—	—	+
Subarachnoid hemorrhage	—	—	—	—	—	—	—	+	—	—

+—FDA approved; ——not FDA approved; (+)—clinical use not FDA approved.

through a membrane pore termed the *slow channel*. A derivative of **verapamil** was subsequently shown to block the movement of calcium through the slow channel and thereby alter the plateau phase of the cardiac action potential. Although the agents are called calcium antagonists, they do not directly antagonize the effects of calcium, but they inhibit the entry of calcium into cells or its mobilization from intracellular stores. For this reason they are also called calcium channel blockers. Their vasodilatory activity is not specific to the coronary vasculature but is widespread, reflecting their general ability to modulate calcium transport.

The increase in the cytosolic concentration of calcium by electromechanical or pharmacochemical coupling results in enhanced binding of calcium to calmodulin and to troponin (in the heart). This complex promotes the contraction of smooth muscle. As a consequence, intravenous **nifedipine**, for example, increased forearm blood flow but the decrease in arterial pressure elicits sympathetic reflexes with resultant tachycardia and positive inotropy. Thus, blood pressure (BP) is lowered, contractility is improved, and heart rate and cardiac output are increased (Table 8.2). After oral administration, peripheral blood flow increases because of arterial dilatation. The increase in cardiac output is due to a decrease in arteriolar resistance coupled with the positive inotropic effect that results from the sympathetic reflexes. However, the increases in heart rate, plasma renin activity, and catecholamines release may lead to a reduction in the efficacy of the dihydropyridine calcium antagonists.

By increasing the supply of oxygen to the potentially ischemic myocardium by coronary dilatation or by decreasing the demand secondary to a decrease in BP, calcium antagonists clearly benefit the ischemic patient.

Verapamil and **diltiazem** slow the spontaneous firing of pacemaker cells in the sinus node, leading to a slowing of heart rate that is partially nullified by increased sympathetic activity due to arterial vasodilatation. Nevertheless, unlike the dihydropyridines, **verapamil** and **diltiazem** produce a net 10% to 15% decrease in heart rate. Furthermore, they decrease conduction velocity through the atrioventricular node and significantly increase the functional refractory period. The effect on atrioventricular nodal conduction is presumably a direct result of calcium channel blockade. However, this effect is not prominent at clinically achieved concentrations of other calcium antagonists such as the dihydropyridines. For these reasons, **verapamil** and **diltiazem**, unlike **nifedipine**, are useful in the treatment of certain arrhythmias.

The antianginal agent **bepridil** inhibits slow calcium as well as fast sodium channels by interfering with calcium binding to calmodulin and blocking both voltage and receptor-operated calcium channels.

AMLODIPINE (Norvasc®)

Amlodipine is a calcium antagonist of the dihydropyridine group. Because of its long elimination half-life, it is suitable for once daily administration in hypertension and angina. In contrast to other dihydropyridines, its pharmacodynamic effects are gradual in onset and offset, giving a smooth vascular effect. The slow onset of action and prolonged effect also minimize or abolish stimulation of cardiovascular reflex mechanisms. It invokes beneficial changes in vascular resistance, stroke volume, and cardiac index. Amlodipine may increase heart rate, noradrenaline, and plasma renin activity to a lesser degree than nifedipine. Its natriuretic properties may contribute to its effect in hypertension in which it provides smooth 24 hour BP control without postural hypotension. Amlodipine is clearly superior to placebo, produces slightly greater reductions in blood pressure than verapamil, and has similar efficacy to hydrochlorothiazide, atenolol, and captopril. Coadministration with diuretics, beta blockers, and ACE inhibitors also achieves further reductions in BP. A particularly useful combination is amlodipine with benazepril. When this combination was used, BP was reduced to a greater extent compared to when either agent was used alone. Further, this combination therapy was associated with a lower incidence of adverse effects, especially edema, than amlodipine alone. In angina, amlodipine is more effective than placebo and as effective as diltiazem and nadolol. The results from the PRAISE study demonstrated that amlodipine did not increase cardiovascular morbidity or mortality in patients with severe heart failure. In fact, amlodipine was shown to reduce the risk of death by 46% in patients with nonischemic cardiomyopathy. An ongoing large randomized clinical trial, ALLHAT, is now in progress to determine whether cardiovascular events differ between hypertensive patients randomized to chlorthalidone and alternative treatments such as amlodipine, lisinopril, or doxazosin.

SPECIAL GROUPS

Race: no differences in response
Children: safety and effectiveness have not been established
Elderly: initiate at lower dose
Renal impairment: normal dosage recommended; amlodipine is not dialyzable
Hepatic impairment: administer with caution; use lower dose
Pregnancy: category C; not recommended
Breast-feeding: not recommended; amlodipine may be excreted in breast milk

DOSAGE

Hypertension: Initially, give 5 mg once daily. May be increased to a maximum dose of 10 mg once daily, depending on individual response. In elderly patients or patients with hepatic insufficiency, initiate with 2.5 mg once daily.
Angina: Usual dose is 5–10 mg once daily. Use lower dose for elderly and patients with hepatic insufficiency.

IN BRIEF

INDICATIONS
Hypertension
Chronic stable angina
Vasospastic (Prinzmetal's or variant) angina

CONTRAINDICATIONS
Hypersensitivity

DRUG INTERACTIONS
Beta blockers
Cyclosporine
Hepatic enzyme inhibitors
Fentanyl

ADVERSE EFFECTS
Cardiovascular: peripheral edema (1%–15%), palpitations (≤1%–5%)
CNS: dizziness/lightheadedness(1%–4%), headache (7%), somnolence(1%–2%), asthenia (1%–2%), fatigue/lethargy (4%–5%)
GI: nausea (3%), abdominal discomfort (1%–2%)
Dermatologic: rash/dermatitis (1%–2%), pruritus/urticaria (1%–2%)
Others: flushing (≤1%–5%), sexual difficulties (1%–2%), shortness of breath (1%–2%), muscle cramps (1%–2%)

PHARMACOKINETICS AND PHARMACODYNAMICS
Duration of action: 24 h
Onset of action: 30–50 min
Time to peak plasma concentration: 6–12 h
Bioavailability: 64%–90%
Effect of food: none
Metabolism: hepatic, extensive, to inactive metabolites
Elimination: metabolite and parent drug excreted renally
Half-life: 30–50 h
Protein binding: 93%

MONITORING
BP, heart rate, hepatic function.

OVERDOSE
If the patient is found shortly after oral ingestion, administer emetics or lavage and cathartics. Treatment is supportive.
For symptomatic hypotension, administer fluids intravenously, dopamine or dobutamine intravenously, calcium chloride, isoproterenol, metaraminol, or norepinephrine.
For tachycardia, rapid ventricular rate in patients with antegrade conduction in atrial flutter/fibrillation, and accessory pathway with Wolff-Parkinson-White or Lown-Ganong-Levine syndrome, administer direct current cardioversion, intravenous lidocaine, or intravenous procainamide. Intravenous fluids should be given by slow drip.
For bradycardia, 2° or 3° atrioventricular block, with a few patients progressing to asystole, administer intravenous atropine, isoproterenol, norepinephrine, or calcium chloride, or use electronic cardiac pacemaker. Intravenous fluids should be given by slow drip.

PATIENT INFORMATION
This medication may cause palpitations, headache, flushing, ankle edema, and cramps. Notify physician if persistent or unusual side effects occur. Do not discontinue therapy without your physician's advice.

AVAILABILITY
Tablets—2.5 mg, 5 mg, 10 mg
Combination formulations:
Lotrel—amlodipine/benazepril hydrochloride combination capsules
2.5 mg/10 mg
5 mg/10 mg
5 mg/20 mg

BEPRIDIL

(Vascor®)

Bepridil hydrochloride is an antianginal agent that inhibits slow calcium as well as fast sodium channels. In addition, bepridil demonstrates electrophysiologic effects such as prolongation of QT and QTc intervals that are characteristic of class I antiarrhythmic agents. Structurally, bepridil is a diarylaminopropylamine-derivative that is unrelated to other currently available calcium-channel blockers. Its precise mechanism of action as an antianginal agent is not fully known. However, the drug is believed to reduce heart rate and arterial pressure at rest and at a given level of exertion by dilating peripheral arterioles and reducing total peripheral resistance (afterload) against which the heart works. Bepridil may be used alone or with beta blockers or nitrates. An added effect occurs when it is administered to patients already receiving propranolol. Because of bepridil's arrhythmogenic potential and case reports of agranulocytosis associated with this agent, bepridil generally is reserved for patients who have fail to respond or are intolerant to other antianginal agents.

SPECIAL GROUPS

Race: no differences in response
Children: safety and effectiveness have not been established
Elderly: normal dosing with caution
Renal impairment: administer with caution; specific dosage has not been established. Bepridil is not removable by hemodialysis
Hepatic impairment: use with caution
Pregnancy: category C; use only if potential benefit justifies the potential risk
Breast-feeding: not recommended; bepridil is excreted in breast milk

DOSAGE

Adult: Individualize therapy according to clinical judgment and each patient's response. Usual initial dose is 200 mg once daily. Upward adjustment may be made after 10 d depending on patient's response. Usual maintenance dose is 300 mg once daily. Maximum daily dose is 400 mg. Minimum effective dose is 200 mg.
Elderly: Same initial dose as above. However, careful monitoring must be done after therapeutic response is demonstrated.
Note: If nausea occurs, administer the drug with meals or at bedtime.

IN BRIEF

INDICATIONS
Chronic stable angina

CONTRAINDICATIONS
Hypersensitivity; History of serious ventricular or atrial arrhythmias (especially tachycardia or those associated with accessory conduction pathways); Uncompensated cardiac insufficiency; Congenital QT interval prolongation; Use with other drugs that prolong QT interval

DRUG INTERACTIONS
Antiarrhythmic agents
Beta blockers
Cyclosporine
Digitalis glycosides
Fentanyl
Hypokalemia-producing medications (eg, sodium phosphates)
Ritonavir

ADVERSE EFFECTS
Cardiovascular: palpitation (≤7%), peripheral edema (≤2%), bradycardia (≤2%), tachycardia (≤2%) ,prolonged QT interval
CNS: dizziness/lightheadedness(12%–27%), headache (7%–14%), nervousness (7%–12%), asthenia (6%–14%), tremor (≤ 9%), drowsiness (>7%), tinnitus (0%–7%), insomnia (2%–3%), paresthesia (2%–3%)
GI: nausea (7%–26%), diarrhea (0%–11%), abdominal discomfort (≤7%), dry mouth (3%–4%), constipation (2%–3%)
Dermatologic: rash/dermatitis (≤2%)
Others: nasal or chest congestion (≤2%), shortness of breath (≤9%), respiratory infection (2%–3%), sexual difficulties (≤2%)

PHARMACOKINETICS AND PHARMACODYNAMICS
Duration of action: 24 h
Onset of action: 1 h
Time to peak effect: 8 d
Time to peak plasma concentration: 2–3 h
Bioavailability: 60%
Effect of food: none
Metabolism: highly metabolized by the liver
Elimination: renal, 70% (none unchanged); biliary/fecal, 22% (none unchanged)
Half-life: 24 h
Protein binding: > 99%

MONITORING
BP, electrocardiogram (EKG) and serum electrolytes, hepatic function, signs and symptoms of congestive heart failure. Elderly may need close monitoring due to underlying cardiac and organ system insufficiencies.

OVERDOSE
Closely observe patient in cardiac care facility for a minimum of 48 h. Gastric lavage may be used.
For symptomatic hypotension, administer fluids intravenously, dopamine or dobutamine intravenously, calcium chloride, isoproterenol, metaraminol, or norepinephrine.
For tachycardia, rapid ventricular rate in patients with antegrade conduction in atrial flutter/fibrillation, and accessory pathway with Wolff-Parkinson-White or Lown-Ganong-Levine syndrome, administer direct current cardioversion, intravenous lidocaine, or intravenous procainamide. Intravenous fluids should be given by slow drip.
For bradycardia, 2° or 3° atrioventricular block, with a few patients progressing to asystole, administer intravenous atropine, isoproterenol, norepinephrine, or calcium chloride, or use electronic cardiac pacemaker. Intravenous fluids should be given by slow drip.

PATIENT INFORMATION
This medication may cause cardiac arrhythmias if potassium concentration in body is low; maintain potassium supplementation as directed by physician. Notify physician if persistent or unusual side effects occur. Follow-up visits must be taken seriously.

AVAILABILITY
Tablets—200 mg, 300 mg, 400 mg

DILTIAZEM
(Diltiazem, Cardizem®, Cardizem® SR, Cardizem® CD, Dilacor™ XR, Tiazac™)

Diltiazem is a benzothiazepine calcium ion influx inhibitor that is extensively metabolized and consequently short acting. When administered orally, diltiazem has been used either alone or in combination with other antihypertensive agents for the management of hypertension. Diltiazem increases exercise capacity and improves all indices of myocardial ischemia in patients with angina; it relieves spasm and vasospastic (Prinzmetal's) angina. It is effective in the treatment of chronic stable angina, with effects equal to those of propranolol, nifedipine, and verapamil, but additional benefit could be obtained by combining the drug with propranolol. Diltiazem is also effective in the treatment of variant angina and unstable angina.

Diltiazem has an inhibitory effect on the cardiac conduction system, acting primarily at the atrioventricular (AV) node, with some effects at the sinus node. This allows diltiazem to be useful in the management of paroxysmal supraventricular tachycardia and atrial fibrillation. Diltiazem also reduces left ventricular hypertrophy. Diltiazem may protect the myocardium against the effects of ischemia and reduces the damage produced by excessive entry of calcium into the myocardial cell during reperfusion (ie, angioplasty). An overview of postinfarction studies with calcium antagonists showed that diltiazem reduced the incidence of reinfarction but it did not reduce mortality. The benefit of reinfarction was only seen in patients with uncompromised left ventricular function, and mainly in patients with non–Q-wave MI.

A greater effect on BP lowering was observed when diltiazem was administered with enalapril and a combination formulation is available. Concomitant use of diltiazem with beta blockers or digitalis may result in additive effects on cardiac conduction. The use of diltiazem with a beta blocker may reduce the frequency of attacks and increase exercise tolerance in patients with chronic stable angina pectoris as suggested by controlled study results; however, additional study is needed to confirm the safety and efficacy of this combination therapy, especially in patients with compromised left ventricular function or cardiac conduction abnormalities. Major side effects of diltiazem include vasodilatory reactions (headache, flushing, hypotension), sinus bradycardia, and atrioventricular block, although these side effects are relatively infrequent.

SPECIAL GROUPS

Race: no differences in response
Children: safety and effectiveness have not been established
Elderly: half-life may be increased; also, more likely to have age-related renal impairment
Renal impairment: use with caution; diltiazem is excreted renally. It is not removed by hemodialysis
Hepatic impairment: use with caution; diltiazem is extensively metabolized by the liver
Pregnancy: category C; use diltiazem in pregnant women only if potential benefit justifies potential risk to fetus
Breast-feeding: not recommended; diltiazem is excreted in breast milk

IN BRIEF

INDICATIONS
Angina (Cardizem, Cardizem CD, Dilacor XR)
Hypertension (Cardizem SR, Cardizem CD, Dilacor XR, Tiazac)
Arrhythmias
Paroxysmal supraventricular tachycardia (Cardizem injectable)
Atrial fibrillation or flutter (Cardizem injectable)

CONTRAINDICATIONS
Hypersensitivity; Severe hypotension (<90 mmHg systolic); Sick sinus syndrome or second- or third- degree AV block except with a functioning pace maker; Acute MI; Pulmonary congestion

DRUG INTERACTIONS
Amiodarone	Cyclosporine	Histamine H_2
Beta blockers	Disopyramide	antagonists
Carbamazepine	Digitalis glycosides	Lithium
Cimetidine	Encainide	Moricizine
Cisapride	Fentanyl	Quinidine
		Theophylline

ADVERSE EFFECTS
Cardiovascular: peripheral edema (2%–9%), AV block (≤1%–8%), bradycardia (1%–6%), abnormal ECG (4%)
CNS: headache (2%–12%), dizziness/lightheadedness (1%–7%), asthenia (2%–5%)
GI: abdominal discomfort(1%–2%), nausea (1%–2%), constipation (1%–2%)
Dermatologic: rash/dermatitis (1%–2%)
Others: flushing (1%–3%), micturition disorder (1%–2%)

PHARMACOKINETCIS AND PHARMACODYNAMICS
Duration of action: 4–8 h (short-acting); 12–24 h (sustained-release)
Onset of action: 30–60 min
Time to peak serum concentration: 2–3 h (short- acting); 6–11 h (sustained release)
Bioavailability: ≈40%–60%
Effect of food: none
Metabolism: extensive, hepatic
Elimination: in urine and bile mostly as metabolites
Half-life: 4–6 h (short-acting), 5–7 h (sustained-release)
Protein binding: 70%–80%

MONITORING
BP, EKG, liver function tests.

OVERDOSE
For symptomatic hypotension, administer fluids intravenously, dopamine or dobutamine intravenously, calcium chloride, isoproterenol, metaraminol, or norepinephrine.
For tachycardia, rapid ventricular rate in patients with antegrade conduction in atrial flutter/fibrillation, and accessory pathway with Wolff-Parkinson-White or Lown-Ganong-Levine syndrome, administer direct current cardioversion, intravenous lidocaine, or intravenous procainamide. Intravenous fluids should be given by slow drip.
For bradycardia, 2° or 3° atrioventricular block, with a few patients progressing to asystole, administer intravenous atropine, isoproterenol, norepinephrine, or calcium chloride, or use electronic cardiac pacemaker. Intravenous fluids should be given by slow drip.

DOSAGE

Short-acting (Diltiazem, Cardizem): As an antianginal agent, usual initial dose is 30 mg four times daily (before meals and at bedtime). Dosage should be increased gradually at 1–2 d intervals. Maximum daily dose is 360 mg.

Sustained-Release (Cardizem SR): As monotherapy for hypertension, start with 60–120 mg twice daily, although some patients may respond well to lower doses. Usual dose range is 240–360 mg/d.

Sustained-Release (Cardizem CD): As monotherapy for hypertension, initially, 180–240 mg once daily. The usual dose range in clinical trials was 240–360 mg/d. Individual patients may respond to higher doses of up to 480 mg once daily. For angina, start with 120 or 180 mg once daily. Dose may be titrated upward every 7–14 d up to a maximum of 480 mg once daily if necessary.

Sustained-Release (Dilacor XR): For hypertension, start with 180–240 mg once daily. Adjust dose as needed depending on antihypertensive response. In clinical trials, the therapeutic dose range is 180–540 mg once daily. For angina, start with 120 mg once daily. Dose may be titrated upward every 7–14 d up to a maximum of 480 mg once daily if needed.

Sustained-Release (Tiazac): Usual starting dose is 120–240 mg once daily. Maximum effect is observed after 14 d. In clinical trials doses up to 540 mg daily were effective.

Injection (Diltiazem I.V., Cardizem I.V.): Direct intravenous single injections (bolus): Initial 0.25 mg/kg body weight administered as a bolus over 2 min (20 mg is a reasonable dose for an average patient). If response is inadequate, a second dose may be administered after 15 min (25 mg is a reasonable dose or 0.35 mg/kg body weight).

Intravenous infusion—An intravenous infusion may be administered for continued reduction of the heart rate (up to 24 h) in patients with atrial fibrillation or atrial flutter. Start an infusion at a rate of 10 mg/h immediately after bolus administration of 0.25 or 0.35 mg/kg. Some patients may maintain response to an initial rate of 5 mg/h. The infusion rate may be increased in 5 mg/h increments up to 15 mg/h as needed. Infusion duration longer than 24 h and infusion rate > 15 mg/h are not recommended (refer to package insert for proper dilution of diltiazem for continuous infusion).

PATIENT INFORMATION
The sustained-released capsules should be swallowed whole, without breaking, crushing, or chewing. This medication may cause a slowing of the heart rate, headache, ankle edema, or constipation. Notify physician if persistent or unusual side effects occur. Do not discontinue therapy without your physician's advice.

AVAILABILITY
Tablets (Diltiazem, Cardizem)—30 mg, 60 mg, 90 mg, 120 mg
Capsules (Cardizem SR)—60 mg, 90 mg, 120 mg
Capsules (Cardizem CD)—120 mg, 180 mg, 240 mg, 300 mg
Capsules (Dilacor XR)—180 mg, 240 mg
Capsules (Tiazac)—120 mg, 180 mg, 240 mg, 300 mg, 360 mg
Injection (as hydrochloride)—5 mg/mL (5 mL, 10 mL)
Injection (Cardizem I.V.)—5 mg/mL (5 mL, 10 mL)
Combination formulations:
  Teczem—enalapril maleate/ diltiazem malate ER (extended-release) combination tablets—5 mg/ 180 mg

FELODIPINE
(Plendil®)

Felodipine is a dihydropyridine calcium antagonist that is extensively metabolized. It is supplied as an extended-release formulation based on the hydrophilic gel principle. This allows once-daily administration with smooth control of BP throughout the 24 hours. Its terminal half-life ranges from 11 to 16 hours in young healthy people to about 20 to 27.5 hours in middle aged hypertensive patients. It is vascularly selective and reduces BP in mild, moderate, and severe hypertension. It causes a fall in BP similar to or greater than that of other antihypertensive agents as monotherapy. Felodipine is also available in a fixed combination with enalapril. This fixed combination therapy has been shown to reduce BP to a greater extent than with felodipine or enalapril alone.

Adverse effects from felodipine are few except for a constellation of symptoms related to its vasodilator ability. These effects include palpitations, flushing, fatigue, dizziness, and headaches. Ankle edema, however, is the most frequent observed unwanted effect. This agent may produce less reflex tachycardia and a less significant rise in plasma renin activity than does nifedipine. Felodipine has been evaluated in a large international placebo-controlled clinical outcomes study, HOTS, in patients with systemic hypertension. The results of this study showed that intensive lowering of BP (down to a mean diastolic BP of 82.6 mmHg) in patients with hypertension was associated with a low rate of cardiovascular events.

SPECIAL GROUPS

Race: no differences in response
Children: safety and effectiveness have not been established
Elderly: initiate at lower dose
Renal impairment: normal dosage recommended
Hepatic impairment: administer with caution; use lower dose
Pregnancy: category C; not recommended
Breast-feeding: not recommended; felodipine may be excreted in breast milk

DOSAGE

Adults: Usual initial dose is 5 mg once daily. Dosage may be increased by 5 mg at 2 wk intervals according to response. Maintenance dose range from 2.5–10 mg once daily.
Elderly: Treatment should be initiated at 2.5 mg once daily because of possible accumulation. Maximum dose is 10 mg once daily. Monitor BP closely.

IN BRIEF

INDICATIONS
Hypertension (felodipine may be used alone or concomitantly with other antihypertensives)

CONTRAINDICATIONS
Hypersensitivity

DRUG INTERACTIONS
Barbiturates	Erythromycin	Histamine H_2 antagonists
Beta blockers	Fentanyl	Hydantoins
Carbamazepine	Grapefruit juice	Theophylline
Digitalis glycosides		

ADVERSE EFFECTS
Cardiovascular: peripheral edema (22%), palpitations (1%–2%), hypotension (≤1.5%), syncope (≤1.5%), AV block (≤1.5%), arrhythmia (≤1.5%), angina (≤1.5%)
CNS: headache (19%), Dizziness/lightheadedness (6%), asthenia (5%), paresthesia (2%–3%), nervousness (≤1.5%), psychiatric disturbances (≤1.5%), insomnia (≤1.5%)
GI: nausea (1%–2%), abdominal discomfort (1%–2%), diarrhea (1%–2%), constipation (1%–2%), dry mouth/thirst (≤1.5%)
Dermatologic: rash/dermatitis (1%–2%), pruritus/urticaria (1%–2%)
Others: flushing (6%), cough (3%), respiratory infection (≤5.5%), nasal or chest congestion (≤1.5%), sexual difficulties (1%–2%), shortness of breath (1%–2%), muscle cramps (1%–2%), anemia (≤1.5%), micturition disorder (≤1.5%), gingival hyperplasia (rare)

PHARMACOKINETICS AND PHARMACODYNAMICS
Duration of action: 16–24 h
Onset of action: 2–5 h
Time to peak plasma concentration: 2.5–5 h
Bioavailability: 20%
Effect of food: bioavailability increased more than twofold when taken with doubly concentrated grapefruit juice compared to water or orange juice
Metabolism: hepatic, extensive, to inactive metabolites
Elimination: renal, 70% (less than 0.5% unchanged); biliary/fecal, 10% (less than 0.5% unchanged)
Half-life: 11–16 h
Protein binding: >99%

MONITORING
BP, heart rate, hepatic function.

OVERDOSE
For symptomatic hypotension, administer fluids intravenously, dopamine or dobutamine intravenously, calcium chloride, isoproterenol, metaraminol, or norepinephrine.
For tachycardia, rapid ventricular rate in patients with antegrade conduction in atrial flutter/fibrillation, and accessory pathway with Wolff-Parkinson-White or Lown-Ganong-Levine syndrome, administer direct current cardioversion, intravenous lidocaine, or intravenous procainamide. Intravenous fluids should be given by slow drip.
For bradycardia, 2° or 3° atrioventricular block, with a few patients progressing to asystole, administer intravenous atropine, isoproterenol, norepinephrine, or calcium chloride, or use electronic cardiac pacemaker. Intravenous fluids should be given by slow drip.

PATIENT INFORMATION
Swallow tablet whole; do not crush or chew tablets.
This medication may cause palpitations, headache, flushing, ankle edema, and cramps. Notify physician if persistent or unusual side effects occur. Do not discontinue therapy without your physician's advice.

AVAILABILITY
Tablets (extended release)—2.5 mg, 5 mg, 10 mg
Combination formulation:
Lexxel—enalapril maleate/ felodipine ER (extended-release) combination tablets—5 mg/ 5 mg

ISRADIPINE (DynaCirc®, DynaCirc CR®)

Isradipine, a typical dihydropyridine and a highly potent drug (milligram for milligram), is extensively metabolized by the liver and has a relatively short half-life, necessitating twice daily administration for hypertension. Unlike other dihydropyridines, chronic therapy with isradipine does not increase heart rate. The efficacy of isradipine is similar to that of nifedipine, propranolol, atenolol, prazosin, hydrochlorothiazide, and diltiazem. It can be safely combined with beta blockers, ACE inhibitors, and diuretics. Adverse effects are secondary to vasodilatation. The antiatherosclerotic effect of isradipine has been evaluated in the MIDAS trial. Over 36 months, no difference in the rate of progression of mean maximum intimal-medial thickness in carotid arteries was observed between patients treated with isradipine and patients treated with hydrochlorothiazide. However, there was a higher incidence of major cardiovascular events in the isradipine group compared to the hydrochorothiazide group (p = 0.07).

SPECIAL GROUPS

Race: no differences in response
Children: safety and effectiveness have not been established
Elderly: bioavailability may be increased
Renal impairment: bioavailability may be increased
Hepatic impairment: administer with caution; use lower dose
Pregnancy: category C; not recommended
Breast-feeding: not recommended; isradipine may be excreted in breast milk

DOSAGE

Immediate-release (DynaCirc): Initially, give 2.5 mg twice daily alone or in combination with a thiazide diuretic. If necessary, adjust in increments of 2.5–5 mg/d at 2–4 wk intervals. The maximum daily dose is 20 mg.
Note: Most patients show no improvement with doses >10 mg/d; adverse reactions are increased in frequency above 10 mg/d.
Controlled-release (DynaCirc CR): Initially, give 5 mg once daily alone or in combination with a thiazide diuretic. If necessary, the dose may be adjusted in increments of 5 mg at 2–4 wk intervals up to a maximum dose of 20 mg/d. Adverse experiences are increased in frequency above 10 mg/d.

IN BRIEF

INDICATIONS
Hypertension (isradipine may be used alone or concomitantly with thiazide-type diuretics)

CONTRAINDICATIONS
Hypersensitivity

DRUG INTERACTIONS
Beta blockers
Fentanyl
Lovastatin
Nonsteroidal anti-inflammatory drugs (NSAIDS) (eg, diclofenac)

ADVERSE EFFECTS
Cardiovascular: peripheral edema (7%), palpitations (4%), angina (2%–3%), tachycardia (1%–2%)
CNS: headache (14%), Dizziness/lightheadedness (7%), fatigue/lethargy (4%)
GI: nausea (2%), vomiting (1%), abdominal discomfort (1%–2%), diarrhea (1%)
Dermatologic: rash/dermatitis (1%–2%), pruritus/urticaria (≤1%)
Others: flushing (2%–3%), sexual difficulties (≤1%), shortness of breath (1%–2%), pollakiuria (1.5%)

PHARMACOKINETICS AND PHARMACODYNAMICS
Duration of action: 12 h (immediate-release); 24 h (controlled-release)
Onset of action: 2 h
Time to peak plasma concentration: 1.5 h (immediate-release)
Time to peak effect: multiple doses (2–4 wk)
Bioavailability: 15%–24%
Effect of food: administration of isradipine (DynaCirc) with food significantly increases the time to peak by about an hour, but has no effect on the total bioavailability of the drug. Food has been shown to decrease the extent of bioavailability of DynaCirc CR by up to 25%
Metabolism: extensive first-pass metabolism by liver
Elimination: renal 60%–65% (none unchanged); biliary/fecal 25%–30% (none unchanged)
Half-life: 8 h (immediate-release)
Protein binding: 95%

MONITORING
BP, heart rate, hepatic function.

OVERDOSE
If the patient is found shortly after oral ingestion, administer emetics or lavage and cathartics. Treatment is supportive.
For symptomatic hypotension, administer fluids intravenously, dopamine or dobutamine intravenously, calcium chloride, isoproterenol, metaraminol, or norepinephrine.
For tachycardia, rapid ventricular rate in patients with antegrade conduction in atrial flutter/fibrillation, and accessory pathway with Wolff-Parkinson-White or Lown-Ganong-Levine syndrome, administer direct current cardioversion, intravenous lidocaine, or intravenous procainamide. Intravenous fluids should be given by slow drip.
For bradycardia, 2° or 3° atrioventricular block, with a few patients progressing to asystole, administer intravenous atropine, isoproterenol, norepinephrine, or calcium chloride, or use electronic cardiac pacemaker. Intravenous fluids should be given by slow drip.

PATIENT INFORMATION
The controlled-release tablets (DynaCirc CR) should be swallowed whole and should not be bitten or divided.
This medication may cause palpitations, headache, flushing, ankle edema, and dizziness. Notify physician if persistent or unusual side effects occur. Do not discontinue therapy without your physician's advice.

AVAILABILITY
Capsules (DynaCirc)—2.5 mg, 5 mg
Tablets (DynaCirc CR)—5 mg, 10 mg

NICARDIPINE
(Cardene®, Cardene® SR)

Nicardipine is a typical dihydropyridine calcium antagonist that is extensively metabolized and has a short half-life, necessitating three times daily administration in the oral form. A sustained-release formulation is available for twice daily dosing in hypertension. It is useful in the treatment of angina pectoris and hypertension. An intravenous formulation is available for short-term management of hypertension. Although no lifesaving benefits after infarction and during unstable angina have been found with nicardipine, studies with other dihydropyridine calcium antagonists have indicated the possibility of benefit when added to or supplementing treatment with beta blockers. Nicardipine's potential as an antiatherosclerotic agent has been investigated. However, there is no evidence of a reduction in mortality with nicardipine and other dihydropyridines similarly evaluated in patients with coronary disease or peripheral atherosclerosis. Nicardipine is as effective in the management of chronic stable angina pectoris as either diltiazem or verapamil. In hypertension, it is as effective as nifedipine, but perhaps without the reflex tachycardia at lower doses. It may be successfully combined with atenolol or propranolol. Side effects are typical of those seen with vasodilating drugs. Note must be taken of the relatively large peak-to-trough differences in BP effect. However, this does not pertain to the sustained-release formulation.

SPECIAL GROUPS

Race:	no differences in response
Children:	safety and effectiveness have not been established
Elderly:	no change in half-life or protein binding
Renal impairment:	titrate dose carefully
Hepatic impairment:	use with caution. Initiate with lower doses; titrate dose carefully
Pregnancy:	category C; not recommended
Breast-feeding:	not recommended; nicardipine may be excreted in breast milk

IN BRIEF

INDICATIONS
Hypertension (Cardene, Cardene SR)
Short-term treatment of hypertension when oral therapy cannot be given (Cardene I.V.)
Angina (Cardene)

CONTRAINDICATIONS
Hypersensitivity; Advanced aortic stenosis.

DRUG INTERACTIONS
Beta blockers
Cyclosporine
Fentanyl
Histamine H_2 antagonists

ADVERSE EFFECTS
Cardiovascular: peripheral edema (7%–8%), angina (6%), palpitations (3%–4%), tachycardia (1%–4%)
CNS: headache (6%–8%), dizziness/lightheadedness (4%–7%), asthenia (4%–6%)
GI: abdominal discomfort(1%–2%), nausea (1%–2%), dry mouth/thirst (1%–2%)
Dermatologic: rash/dermatitis (1%)
Others: flushing (5%–10%)

PHARMACOKINETICS AND PHARMACODYNAMICS
Duration of action:	8 h (immediate-release);12 h (sustained-release)
Onset of action:	20 min
Time to peak serum concentration:	0.5–2 h
Bioavailability:	35%
Effect of food:	the mean maximum concentration and AUC were 20%–30% lower compared to fasting subjects when nicardipine was given 1 – 3 h after a high-fat meal
Metabolism:	hepatic; extensive first-pass metabolism
Elimination:	renal, 60% (<1% unchanged); biliary/fecal, 35%
Half-life:	2–4 h (early); 8 h (terminal)
Protein binding:	>95%

The information here is provided as guidance only. Prescribers should always consult the manufacturer's current prescribing information.

157

NICARDIPINE (CONTINUED)

DOSAGE

Immediate-Release (Cardene): As an antianginal or antihypertensive agent, administer 20 mg in capsules three times daily. Usual maintenance dose is 20–40 mg three times daily. Allow at least 3 d between dose increases. For patients with renal impairment, titrate dose beginning with 20 mg three times daily. For patients with hepatic impairment, titrate dose starting with 20 mg twice daily.

Sustained-Release (Cardene SR): Initiate treatment with 30 mg twice daily. The effective dose ranges from 30–60 mg twice daily. For patients with renal impairment, carefully titrate dose beginning with 30 mg twice daily. The total daily dose of immediate-release product may not automatically be equivalent to the daily sustained-release dose; use caution in converting.

Injection (Cardene I.V.): Intravenously administered nicardipine injection must be diluted before infusion. Administer (concentration of 0.1 mg/mL) by slow, continuous infusion. BP lowering effect is seen within minutes. For gradual BP lowering, initiate at 50 mL/h (5 mg/h). Infusion rate may be increased by 25 mL/h (2.5 mg/h) every 15 min to a maximum of 150 mL/h (15 mg/h). For rapid BP reduction, initiate at 50 mL/h. Increase infusion rate by 25 mL/h every 5 min to a maximum of 150 mL/h until desirable BP lowering is reached. Infusion rate must be decreased to 30 mL/h (3 mg/h) when desirable BP is achieved. Conditions requiring infusion adjustment include hypotension and tachycardia. The intravenous infusion rate required to produce an average plasma concentration equivalent to a given oral dose at steady state is as follows:

Oral dose (immediate-release)	Equivalent intravenous infusion rate
20 mg every 8 h	0.5 mg/h
30 mg every 8 h	1.2 mg/h
40 mg every 8 h	2.2 mg/h

Intravenous nicardipine should be transferred to oral medication for prolonged control of BP as soon as the clinical condition permits. If treatment includes transfer to an oral antihypertensive agent other than nicardipine, generally initiate therapy upon discontinuation of the infusion. If oral nicardipine is to be used, administer the first dose of a three times daily regimen 1 h before discontinuation of the infusion.

MONITORING

BP, heart rate, liver function tests.

OVERDOSE

Monitor cardiac and respiratory functions. Position patient to avoid cerebral anoxia. Frequent BP determinations are essential.

For symptomatic hypotension, administer fluids intravenously, dopamine or dobutamine intravenously, calcium chloride, isoproterenol, metaraminol, or norepinephrine.

For tachycardia, rapid ventricular rate in patients with antegrade conduction in atrial flutter/fibrillation, and accessory pathway with Wolff-Parkinson-White or Lown-Ganong-Levine syndrome, administer direct current cardioversion, intravenous lidocaine, or intravenous procainamide. Intravenous fluids should be given by slow drip.

For bradycardia, 2° or 3° atrioventricular block, with a few patients progressing to asystole, administer intravenous atropine, isoproterenol, norepinephrine, or calcium chloride, or use electronic cardiac pacemaker. Intravenous fluids should be given by slow drip.

PATIENT INFORMATION

The sustained-released capsules should be swallowed whole, without breaking, crushing, or chewing. This medication may cause headache, flushing, dizziness, and ankle edema. Discuss exertion limits with physician. Notify physician if persistent or unusual side effects occur. Do not discontinue therapy without your physician's advice.

AVAILABILITY

Capsules (Cardene)—20 mg, 30 mg
Capsules (Cardene SR)—30 mg 45 mg, 60 mg
Injection (Cardene I.V.)—2.5 mg/mL, 10 mL ampules

NIFEDIPINE (Nifedipine, Adalat®, Adalat® CC, Procardia®, Procardia XL®)

Nifedipine, the benchmark dihydropyridine calcium antagonist, is widely prescribed. It undergoes almost complete hepatic oxidation to three pharmacologically inactive metabolites and its half-life is thus short, necessitating three times daily administration. An extended-release formulation has been developed to allow once or twice daily administration. It can be used as a first-, second- or third- line agent in mild to moderate hypertension, with an efficacy similar to that of beta blockers and diuretics. An added effect is obtained when it is combined with beta blockers, methyldopa, clonidine, and captopril. Side effects are typical of a peripheral vasodilator and include flushing, headaches, and palpitations. In some trials, ankle edema has proved to be troublesome. Serious adverse cardiovascular effects such as cerebrovascular ischemia, stroke, and MI have also been reported for the short-acting formulation of nifedipine. Therefore, short-acting nifedipine is no longer recommended for the management of any form of hypertension, including hypertensive crises. Currently, only extended-release formulations of nifedipine are recommended for the treatment of hypertension.

The antianginal efficacy of nifedipine has been seen during acute and chronic administration, but the effect may be reduced in those who smoke. It is less effective than some beta blockers, but the combination appears to be more effective than either therapy alone. Nifedipine is particularly beneficial in the treatment of rare variant (Prinzmetal) angina. An overview of trials with nifedipine and other dihydropyridines in the treatment of unstable angina and acute and post-MI indicates that the combined endpoints of mortality and re-infarction may be increased with treatment. A large randomized trial, INSIGHT, is now in progress to compare nifedipine GITS (gastrointestinal therapeutic system) with a combination of thiazide and potassium-sparing diuretics in the treatment of hypertensive patients with concomitant coronary artery disease (CAD) risk factors.

SPECIAL GROUPS

Race: no differences in response
Children: safety and effectiveness have not been established
Elderly: nifedipine may cause a greater hypotensive effect than that seen in younger patients, probably due to age-related alterations in drug disposition
Renal impairment: dosage adjustment is usually not necessary; it is not removed by hemodialysis
Hepatic impairment: use with caution; nifedipine is extensively metabolized by the liver
Pregnancy: category C; not recommended
Breast-feeding: not recommended; nifedipine is excreted in breast milk

IN BRIEF

INDICATIONS
Vasospastic angina (Nifedipine, Adalat, Procardia, Procardia XL)
Chronic stable angina (Nifedipine, Adalat, Procardia, Procardia XL)
Hypertension (Adalat CC, Procardia XL)

CONTRAINDICATIONS
Hypersensitivity
Acute MI (short-acting formulation)

DRUG INTERACTIONS
Anticoagulants	Magnesium sulfate, parenteral
Beta blockers	Phenobarbital
Digitalis glycosides	Quinidine
Disopyramide	Rifampin
Fentanyl	Theophylline
Histamine H2 antagonists	Vincristine

ADVERSE EFFECTS
Cardiovascular: peripheral edema (10%–30%), pulmonary edema (7%), palpitations (≤7%), hypotension (≤5%), MI (4%–7%), CHF (2%–7%)
CNS: headache (19%), dizziness/lightheadedness (4%), nervousness (≤ 7 %), fatigue/asthenia (4%), paresthesia (<3%), somnolence (<3%), insomnia (<3%)
GI: nausea (2%), abdominal discomfort (≤3%), constipation (1%), diarrhea (<3%), dry mouth/thirst (< 3%)
Dermatologic: rash/dermatitis (≤3%), pruritus/urticaria (≤3%)
Others: giddiness, flushing/heat sensation (4%), shortness of breath (≤8%), Muscle cramps (≤8%), cough (6%), nasal or chest congestion (≤6%), fever, chills (≤3%), micturition disorder (<3%), gingival hyperplasia (≤1%)

PHARMACOKINETICS AND PHARMACODYNAMICS
Duration of action: 8 h (short-acting); up to 24 h (extended-release)
Onset of action: 20 min
Time to peak serum concentration: 0.5 h (short-acting); 6 h (extended-release)
Bioavailability: 45%-70% (short-acting); 86% (extended-release)
Effect of food: food may slow the rate but not the extent of nifedipine absorption
Metabolism: extensively metabolized by the liver to three pharmacologically inactive metabolites
Elimination: renal, 80% (as metabolites); biliary/fecal, 20% (as metabolites)
Half-life: 2–5 h
Protein binding: 92%–98%

MONITORING
BP, heart rate, liver function tests, signs and symptoms of CHF, peripheral edema.

OVERDOSE
Perform gastric lavage and charcoal instillation.
For symptomatic hypotension, administer fluids intravenously, dopamine or dobutamine intravenously, calcium chloride, isoproterenol, metaraminol, or norepinephrine.
For tachycardia, rapid ventricular rate in patients with antegrade conduction in atrial flutter/fibrillation, and accessory pathway with Wolff-Parkinson-White or Lown-Ganong-Levine syndrome, administer direct current cardioversion, intravenous lidocaine, or intravenous procainamide. Intravenous fluids should be given by slow drip.
For bradycardia, 2° or 3° atrioventricular block, with a few patients progressing to asystole, administer intravenous atropine, isoproterenol, norepinephrine, or calcium chloride, or use electronic cardiac pacemaker. Intravenous fluids should be given by slow drip.

The information here is provided as guidance only. Prescribers should always consult the manufacturer's current prescribing information.

159

DOSAGE

Short-acting (Nifedipine, Adalat, Procardia): As an antianginal, initiate capsules at 10 mg three times daily, gradually increasing over 7–14 d as needed. For hospitalized patients under close supervision, dosage may be increased by 10 mg increments over 4–6 h periods until symptoms are controlled. For elderly patients and patients with hepatic impairment, initiate treatment at 10 mg twice daily, with careful monitoring.

Note: New labeling states that the short-acting product should not be used for hypertension, hypertensive crisis, acute MI, and some forms of unstable angina and chronic stable angina.

Extended-Release (Adalat CC): Initiate with 30 mg once daily, titrate over a 7–14 d period according to response. Usual maintenance dose is 30–60 mg once daily. Titration to doses >90 mg daily is not recommended.

Extended-Release (Procardia XL): Initiate with 30 or 60 mg once daily, titrate over a period of 7–14 d according to response. Titration may proceed more rapidly if the patient is frequently assessed. Titration to doses >120 mg daily is not recommended. Angina patients maintained on the short-acting formulation (nifedipine capsule) may be switched to the extended-release tablet at the nearest equivalent total daily dose. Experience with doses >90 mg daily in patients with angina is limited.

PATIENT INFORMATION

The extended-released tablets should be swallowed whole, without breaking, crushing, or chewing. This medication may cause headache, dizziness, flushing, palpitation, and ankle edema. Discuss exertion limits with physician. Notify physician if persistent or unusual side effects occur. Do not discontinue therapy without your physician's advice.

AVAILABILITY

Capsules, liquid-filled (Nifedipine, Adalat, Procardia)—10 mg, 20 mg
Tablets (Adalat CC)—30 mg, 60 mg, 90 mg
Tablets (Procardia XL)—30 mg, 60 mg, 90 mg

NIMODIPINE (Nimotop®)

Nimodipine is a dihydropyridine calcium antagonist that has been approved for use in patients with acute subarachnoid hemorrhage to improve associated neurologic deficits. Nimodipine is lipophilic and can cross the blood-brain barrier easily. It appears to have a greater effect on the cerebral arteries than arteries elsewhere in the body. The drug may prevent cerebral arterial spasm following subarachnoid hemorrhage, but this mechanism has not been confirmed conclusively. Nimodipine's exact mechanism of action in treating neurologic deficits associated with subarachnoid hemorrhage is not known. Nimodipine has also been used in the management of migraine headache, although this indication has not been approved by the Food and Drug Administration (FDA).

SPECIAL GROUPS

Race: no differences in response
Children: safety and effectiveness have not been established
Elderly: risk of hypotension may be increased; lower doses may be needed
Renal impairment: normal dosage recommended; nimodipine is not likely to be dialyzable
Hepatic impairment: administer with caution; use lower doses
Pregnancy: category C; not recommended
Breast-feeding: not recommended; nimodipine may be excreted in breast milk

DOSAGE

Usual dose is 60 mg every 4 h, beginning within 96 h of subarachnoid hemorrhage and continuing for 21 d. In patients with hepatic cirrhosis, dosage should be reduced to 30 mg every 4 h, with close monitoring of BP and heart rate.

Note: This medication is given preferably not less than 1 h before or 2 h after meals. If the capsule cannot be swallowed (*e.g.*, time of surgery, unconscious patient), make a hole in both ends of the capsule with an 18 gauge needle and extract the contents into a syringe. Empty the contents into the patient's in situ nasogastric tube and wash down the tube with 30 ml of normal saline.

CALCIUM ANTAGONISTS

IN BRIEF

INDICATIONS
Subarachnoid hemorrhage (nimodipine is indicated for the improvement of neurological outcome by reducing the incidence and severity of ischemic deficits in patients with subarachnoid hemorrhage from ruptured congenital aneurysms who are in good neurological condition post-ictus (eg, Hunt and Hess Grades I-III).

CONTRAINDICATIONS
Hypersensitivity

DRUG INTERACTIONS
Beta blockers
Cimetidine
Fentanyl
Omeprazole

ADVERSE EFFECTS
Cardiovascular: hypotension (1%–8%), peripheral edema (1%), abnormal ECG (1%), bradycardia (≤1%)
CNS: headache (1%–4%), psychiatric disturbances (1%), dizziness/lightheadedness (<1%)
GI:diarrhea (1%–4%), abdominal discomfort (2%), nausea (1%)
Dermatologic: rash/dermatitis (1%–2%), pruritus/urticaria (<1%)
Others: flushing (1%–2%), shortness of breath (1%–2%), muscle cramps (1%–2%)

PHARMACOKINETICS AND PHARMACODYNAMICS
Duration of action: 4 h
Onset of action: rapid
Time to peak plasma concentration: ≤1 h
Bioavailability: 13%, increased in patients with hepatic impairment.
Effect of food: administration of nimodipine following a standard breakfast resulted in a 68% lower peak plasma concentration and a 38% lower bioavailability relative to dosing under fasted conditions in a study of 24 healthy male volunteers
Metabolism: hepatic, extensive, to inactive metabolites
Elimination: renal (<1% unchanged); biliary/fecal
Half-life: 1–2 h (early), 8–9 h (terminal)
Protein binding: >95%

MONITORING
BP, heart rate, hepatic function.

OVERDOSE
For symptomatic hypotension, administer fluids intravenously, dopamine or dobutamine intravenously, calcium chloride, isoproterenol, metaraminol, or norepinephrine.
For tachycardia, rapid ventricular rate in patients with antegrade conduction in atrial flutter/fibrillation, and accessory pathway with Wolff-Parkinson-White or Lown-Ganong-Levine syndrome, administer direct current cardioversion, intravenous lidocaine, or intravenous procainamide. Intravenous fluids should be given by slow drip.
For bradycardia, 2° or 3° atrioventricular block, with a few patients progressing to asystole, administer intravenous atropine, isoproterenol, norepinephrine, or calcium chloride, or use electronic cardiac pacemaker. Intravenous fluids should be given by slow drip.

PATIENT INFORMATION
Take this medication at least 1 h before or 2 h after meals. This medication may cause dizziness, headache, flushing, ankle edema, and cramps. Notify physician if persistent or unusual side effects occur. Do not discontinue therapy without your physician's advice.

AVAILABILITY
Capsules, liquid-filled—30 mg

NISOLDIPINE
(Sular®)

Nisoldipine is a dihydropyridine calcium antagonist that is structurally related to nifedipine. Due to its vascular selectivity, nisoldipine is capable of lowering BP without affecting the functioning of the myocardium and skeletal muscle. This drug has been used as monotherapy, or in combination with other classes of antihypertensive agents, in the management of hypertension. Nisoldipine currently is available in the United States only as extended-release tablets, nisoldipine coat core (nisoldipine CC), which consist of an external coat and an internal core. Both coat and core contain nisoldipine; the coat as a slow release formulation and the core as a fast release formulation. This allows the drug to be released gradually over 24 hours, minimizing fluctuations in plasma concentration and providing a good trough to peak ratio.

Nisoldipine's efficacy in hypertensive patients has been demonstrated to be similar to that of thiazide diuretics, beta blockers, ACE inhibitors, and other calcium antagonists, without adverse effects on metabolic parameters. Further, nisoldipine was shown to reduce early morning rise in BP without reflex tachycardia in a large, South African multicenter trial. Similar to other calcium antagonists, nisoldipine works equally well as an antihypertensive agent in both black and white patients. Regression of left ventricular hypertrophy was demonstrated in black patients with severe diastolic hypertension in another South African study. Recently, nisoldipine CC was demonstrated to be safe and had no adverse effect on mortality when given to post-infarction patients with impaired left ventricular function in the DEFIANT-II study. In addition, nisoldipine CC was shown to be well tolerated in all groups of patients. The most frequently reported adverse effects were headache and peripheral edema, which were usually mild and transient.

SPECIAL GROUPS

Race: no differences in response
Children: safety and effectiveness have not been established
Elderly: initiate at lower dose
Renal impairment: normal dosage recommended in patients with mild to moderate renal impairment
Hepatic impairment: administer with caution; use lower initial and maintenance doses
Pregnancy: category C; use only if the potential benefit justifies the potential risk to the fetus
Breast-feeding: not recommended; nisoldipine may be excreted in breast milk

DOSAGE

Initiate therapy with 20 mg orally once daily, then increase by 10 mg/wk, or longer intervals, to attain adequate response. The usual maintenance dose is 20–40 mg once daily. Doses greater than 60 mg daily are not recommended. For elderly patients and patients with hepatic function impairment, initiate with a dose not exceeding 10 mg daily. Monitor BP closely during any dosage adjustment.
Note: Nisoldipine has been used safely with diuretics, ACE inhibitors, and beta blockers. Administration of this medication with a high fat meal can lead to excessive peak drug concentration and should be avoided. In addition, grapefruit products should be avoided before and after dosing.

IN BRIEF

INDICATIONS
Hypertension (Nisoldipine can be used alone or in combination with other antihypertensive agents)

CONTRAINDICATIONS
Hypersensitivity

DRUG INTERACTIONS
Beta blockers	Histamine H$_2$ antagonists (cimetidine)
Fentanyl	Ketoconazole
Grapefruit juice	Omeprazole
	Quinidine

ADVERSE EFFECTS
Cardiovascular: peripheral edema (22%), palpitations (3%), chest pain (2%)
CNS: headache (22%), dizziness/lightheadedness (5%)
GI: nausea (2%), abdominal discomfort (≤1%)
Dermatologic: rash/dermatitis (2%)
Others: pharyngitis (5%), vasodilation (4%), sinusitis (3%), sexual difficulties (≤1%), shortness of breath (≤1%)

PHARMACOKINETICS AND PHARMACODYNAMICS
Duration of action: 24 h (extended-release)
Onset of action: no data
Time to peak plasma concentration: 6–12 h
Bioavailability: 5%
Effect of food: food with a high fat content has a pronounced effect on the release of nisoldipine from the coat-core formulation and results in a significant increase in peak plasma concentration by up to 300%. Total exposure, however, is decreased about 25%. Grapefruit juice can interfere with nisoldipine metabolism, resulting in a mean increase in peak plasma concentration of about three-fold and AUC of almost two-fold
Metabolism: extensive presystemic metabolism in the intestinal wall and the liver; hepatically metabolized to inactive metabolites
Elimination: urinary excretion (60%–80%); only traces of unchanged drug are found in the urine
Half-life: 7–12 hours
Protein binding: >99%

MONITORING
BP, heart rate, hepatic function.

OVERDOSE
For symptomatic hypotension, administer fluids intravenously, dopamine or dobutamine intravenously, calcium chloride, isoproterenol, metaraminol, or norepinephrine.
For tachycardia, rapid ventricular rate in patients with antegrade conduction in atrial flutter/fibrillation, and accessory pathway with Wolff-Parkinson-White or Lown-Ganong-Levine syndrome, administer direct current cardioversion, intravenous lidocaine, or intravenous procainamide. Intravenous fluids should be given by slow drip.
For bradycardia, 2° or 3° atrioventricular block, with a few patients progressing to asystole, administer intravenous atropine, isoproterenol, norepinephrine, or calcium chloride, or use electronic cardiac pacemaker. Intravenous fluids should be given by slow drip.

PATIENT INFORMATION
Nisoldipine (Sular) is an extended-release formulation; swallow whole, do not bite or divide tablets. Avoid taking this medication with high fat meals. Grapefruit products should also be avoided before and after dosing. This medication may cause dizziness, palpitations, headache, flushing, and ankle edema. Notify physician if persistent or unusual side effects occur. Do not discontinue therapy without your physician's advice.

AVAILABILITY
Tablets (extended-release)—10 mg, 20 mg, 30 mg, 40 mg

VERAPAMIL

(Verapamil, Sustained-release Verapamil, Calan®, Calan® SR, Isoptin®, Isoptin® SR, Verelan®, Verelan®PM, Covera-HS™, Verapamil I.V., Isoptin® I.V.)

Verapamil hydrochloride is a phenylalkylamine calcium antagonist. It exerts its pharmacologic effects by modulating ionic calcium across the cell membrane of the arterial smooth muscle as well as in conductile and contractile myocardial cells. Verapamil lowers peripheral vascular resistance with little or no reflex tachycardia and may, in fact, reduce heart rate. The decrease in systemic and coronary vascular resistance and the sparing effect on intracellular oxygen consumption appear to explain its powerful antianginal properties. In the treatment of angina, verapamil is at least as effective as beta blockers and probably more so than nifedipine. As monotherapy, it can control BP for 24 hours in patients with uncomplicated hypertension given the sustained-release preparations. Verapamil has been combined with beta blockers, diuretics, ACE inhibitors, and reserpine successfully. Caution should be exercised when coadministering verapamil with a beta blocker, particularly in patients with myocardial conduction disease, because heart block may result. A particularly useful fixed combination available commercially is verapamil sustained-release and trandolapril (verapamil SR/trandolapril). This combination has been shown to reduce BP to a greater extent than when verapamil SR or trandolapril was used alone. Verapamil SR/trandolapril was demonstrated to reduce proteinuria to a greater extent than the individual agents in patients with diabetic or non-diabetic proteinuria. In a double-blind, randomized trial involving 100 post-acute MI patients with CHF, cardiac events occurred less frequently after verapamil SR/trandolapril than after monotherapy with trandolapril. Further, verapamil SR/trandolapril does not adversely influence glucose, insulin or lipid parameters in patients with mild to moderate essential hypertension and type II diabetes mellitus.

Verapamil is very effective in suppressing supraventricular arrhythmias and it slows the ventricular rate in patients with chronic atrial flutter or atrial fibrillation. However, this drug should not be used when these arrhythmias are associated with an accessory bypass tract (eg, Wolff-Parkinson-White). Verapamil is the only calcium antagonist for which a protective effect has been shown in patients who endured an acute coronary event. Decreased mortality and a lower rate of reinfarction was found in the DAVIT II study among patients treated with verapamil for 12 to 18 months after a MI. However, mortality rate was only significantly reduced in patients without heart failure who were in the verapamil group. A large, randomized clinical trial, CONVINCE, is now in progress to compare controlled onset-extended release verapamil with hydrochlorothiazide and/or atenolol for the management of hypertensive patients who have an established second risk factor for cardiovascular disease. The results of this study may clarify the safety and efficacy of these medications in preventing cardiovascular events.

IN BRIEF

INDICATIONS

Hypertension (all oral formulations)

Angina (all oral immediate-release formulations and Covera-HS)

Arrhythmias (all oral immediate-release formulations)

Supraventricular tachyarrhythmias (intravenous formulations)

CONTRAINDICATIONS

Hypersensitivity

Severe left ventricular dysfunction

Hypotension (systolic pressure less than 90 mm Hg)

Sick sinus syndrome (except in patients with a functioning artificial ventricular pacemaker)

Second- or third-degree AV block (except in patients with a functioning artificial ventricular pacemaker)

Patients with atrial flutter or atrial fibrillation and an accessory bypass tract (eg, Wolff-Parkinson- White, Lown-Ganong-Levine syndromes)

Cardiogenic shock and severe CHF, unless secondary to a supraventricular tachycardia amenable to verapamil therapy

Ventricular tachycardia (the use of intravenous verapamil in patients with wide-complex ventricular tachycardia (QRS ≥0.12 sec) can result in marked hemodynamic deterioration and ventricular fibrillation

DRUG INTERACTIONS

Barbiturates	Disopyramide	Prazosin
Beta blockers	Fentanyl	Procainamide
Calcium salts	Flecainide	Quinidine
Carbamazepine	Histamine H$_2$	Rifampin
Cyclosporine	antagonists	Sulfinpyrazone
Dantrolene	Hydantoins	Theophylline
Digitalis glycosides	Lithium	Vitamin D
Etomidate	Nondepolarizing muscle relaxants	

ADVERSE EFFECTS

Cardiovascular: peripheral edema (2%), hypotension (2%), CHF (2%), pulmonary edema (2%), AV block (1%), bradycardia (1%–2%)

CNS: dizziness/lightheadedness (3%–4%), headache (2%), asthenia (2%)

GI: constipation (7%), nausea (2%–3%)

Dermatologic: rash/dermatitis (1%–2%)

Others: shortness of breath (1%–2%), flushing (<1%), micturition disorder (<1%), sexual difficulties (<1%), muscle cramps (<1%)

PHARMACOKINETICS AND PHARMACODYNAMICS

Duration of action: 8 h (immediate-release); 24 h (sustained-release); 10–20 min (duration of hemodynamic effects after a single intravenous dose)

Onset of action: 30 min (oral); 1–5 min (intravenous)

Time to peak serum concentration: 1–2 h (immediate-release); 4–9 h (sustained- release)

Bioavailability: 20%–35%

Effect of food: food decreases the rate and extent of absorption of sustained-release verapamil tablets but produces smaller differences between peak and trough plasma concentrations of the drug; food does not appear to substantially affect the absorption of immediate-release tablets, extended-release tablets, or sustained-release capsules.

Metabolism: extensive; principle metabolite is norverapamil, which has approximately 20% of the cardiovascular activity of verapamil

Elimination: renal, 70% (3%–4% as unchanged drug); biliary/fecal, 9%–16 %

Half-life: single oral dose (3–7 h), repetitive oral dose (4.5–12 h), intravenous (4 min, early; 2–5 h, terminal)

Protein binding: 90%

SPECIAL GROUPS

Race: no differences in response

Children: safety and effectiveness have not been established. However, verapamil has been used in the pediatric population

Elderly: verapamil may cause a greater hypotensive effect compared to that seen in younger patients, probably due to age-related alterations in drug disposition. Lower doses may be required

Renal impairment: use with caution; lower doses may be required. Verapamil is not removed by hemodialysis

Hepatic impairment: use with caution; verapamil is extensively metabolized by the liver. Use lower doses

Pregnancy: category C; use verapamil in pregnant women only if potential benefit justifies potential risk to the fetus

Breast-feeding: not recommended; verapamil is excreted in breast milk

DOSAGE

Immediate-release Tablets (Verapamil, Calan, Isoptin): Adults— As an antianginal, antiarrhythmic, and antihypertensive, initiate at 80–120 mg three times daily, increase at daily or weekly intervals as needed and tolerated. Limit to 480 mg daily in divided doses.

Elderly—Initiate at 40 mg three times daily; adjust as needed.

Children— For infants less than 1 y of age and children 1 – 15 y, give 4–8 mg/kg body weight daily in divided doses.

Sustained-Release Capsules (Verelan): Adults—As an antihypertensive, initiate at 240 mg once daily; increase in increments of 120 mg /d at daily or weekly intervals as needed and tolerated.

Note: Initiate dose at 120 mg/d for patients who may have an increased response to verapamil. Usual total daily dose range, 240–480 mg

Sustained-Release Tablets(Verapamil SR, Calan SR, Isoptin SR): Adults— As an antihypertensive, initiate at 120–240 mg once daily with food; increase in increments of 40–120 mg/d at daily or weekly intervals as needed and as tolerated. Usual total daily dose range is 240–480 mg.

Extended-Release Tablets, Controlled Onset (Covera-HS): Adults— Initiate with 180 mg dose at bedtime for both hypertension and angina; if response is inadequate, the dose may be titrated upward to 540 mg/d given at bedtime.

Extended-Release Capsules, Controlled Onset (Verelan PM): Adults— Initiate with 200 mg dose at bedtime for hypertension; if response is inadequate, the dose may be titrated upward to 300 or 400 mg/d given at bedtime.

MONITORING
BP, EKG, liver function tests.

OVERDOSE
If acute complications occur after intravenous injection, apply cardiac massage, mechanical ventilation, adrenaline, and calcium gluconate.
For symptomatic hypotension, administer fluids intravenously, dopamine or dobutamine intravenously, calcium chloride, isoproterenol, metaraminol, or norepinephrine.
For tachycardia, rapid ventricular rate in patients with antegrade conduction in atrial flutter/fibrillation, and accessory pathway with Wolff-Parkinson-White or Lown-Ganong-Levine syndrome, administer direct current cardioversion, intravenous lidocaine, or intravenous procainamide. Intravenous fluids should be given by slow drip.
For bradycardia, 2° or 3° atrioventricular block, with a few patients progressing to asystole, administer intravenous atropine, isoproterenol, norepinephrine, or calcium chloride, or use electronic cardiac pacemaker. Intravenous fluids should be given by slow drip.

PATIENT INFORMATION
Take sustained-release tablets (Verapamil SR, Calan SR, Isoptin SR) with food. The sustained- or extended-released formulation of this medication should be swallowed whole, without breaking, crushing, or chewing. Verapamil may cause a slowing of the heart rate, headache, dizziness, ankle edema, or constipation. Discuss exertion limits with physician. Notify physician if persistent or unusual side effects occur. Do not discontinue therapy without your physician's advice.

AVAILABILITY
Tablets, immediate release (Verapamil, Calan, Isoptin)—40 mg, 80 mg, 120 mg
Capsules, sustained-release (Verelan)—120 mg, 180 mg, 240 mg, 360 mg
Tablets, extended-release and controlled onset (Covera- HS)—180 mg, 240 mg
Capsules, extended-release and controlled onset (Verelan PM)—100 mg, 200 mg, 300 mg
Tablets, sustained-release (Verapamil)—180 mg, 240 mg
Tablets,sustained-release(Calan SR, Isoptin SR)—120 mg, 180 mg, 240 mg
Injection (Verapamil I.V., Isoptin I.V.)—5 mg/2 ml (2 and 4 ml ampules and vials; syringes)
Combination formulations:
Tarka—trandolapril/ verapamil hydrochloride ER combination tablets
2 mg/ 180 mg
1 mg/ 240 mg
2 mg/ 240 mg
4 mg/ 240 mg

DOSAGE (CONTINUED)

Injection (Verapamil I.V., Isoptin I.V.): Adults—Initiate as 5–10 mg [or 75–150 µg/kg body weight (0.075–0.15 mg/kg)] slowly over at least 2 minutes with continuous electrocardiographic and blood pressure monitoring. If response is inadequate, 10 mg [or 150 µg/kg body weight (0.15 mg/kg)] may be administered 30 min after completion of the initial dose.

Elderly—Administer intravenous dose slowly over 3 min to minimize undesired effects.

Children—In infants up to 1 y of age, initiate at 100–200 µg/kg body weight (0.1–0.2 mg/kg) as an intravenous bolus over at least 2 min. Usual range is 0.75–2 mg. In children 1–15 y, initiate at 100–300 µg/kg body weight (0.1–0.3 mg/kg) as an intravenous bolus over at least 2 min. Usual range is 2–5 mg (not to exceed 5 mg). Repeat above dose 30 minutes after the first dose if the initial response is not adequate. Do not exceed 10 mg as a single dose in patients 1–15 y of age.

Note: A small fraction (<1%) of patients may have life-threatening adverse responses (rapid ventricular rate in atrial flutter/fibrillation, marked hypotension or extreme bradycardia/ asystole); monitor initial use of intravenous verapamil and have resuscitation facilities available. An intravenous infusion has been used (5 mg/h); precede the infusion with an intravenous loading dose. See package insert for information on compatibility.

The information here is provided as guidance only. Prescribers should always consult the manufacturer's current prescribing information.

165

Selected bibliography

Antonios TFT, MacGregor GA: Some similarities and differences between verapamil and the dihydropyridines. *J Hypertens* 1998, 16(Suppl 1):S31–S34.

Black HR, Elliott WJ, Neaton JD, *et al.*: Rationale and design for the Controlled ONset Verapamil INvestigation of Cardiovascular Endpoints (CONVINCE) Trial. *Controlled Clin Trials* 1998; 19(4):370–90.

Borhani NO, Mercuri M, Borhani PA, *et al.*: Final outcome results of the Multicenter Isradipine Diuretic Atherosclerosis study (MIDAS). A randomized controlled trial. *JAMA* 1996;276(10):785–91.

Conlin PR, Williams GH: Use of calcium channel blockers in hypertension. *Adv Intern Med* 1998;43:533–62.

Davis BR, Cutler JA, Gordon DJ, *et al.*: Rationale and design for the antihypertensive and lipid lowering treatment to prevent heart attack trial (ALLHAT). ALLHAT Research Group. *Am J Hypertens* 1996;9(4 Pt 1):342–60.

Dooley M, Goa KL: Fixed combination Verapamil SR/Trandolapril. *Drugs* 1998; 56:837–844.

Fodor JG: Nisoldipine CC: Efficacy and tolerability in hypertension and ischemic heart disease. *Cardiovasc Drugs Ther* 1997;10(Suppl 3):873–9.

Freher M, Challapalli S, Pinto JV, *et al.*: Current status of calcium channel blockers in patients with cardiovascular disease. *Curr Probl Cardiol* 1999; 24:229–340.

Frishman WH; Comparative efficacy and concomitant use of bepridil and beta blockers in the management of angina pectoris. *Am J Cardiol* 1992; Suppl 69:50D–60D.

Frishman WH: Current status of calcium channel blockers. *Curr Probl Cardiol* 19(11):637–88, 1994.

Frishman WH: Calcium channel blockers. In *Cardiovascular Pharmacotherapeutics*. Edited by Frishman WH, Sonnenblick EH. New York: McGraw Hill 1997; 101–30.

Frishman WH: Calcium channel blockers. In *Cardiovascular Pharmacotherapeutics Companion Handbook*. Edited by Frishman WH, Sonnenblick EH. New York: McGraw Hill 1998; 73–106.

Frishman WH, Hershman D: Amlodipine. In *Cardiovascular Drug Therapy* 2nd ed. Edited by Messerli FH. Philadelphia: WB Saunders, 1996:1024–40.

Frishman WH, Rosenberg A, Katz B: Calcium antagonists in the management of systemic hypertension: the impact of sustained-release drug delivery systems. *Coronary Art Dis* 1994; 5:4–13.

Frishman WH, Sonnenblick EH: Cardiovascular uses of calcium antagonists. In *Cardiovascular Drug Therapy* 2nd ed. Edited by Messerli FH. Philadelphia: WB Saunders, 1996:891–901.

Frishman WH, Sonnenblick EH: Beta-Adrenergic blocking drugs and calcium channel blockers. In *Hurst's The Heart* 9th ed. Edited by Alexander RW, Schlant RC, Fuster V. New York: McGraw Hill, 1998:1583–1618.

Hansson L, Zanchetti A, Carruthers SG, *et al.*: Effects of intensive blood-pressure lowering and low-dose aspirin in patients with hypertension: principal results of the Hypertension Optimal Treatment (HOT) randomised trial. HOT study Group. *Lancet* 1998;351(9118):1755–62.

Lopez LM, Santiago TM: Isradipine-Another calcium-channel blocker for the treatment of hypertension and angina. *Ann Pharmacother* 1992;26:789–99.

Mancia G, Grassi G: The International Nifedipine GITS Study of Intervention as a Goal in Hypertension Treatment (INSIGHT) trial. *Am J Cardiol* 1998;82(9B):23R–28R.

Messerli FH, Weiner DA: Are all calcium antagonists equally effective for reducing reinfarction rate? *Am J Cardiol* 1993; 72:818–20.

Messerli FH: What, if anything, is controversial about calcium antagonists? *Am J Hypertens* 1996; 9(12 Pt 2):177S–181S.

Opie LH: What does Nisoldipine Coat Core (CC) add to current therapy that is clinically meaningful? *Am J Cardiol* 1997;79(10A):29–32.

Packer M: Combined beta-adrenergic and calcium-entry blockade in angina pectoris. *N Engl J Med* 1989; 302:709–718.

Packer M: Calcium channel blockers in chronic heart failure. *Circulation* 1990; 82:2254–56.

Packer M, Frishman WH: Calcium Channel Antagonists in Cardiovascular Disease. Norwalk: Appleton Century Crofts, 1984.

Packer M, O'Connor CM, Ghali JK, *et al.*: Effect of amlodipine on morbidity and mortality in severe chronic heart failure. Prospective Randomized Amlodipine Survival Evaluation Study Group. *New Engl J Med* 1996;335(15):1107–14.

Rich S, Kaufmann E, Levy PS: The effect of high doses of calcium-channel blockers on survival in primary pulmonary hypertension. *N Engl J Med* 1992; 327:76–81.

Singh V, Frishman WH: Calcium antagonists. In *The ABCs of Antihypertensive Therapy*. Edited by Messerli FH. New York: Authors Publishing House 1999, in press.

The DEFIANT-II Research Group: Doppler flow and echocardiography in functional cardiac insufficiency: assessment of nisoldipine therapy. Results of the DEFIANT-II Study. *European Heart Journal* 1997;18(1):31–40.

The Multicentre Diltiazem Postinfarction Trial Research Group: The effect of diltiazem on mortality and reinfarction after myocardial infarction. *N Engl J Med* 1988; 319:386–392.

Waters D: Calcium channel blockers: An evidence-based review. *Can J Cardiol* 1997;13(8):757–766.

Yusuf S, Held P, Furberg C: Update of effects of calcium antagonists in myocardial infarction or angina in light of the second Danish Infarction Trial (DAVIT-II) and other recent studies (editorial). *Am J Cardiol* 1991; 67:1295–97.

9

DIURETICS

Diuretics have been in widespread use for more than 40 years and have been the mainstay of treatment of hypertension and congestive heart failure (CHF). Despite the advent of newer agents, they continue to enjoy a large clinical demand and remain among the most widely prescribed drugs. Although originally intended for the treatment of edematous conditions, the most common application of diuretics is in the management of hypertension, and their efficacy as antihypertensive agents in mild to moderate hypertension is impressive. They remain the cornerstone of treatment for conditions in which the presence of edema is a feature, notably CHF.

Diuretics are classified into three main categories, and are defined by their structures, their sites of action, and their effects on electrolyte excretion. The three main types of diuretics are the thiazides (and related drugs), the loop diuretics, and the potassium-sparing diuretics.

The thiazides (benzothiadiazines) and loop diuretics act predominantly at the luminal face of the distal tubule. Differences in their diuretic potency and electrolyte effects are attributable to their actions at different functional loci in the renal tubular apparatus.

MODE OF ACTION

By definition, diuretics are drugs that increase urine output. Their primary effect, however, is to inhibit tubular electrolyte reabsorption. This inhibition leads to an increase in the osmolar pressure, resulting in depressed fluid reabsorption so that an increase in urine output occurs. The individual segments of the nephron differ in selectivity of ion reabsorption.

The main action of the thiazide diuretics is to inhibit sodium-chloride cotransport in the distal tubule. Loop diuretics, which can achieve urine output of about 25% of glomerular filtration rate, inhibit sodium-potassium-chloride cotransport in the medullary portion of the ascending limb of the loop of Henle, although they may also have a minor effect on the proximal tubule. The potassium-sparing diuretics act on a sodium channel in the distal tubule. The result is a reduction of the membrane potential that drives potassium secretion, and the end result is a mild natriuretic action combined with potassium retention (Figure 9.1).

All diuretics increase the excretion of sodium as the main cation and are effective in lowering blood pressure (BP) in hypertensive patients and animals. They are effective antihypertensive agents at doses that are not overtly diuretic. Their initial effect is to reduce the plasma volume, although later this change is largely compensated for and the peripheral vascular resistance falls. There is usually a fall in plasma volume, which in turn may result in increased plasma renin activity; this may or may not be accompanied by a rise in plasma catecholamines. The action of diuretics in stimulating renin responsiveness makes them particularly useful for treating elderly and black patients.

In addition to the three groups of diuretics in common use, organomercurials and carbonic anhydrase inhibitors were once used. Because of the toxicity of the former and the poor efficacy of the latter, neither type of compound is now viewed as useful. (Carbonic anhydrase inhibitors, however, have retained a role in the topical treatment of glaucoma.) Further discussion

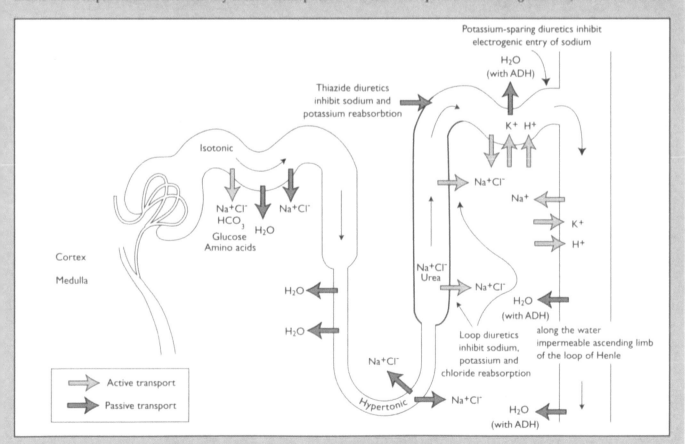

FIGURE 9.1 A simplified schema of the functional divisions of a mammalian nephron.

will therefore be confined to the three types of drugs in current use: the thiazides, the loop diuretics, and the potassium-sparing agents.

LOOP DIURETICS

Loop diuretics are one of the mainstays in the treatment of CHF and other edematous conditions. The group comprises **furosemide, ethacrynic acid, bumetanide, and torsemide**. All have similar efficacies and modes of action, but differ in their pharmacokinetic profiles.

EFFICACY AND USE

Loop diuretics are of particular value in treating CHF. They not only relieve the symptoms of congestion, but may also increase exercise capacity. Clinical signs, such as edema, are rarely refractory to treatment, except in the terminal stage; apparent resistance may reflect inadequate dosage or failure to combine the actions of drugs that act on different segments of the renal tubule. Intermittent administration has proved more efficacious in promoting fluid loss than has continuous treatment.

Some loop diuretics may have a useful antihypertensive effect, particularly in patients resistant to thiazides or with severe renal impairment. Loop diuretics have an adjunctive place in the treatment of acute pulmonary edema. Intravenous furosemide or ethacrynic acid produce rapid losses of salt and water. A reduction in BP may be apparent before diuresis occurs; this benefit has been attributed to venodilatation and a reduced cardiac filling pressure.

MODE OF ACTION

Loop diuretics exert their main action in the thick ascending limb of the loop of Henle. Although their chemical structures are diverse, they are all actively secreted by the proximal tubule in the lumen; their concentration in the loop of Henle is thus high. This high concentration appears to be a prerequisite for their inhibitory effect on ion reabsorption. They appear to inhibit the sodium-chloride cotransport system at the luminal membrane of the loop of Henle. The excretion of calcium and potassium is also increased.

Loop diuretics are sometimes referred to as high-ceiling diuretics because a good correlation is observed between the diuretic effect and the dose administered. How much of the diuretic response can be attributed solely to direct interference with transport systems at specific membrane sites, and how much can be attributed to secondary effects resulting from the release of intrarenal mediators and the associated redistribution of blood flow in the kidneys remains unclear.

INDICATIONS

	Bumetanide	Ethacrynic Acid	Furosemide	Torsemide
CHF	+	+	+	+
Edema	+	+	+	+
Hypertension	–	–	+	+

+—FDA approved; ––—not FDA approved; CHF—congestive heart failure.

BUMETANIDE (Bumetanide, Bumex®)

Bumetanide, similar to furosemide, is a sulfonamide-type loop diuretic. The diuretic potency of bumetanide is approximately 40 times that of furosemide. In addition to the inhibition of sodium reabsorption in the ascending limb of the loop of Henle, bumetanide also acts in the proximal tubule by blocking the reabsorption of phosphate. Bumetanide enhances renal blood flow via renal vascular dilation. However, its effect on glomerular filtration rate is variable. Bumetanide therapy is indicated for the management of excessive fluid overload or edema in various clinical conditions. Bumetanide may be effective in some patients who are unresponsive or refractory to other diuretics. Chronic bumetanide therapy has been associated with increases in plasma renin activity.

SPECIAL GROUPS

Race: no differences in response

Children: safety and effectiveness have not been established

Elderly: use with caution; no dosage adjustment is required

Renal impairment: use with caution; higher doses may be required to enhance diuresis; contraindicated in patients with anuria or progressive oliguric renal failure unresponsive to diuretic therapy

Hepatic impairment: use with caution; dosage adjustment is probably not required

Pregnancy: category C; should only be used if clearly indicated

Breast-feeding: use with caution; not known if the drug is excreted in human milk

DOSAGE

Oral: Usual dose range—0.5–2 mg/day as a single dose*

In patients with edema, if the initial diuresis is inadequate, repeated doses may be administered every 4–6 h until the desired diuretic response or a **maximum daily dosage of 10 mg** is achieved. Intermittent dosing schedule—Bumetanide is administered on alternate days or daily for 3–4 days with a drug holiday of 1–2 d in between.

Intravenous or Intramuscular: Usual dose range—0.5–1 mg*

In patients with edema, if the initial diuresis is inadequate, repeated doses may be administered every 2–3 h until the desired diuretic response or a **maximum daily dosage of 10 mg** is achieved.

* Higher dosage (>1–2 mg daily) may be required to achieve the desired therapeutic response in patients with renal insufficiency.

IN BRIEF

INDICATIONS

Edema associated with CHF, hepatic or renal disease, including the nephrotic syndrome.

CONTRAINDICATIONS

Known hypersensitivity to bumetanide, furosemide (has been used safely in patients with furosemide allergy), torsemide or sulfur

Anuria or severe, progressive oliguria unresponsive to diuretic therapy

Hepatic coma

Severe electrolyte depletion

DRUG INTERACTIONS

Other diuretics

Antihypertensive agents

Cardiac glycosides

Other potassium-depleting agents (corticosteroids, amphotericin B)

NSAIDs

Agents with high sodium content (ticarcillin)

Probenecid

Lithium

Other ototoxic agents (aminoglycosides, erythromycin, cisplatin)

Non-depolarizing neuromuscular blockers

ADVERSE EFFECTS

CV: hypotension, arrhythmias, chest pain

CNS: dizziness, headache, fatigue, ototoxicity, encephalopathy (in patients with liver disease)

Blood: volume and electrolyte depletion ($\downarrow$ K,$\downarrow$ Cl,$\downarrow$ Na,$\downarrow$ Ca, $\downarrow$ Mg, $\uparrow$ uric acid), metabolic alkalosis, azotemia, $\uparrow$ serum creatinine, hyperglycemia, dyslipidemia, leukopenia, thrombocytopenia

GI: nausea, elevated liver function test

GU: sexual dysfunction, polyuria

Skin: pruritus, urticaria, rash

Other: dehydration, muscle cramps

PHARMACOKINETICS AND PHARMACODYNAMICS

Duration of action: (po/IM) 4–6 h; (IV) 2–3 h

Onset of action: (po/IM) 30–60 min; (IV) few min

Peak effect: (po/IM) 1–2 h; (IV) 15–30 min

Bioavailability: (po) 85%–95%; (IV/IM) 100%

Effect of food: insignificant, delays the absorption

Metabolism: partially metabolized in liver

Excretion: urine—80% (50% unchanged); feces—10%–20% (< 2% unchanged); $\uparrow$ nonrenal clearance in renal insufficiency

Plasma half-life: 1–3 h

Protein binding: 94%–96%

MONITORING

BP, urine output, weight, hearing acuity;
Lab: serum electrolytes/BUN/CO_2.

OVERDOSE

Supportive: replace fluid and electrolyte losses.

PATIENT INFORMATION

Bumetanide is used to reduce excessive water in the body. Take the medication as instructed. Avoid excessive dietary sodium intake while maintaining on this therapy. Potassium-rich diet is encouraged to avoid potassium depletion. Sit or lie down if dizziness occurs and rise slowly from a sitting or lying position.

AVAILABILITY

Tablets—0.5, 1, 2 mg
Ampules—0.25 mg/mL, 2 mL

The information here is provided as guidance only. Prescribers should always consult the manufacturer's current prescribing information.

169

ETHACRYNIC ACID
ETHNACRYNATE
SODIUM

(Edecrin®)
(Sodium Edecrin®)

Ethacrynic acid is a loop diuretic with similar pharmacologic effects to furosemide. It is metabolized to a cysteine conjugate, which may contribute to its diuretic effects. Ethacrynic acid enhances the excretion of sodium, chloride, potassium, hydrogen, calcium, and magnesium, but has no effect on urinary phosphate content. The agent has little or no direct effect on glomerular filtration rate or renal blood flow except in severe intravascular volume depletion associated with aggressive diuresis. Ethacrynic acid is mainly used for the treatment of refractory edema or fluid overload when response to other diuretic therapy is inadequate. Although ethacrynic acid is effective even in patients with significant renal insufficiency, its use has been limited by ototoxicity. The problem is manifested as deafness, tinnitus, and vertigo with a sense of fullness in the ears. Ototoxicity associated with ethacrynic acid therapy can be irreversible and has been reported most frequently in patients with severe renal insufficiency, especially after receiving high IV doses. To alleviate the problem, it is recommended that a single dose should not exceed 100 mg and rapid IV administration should be avoided. Ethacrynic acid, structurally free of sulfur, may be used safely in patients with a known allergy to sulfonamides or thiazide diuretics.

SPECIAL GROUPS

Race: no differences in response

Children: safety and effectiveness have not been established in children for IV administration and in infants for oral administration

Elderly: use with caution; no dosage adjustment is required

Renal impairment: use with caution; higher doses may be required to enhance diuresis; contraindicated in patients with anuria or progressive oliguric renal failure unresponsive to diuretic therapy

Hepatic impairment: use with caution; titrate dose based on clinical assessment

Pregnancy: category B; should only be used if clearly indicated

Breast-feeding: not recommended; not known if the drug is excreted in human milk

IN BRIEF

INDICATIONS
Edema associated with CHF, liver cirrhosis, and renal disease, including the nephrotic syndrome

Ascites associated with malignancy, idiopathic edema, and lymphedema

Hospitalized pediatric patients with congenital heart disease or the nephrotic syndrome (not indicated for infants)

CONTRAINDICATIONS
Known hypersensitivity

Infants

Anuria or severe, progressive oliguria unresponsive to diuretic therapy

Hepatic coma

Severe electrolyte depletion

DRUG INTERACTIONS
Other diuretics

Antihypertensive agents

Cardiac glycosides

Other potassium-depleting agents (corticosteroids, amphotericin B)

NSAIDs

Agents with high sodium content (ticarcillin)

Lithium

Probenecid

Other ototoxic agents (aminoglycosides, erythromycin, cisplatin)

Warfarin

Non-depolarizing neuromuscular blockers

ADVERSE EFFECTS
CV: hypotension, orthostatic symptoms, arrhythmias, chest pain

CNS: dizziness, headache, fatigue, ototoxicity, encephalopathy (in patients with liver disease)

Blood: volume and electrolyte depletion ($\downarrow$ K, $\downarrow$ Cl, $\downarrow$ Na, $\downarrow$ Ca, $\downarrow$ Mg, $\uparrow$ uric acid), metabolic alkalosis, azotemia, $\uparrow$ serum creatinine, hyperglycemia, hypoglycemia (high dose in uremic patients), agranulocytosis, thrombocytopenia

GI: anorexia, nausea, vomiting, constipation, diarrhea, elevated liver function test, hepatocellular injury, pancreatitis

GU: sexual dysfunction, polyuria

Skin: rash

Other: dehydration, muscle cramps, fever, chills

PHARMACOKINETICS AND PHARMACODYNMAICS
Duration of action: (po) 6–8 h or longer; (IV) 2–7 h

Onset of action: (po) <30 min; (IV) <5 min

Peak effect: (po) 2 h; (IV) 15–30 min

Bioavailability: 100%

Effect of food: no data

Metabolism: partially metabolized in liver; with one active metabolite

Excretion: (IV) 30%–65% in urine (partly unchanged); 35%–40% in bile

Plasma half-life: 1–4 h

Protein binding: 90%

MONITORING
BP, urine output, weight, hearing acuity;

Lab—serum electrolytes/BUN/CO_2, CBC/WBC with differential, liver function test.

OVERDOSE
Supportive: replace fluid and electrolyte losses.

ETHACRYNIC ACID (*CONTINUED*)

DOSAGE

Oral (ethacrynic acid): Usual dose range—50–200 mg/d in 1–2 divided doses taken after a meal

The initial dose is 25–50 mg* once daily administered after a meal. The dose may be increased in 25–50 mg* increments daily until the desired diuresis or a maximum dose of 100 mg twice daily is achieved. In patients with severe, refractory edema, a dose of 200 mg twice daily may be required to maintain adequate diuresis.

Intermittent dosing schedule: After an effective diuresis or an ideal dry weight is achieved, ethacrynic acid can be administered on alternate days, or daily for a few days interspersed with a drug holiday of 1–2 d.

* Lower dose is recommended in patients who receive other diuretic therapy concurrently.

IV (ethacrynate sodium): indicated when a rapid onset of diuresis is desired such as in acute pulmonary edema, or when oral administration is not practical

Usual dose—50 mg (0.5–1 mg/kg, up to 100 mg) as a single dose infused over a few minutes (or, over 20—30 min), may be repeated once after 2—3 h if the desired diuresis is not achieved.

PATIENT INFORMATION

Ethacrynic acid is used to reduce excessive water in the body. Take the medication as instructed. Avoid excessive dietary sodium intake while maintaining on this therapy. Potassium-rich diet is encouraged to avoid potassium depletion. Sit or lie down if dizziness occurs and rise slowly from a sitting or lying position.

AVAILABILITY

Tablets—25, 50 mg
Vials—50 mg

The information here is provided as guidance only. Prescribers should always consult the manufacturer's current prescribing information.

171

FUROSEMIDE (Furosemide, Lasix®)

Furosemide is the most widely used loop diuretic. It is useful in the management of edema associated with various cardiac, hepatic and renal dysfunctions. Furosemide has also been used in the treatment of hypertension, especially in patients with concurrent clinical evidence of fluid overload. Furosemide therapy enhances renal excretion of sodium, chloride, potassium, hydrogen, calcium, magnesium, ammonium, bicarbonate and possibly phosphate. Its calcium lowering effect has been utilized, along with normal saline hydration, to increase renal calcium excretion in patients with hypercalcemia.

SPECIAL GROUPS

Race: no differences in response

Children: recommended in children for the management of edema, but not for hypertension

Elderly: use with caution; no dosage adjustment is required

Renal impairment: use with caution; higher doses may be required to enhance diuresis; contraindicated in patients with anuria or progressive oliguric renal failure unresponsive to diuretic therapy

Hepatic impairment: use with caution; titrate dose based on clinical assessment

Pregnancy: category C; should only be used if clearly indicated

Breast-feeding: use with caution; excreted in human milk

DOSAGE

Edema: Oral—The usual dose is 20–80 mg given as a single dose. The same dose may be repeated, or increased in 20–40 mg increments every 6–8 h until the desired diuresis is achieved. The effective dose may then be given once or twice daily to maintain adequate fluid balance. For chronic maintenance therapy, furosemide given on alternate days or on 2–4 consecutive days each week is preferred. Maximum oral dose of 600 mg/d has been used in patients with severe fluid overload.

IV/IM—The usual dose is 20–40 mg given as a single injection. The IV route is preferred when rapid diuresis is indicated. The same dose may be repeated, or increased in 20–40 mg increments every 1–2 h until the desired response is achieved. Each IV dose should be **administered over a few minutes.**

Furosemide has been administered as a continuous IV infusion in some patients to maintain adequate urine flow. A bolus of 20–40 mg should be given first, followed by an infusion of 0.25–0.5 mg/min. The rate should be titrated, up to **a maximum of 4 mg/min,** based on clinical response.

Hypertension: The usual initial dose is 40 mg twice daily. Dosage should then be adjusted based on response. The maximum dose is 240 mg/d in 2–3 divided doses.

Higher dosages may be required for the management of edema or hypertension in patients with renal insufficiency or CHF. These patients should be monitored closely to ensure efficacy and avoid undesired toxicity.

IN BRIEF

INDICATIONS
Edema associated with CHF, liver cirrhosis, and renal disease including the nephrotic syndrome (both adults and children)
Hypertension (adults only)

CONTRAINDICATIONS
Known hypersensitivity to furosemide, bumetanide, torsemide, or sulfur
Anuria or severe, progressive oliguria unresponsive to diuretic therapy
Hepatic coma
Severe electrolyte depletion

DRUG INTERACTIONS
Other diuretics
Antihypertensive agents
Cardiac glycosides
Other potassium-depleting agents (corticosteroids, amphotericin B)
NSAIDs
Agents with high sodium content (ticarcillin)
Probenecid
Lithium
Other ototoxic agents (aminoglycosides, erythromycin, cisplatin)
Sucralfate
Non-depolarizing neuromuscular blockers

ADVERSE EFFECTS
CV: hypotension, orthostatic symptoms, arrhythmias, chest pain
CNS: dizziness, headache, fatigue, ototoxicity
Blood: volume and electrolyte depletion ($\downarrow$ K, $\downarrow$ Cl, $\downarrow$ Na, $\downarrow$ Ca, $\downarrow$ Mg, $\uparrow$ uric acid), metabolic alkalosis, azotemia, $\uparrow$ serum creatinine, hyperglycemia, dyslipidemia, blood dyscrasias
GI: anorexia, nausea, vomiting, constipation, diarrhea, jaundice, pancreatitis
GU: sexual dysfunction, polyuria
Skin: rash, pruritus, urticaria, photosensitivity, exfoliative dermatitis, erythema multiforme
Other: dehydration, muscle cramps, fever, vasculitis, interstitial nephritis

PHARMACOKINETICS AND PHARMACODYNAMICS
Duration of action: (po) 6–8 h; (IV) $\geq$2 h
Onset of action: (po) 30–60 min; (IV) 2–5 min
Peak effect: (po) 1–2 h; (IV) <30 min
Bioavailability: (po) 60%–70%
Effect of food: may slow down the rate and reduce the amount of absorption
Metabolism: 10% ($\uparrow$ in renal failure)
Excretion: urine—60%–90% (>50% unchanged); bile/feces—6%–9%
Plasma half-life: 0.5–2 h ($\uparrow$ renal and/or hepatic dysfunction)
Protein binding: 91%–99%

MONITORING
BP, urine output, weight, hearing acuity;
Lab—serum electrolytes/ BUN/CO_2.

OVERDOSE
Supportive: replace fluid and electrolyte losses.

PATIENT INFORMATION
Furosemide is used to lower BP or reduce excessive water in the body. Take the medication as instructed. Avoid excessive dietary sodium intake while maintaining on this therapy. Potassium-rich diet is encouraged to avoid potassium depletion. Sit or lie down if dizziness occurs and rise slowly from a sitting or lying position.

AVAILABILITY
Tablets—20, 40, 80 mg
Ampules/Syringes/Vials—10 mg/mL in 2, 4, 8, 10 mL
Oral Solution—8 mg/mL, 10 mg/mL

TORSEMIDE (Demadex®)

Similar to furosemide and bumetanide, torsemide is a sulfonamide-type loop diuretic. It inhibits sodium and chloride reabsorption in the ascending limb of the loop of Henle, which is mainly responsible for its diuretic activity. Torsemide lowers BP via an unknown mechanism of action in low doses, 2.5 to 10 mg/day, that have little diuretic effect. Torsemide is available for oral and IV administration. The absorption is reliable and nearly complete, 80% to 90%, after an oral dose. Oral and IV doses of torsemide are equivalent. After entering the systemic circulation, 80% of torsemide is metabolized in the liver. As a result, there is less drug accumulation in patients with renal failure. This may account for the lower risk of ototoxicity reported with torsemide therapy. It is an effective, but a relatively more expensive alternative for the management of edema and hypertension.

SPECIAL GROUPS

Race: no differences in response

Children: safety and effectiveness have not been established

Elderly: no dosage adjustment is required

Renal impairment: use with caution; higher doses may be required to enhance diuresis; contraindicated in patients with anuria or progressive oliguric renal failure unresponsive to diuretic therapy

Hepatic impairment: use with caution; titrate dose based on clinical assessment

Pregnancy: category B; should only be used if clearly indicated

Breast-feeding: use with caution; not known if the drug is excreted in human milk

DOSAGE

CHF/ Chronic renal failure: Usual dose range—10–200 mg/d

The usual initial dose is 10–20 mg once daily via oral or IV administration. If the diuretic response is inadequate, the dose may be doubled until the desired response or the maximum single dose of 200 mg is achieved.

Hepatic cirrhosis: Usual dose range—5–40 mg/d

The usual initial dose is 5–10 mg once daily administered orally or IV along with an aldosterone antagonist or a potassium-sparing diuretic. If the diuretic response is inadequate, the dose may be doubled until the desired response or the maximum single dose of 40 mg is achieved.

Hypertension: Usual dose range—5–10 mg/d

The usual initial dose is 5 mg once daily administered orally. If adequate reduction in BP is not achieved in 4–6 wk, the dose may be increased up to 10 mg once daily. If the response is still inadequate, an additional antihypertensive agent should be added.

IN BRIEF

INDICATIONS
Edema associated with CHF, liver cirrhosis, and renal disease
Hypertension

CONTRAINDICATIONS
Known hypersensitivity to torsemide, sulfonylureas, or other sulfur-containing agents
Anuria or severe, progressive oliguria unresponsive to diuretic therapy
Hepatic coma
Severe electrolyte depletion

DRUG INTERACTIONS
Other diuretics
Antihypertensive agents
Cardiac glycosides
Other potassium-depleting agents (corticosteroids, amphotericin B)
NSAIDs
Agents with high sodium content (ticarcillin)
Probenecid
Lithium
Other ototoxic agents (aminoglycosides, erythromycin, cisplatin)
Cholestyramine
Non-depolarizing neuromuscular blockers

ADVERSE EFFECTS
CV: hypotension, orthostatic symptoms, arrhythmias, chest pain
CNS: dizziness, headache, fatigue, ototoxicity
Blood: volume and electrolyte depletion ($\downarrow$ K, $\downarrow$ Cl, $\downarrow$ Na, $\downarrow$ Ca, $\downarrow$ Mg, $\uparrow$ uric acid), metabolic alkalosis, azotemia, $\uparrow$ serum creatinine, hyperglycemia, dyslipidemia
GI: anorexia, nausea, vomiting, constipation, diarrhea
GU: sexual dysfunction, polyuria
Skin: rash
Other: dehydration, thirst, arthralgia, angioedema

PHARMACOKINETICS AND PHARMACODYNAMICS
Duration of action: (po) 8–12 h; (IV) 6 h
Onset of action: (po) <1 h ; (IV) <10 min
Peak effect: (po) 1–2 h; (IV) <1 h
Bioavailability: 75%–90%
Effect of food: delayed absorption but no effect on bioavailability and diuretic activity
Metabolism: 80% metabolized in liver
Excretion: renal (20% unchanged)
Plasma half-life: 3.5 h
Protein binding: >99%

MONITORING
BP, urine output, weight, hearing acuity;
Lab—serum electrolytes/ BUN/CO_2.

OVERDOSE
Supportive: replacement of fluid and electrolyte losses.

PATIENT INFORMATION
Torsemide is used to lower BP or reduce excessive water in the body. Take the medication as instructed. Avoid excessive dietary sodium intake while maintaining on this therapy. Potassium-rich diet is encouraged to avoid potassium depletion. Sit or lie down if dizziness occurs and rise slowly from a sitting or lying position.

AVAILABILITY
Tablets—5, 10, 20, 100 mg
Ampules—10 mg/mL in 2 mL and 5 mL

THIAZIDE DIURETICS

Thiazide diuretics remain the most commonly used agents in the initial treatment of essential hypertension and are recognized as the preferred diuretic for this condition. They are very effective in lowering BP in up to 60% of patients with mild-to-moderate essential hypertension. During the first few days after administration, systolic and diastolic pressures are significantly reduced, and this effect is sustained during continued treatment. The longer-acting thiazides and their congeners are distinctly superior to loop diuretics in treating uncomplicated hypertension. In comparative studies, the benzothiazides have been shown to be as effective as other classes of drugs commonly used for the treatment of uncomplicated hypertension. Their effect adds to that of beta blockers and ACE inhibitors, but is not as additive with calcium antagonists.

EFFICACY AND USE

The Medical Research Council (MRC) trial identified several side effects of thiazide diuretics, particularly impotence. The metabolic effects of these drugs (increases in uric acid levels, decreases in serum potassium levels, the appearance of insulin resistance, and changes in the blood lipid profile) are well established. Left ventricular hypertrophy may be reversed, an effect also seen in the Trial of Mild Hypertension Study. The risk of stroke in middle-aged and older patients is significantly reduced (Figure 9.2).

Thiazide diuretics were used as initial therapy in the specially-treated group in the Hypertension Detection and Follow-Up Program. Overall death rate fell by 17%, cerebrovascular deaths fell by 45%, and deaths from heart disease fell by 20%, compared with a less aggressively-treated group. The Australian Therapeutic Trial in Mild Hypertension demonstrated a significant reduction in cardiovascular events when thiazide diuretics were compared with placebo. In the Oslo Study, however, which compared no active treatment with thiazide diuretic therapy over 10 years, significantly more deaths resulting from MI occurred in the active-treatment group. This finding has led to the suggestion that the metabolic effects of diuretics may reduce the potential benefit derived from the lowering of BP. The MRC showed a beneficial effect with stroke prevention, but failed to detect a benefit with deaths caused by MI (Figure 9.3). In a subsequent analysis, significant increases in MI (Q waves on the ECG, including silent and overt MI) and sudden death were noted in patients treated with diuretics. These findings lend some support to those of the Multiple Risk Factor Intervention Trial.

Nevertheless, in the Systolic Hypertension in the Elderly Program of elderly patients with isolated systolic hypertension, treatment with low dose chlorthalidone (12.5 to 25 mg) was shown to reduce stroke and heart attack significantly.

A study examining the association between thiazide diuretic therapy and the risk of primary cardiac death found a direct correlation between the daily thiazide dose and the risk of primary cardiac arrest in patients with hypertension. Low-dose thiazide treatment and the presence of a potassium-sparing diuretic in the regimen were associated with lower risk as compared with moderate- or high-dose thiazide therapy and the absence of a potassium-sparing component in the regimen.

These findings may partially explain the results of some earlier clinical trials (as mentioned above) in which diuretic therapy was associated with no improvement or increase in the number of cardiac events.

MODE OF ACTION

The precise mechanisms that underlie the antihypertensive action of thiazide diuretics have not been defined. As with other diuretics, however, their effect on BP presumably results

INDICATIONS

	Bendroflume	Benz	Chloro	Chlorthal	Hydrochloro	Hydroflum	Indap	Methyclo	Metola	Poly	Quineth	Trichlor
Hypertension	+	+	+	+	+	+	+	+	+	+	+	+
Mild CHF (adjunctive)	+	+	+	+	+	+	+	+	+	+	+	+
Edema	+	+	+	+	+	+	+	+	+	+	+	+

+—FDA approved; CHF—congestive heart failure; bendroflume—bendroflumethiazide; benz—benzthiazide; chloro—chlorothiazide; chlorthal—chlorthalidone; hydrochloro—hydrochlorothiazide; hydroflum—hydroflumethiazide; indap—indapamide; methyclo—methyclothiazide; metola—metolazone; poly—polythiazide; quineth—quinethazone; trichlor—trichlormethaizide.

from their action in producing a negative sodium balance. Thiazide diuretics may have a weak potassium-channel-opening action, similar to that of diazoxide, and this weak action may cause smooth muscle relaxation and may also explain their diabetogenic effect because of the reverse of the action of glyburide on the pancreatic islet cells. Thiazide diuretics gain access to tubular fluid via the organic secretory pathway in the proximal tubules. During diuresis, in addition to enhanced sodium and chloride excretion, potassium loss is also promoted. Urinary calcium excretion is decreased, in contrast to what is seen with loop diuretics. This decrease may reduce the risk of hip fractures, and thus may benefit elderly patients.

Natriuretic effects of thiazide diuretics last only 3 to 5 days with chronic administration. Sodium concentrations and extracellular fluid volumes remain steady and lower than baseline values thereafter.

The antihypertensive effects of thiazide diuretics may be noted after 3 to 4 days, although up to 3 to 4 weeks may be required for the optimal effect. Antihypertensive effects persist for up to 1 week after therapy withdrawal.

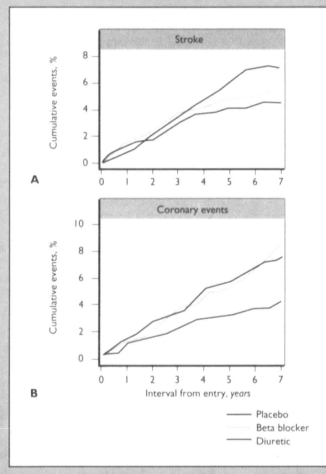

FIGURE 9.2 Cumulative percentage of patients experiencing stroke (a) and coronary events (b) according to randomized treatment in the MRC trial of hypertension in older adults. (*Adapted from* Medical Research Council Working Party. *Br Med J* 1985; 29:97–104.)

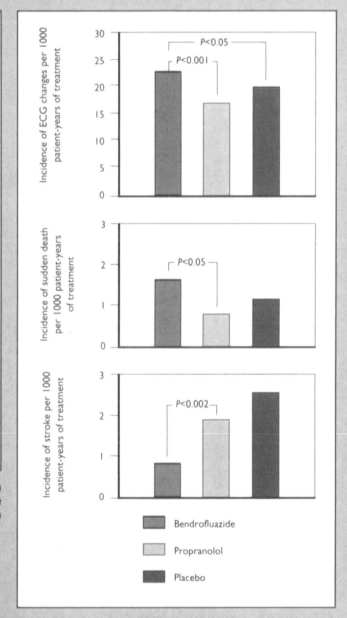

FIGURE 9.3 Close analysis of the MRC trial showed an increased frequency of infarction, as gauged by abnormalities on the electrocardiogram, after diuretic treatment and by an increase in the incidence of sudden death compared with beta-blocker treatment. (*Adapted from* Medical Research Council Working Party. *Br Med J* 1985; 29:97–104.)

BENDROFLUMETHIAZIDE
(Bendroflumethiazide, Naturetin®)

Bendroflumethiazide is a thiazide diuretic. All thiazide diuretics share similar pharmacological activity and adverse effect profile when equivalent dosages are employed clinically. In addition to enhancing diuresis, thiazide diuretics are effective antihypertensive agents. Diuresis usually occurs within 2 hours, peaks within 2 to 6 hours, and lasts for 6 to 12 hours or longer. The onset of antihypertensive effect requires several days. Two to 4 weeks are usually required to achieve optimal BP effect for a given dose. The antihypertensive effect persists longer than the diuretic effect after an oral dose and the effect may last up to 7 days after discontinuing a chronic thiazide diuretic regimen. For more information, please refer to "Hydrochlorothiazide" monograph.

SPECIAL GROUPS

Race: no differences in response
Children: safety and effectiveness have not been established
Elderly: use with caution; no dosage adjustment is required
Renal impairment: use with caution; may be ineffective in severe renal failure and may exacerbate azotemia; contraindicated in anuria
Hepatic impairment: use with caution; dosage adjustment is probably not required
Pregnancy: category C; should only be used if clearly indicated
Breast-feeding: use with caution; excreted in human milk in low concentrations

DOSAGE

Edema: Initial dose—5–20 mg/day once daily in the morning or in two divided doses
Maintenance—2.5–5 mg once daily in the morning; intermittent therapy may be preferred by giving the dose every other day or on a 3– 5 d/wk schedule
Hypertension: Initial dose—5–20 mg/d once daily in the morning or in two divided doses
Maintenance—2.5–15 mg once daily in the morning

IN BRIEF

INDICATIONS
Hypertension
Edema

CONTRAINDICATIONS
Known hypersensitivity to thiazides, other related diuretics or sulfonamide-derived agents
Anuria or severe renal insufficiency
Hepatic coma

DRUG INTERACTIONS
Other diuretics
Hypotensive agents
Cardiac glycosides
Other potassium-depleting agents (corticosteroids, amphotericin B)
NSAIDs
Agents with high sodium content (ticarcillin)
Lithium
Antidiabetic agents
Cholestyramine, colestipol
Non-depolarizing neuromuscular blockers

ADVERSE EFFECTS
CV: hypotension, orthostatic symptoms, arrhythmias, angina, transient ischemic attack
CNS: dizziness, headache, fatigue, vertigo
Blood: volume and electrolyte depletion ($\downarrow$ K, $\downarrow$ Cl, $\downarrow$ Na, $\downarrow$ Mg, $\uparrow$ Ca, $\uparrow$ uric acid), dilutional hyponatremia, metabolic alkalosis, azotemia, $\uparrow$ serum creatinine, hyperglycemia, dyslipidemia, hematologic abnormalities
GI: anorexia, nausea, vomiting, constipation, diarrhea, cholestatic jaundice, pancreatitis
GU: sexual dysfunction, polyuria
Skin: rash, pruritus, urticaria, photosensitivity, exfoliative dermatitis, erythema multiforme
Other: dehydration, muscle cramps, allergic reaction, interstitial nephritis

PHARMACOKINETICS AND PHARMACODYNAMICS
Duration of action: 6–12 h
Onset of action: 2 h
Peak effect: 4 h
Bioavailability: 100%
Effect of food: not known
Clearance: not clear; mainly excreted unchanged in the urine
Plasma half-life: 3–4 hrs
Protein binding: not known

MONITORING
BP, urine output, weight, serum electrolytes.

OVERDOSE
Supportive: replacement of fluid and electrolyte losses.

PATIENT INFORMATION
Bendroflumethiazide is used to lower BP or to reduce excessive water in the body. Take the medication as instructed. Avoid excessive dietary sodium intake while maintaining on this therapy. Potassium-rich diet is encouraged to avoid potassium depletion. Sit or lie down if dizziness occurs and rise slowly from a sitting or lying position.

AVAILABILITY
Tablets—5, 10 mg
Combination Formulations:
Bendroflumethiazide 4 mg/Rauwolfia Serpentina 50 mg
Corzide® 80/5—Bendroflumethiazide 5 mg/Nadolol 80 mg
Corzide® 40/5—Bendroflumethiazide 5 mg/Nadolol 40 mg

BENZTHIAZIDE (Exna®)

Benzthiazide is a thiazide diuretic. All thiazide diuretics share similar pharmacological activity and adverse effect profile when equivalent dosages are employed clinically. In addition to enhancing diuresis, thiazide diuretics are effective antihypertensive agents. Diuresis usually occurs within 2 hours, peaks within 2 to 6 hours, and lasts for 6 to 12 hours or longer. The onset of antihypertensive effect requires several days. Two to 4 weeks are usually required to achieve optimal BP effect for a given dose. The antihypertensive effect persists longer than the diuretic effect after an oral dose and the effect may last up to 7 days after discontinuing a chronic thiazide diuretic regimen. For more information, please refer to "Hydrochlorothiazide" monograph.

SPECIAL GROUPS

Race: no differences in response
Children: safety and effectiveness have not been established
Elderly: use with caution; no dosage adjustment is required
Renal impairment: use with caution; may be ineffective in severe renal failure and may exacerbate azotemia; contraindicated in anuria
Hepatic impairment: use with caution; dosage adjustment is probably not required
Pregnancy: category C; should only be used if clearly indicated
Breast-feeding: use with caution; excreted in human milk in low concentrations

DOSAGE

Edema: Initial dose—50–200 mg/d administered in 1–2 doses for a few days until the desired diuresis/weight is achieved (dosages above 100 mg/d, divide and administer in two doses after breakfast and lunch)
Maintenance—50–150 mg/d; intermittent therapy may be preferred by giving the dose every other day or on a 3–5 d/wk schedule
Hypertension: Initial dose—25–50 mg twice daily after breakfast and lunch
Maintenance—up to 100 mg twice daily

IN BRIEF

INDICATIONS
Hypertension
Edema

CONTRAINDICATIONS
Known hypersensitivity to thiazides, other related diuretics, sulfonamide-derived agents, or tartrazine
Anuria or severe renal insufficiency
Hepatic coma

DRUG INTERACTIONS
Other diuretics
Hypotensive agents
Cardiac glycosides
Other potassium-depleting agents (corticosteroids, amphotericin B)
NSAIDs
Agents with high sodium content (ticarcillin)
Lithium
Antidiabetic agents
Cholestyramine, colestipol
Non-depolarizing neuromuscular blockers

ADVERSE EFFECTS
CV: hypotension, orthostatic symptoms, arrhythmias, angina, transient ischemic attack
CNS: dizziness, headache, fatigue, vertigo
Blood: volume and electrolyte depletion ($\downarrow$ K, $\downarrow$ Cl, $\downarrow$ Na, $\downarrow$ Mg, $\uparrow$ Ca, $\uparrow$ uric acid), dilutional hyponatremia, metabolic alkalosis, azotemia, $\uparrow$ serum creatinine, hyperglycemia, dyslipidemia, hematologic abnormalities
GI: anorexia, nausea, vomiting, constipation, diarrhea, cholestatic jaundice, pancreatitis
GU: sexual dysfunction, polyuria
Skin: rash, pruritus, urticaria, photosensitivity, exfoliative dermatitis, erythema multiforme
Other: dehydration, muscle cramps, allergic reaction, interstitial nephritis

PHARMACOKINETICS AND PHARMACODYNAMICS
Duration of action: 6–18 h
Onset of action: 2 h
Peak effect: 4–6 h
Bioavailability: 25% or less
Effect of food: not known
Clearance: not clear, partially cleared renally as unchanged drug
Plasma half-life: not known
Protein binding: not known

MONITORING
BP, urine output, weight, serum electrolytes.

OVERDOSE
Supportive: replacement of fluid and electrolyte losses.

PATIENT INFORMATION
Benzthiazide is used to lower BP or to reduce excessive water in the body. Take the medication as instructed. Avoid excessive dietary sodium intake while maintaining on this therapy. Potassium-rich diet is encouraged to avoid potassium depletion. Sit or lie down if dizziness occurs and rise slowly from a sitting or lying position.

AVAILABILITY
Tablets —50 mg

CHLOROTHIAZIDE (Chlorothiazide, Diuril®, Diurigen®)

Chlorothiazide is the only thiazide diuretic available in both oral and IV formulations in the United States. All thiazide diuretics share similar pharmacological activity and adverse effect profile when equivalent dosages are employed clinically. In addition to enhancing diuresis, thiazide diuretics are effective antihypertensive agents. Diuresis usually occurs within 2 hours, peaks within 2 to 6 hours, and lasts for 6 to 12 hours or longer. The onset of antihypertensive effect requires several days. Two to 4 weeks are usually required to achieve optimal BP effect for a given dose. The antihypertensive effect persists longer than the diuretic effect after an oral dose and the effect may last up to 7 days after discontinuing a chronic thiazide diuretic regimen. For more information, please refer to "Hydrochlorothiazide" monograph.

SPECIAL GROUPS

Race: no differences in response

Children: only oral administration is indicated; IV use is not recommended

Elderly: use with caution; no dosage adjustment is required

Renal impairment: use with caution; may be ineffective in severe renal failure and may exacerbate azotemia; contraindicated in anuria

Hepatic impairment: use with caution; dosage adjustment is probably not required

Pregnancy: category B; should only be used if clearly indicated

Breast-feeding: use with caution; excreted in human milk in low concentrations

DOSAGE

Edema: Adults—500–1000 mg once daily in the morning or twice daily, administered orally or IV (only for patients who are unable to take oral medication or for emergency)

Intermittent therapy may be preferred by giving the dose every other day or on a 3–5 d/wk schedule

Hypertension: Adults—250–500 mg once daily in the morning or twice daily, up to 2 g/d in divided doses

IN BRIEF

INDICATIONS
Hypertension
Edema

CONTRAINDICATIONS
Known hypersensitivity to thiazides, other related diuretics, or sulfonamide-derived agents
Anuria or severe renal insufficiency
Hepatic coma

DRUG INTERACTIONS
Other diuretics
Hypotensive agents
Cardiac glycosides
Other potassium-depleting agents (corticosteroids, amphotericin B)
NSAIDs
Agents with high sodium content (ticarcillin)
Lithium
Antidiabetic agents
Cholestyramine, colestipol
Non-depolarizing neuromuscular blockers

ADVERSE EFFECTS
CV: hypotension, orthostatic symptoms, arrhythmias, angina, transient ischemic attack
CNS: dizziness, headache, fatigue, vertigo
Blood: volume and electrolyte depletion ($\downarrow$ K, $\downarrow$ Cl, $\downarrow$ Na, $\downarrow$ Mg, $\uparrow$ Ca, $\uparrow$ uric acid), dilutional hyponatremia, metabolic alkalosis, azotemia, $\uparrow$ serum creatinine, hyperglycemia, dyslipidemia, hematologic abnormalities
GI: anorexia, nausea, vomiting, constipation, diarrhea, cholestatic jaundice, pancreatitis
GU: sexual dysfunction, polyuria
Skin: rash, pruritus, urticaria, photosensitivity, exfoliative dermatitis, erythema multiforme
Other: dehydration, muscle cramps, allergic reaction, interstitial nephritis

PHARMACOKINETICS AND PHARMACODYNAMICS
Duration of action: 6–12 h
Onset of action: (po) 2 h; (IV) 15 min
Peak effect: (po) 4 h; (IV) 30 min
Bioavailability: 10%–20%
Effect of food: increases absorption (doubled)
Clearance: mainly cleared renally as unchanged drug (96% after an IV dose; only 10%–15% after an oral dose due to the low bioavailability)
Plasma half-life: 45–120 min
Protein binding: not known

MONITORING
BP, urine output, weight, serum electrolytes.

OVERDOSE
Supportive: replacement of fluid and electrolyte losses.

PATIENT INFORMATION
Chlorothiazide is used to lower BP or to reduce excessive water in the body. Take the medication as instructed. Avoid excessive dietary sodium intake while maintaining on this therapy. Potassium-rich diet is encouraged to avoid potassium depletion. Sit or lie down if dizziness occurs and rise slowly from a sitting or lying position.

AVAILABILITY
Tablets—250, 500 mg
Suspension—250 mg/5 mL in 237 mL
Vials — 500 mg powder
Combination Formulations:
Diupres®-500 and -250 Tablets, various sources—
Chlorothiazide 500 mg/ Reserpine 0.125 mg
Chlorothiazide 250 mg/ Reserpine 0.125 mg
Aldoclor®-250 and -150 Tablets—
Chlorothiazide 250 mg/ Methyldopa 250 mg
Chlorothiazide 150 mg/ Methyldopa 250 mg

CHLORTHALIDONE

(Chlorthalidone,
Hygroton®, Thalitone®)

Chlorthalidone is a thiazide diuretic. All thiazide diuretics share similar pharmacological activity and adverse effect profile when equivalent dosages are employed clinically. In addition to enhancing diuresis, thiazide diuretics are effective antihypertensive agents. Diuresis usually occurs within 2 hours, peaks within 2 to 6 hours, and lasts for 6 to 12 hours or longer. The onset of antihypertensive effect requires several days. Two to 4 weeks are usually required to achieve optimal BP effect for a given dose. The antihypertensive effect persists longer than the diuretic effect after an oral dose and the effect may last up to 7 days after discontinuing a chronic thiazide diuretic regimen. For more information, please refer to "Hydrochlorothiazide" monograph.

SPECIAL GROUPS

Race: no differences in response

Children: safety and effectiveness have not been established

Elderly: use with caution; no dosage adjustment is required

Renal impairment: use with caution; may be ineffective in severe renal failure and may exacerbate azotemia; contraindicated in anuria

Hepatic impairment: use with caution; dosage adjustment is probably not required

Pregnancy: category B; should only be used if clearly indicated

Breast-feeding: not recommended; excreted in human milk with significant concentrations reported

DOSAGE

Edema: Usual dose—30–100 mg/d administered as a single dose with breakfast; dosage may be gradually increased up to 200 mg once daily if indicated (or, 120 mg as Thalitone®)until the desired diuresis / weight is achieved

Intermittent therapy may be preferred by giving the dose every other day or on a 3–5 d/wk

Hypertension: Usual dose*—15–25 mg once daily with breakfast; dosage may be gradually increased up to 100 mg once daily if indicated (or, 50 mg as Thalitone®)

* Dosages above 25 mg/d are likely to potentiate potassium waste, but provide no further benefit in BP reduction.

IN BRIEF

INDICATIONS
Hypertension
Edema

CONTRAINDICATIONS
Known hypersensitivity to thiazides, other related diuretics, or sulfonamide-derived agents
Anuria or severe renal insufficiency
Hepatic coma

DRUG INTERACTIONS
Other diuretics
Hypotensive agents
Cardiac glycosides
Other potassium-depleting agents (corticosteroids, amphotericin B)
NSAIDs and Agents with high sodium content (ticarcillin)
Lithium
Antidiabetic agents
Cholestyramine, colestipol
Non-depolarizing neuromuscular blockers

ADVERSE EFFECTS
CV: hypotension, orthostatic symptoms, arrhythmias, angina, transient ischemic attack
CNS: dizziness, headache, fatigue, vertigo
Blood: volume and electrolyte depletion ($\downarrow$ K, $\downarrow$ Cl, $\downarrow$ Na, $\downarrow$ Mg, $\uparrow$ Ca, $\uparrow$ uric acid), dilutional hyponatremia, metabolic alkalosis, azotemia, $\uparrow$ serum creatinine, hyperglycemia, dyslipidemia, hematologic abnormalities
GI: anorexia, nausea, vomiting, constipation, diarrhea, cholestatic jaundice, pancreatitis
GU: sexual dysfunction, polyuria
Skin: rash, pruritus, urticaria, photosensitivity, exfoliative dermatitis, erythema multiforme
Other: dehydration, muscle cramps, allergic reaction, interstitial nephritis

PHARMACOKINETICS AND PHARMACODYNAMICS
Duration of action: up to 72 h
Onset of action: 2–3 h
Peak effect: 2–6 h
Bioavailability: 65%
Effect of food: not known
Clearance: 50%–74 % cleared renally as unchanged drug: some is metabolized in liver
Plasma half-life: 40–60 h
Protein binding: 75%

MONITORING
BP, urine output, weight, serum electrolytes.

OVERDOSE
Supportive: replacement of fluid and electrolyte losses.

PATIENT INFORMATION
Chlorthalidone is used to lower BP or to reduce excessive water in the body. Take the medication as instructed. Avoid excessive dietary sodium intake while maintaining on this therapy. Potassium-rich diet is encouraged to avoid potassium depletion. Sit or lie down if dizziness occurs and rise slowly from a sitting or lying position.

AVAILABILITY
Tablets—15, 25, 50, 100 mg
Combination Formulations:
Combipres® 0.1, 0.2, and 0.3 Tablets, various sources—
Chlorthalidone 15 mg/ Clonidine 0.1 mg
Chlorthalidone 15 mg/ Clonidine 0.2 mg
Chlorthalidone 15 mg/ Clonidine 0.3 mg
Tenoretic® 50, and 100 Tablets, various sources—
Chlorthalidone 25 mg/ Atenolol 50 mg
Chlorthalidone 25 mg/ Atenolol 100 mg
Regroton® and Demi-Regroton® Tablets—
Chlorthalidone 50 mg/ Reserpine 0.25 mg
Chlorthalidone 25 mg/ Reserpine 0.125 mg

HYDROCHLOROTHIAZIDE
(Various sources)

Hydrochlorothiazide (HCTZ) is the most widely used thiazide diuretic. Thiazide diuretics act primarily by blocking sodium and chloride reabsorption, therefore blocking water reabsorption, in the cortical thick ascending limb of the loop of Henle and the early distal renal tubule. The natriuretic effect of thiazide diuretics is determined by the amount of sodium reaching the distal renal tubule. Sodium delivery to the site is compromised in patients with severe renal dysfunction (ie. with serum creatinine or BUN concentrations greater than about twice normal), CHF, or liver cirrhosis. As a result, thiazide and thiazide-like diuretics (except metolazone) may not be effective in enhancing diuresis in these patients and a more potent diuretic therapy may be required. Thiazide diuretics have an antihypertensive effect and work synergistically with other antihypertensive agents. Although the exact antihypertensive mechanism is not clear, both direct arteriolar dilation and sodium depletion contribute to the effect.

HCTZ is available in combination with different antihypertensive agents for the management of hypertension. When used alone, BP reduction is usually observed after 3–4 d of therapy, which lags behind its diuretic effect. While the diuretic effect occurs within 2 h after an oral dose and may last for 6–12 h, the antihypertensive effect may last up to 7 d after discontinuing chronic HCTZ therapy.

SPECIAL GROUPS

Race: no differences in response

Children: dose based on weight or body surface area and clinical response

Elderly: use with caution; no dosage adjustment is required

Renal impairment: use with caution; may be ineffective in severe renal failure and may exacerbate azotemia; contraindicated in anuria

Hepatic impairment: use with caution; dosage adjustment is probably not required

Pregnancy: category B; should only be used if clearly indicated

Breast-feeding: use with caution; excreted in human milk in low concentrations

IN BRIEF

INDICATIONS
Hypertension
Edema

CONTRAINDICATIONS
Known hypersensitivity to thiazides, other related diuretics, sulfonamide-derived agents, or sulfites (some products contain sulfites)
Anuria or severe renal insufficiency
Hepatic coma

DRUG INTERACTIONS
Other diuretics
Hypotensive agents
Cardiac glycosides
Other potassium-depleting agents (corticosteroids, amphotericin B)
NSAIDs
Agents with high sodium content (ticarcillin)
Lithium
Antidiabetic agents
Cholestyramine, colestipol
Non-depolarizing neuromuscular blockers

ADVERSE EFFECTS
CV: hypotension, orthostatic symptoms, arrhythmias, angina, transient ischemic attack
CNS: dizziness, headache, fatigue, vertigo
Blood: volume and electrolyte depletion ($\downarrow$ K, $\downarrow$ Cl, $\downarrow$ Na, $\downarrow$ Mg, $\uparrow$ Ca, $\uparrow$ uric acid), dilutional hyponatremia, metabolic alkalosis, azotemia, $\uparrow$ serum creatinine, hyperglycemia, dyslipidemia, hematologic abnormalities
GI: anorexia, nausea, vomiting, constipation, diarrhea, cholestatic jaundice, pancreatitis
GU: sexual dysfunction, polyuria
Skin: rash, pruritus, urticaria, photosensitivity, exfoliative dermatitis, erythema multiforme
Other: dehydration, muscle cramps, allergic reaction, interstitial nephritis

PHARMACOKINETICS AND PHARMACODYNAMICS
Duration of action: 6–12 h (up to a week for hypotensive effect)
Onset of action: 2 h
Peak effect: 4–6 h
Bioavailability: 65%–75%
Effect of food: reduced plasma levels
Clearance: mainly in the urine as unchanged drug
Plasma half-life: 6–15 h ($\uparrow$ in heart or renal failure)
Protein binding: 40%

MONITORING
BP, urine output, weight, serum electrolytes.

OVERDOSE
Supportive: replacement of fluid and electrolyte losses.

PATIENT INFORMATION
Hydrochlorothiazide is used to lower BP or to reduce excessive water in the body. Take the medication as instructed. Avoid excessive dietary sodium intake while maintaining on this therapy. Potassium-rich diet is encouraged to avoid potassium depletion. Sit or lie down if dizziness occurs and rise slowly from a sitting or lying position.

DOSAGE

Edema: Initial dose—25–200 mg/d administered in 1–3 divided doses for a few days until the desired diuresis / weight is achieved
Maintenance—25–100 mg/d*; intermittent therapy may be preferred by giving the dose every other day or on a 3–5 d/wk schedule

Hypertension: Initial dose—12.5–25 mg once daily in the morning
Maintenance*—up to 50 mg once daily in the morning
* Higher doses have been used, but the benefits should be assessed carefully against the potential risks of high dose diuretic therapy.

AVAILABILITY

Tablets—25, 50, 100 mg
Solution—50 mg/5 mL
Combination Formulations:
 Various sources—
    HCTZ 50 mg/ Reserpine 0.125 mg Tablets
    HCTZ 25 mg/ Reserpine 0.125 mg Tablets
 Hydrap-ES®, Marpres®, Ser-Ap-Es® Tablets—
    HCTZ 15 mg/ Reserpine 0.1 mg/ Hydralazine 25 mg
 Apresazide® Capsules and various sources—
    HCTZ 50 mg/ Hydralazine 100 mg
    HCTZ 50 mg/ Hydralazine 50 mg
    HCTZ 25 mg/ Hydralazine 25 mg
 Ziac® Tablets—
    HCTZ 6.25 mg/ Bisoprolol 2.5 mg
    HCTZ 6.25 mg/ Bisoprolol 5 mg
    HCTZ 6.25 mg/ Bisoprolol 10 mg
 Timolide 10-25® Tablets—
    HCTZ 25 mg/ Timolol 10 mg
 Inderide LA® 160/50, 120/50, and 80/50 Capsules—
    HCTZ 50 mg/ Propranolol 160 mg
    HCTZ 50 mg/ Propranolol 120 mg
    HCTZ 50 mg/ Propranolol 80 mg
 Inderide® Tablets and various sources—
    HCTZ 25 mg/ Propranolol 80 mg
    HCTZ 25 mg/ Propranolol 40 mg
 Aldoril® Tablets and various sources—
    HCTZ 50 mg/ Methyldopa 500 mg
    HCTZ 30 mg/ Methyldopa 500 mg
    HCTZ 25 mg/ Methyldopa 250 mg
    HCTZ 15 mg/ Methyldopa 250 mg
 Lopressor HCT® 100/50, 100/25, and 50/25 Tablets—
    HCTZ 50 mg/ Metoprolol 100 mg
    HCTZ 25 mg/ Metoprolol 100 mg
    HCTZ 25 mg/ Metoprolol 50 mg
 Capozide® 50/25, 25/25, 50/15, and 25/15 Tablets—
    HCTZ 25 mg/ Captopril 50 mg
    HCTZ 25 mg/ Captopril 25 mg
    HCTZ 15 mg/ Captopril 50 mg
    HCTZ 15 mg/ Captopril 25 mg
 Lotensin HCT® 20/25, 20/12.5, 10/12.5, and 5/6.25 Tablets—
    HCTZ 25 mg/ Benazepril 20 mg
    HCTZ 12.5 mg/ Benazepril 20 mg
    HCTZ 12.5 mg/ Benazepril 10 mg
    HCTZ 6.25 mg/ Benazepril 5 mg
 Vaseretic® 10-25 Tablets—
    HCTZ 25 mg/ Enalapril 10 mg
 Prinzide® and Zestoretic® Tablets—
    HCTZ 25 mg / Lisinopril 20 mg
    HCTZ 12.5 mg/ Lisinopril 20 mg
 Esimil® Tablets—
    HCTZ 25 mg/ Guanethidine 10 mg

HYDROFLUMETHIAZIDE
(Hydroflumethiazide, Diucardin®, Saluron®)

Hydroflumethiazide is a thiazide diuretic. All thiazide diuretics share similar pharmacological activity and adverse effect profile when equivalent dosages are employed clinically. In addition to enhancing diuresis, thiazide diuretics are effective antihypertensive agents. Diuresis usually occurs within 2 hours, peaks within 2 to 6 hours, and lasts for 6 to 12 hours or longer. The onset of antihypertensive effect requires several days. Two to 4 weeks are usually required to achieve optimal BP effect for a given dose. The antihypertensive effect persists longer than the diuretic effect after an oral dose and the effect may last up to 7 days after discontinuing a chronic thiazide diuretic regimen. For more information, please refer to "Hydrochlorothiazide" monograph.

SPECIAL GROUPS

Race: no differences in response
Children: safety and effectiveness have not been established
Elderly: use with caution; no dosage adjustment is required
Renal impairment: use with caution; may be ineffective in severe renal failure and may exacerbate azotemia; contraindicated in anuria
Hepatic impairment: use with caution; dosage adjustment is probably not required
Pregnancy: category C; should only be used if clearly indicated
Breast-feeding: not recommended; excreted in human milk

DOSAGE

Edema: Usual dose range—25–200 mg/d once daily in the morning, or given in two divided doses
For dosages above 100 mg/d, divide and administer in two doses. Intermittent therapy may be preferred by giving the dose every other day or on a 3–5 d/wk schedule
Hypertension: Usual dose range—12.5–100 mg/d once daily in the morning, or given in two divided doses

IN BRIEF

INDICATIONS
Hypertension
Edema

CONTRAINDICATIONS
Known hypersensitivity to thiazides, other related diuretics or sulfonamide-derived agents
Anuria or severe renal insufficiency
Hepatic coma

DRUG INTERACTIONS
Other diuretics
Hypotensive agents
Cardiac glycosides
Other potassium-depleting agents (corticosteroids, amphotericin B)
NSAIDs
Agents with high sodium content (ticarcillin)
Lithium
Antidiabetic agents
Cholestyramine, colestipol
Non-depolarizing neuromuscular blockers

ADVERSE EFFECTS
CV: hypotension, orthostatic symptoms, arrhythmias, angina, transient ischemic attack
CNS: dizziness, headache, fatigue, vertigo
Blood: volume and electrolyte depletion ($\downarrow$ K, $\downarrow$ Cl, $\downarrow$ Na, $\downarrow$ Mg, $\uparrow$ Ca, $\uparrow$ uric acid), dilutional hyponatremia, metabolic alkalosis, azotemia, $\uparrow$ serum creatinine, hyperglycemia, dyslipidemia, hematologic abnormalities
GI: anorexia, nausea, vomiting, constipation, diarrhea, cholestatic jaundice, pancreatitis
GU: sexual dysfunction, polyuria
Skin: rash, pruritus, urticaria, photosensitivity, exfoliative dermatitis, erythema multiforme
Other: dehydration, muscle cramps, allergic reaction, interstitial nephritis

PHARMACOKINETICS AND PHARMACODYNAMICS
Duration of action: 12–24 h
Onset of action: <2 h
Peak effect: 4 h
Bioavailability: 50%
Effect of food: not known
Clearance: not clear; mainly excreted in the urine
Plasma half-life: 17 h
Protein binding: not known

MONITORING
BP, urine output, weight, serum electrolytes.

OVERDOSE
Supportive: replacement of fluid and electrolyte losses.

PATIENT INFORMATION
Hydroflumethiazide is used to lower BP or to reduce excessive water in the body. Take the medication as instructed. Avoid excessive dietary sodium intake while maintaining on this therapy. Potassium-rich diet is encouraged to avoid potassium depletion. Sit or lie down if dizziness occurs and rise slowly from a sitting or lying position.

AVAILABILITY
Tablets —50 mg
Combination Formulations:
Salutensin® Tablets—
Hydroflumethiazide 50 mg/ Reserpine 0.125 mg

INDAPAMIDE (Indapmide, Lozol®)

Indapamide, a methylindoline derivative, is a sulfonamide diuretic. Although structurally different from thiazide diuretics, it has similar pharmacologic activity. Indapamide lowers BP in hypertensive patients via unclear mechanism. It reduces BP probably by reducing plasma and extracellular fluid volume, by decreasing peripheral vascular resistance, and by causing direct arteriolar dilation. Indapamide acts synergistically with other antihypertensive agents. Similar to thiazide diuretics, the diuretic effect of indapamide diminishes as renal function declines. However, the hypotensive effect remains in patients with an estimated creatinine clearance above 15 ml/min. Different from thiazide diuretics, indapamide has less of an adverse effect on serum levels of triglyceride, total cholesterol, low-density lipoprotein, very low-density lipoprotein, and high-density lipoprotein. The clinical significance of these differences is not known. As a general rule, thiazide-induced mild changes in serum lipid profile can be managed by a diet low in saturated fat and cholesterol. For more information, please refer to "Hydrochlorothiazide" monograph.

SPECIAL GROUPS

Race: no differences in response
Children: safety and effectiveness have not been established
Elderly: use with caution; no dosage adjustment is required
Renal impairment: use with caution; may be ineffective in severe renal failure and may exacerbate azotemia; contraindicated in anuria
Hepatic impairment: use with caution; dosage adjustment may be required
Pregnancy: category B; should only be used if clearly indicated
Breast-feeding: not recommended; not known if the drug is excreted in human milk

DOSAGE

Edema: Usual dose range—2.5–5 mg once daily in the morning
Intermittent therapy may be preferred by giving the dose every other day or on a 3–5 d/wk schedule
Hypertension: Usual dose range—1.25–5 mg once daily in the morning

IN BRIEF

INDICATIONS
Hypertension
Edema

CONTRAINDICATIONS
Known hypersensitivity to thiazides, other related diuretics or sulfonamide-derived agents
Anuria or severe renal insufficiency
Hepatic coma

DRUG INTERACTIONS
Other diuretics
Hypotensive agents
Cardiac glycosides
Other potassium-depleting agents (corticosteroids, amphotericin B)
NSAIDs
Agents with high sodium content (ticarcillin)
Lithium
Antidiabetic agents
Cholestyramine, colestipol
Non-depolarizing neuromuscular blockers

ADVERSE EFFECTS
CV: hypotension, orthostatic symptoms, arrhythmias, angina, transient ischemic attack
CNS: dizziness, headache, fatigue, vertigo
Blood: volume and electrolyte depletion ($\downarrow$ K, $\downarrow$ Cl, $\downarrow$ Na, $\downarrow$ Mg, $\uparrow$ Ca, $\uparrow$ uric acid), dilutional hyponatremia, metabolic alkalosis, azotemia, $\uparrow$ serum creatinine, hyperglycemia, hematologic abnormalities
GI: anorexia, nausea, vomiting, constipation, diarrhea, cholestatic jaundice, pancreatitis
GU: sexual dysfunction, polyuria
Skin: rash, pruritus, urticaria, photosensitivity, exfoliative dermatitis, erythema multiforme
Other: dehydration, muscle cramps, allergic reaction, interstitial nephritis

PHARMACOKINETICS AND PHARMACODYNAMICS
Duration of action: up to 36 h
Onset of action: 1–2 h
Peak effect: <2 h
Bioavailability: 93%
Effect of food: no effect
Clearance: extensively metabolized in liver; excreted in urine (mainly as metabolites, 5% as unchanged) and in feces (16%–23%)
Plasma half-life: 14 hrs or longer
Protein binding: 75%

MONITORING
BP, urine output, weight, serum electrolytes.

OVERDOSE
Supportive: replacement of fluid and electrolyte losses.

PATIENT INFORMATION
Indapamide is used to lower BP or to reduce excessive water in the body. Take the medication as instructed. Avoid excessive dietary sodium intake while maintaining on this therapy. Potassium-rich diet is encouraged to avoid potassium depletion. Sit or lie down if dizziness occurs and rise slowly from a sitting or lying position.

AVAILABILITY
Tablets—1.25, 2.5 mg

METHYCLOTHIAZIDE (Aquatensen®, Enduron®)

Methyclothiazide is a thiazide diuretic. All thiazide diuretics share similar pharmacological activity and adverse effect profile when equivalent dosages are employed clinically. In addition to enhancing diuresis, thiazide diuretics are effective antihypertensive agents. Diuresis usually occurs within 2 hours, peaks within 2 to 6 hours, and lasts for 6 to 12 hours or longer. The onset of antihypertensive effect requires several days. Two to 4 weeks are usually required to achieve optimal BP effect for a given dose. The antihypertensive effect persists longer than the diuretic effect after an oral dose and the effect may last up to 7 days after discontinuing a chronic thiazide diuretic regimen. For more information, please refer to "Hydrochlorothiazide" monograph.

SPECIAL GROUPS

Race: no differences in response
Children: safety and effectiveness have not been established
Elderly: use with caution; no dosage adjustment is required
Renal impairment: use with caution; may be ineffective in severe renal failure and may exacerbate azotemia; contraindicated in anuria
Hepatic impairment: use with caution; titrate the dose based on clinical response
Pregnancy: category B; should only be used if clearly indicated
Breast-feeding: not recommended; excreted in human milk

DOSAGE

Edema: Initial dose—2.5–10 mg/d once daily in the morning
Maintenance—2.5–5 mg once daily in the morning; intermittent therapy may be preferred by giving the dose every other day or on a 3–5 d/wk schedule
Hypertension: Usual dose range—2.5–5 mg once daily in the morning

IN BRIEF

INDICATIONS
Hypertension
Edema

CONTRAINDICATIONS
Known hypersensitivity to thiazides, other related diuretics or sulfonamide-derived agents
Anuria or severe renal insufficiency
Hepatic coma

DRUG INTERACTIONS
Other diuretics
Hypotensive agents
Cardiac glycosides
Other potassium-depleting agents (corticosteroids, amphotericin B)
NSAIDs
Agents with high sodium content (ticarcillin)
Lithium
Antidiabetic agents
Cholestyramine, colestipol
Non-depolarizing neuromuscular blockers

ADVERSE EFFECTS
CV: hypotension, orthostatic symptoms, arrhythmias, angina, transient ischemic attack
CNS: dizziness, headache, fatigue, vertigo
Blood: volume and electrolyte depletion ($\downarrow$ K, $\downarrow$ Cl, $\downarrow$ Na, $\downarrow$ Mg, $\uparrow$ Ca, $\uparrow$ uric acid), dilutional hyponatremia, metabolic alkalosis, azotemia, $\uparrow$ serum creatinine, hyperglycemia, dyslipidemia, hematologic abnormalities
GI: anorexia, nausea, vomiting, constipation, diarrhea, cholestatic jaundice, pancreatitis
GU: sexual dysfunction, polyuria
Skin: rash, pruritus, urticaria, photosensitivity, exfoliative dermatitis, erythema multiforme
Other: dehydration, muscle cramps, allergic reaction, interstitial nephritis

PHARMACOKINETICS AND PHARMACODYNAMICS
Duration of action: ≥24 h
Onset of action: 2 h
Peak effect: 6 h
Bioavailability: not known
Effect of food: not known
Clearance: not clear; mainly excreted unchanged in the urine
Plasma half-life: not known
Protein binding: not known

MONITORING
BP, urine output, weight, serum electrolytes.

OVERDOSE
Supportive: replacement of fluid and electrolyte losses.

PATIENT INFORMATION
Methyclothiazide is used to lower BP or to reduce excessive water in the body. Take the medication as instructed. Avoid excessive dietary sodium intake while maintaining on this therapy. Potassium-rich diet is encouraged to avoid potassium depletion. Sit or lie down if dizziness occurs and rise slowly from a sitting or lying position.

AVAILABILITY
Tablets—2.5, 5 mg
Combination formulations:
Enduronyl® Tablets—Methyclothiazide 5 mg/ Deserpidine 0.25 mg
Enduronyl Forte® Tablets—Methyclothiazide 5 mg/ Deserpidine 0.5 mg
Diutensen-R® Tablets—Methyclothiazide 2.5 mg/ Reserpine 0.1 mg

METOLAZONE
(Metolazone, Mykrox®, Zaroxolyn®)

Metolazone is a quinazoline diuretic with similar structure and pharmacologic activity to thiazide diuretics. It acts primarily to inhibit sodium reabsorption at the cortical diluting site and to a lesser extent in the proximal convoluted tubule. Its diuretic potency at maximum therapeutic dosage is comparable to thiazide diuretics. However, different from thiazide diuretics, metolazone continues to promote diuresis in patients with glomerular filtration rates below 20 mL/min. Metolazone has been used together with a loop diuretic in the management of edema in patients with impaired renal function who failed to respond to either agent alone. For more information, please refer to "Hydrochlorothiazide" monograph.

SPECIAL GROUPS

Race: no differences in response
Children: safety and effectiveness have not been established
Elderly: use with caution; no dosage adjustment is required
Renal impairment: use with caution; may exacerbate azotemia; contraindicated in anuria
Hepatic impairment: use with caution; dosage adjustment is probably not required
Pregnancy: category B; should only be used if clearly indicated
Breast-feeding: not recommended; excreted in human milk

DOSAGE*

Edema: Initial dose—5–10 mg/day of Zaroxolyn® once daily in the morning; dosage up to 20 mg once daily may be used in patients with renal insufficiency
Maintenance—2.5–10 mg of Zaroxolyn® once daily in the morning; intermittent therapy may be preferred by giving the dose every other day or on a 3–5 d/wk schedule
Hypertension: Usual dose range—2.5–10 mg of Zaroxolyn®, or 0.5–1 mg of Mykrox®once daily in the morning
* Note—Because of the difference in formulations, different products have different dosage recommendations and should not be used interchangeably.

IN BRIEF

INDICATIONS
Hypertension (both Zaroxolyn® and Mykrox®)
Edema (Zaroxolyn® only)

CONTRAINDICATIONS
Known hypersensitivity to thiazides, other related diuretics or sulfonamide-derived agents
Anuria or severe renal insufficiency
Hepatic coma

DRUG INTERACTIONS
Other diuretics
Hypotensive agents
Cardiac glycosides
Other potassium-depleting agents (corticosteroids, amphotericin B)
NSAIDs
Agents with high sodium content (ticarcillin)
Lithium
Antidiabetic agents
Cholestyramine, colestipol
Non-depolarizing neuromuscular blockers

ADVERSE EFFECTS
CV: hypotension, orthostatic symptoms, arrhythmias, angina, transient ischemic attack
CNS: dizziness, headache, fatigue, vertigo
Blood: volume and electrolyte depletion ($\downarrow$ K,$\downarrow$ Cl, $\downarrow$ Na, $\downarrow$ Mg, $\uparrow$ Ca, $\uparrow$ uric acid), dilutional hyponatremia, metabolic alkalosis, azotemia, $\uparrow$ serum creatinine, hyperglycemia, dyslipidemia, hematologic abnormalities
GI: anorexia, nausea, vomiting, constipation, diarrhea, cholestatic jaundice, pancreatitis
GU: sexual dysfunction, polyuria
Skin: rash, pruritus, urticaria, photosensitivity, exfoliative dermatitis, erythema multiforme
Other: dehydration, muscle cramps, allergic reaction, interstitial nephritis

PHARMACOKINETICS AND PHARMACODYNAMICS
Duration of action: 12–24 h or longer
Onset of action: <1 h
Peak effect: 1–2 h
Bioavailability: 40%–65% (Mykrox® has better absorption)
Effect of food: not known
Clearance: some is metabolized; 70%–95% is excreted unchanged in urine; the rest is excreted in bile
Plasma half-life: 8–14 h
Protein binding: 95%

MONITORING
BP, urine output, weight, serum electrolytes.

OVERDOSE
Supportive: replacement of fluid and electrolyte losses.

PATIENT INFORMATION
Metolazone is used to lower BP or to reduce excessive water in the body. Take the medication as instructed. Avoid excessive dietary sodium intake while maintaining on this therapy. Potassium-rich diet is encouraged to avoid potassium depletion. Sit or lie down if dizziness occurs and rise slowly from a sitting or lying position.

AVAILABILITY*
Zaroxolyn® Tablets—2.5, 5, 10 mg
Mykrox® Tablets— 0.5 mg

POLYTHIAZIDE (Renese®)

Polythiazide is a thiazide diuretic. All thiazide diuretics share similar pharmacological activity and adverse effect profile when equivalent dosages are employed clinically. In addition to enhancing diuresis, thiazide diuretics are effective antihypertensive agents. Diuresis usually occurs within 2 hours, peaks within 2 to 6 hours, and lasts for 6 to 12 hours or longer. The onset of antihypertensive effect requires several days. Two to 4 weeks are usually required to achieve optimal BP effect for a given dose. The antihypertensive effect persists longer than the diuretic effect after an oral dose and the effect may last up to 7 days after discontinuing a chronic thiazide diuretic regimen. For more information, please refer to "Hydrochlorothiazide" monograph.

SPECIAL GROUPS

Race: no differences in response

Children: safety and effectiveness have not been established

Elderly: use with caution; no dosage adjustment is required

Renal impairment: use with caution, may be ineffective in severe renal failure and may exacerbate azotemia; contraindicated in anuria

Hepatic impairment: use with caution; titrate the dose based on clinical response

Pregnancy: category C; should only be used if clearly indicated

Breast-feeding: use with caution; excreted in human milk

DOSAGE

Edema: Usual dose range—1–4 mg once daily in the morning. Intermittent therapy may be preferred by giving the dose every other day or on a 3–5 d/wk schedule.

Hypertension: Usual dose range—2–4 mg once daily in the morning

IN BRIEF

INDICATIONS
Hypertension
Edema

CONTRAINDICATIONS
Known hypersensitivity to thiazides, other related diuretics or sulfonamide-derived agents
Anuria or severe renal insufficiency
Hepatic coma

DRUG INTERACTIONS
Other diuretics
Hypotensive agents
Cardiac glycosides
Other potassium-depleting agents (corticosteroids, amphotericin B)
NSAIDs
Agents with high sodium content (ticarcillin)
Lithium
Antidiabetic agents
Cholestyramine, colestipol
Non-depolarizing neuromuscular blockers

ADVERSE EFFECTS
CV: hypotension, orthostatic symptoms, arrhythmias, angina, transient ischemic attack
CNS: dizziness, headache, fatigue, vertigo
Blood: volume and electrolyte depletion ($\downarrow$ K, $\downarrow$ Cl, $\downarrow$ Na, $\downarrow$ Mg, $\uparrow$ Ca, $\uparrow$ uric acid), dilutional hyponatremia, metabolic alkalosis, azotemia, $\uparrow$ serum creatinine, hyperglycemia, dyslipidemia, hematologic abnormalities
GI: anorexia, nausea, vomiting, constipation, diarrhea, cholestatic jaundice, pancreatitis
GU: sexual dysfunction, polyuria
Skin: rash, pruritus, urticaria, photosensitivity, exfoliative dermatitis, erythema multiforme
Other: dehydration, muscle cramps, allergic reaction, interstitial nephritis

PHARMACOKINETICS AND PHARMACODYNAMICS
Duration of action: 24–48 h
Onset of action: <2 h
Peak effect: 6 h
Bioavailability: no data, but absorbed rapidly
Effect of food: not known
Clearance: not clear; 25% excreted unchanged in the urine
Plasma half-life: 26 h
Protein binding: not known

MONITORING
BP, urine output, weight, serum electrolytes.

OVERDOSE
Supportive: replacement of fluid and electrolyte losses.

PATIENT INFORMATION
Polythiazide is used to lower BP or to reduce excessive water in the body. Take the medication as instructed. Avoid excessive dietary sodium intake while maintaining on this therapy. Potassium-rich diet is encouraged to avoid potassium depletion. Sit or lie down if dizziness occurs and rise slowly from a sitting or lying position.

AVAILABILITY
Tablets—1, 2, 4 mg
Combination formlations:
Minizide® Capsules—
Polythiazide 0.5 mg/ Prazosin 1 mg
Polythiazide 0.5 mg/ Prazosin 2 mg
Polythiazide 0.5 mg/ Prazosin 5 mg
Renese-R® Tablets—
Polythiazide 2 mg/ Reserpine 0.25 mg

QUINETHAZONE (Hydromox®)

Quinethazone is a thiazide diuretic. All thiazide diuretics share similar pharmacological activity and adverse effect profile when equivalent dosages are employed clinically. In addition to enhancing diuresis, thiazide diuretics are effective antihypertensive agents. Diuresis usually occurs within 2 hours, peaks within 2 to 6 hours, and lasts for 6 to 12 hours or longer. The onset of antihypertensive effect requires several days. Two to 4 weeks are usually required to achieve optimal BP effect for a given dose. The antihypertensive effect persists longer than the diuretic effect after an oral dose and the effect may last up to 7 days after discontinuing a chronic thiazide diuretic regimen. For more information, please refer to "Hydrochlorothiazide" monograph.

SPECIAL GROUPS

Race: no differences in response

Children: safety and effectiveness have not been established

Elderly: use with caution; no dosage adjustment is required

Renal impairment: use with caution; may be ineffective in severe renal failure and may exacerbate azotemia; contraindicated in anuria

Hepatic impairment: use with caution; titrate the dose based on clinical response

Pregnancy: category C; should only be used if potential benefit outweighs risk

Breast-feeding: use with caution; excreted in human milk

DOSAGE

Edema: Usual dose range—25–200 mg/day as a single dose in the morning or in two divided doses

Intermittent therapy may be preferred by giving the dose every other day or on a 3–5 d/wk schedule.

Hypertension: Usual dose range—25–100 mg/d as a single dose in the morning or in two divided doses

IN BRIEF

INDICATIONS
Hypertension
Edema

CONTRAINDICATIONS
Known hypersensitivity to thiazides, other related diuretics or sulfonamide-derived agents
Anuria or severe renal insufficiency
Hepatic coma

DRUG INTERACTIONS
Other diuretics
Hypotensive agents
Cardiac glycosides
Other potassium-depleting agents (corticosteroids, amphotericin B)
NSAIDs
Agents with high sodium content (ticarcillin)
Lithium
Antidiabetic agents
Cholestyramine, colestipol
Non-depolarizing neuromuscular blockers

ADVERSE EFFECTS
CV: hypotension, orthostatic symptoms, arrhythmias, angina, transient ischemic attack
CNS: dizziness, headache, fatigue, vertigo
Blood: volume and electrolyte depletion ($\downarrow$ K, $\downarrow$ Cl, $\downarrow$ Na, $\downarrow$ Mg, $\uparrow$ Ca, $\uparrow$ uric acid), dilutional hyponatremia, metabolic alkalosis, azotemia, $\uparrow$ serum creatinine, hyperglycemia, dyslipidemia, hematologic abnormalities
GI: anorexia, nausea, vomiting, constipation, diarrhea, cholestatic jaundice, pancreatitis
GU: sexual dysfunction, polyuria
Skin: rash, pruritus, urticaria, photosensitivity, exfoliative dermatitis, erythema multiforme
Other: dehydration, muscle cramps, allergic reaction, interstitial nephritis

PHARMACOKINETICS AND PHARMACODYNAMICS
Duration of action: 18–24 h
Onset of action: 2 h
Peak effect: 6 h
Bioavailability: not known
Effect of food: not known
Clearance: not known
Plasma half-life: not known
Protein binding: not known

MONITORING
BP, urine output, weight, serum electrolytes.

OVERDOSE
Supportive: replacement of fluid and electrolyte losses.

PATIENT INFORMATION
Quinethazone is used to lower BP or to reduce excessive water in the body. Take the medication as instructed. Avoid excessive dietary sodium intake while maintaining on this therapy. Potassium-rich diet is encouraged to avoid potassium depletion. Sit or lie down if dizziness occurs and rise slowly from a sitting or lying position.

AVAILABILITY
Tablets—50 mg

The information here is provided as guidance only. Prescribers should always consult the manufacturer's current prescribing information.

187

TRICHLORMETHIAZIDE (Aquazide®, Diurese®, Naqua®, etc.)

Trichlormethiazide is a thiazide diuretic. All thiazide diuretics share similar pharmacological activity and adverse effect profile when equivalent dosages are employed clinically. In addition to enhancing diuresis, thiazide diuretics are effectice antihypertensive agents. Diuresis usually occurs within 2 hours, peaks within 2 to 6 hours, and lasts for 6 to 12 hours or longer. The onset of antihypertensive effect requires several days. Two to 4 weeks are usually required to achieve optimal BP effect for a given dose. The antihypertensive effect persists longer than the diuretic effect after an oral dose and the effect may last up to 7 days after discontinuing a chronic thiazide diuretic regimen. For more information, please refer to "Hydrochlorothiazide" monograph.

SPECIAL GROUPS

Race: no differences in response
Children: safety and effectiveness have not been established
Elderly: use with caution; no dosage adjustment is required
Renal impairment: use with caution; may be ineffective in severe renal failure and may exacerbate azotemia; contraindicated in anuria
Hepatic impairment: use with caution; titrate the dose based on clinical response
Pregnancy: category C; should only be used if potential benefit outweighs risk
Breast-feeding: use with caution; excreted in human milk

DOSAGE

Edema: Usual dose range—1–4 mg once daily in the morning
Intermittent therapy may be preferred by giving the dose every other day or on a 3–5 d/ wk schedule.
Hypertension: Usual dose range—1–4 mg/d as a single dose in the morning or in two divided doses

IN BRIEF

INDICATIONS
Hypertension
Edema

CONTRAINDICATIONS
Known hypersensitivity to thiazides, other related diuretics, sulfonamide-derived agents, or tartrazine (contained in some products)
Anuria or severe renal insufficiency
Hepatic coma

DRUG INTERACTIONS
Other diuretics
Hypotensive agents
Cardiac glycosides
Other potassium-depleting agents (corticosteroids, amphotericin B)
NSAIDs
Agents with high sodium content (ticarcillin)
Lithium
Antidiabetic agents
Cholestyramine, colestipol
Non-depolarizing neuromuscular blockers

ADVERSE EFFECTS
CV: hypotension, orthostatic symptoms, arrhythmias, angina, transient ischemic attack
CNS: dizziness, headache, fatigue, vertigo
Blood: volume and electrolyte depletion ($\downarrow$ K, $\downarrow$ Cl, $\downarrow$ Na, $\downarrow$ Mg, $\uparrow$ Ca, $\uparrow$ uric acid), dilutional hyponatremia, metabolic alkalosis, azotemia, $\uparrow$ serum creatinine, hyperglycemia, dyslipidemia, hematologic abnormalities
GI: anorexia, nausea, vomiting, constipation, diarrhea, cholestatic jaundice, pancreatitis
GU: sexual dysfunction, polyuria
Skin: rash, pruritus, urticaria, photosensitivity, exfoliative dermatitis, erythema multiforme
Other: dehydration, muscle cramps, allergic reaction, interstitial nephritis

PHARMACOKINETICS AND PHARMACODYNAMICS
Duration of action: 24 h
Onset of action: 1–2 h
Peak effect: 3–6 h
Bioavailability: not clear, but absorbed rapidly
Effect of food: not known
Clearance: not clear, but excreted renally and half-life is prolonged in renal impairment
Plasma half-life: 2.5–7.5 h
Protein binding: not known

MONITORING
BP, urine output, weight, serum electrolytes.

OVERDOSE
Supportive: replacement of fluid and electrolyte losses.

PATIENT INFORMATION
Trichlormethiazide is used to lower BP or to reduce excessive water in the body. Take the medication as instructed. Avoid excessive dietary sodium intake while maintaining on this therapy. Potassium-rich diet is encouraged to avoid potassium depletion. Sit or lie down if dizziness occurs and rise slowly from a sitting or lying position.

AVAILABILITY
Tablets—2, 4 mg
Combination formulations:
Metatensin® #4 and #2 Tablets—
Trichlormethiazide 4 mg/ Reserpine 0.1 mg
Trichlormethiazide 2 mg/ Reserpine 0.1 mg

POTASSIUM-SPARING DIURETICS

Although potassium-sparing diuretics have some diuretic capability, this action is relatively weak. Three drugs are recognized as having a potassium-sparing action: amiloride, spironolactone, and triamterene. They are generally used in fixed-ratio combinations with the more powerful diuretics, which tend to cause excessive potassium loss. Nevertheless, amiloride is regarded in some countries as a single-entity diuretic agent.

EFFICACY AND USE

The main applications of the potassium-sparing diuretics are in the treatment of hypertension and edematous states arising from cardiac, renal, and hepatic failure. They are used in conjunction with a thiazide or a loop diuretic in the management of hypertension or fluid overload to prevent excessive potassium loss associated with the diuresis. Potassium-sparing diuretics can also be used alone to correct hypokalemia from causes other than diuresis. Spironolactone blocks the effect of aldosterone, and thus is indicated for the treatment of hyperaldosteronism.

The European Working Part on Hypertension in the Elderly (EWPHE) study demonstrated that the treatment of elderly patients with a combination of hydrochlorothiazide and triamterene resulted in a significant reduction in fatal cardiac events, but increased nonfatal events, with a trend toward a decrease in the incidence of stroke. The MRC study on older hypertensives compared amiloride plus hydrochlorothiazide, atenolol and placebo in over 4000 patients. The diuretic combination, but not the beta blocker, significantly reduced stroke and MI. A study has also shown that the addition of a potassium-sparing diuretic to thiazide treatment in patients with hypertension was associated with a lower risk of primary cardiac arrest when compared with treatment with a thiazide alone.

MODE OF ACTION

Both amiloride and triamterene act directly on the distal renal tubule of the nephron to inhibit sodium-potassium exchange. They induce only a modest natriuresis but decrease the excretion of potassium. Hydrogen secretion is also reduced, rendering the urine alkaline. Magnesium excretion is decreased, possibly as a consequence of the alkalinization.

Spironolactone acts through competition with the binding sites of aldosterone, a mineralocorticoid. Since these drugs are relatively weak diuretics, their effectiveness can be potentiated by combining any one of them with a diuretic that acts more proximally in the tubule (*ie*, loop or thiazide-type diuretic).

INDICATIONS

	Amiloride	Spironolactone	Triamterene
Hypertension	+*	+*	+*
Edema	+*	+	+*
Hyperaldosteronism	—	+	—
Hypokalemia	+	+	+

* Only use in combination with other diuretics.

+—FDA approved; – —not FDA approved.

The information here is provided as guidance only. Prescribers should always consult the manufacturer's current prescribing information.

189

AMILORIDE (Amiloride, Midamor®)

Amiloride is a weak natriuretic, diuretic and hypotensive agent. It acts directly on the distal renal tubule of the nephron to inhibit sodium-potassium ion exchange and its diuretic activity is independent of aldosterone. When amiloride is combined with a more potent natriuretic agent, they have additive effects on urinary sodium excretion and an antagonistic effect on potassium excretion. In patients with hypertension, amiloride therapy lowers systolic pressure by 10 to 20 mmHg and diastolic pressure by 5 to 10 mmHg. An additive reduction in BP is observed when amiloride is used in combination with a thiazide diuretic. With its potassium-sparing effect, hyperkalemia may be a problem especially in elderly patients or those with underlying renal insufficiency or diabetes mellitus.

SPECIAL GROUPS

Race: no differences in response

Children: safety and effectiveness have not been established

Elderly: use with caution; no dosage adjustment is required

Renal impairment: use with caution; contraindicated in anuria, acute or chronic renal insufficiency

Hepatic impairment: use with caution; dosage adjustment is probably not required

Pregnancy: category B; should only be used if clearly indicated

Breast-feeding: not recommended; not known if the drug is excreted in human milk

DOSAGE

Usual dose range—5–10 mg once daily.

Although dosages exceeding 10 mg/day are usually not necessary, higher dosages have been used occasionally in some patients with persistent hypokalemia.

IN BRIEF

INDICATIONS
As adjunctive therapy with thiazide or other kaliuretic diuretics in CHF or hypertension to prevent excessive potassium loss.

CONTRAINDICATIONS
Known hypersensitivity

Hyperkalemia (>5.5 mEq/L)

Anuria, acute and chronic renal insufficiency, diabetic nephropathy

Concurrent therapy with other potassium-sparing agents or potassium supplements

DRUG INTERACTIONS
Other potassium sparing agents (spironolactone, triamterene, angiotensin converting enzyme (ACE) inhibitors, angiotensin II receptor antagonists)

Potassium-containing products

Other diuretics

Hypotensive agents

Lithium

NSAIDs

Cardiac glycosides

ADVERSE EFFECTS
CV: hypotension, orthostatic symptoms, arrhythmias, angina

CNS: dizziness, headache, fatigue

Blood: hyperkalemia, metabolic acidosis, ↑ glucose, ↑ BUN, ↑ serum creatinine, blood dyscrasias

GI: anorexia, nausea, vomiting, diarrhea, abdominal discomfort, jaundice

GU: sexual dysfunction, polyuria

Skin: rash, pruritus

Other: dehydration, muscle cramps, allergic reaction, interstitial nephritis

PHARMACOKINETICS AND PHARMACODYNAMICS
Duration of action: 24 h

Onset of action: 2 h

Peak effect: 6–10 h

Bioavailability: 50%

Effect of food: ↓ absorption, 30% absorbed

Clearance: not metabolized, mainly excreted unchanged in the urine (50%) and in the stools (unabsorbed, 40%)

Plasma half-life: 6–9 h or longer

Protein binding: not known

MONITORING
BP, urine output, weight, serum electrolytes.

OVERDOSE
Supportive: correct severe, symptomatic hyperkalemia or hypotension.

PATIENT INFORMATION
Amiloride is used to reduce potassium loss from the body. Take the medication as instructed. Avoid excessive dietary sodium and potassium intake while maintaining on this therapy. Sit or lie down if dizziness occurs and rise slowly from a sitting or lying position.

AVAILABILITY
Tablets—5 mg

Combination formulations:
Moduretic® Tablets and various products—
Amiloride 5 mg/ Hydrochlorothiazide 50 mg

SPIRONOLACTONE (Spironolactone, Aldactone®)

Spironolactone is a synthetic steroid aldosterone antagonist. It competitively inhibits the physiologic effects of aldosterone on the distal renal tubules, which enhances the excretion of sodium, chloride, and water, and reduces excretion of potassium, ammonium, phosphate and titratable acid. The weak diuretic effect of spironolactone is determined by the presence of aldosterone and is most pronounced in patients with liver cirrhosis or hyperaldosteronism. It is usually used together with a thiazide or a loop diuretic to enhance diuresis. Recent data indicated that in patients with severe heart failure (NYHA Class IV), adding spironolactone 25 mg daily to standard treatment led to a reduction in long-term mortality. Spironolactone has antiandrogenic effect, which is responsible for the troublesome adverse effects such as gynecomastia, sexual dysfunction, and menstrual irregularities reported in some patients. These side effects may be related to both dosage and duration of the therapy. Spironolactone has been shown to be a tumorigen in chronic toxicity studies in rats at doses much higher than the usual human dose. The long-term effect in patients receiving the drug chronically is not clear.

SPECIAL GROUPS

Race: no differences in response

Children: indicated in the management of edema only

Elderly: use with caution; no dosage adjustment is required

Renal impairment: use with caution; contraindicated in anuria, acute or chronic renal insufficiency

Hepatic impairment: use with caution; dosage should be titrated based on clinical response

Pregnancy: category C; spironolactone and its metabolites may cross the placenta barrier; should only be used if clearly indicated

Breast-feeding: not recommended; canrenone, a metabolite of spironolactone, is excreted in human milk

DOSAGE

Edema: Usual dose range—25–200 mg daily. The usual initial dose is 100 mg administered as a single dose or in divided doses. If used alone, the treatment should be continued for at least 5 d. Then, the dose may be adjusted based on the response or a more potent diuretic may be added.

Diuretic-induced hypokalemia: Usual dose range—25–100 mg daily

Hypertension: Usual dose range—25–100 mg daily administered as a single dose or in divided doses (usually used in combination with another agent such as a thiazide diuretic)

Primary aldosteronism:

As a diagnostic test: Long test—Spironolactone 400 mg is administered daily for 3–4 wk. Correction of hypokalemia and hypertension provides presumptive evidence for the diagnosis

Short test—Spironolactone 400 mg is administered daily for 4 d. If serum potassium levels increase during the therapy but decline after discontinuing the drug, a presumptive diagnosis should be considered.

Treatment:

As a diagnostic test: Spironolactone in doses of 100–400 mg daily may be administered in preparation for surgery. For patients who are not surgical candidates, long-term spironolactone therapy may be used and the dose should be titrated individually.

IN BRIEF

INDICATIONS
Edema associated with CHF, liver cirrhosis, or nephrotic syndrome
Hypokalemia
Hypertension, combine with other agents usually
Primary hyperaldosteronism

CONTRAINDICATIONS
Known hypersensitivity
Hyperkalemia (>5.5 mEq/L)
Anuria, acute and chronic renal insufficiency, diabetic nephropathy
Concurrent therapy with other potassium-sparing agents or potassium supplements

DRUG INTERACTIONS
Other potassium sparing agents (amiloride, triamterene, ACE inhibitors, angiotensin II receptor antagonists)
Potassium-containing products
Other diuretics
Hypotensive agents
Norepinephrine
Indomethacin
Aspirin
Cardiac glycosides

ADVERSE EFFECTS
CV: hypotension, orthostatic symptoms, arrhythmias, angina
CNS: dizziness, headache, fatigue
Blood: hyperkalemia, metabolic acidosis, ↓ Na, ↑ glucose, ↑ BUN, ↑ serum creatinine, agranulocytosis
GI: anorexia, nausea, vomiting, diarrhea, abdominal discomfort, jaundice, hepatocellular injury
GU: sexual dysfunction, amenorrhea or irregular menses, post-menopausal bleeding, polyuria
Skin: rash, urticaria
Other: gynecomastia, muscle cramps, drug fever, dehydration

PHARMACOKINETICS AND PHARMACODYNAMICS
Duration of action: 2–3 d
Onset of action: 2 h
Peak effect: 48–72 h
Bioavailability: not known, but well absorbed
Effect of food: increase absorption
Clearance: extensively metabolized; has 3 three active metabolites, mainly excreted in the urine, and also in the stools
Plasma half-life: spironolactone—1–2 hrs; canrenone (active metabolites)—13–24 h; 7α-thiomethylspirono-lactone—3 h
Protein binding: >90% (spironolactone/metabolites)

MONITORING
BP, urine output, weight, serum electrolytes.

OVERDOSE
Supportive: correct severe, symptomatic hyperkalemia or hypotension.

PATIENT INFORMATION
Spironolactone is used to prevent excessive water accumulation or to reduce potassium loss from the body. Take the medication as instructed. Avoid excessive dietary sodium and potassium intake while maintaining on this therapy. Sit or lie down if dizziness occurs and rise slowly from a sitting or lying position.

AVAILABILITY
Tablets—25, 50, 100 mg
Combination formulations:
Aldactazide® Tablets and various products—
Spironolactone 25 mg/ Hydrochlorothiazide 25 mg
Spironolactone 50 mg/ Hydrochlorothiazide 50 mg

TRIAMTERENE (Triamterene, Dyrenium®)

Similar to amiloride, triamterene inhibits reabsorption of sodium and excretion of potassium and hydrogen in the distal renal tubule. Its activity is independent of aldosterone concentrations in the body. Triamterene alone has little antihypertensive effect. It is usually used in combination with other diuretics to enhance diuresis and to prevent or treat excessive diuretic-induced potassium loss.

SPECIAL GROUPS

Race: no differences in response

Children: safety and effectiveness have not been established

Elderly: use with caution; start with low dose and adjust the dose based on response

Renal impairment: use with caution; contraindicated in anuria, acute or chronic renal insufficiency

Hepatic impairment: use with caution; start with low dose and adjust the dose based on response

Pregnancy: category B; should only be used if clearly indicated

Breast-feeding: not recommended; not known if the drug is excreted in human milk

DOSAGE

As a single agent: The usual initial dose is 100 mg twice daily after meals. Dosage should not exceed 300 mg daily. Once edema is controlled, most patients can be maintained on 100 mg daily or every other day.

In combination with a kaliuretic diuretic: The initial dose is 25 mg once daily. The dose should be titrated based on response to a maximum of 100 mg daily.

IN BRIEF

INDICATIONS
Edema associated with CHF, liver cirrhosis, nephrotic syndrome, steroid use, or secondary hyperaldosteronism

Hypokalemia

Hypertension, combined with other diuretics usually

CONTRAINDICATIONS
Known hypersensitivity

Hyperkalemia (>5.5 mEq/L)

Anuria, acute and chronic renal insufficiency, diabetic nephropathy

Concurrent therapy with other potassium-sparing agents or potassium supplements

DRUG INTERACTIONS
Other potassium sparing agents (amiloride, spironolactone, ACE inhibitors, angiotensin II receptor antagonists)

Potassium-containing products

Other diuretics

Hypotensive agents

Lithium

Indomethacin

NSAIDs

Cardiac glycosides

ADVERSE EFFECTS
CV: arrhythmias, hypotension, orthostatic symptoms, angina

CNS: dizziness, headache, fatigue

Blood: hyperkalemia, metabolic acidosis, $\downarrow$ Na, $\downarrow$ Mg, $\uparrow$ BUN, $\uparrow$ serum creatinine, blood dyscrasias

GI: nausea, vomiting, diarrhea

GU: sexual dysfunction, polyuria, nephrolithiasis

Skin: rash, photosensitivity

Other: dehydration, muscle cramps, anaphylaxis, interstitial nephritis

PHARMACOKINETICS AND PHARMACODYNAMICS
Duration of action: 7–9 h

Onset of action: 2–4 h

Peak effect: several days of therapy

Bioavailability: 30%–70%

Effect of food: not known

Clearance: 80% metabolized in liver, has an active metabolite; excreted in urine as unchanged drug and metabolites

Plasma half-life: 1.5–2.5 h

Protein binding: 55%–67%

MONITORING
BP, urine output, weight, serum electrolytes.

OVERDOSE
Supportive: correct severe, symptomatic hyperkalemia or hypotension.

PATIENT INFORMATION
Triamterene is used to reduce potassium loss and/or to increase water excretion from the body. Take the medication as instructed. Avoid excessive dietary sodium and potassium intake while maintaining on this therapy. Sit or lie down if dizziness occurs and rise slowly from a sitting or lying position.

AVAILABILITY
Capsules—50, 100 mg

Combination formulations:

Dyazide® Capsules, Maxzide® Tablets and various products—
Triamterene 75 mg/ Hydrochlorothiazide 50 mg
Triamterene 50 mg/ Hydrochlorothiazide 25 mg
Triamterene 37.5 mg/ Hydrochlorothiazide 25 mg

SELECTED BIBLIOGRAPHY

Amery A, Birkenhager W, Brixko P, *et al*: Mortality and morbidity results from the European Working Party on High Blood Pressure in the Elderly Trial. *Lancet* 1985; 1: 1349–1354.

Bayliss J, Norell M, Canepa-Anson R, Sutton G, *et al*.: Untreated heart failure: clinical and neuroendocrine effects of introducing diuretics. *Br Heart J* 1987; 57: 17–22.

Channer KS, McLean KA, Lawson-Matthew P, *et al*: Combination diuretic treatment in severe heart failure: a randomized controlled trial. *Br Heart J* 1994; 71: 146–150.

Coope J, Warrender TS: Randomized trial of treatment of hypertension in elderly patients in primary care. *Br Med J* 1986; 293: 1145–1151.

Cutler JA, Neaton JD, Hulley SB, Kullere L, *et al*.: Coronary heart disease and all-cause mortality in the Multiple Risk Factor Intervention Trial: subgroup findings and comparisons with other trials. *Prev Med* 1985; 16: 293–311.

Friedel HA, Buckley MMT: Torasemide. A review of its pharmacological properties and therapeutic potential. *Drugs* 1991; 41: 81–103.

Frishman WH: Diagnosis and treatment of systolic heart failure in the elderly. *Am J Geriatr Cardiol* 1998; 7: 10–16.

Frishman WH, Burris JF, Mroczek WJ, *et al*: First-line therapy option with low-dose bisoprolol fumarate and low-dose hydrochlorothiazide in patients with stage I and stage II systemic hypertension. *J Clin Pharmacol* 1995; 35: 182–88.

Frishman WH, Bryzinski BS, Coulson LR, *et al*: A multifactorial trial design to assess combination therapy in hypertension: treatment with bisoprolol and hydrochlorothiazide. *Arch Intern Med* 1994; 154: 1461–68.

Grossman E, Messerli FH, Goldbourt U: Does diuretic therapy increase the risk of renal cell carcinoma? *Am J Card* 1999; 83:1090–1093.

Hachamovitch R, Strom JA, Sonnenblick EH, *et al*: Left ventricular hypertrophy in hypertension and the effects of antihypertensive drug therapy. *Curr Probl Cardiol* 1988; 13: 371–421.

Kiyingi A, Field MJ, Pawsey CC, *et al*: Metolazone in treatment of severe refractory congestive cardiac failure. *Lancet* 1990; 335: 29–31.

Kramer WG, Smith WB, Ferguson J, *et al*: Pharmacodynamics of torsemide administered as an intravenous injection and as a continuous infusion to patients with congestive heart failure. *J Clin Pharmacol* 1996; 36: 265–270.

LaCroix AZ, Wienpahl J, White LR, *et al*: Thiazide diuretic agents and the incidence of hip fracture. *N Engl J Med* 1990; 322: 286–290.

Lakshman MR, Reda DJ, Materson BJ, *et al*: Diuretics and β-blockers do not have adverse effect at 1 year on plasma lipid and lipoprotein profiles in men with hypertension. *Arch Intern Med* 1999; 159: 551–58.

Lant A: Diuretics: clinical pharmacology and therapeutic use (Part I). *Drugs* 1985; 29: 57–87.

LeJemtel TH, Sonnenblick EH, Frishman WH: Diagnosis and management of heart failure. In, Alexander RW, Schlant RC, Fuster V (eds): *Hurst's The Heart*, 9th ed. New York: McGraw Hill, 1998: 745–81.

Leren P, Helgeland A: Coronary heart disease and treatment of hypertension. Some Oslo study data. *Am J Med* 1986; 80: 3–6.

Levine SD: Diuretics. *Med Clin North Am* 1989; 73: 271–282.

Medical Research Council Working Party: MRC trial of treatment of mild hypertension: principal results. *Br Med J* 1985; 29: 97–104.

Mokrzycki M, Tamirisa P: Diuretic therapy in cardiovascular disease. In, Frishman WH, Sonnenblick EH: *Cardiovascular Pharmacotherapeutics*. New York: McGraw Hill, 1997: 193–222.

Mokrzycki M, Tamirisa P, Frishman WH: Diuretic therapy in cardiovascular disease. In, Frishman WH, Sonnenblick EH: *Cardiovascular Pharmacotherapeutics Companion Handbook*. New York: McGraw Hill, 1998: 152–74.

Neaton JD, Grimm RH, Prineas RJ, *et al*: Treatment of Mild Hypertension Study. Final results. *JAMA* 1993; 270: 713–724.

Parker JD, Parker AB, Farrell B, *et al*: Effects of diuretic therapy on the development of tolerance to nitroglycerin and exercise capacity in patients with chronic stable angina. *Circulation* 1996; 93: 691–696.

Reader R, Bauer GE, Doyle AE, *et al*: The Australian Therapeutic Trial of Mild Hypertension: report by the management committee. *Lancet* 1980; 1: 1261–1267.

Schuller D, Lynch JP, Fine D: Protocol-guided diuretic management: comparison of furosemide by continuous infusion and intermittent bolus. *Crit Care Med* 1997; 25: 1969–75.

Shapiro PA: Five year findings of the Hypertension Detection and Follow-up Program: 1. Reduction in mortality of persons with high blood pressure, including mild hypertension. *JAMA* 1979; 242: 2562–2571.

SHEP Cooperative Research Group: Prevention of stroke by anti-hypertensive drug treatment in older persons with isolated systolic hypertension. Final results of the Systolic Hypertension in the Elderly Program. *JAMA* 1991; 24: 3255–3264.

Siscovick DS, Raghunathan TE, Psaty BM, *et al*: Diuretic therapy for hypertension and the risk of primary cardiac arrest. *N Engl J Med* 1994; 330: 1852–57.

The Sixth Report of the Joint National Committee on Prevention, Detection, Evaluation and Treatment of High Blood Pressure. *Arch Intern Med* 1997; 157: 2413–46.

Velazquez H: Thiazide diuretics. *Renal Physiol* 1987; 10: 184–197.

Weber KT: Aldosterone and spironolactone in heart failure. *N Engl J Med* 1999: 341:753–754.

10

INOTROPIC AND VASOPRESSOR AGENTS

The major aim of inotropic therapy is to improve ventricular contractility of the depressed heart so as to increase cardiac output as needed and reduce elevated ventricular filling pressures. They may be employed intravenously for acute ventricular failure (*eg*, phosphodiesterase (PDE) III inhibitors or catecholamines) or chronically as oral agents (*eg*, digitalis glycosides).

Traditionally, the treatment of congestive heart failure (CHF) has included the use of diuretics, vasodilators, and digitalis. Lack of response has spurred the development of new inotropic drugs. Inotropic agents currently available can be classified into three groups: the PDE inhibitors (**amrinone, milrinone**), the adrenergic receptor agonists (**dobutamine, dopamine, norepinephrine**) for acute, short-term intravenous use, and the inhibitors of sodium-potassium ATPase (the digitalis family) for chronic oral therapy as well as intravenous use (Table 10.1).

Although digitalis has been available for some 200 years, it has only recently been shown to be an effective inotrope for chronic oral use. Short-term inotropic support with newer agents such as PDE inhibitors has been effective when administered intravenously. These agents increase contractility and relax both venous and arterial vasculature. As a result, cardiac output is increased and ventricular filling pressure is decreased. It is unclear if chronic use of these agents can improve mortality. In clinical trials, chronic oral **milrinone** or **vesnarinone** therapy in patients with ventricular dysfunction has been associated with increased mortality.

TABLE 10.1 RELATIVE HEMODYNAMIC EFFECTS OF INOTROPIC AGENTS IN HEART FAILURE					
	Ventricular filling pressure	Peripheral vascular resistance	Cardiac output	Blood pressure	Ejection fraction
Inotropic agents					
Digoxin	↓	↓	↑	—	↑
Dobutamine	↓/NC	↓↓	↑↑	↑/NC	↑↑
Dopamine	↓/NC	↑	↑	↑	↑/NC
Norepinephrine	↓/NC	↑↑	↑/NC	↑↑	↑/NC
Inolators					
Milrinone	↓↓	↓↓	↑↑	↓	↑

↓—decrease; ↑—increase; NC—no change.

Adapted from Sonnenblick EH, LeJemtel TH, Frishman WH: Digitalis preparations and other inotropic agents. In Frishman WH, Sonnenblick EH: Cardiovascular Pharmacotherapeutics. New York: McGraw Hill, 1997: 248.

INOTROPIC AGENTS: PHOSPHODIESTERASE (PDE) INHIBITORS

In addition to their direct cardiac actions, PDE inhibitors also have vasodilatory properties, a combination that theoretically may make them seem ideal for the treatment of CHF. Currently they are only approved for intravenous use, because prolonged oral use in patients with severe left ventricular dysfunction was associated with increased mortality.

EFFICACY AND USE

Administration of the biperidylphosphodiesterase inhibitors, **amrinone** and **milrinone**, to patients with CHF results in a marked increase in cardiac index and substantial reduction in cardiac filling pressures. Systemic blood pressure (BP) only slightly alters. At high doses, a reflexive rise in heart rate and fall in BP can be observed. A rise in contractility observed early in the development of amrinone and milrinone was presumed to be the result of their inotropic action, but this is now attributed to their vasodilatory action.

Due to their vasodilating action, both **amrinone** and **milrinone** are very effective in lowering filling pressures and in-creasing cardiac output. These effects are synergistic with those of dobutamine or other catecholamines.

MODE OF ACTION

Amrinone and **milrinone** inhibit the enzyme responsible for the breakdown of cyclic adenosine monophosphate (AMP) in the target cell. More specifically, they selectively inhibit PDE III, the isoenzyme specific for cyclic AMP. The subsequent increase in cyclic AMP leads to enhanced phosphorylation of protein in the sarcoplasmic reticulum and sarcolemma, which in turn promotes improved calcium uptake, storage and release from the sarcoplasmic reticulum during excitation-contraction coupling. Adenosine receptors have also been implicated in the action of these drugs. **Milrinone** may also increase calcium influx into myocardial cells via the slow calcium channel. In addition to their inotropic effect, **amrinone** and **milrinone** produce vasodilatation and a decrease in both preload and afterload. These agents have a rapid onset and reach a peak hemodynamic effect within 10 minutes when given intravenously.

INDICATIONS

	Amrinone	Milrinone
Short-term support in CHF	+	+

+—FDA approved; CHF—congestive heart failure.

The information here is provided as guidance only. Prescribers should always consult the manufacturer's current prescribing information.

195

AMRINONE (Inocor®)

Amrinone is a PDE inhibitor with positive inotropic and vasodilating activity. Amrinone has different chemical structure and mechanism of action from either digitalis glycosides or catecholamines. Amrinone provides hemodynamic benefits and symptomatic relief in patients not adequately controlled by diuretic, vasodilator and cardioglycoside therapy.

Thrombocytopenia has been a concern with amrinone therapy. The problem may be related to high dose and prolonged administration or high blood concentration of a metabolite, N-acetylamrinone. Bone marrow is not involved and the platelet count is usually normalized after withdrawal of amrinone. Intravenous amrinone is only indicated for short-term management in patients with low output heart failure. Prolonged therapy is generally not recommended. Chronic inotropic therapy, with the exception of digitalis glycosides, may improve symptoms of heart failure transiently but has been associated with excessive increase in mortality.

SPECIAL GROUPS

Race: no differences in response
Children: safety and effectiveness have not been established
Elderly: dose should be adjusted based on renal function
Renal impairment: dose should be adjusted based on renal function
Hepatic impairment: use with caution; dose should be adjusted based on renal function
Pregnancy: category C; should only be used if clearly indicated
Breast-feeding: use with caution; not known if the drug is excreted in human milk

DOSAGE

An IV bolus dose of 750 µg/kg (or, 0.75 mg/kg) should be administered over 2–3 min, followed by a continuous infusion of 5–10 µg/kg/min and titrated to the maximum hemodynamic effect based on close patient monitoring. A second bolus of 750 µg/kg (or, 0.75 mg/kg) may be administered 30 min after the initial bolus. The total dose should not exceed 10 mg/kg/d. Duration of therapy is determined by the responsiveness of the patient.

IN BRIEF

INDICATIONS
CHF, short-term inotropic support.

CONTRAINDICATIONS
Known hypersensitivity to milrinone, amrinone, or bisulfites
Severe obstructive aortic or pulmonic valvular disease
Severe hypotension
Acute MI

DRUG INTERACTIONS
Not clear; any agents that may affect cardiac or hemodynamic system can potentially interact with amrinone.

ADVERSE EFFECTS
CV: arrhythmias, angina, hypotension
CNS: headache
GI: hepatotoxicity, nausea, vomiting
Other: thrombocytopenia, hypokalemia, tremor, hypersensitivity reaction, fever

PHARMACOKINETICS AND PHARMACODYNAMICS
Duration of action: up to 8 h
Onset of action: 5–10 min
Peak effect: within 10 min
Bioavailability: 100%
Effect of food: not applicable
Metabolism: partially metabolized by conjugative pathway
Excretion: renal (10%–40% as unchanged within 24 h)
Plasma half-life: 5.8 h (3–15 h)
Protein binding: 10%–49%

MONITORING
BP, heart rate, electrocardiogram (ECG), platelet count, serum electrolytes, renal function, weight, cardiac index, central venous or pulmonary wedge pressure, and improvement in signs and symptoms of heart failure.

OVERDOSE
Supportive: Fluid therapy and vasopressors may be used in severe hypotension for circulatory support.

PATIENT INFORMATION
Amrinone is used to treat heart failure.

AVAILABILITY
Ampules—100 mg/20 mL (5 mg/mL)

MILRINONE

(Primacor®)

Milrinone is a PDE inhibitor with positive inotropic and vasodilating activity. Similar to amrinone, milrinone has a different mechanism of action from either digitalis glycosides or catecholamines. However, milrinone has rarely been associated with thrombocytopenia, a significant problem reported with amrinone therapy. Milrinone IV is only indicated for short-term management in patients with low output heart failure. Prolonged IV maintenance therapy has been associated with increased risk of arrhythmias and sudden death. Actually, when oral milrinone was investigated as a chronic inotropic support in heart failure patients, the study was terminated because an excessive mortality rate was observed.

SPECIAL GROUPS

Race: no differences in response

Children: safety and effectiveness have not been established

Elderly: dose should be adjusted based on renal function

Renal impairment: dose should be lowered and adjusted based on renal function

Hepatic impairment: use with caution; dosage adjustment is probably not required

Pregnancy: category C; should only be used if clearly indicated

Breast-feeding: use with caution; not known if the drug is excreted in human milk

DOSAGE

A loading dose of 50 µg/kg should be administered IV over 10 min, followed by a continuous infusion of 0.375 µg/kg/min and titrated to the maximum hemodynamic effect based on close patient monitoring*. The total dose should not exceed 1.13 mg/kg/d (or, 0.75 µg/kg/min). Duration of therapy is determined by the responsiveness of the patient.

* Recommended infusion rate in patients with renal impairment:

Creatinine Clearance (mL/min/1.73 m²)	Infusion Rate
50	0.43 µg/kg/min
40	0.38 µg/kg/min
30	0.33 µg/kg/min
<20	0.2–0.28 µg/kg/min

IN BRIEF

INDICATIONS
CHF, short-term inotropic support.

CONTRAINDICATIONS
Known hypersensitivity to milrinone or amrinone
Severe obstructive aortic or pulmonic valvular disease
Severe hypotension
Acute MI

DRUG INTERACTIONS
Not clear; any agents that may affect cardiac and hemodynamic system can potentially interact with milrinone.

ADVERSE EFFECTS
CV: arrhythmias, angina, hypotension
CNS: headache
Other: thrombocytopenia, hypokalemia, tremor, hypersensitivity reaction

PHARMACOKINETICS AND PHARMACODYNAMICS
Duration of action: 3–5 h
Onset of action: immediate
Peak effect: within 5–15 min
Bioavailability: 100%
Effect of food: not applicable
Metabolism: 12% converted to O-glucuronide
Excretion: renal (83%– unchanged)
Plasma half-life: 2.3 hours ($\uparrow$ in renal dysfunction)
Protein binding: 70%

MONITORING
BP, heart rate, electrocardiogram, serum electrolytes, platelet count, renal function, weight, and improvement in signs and symptoms of heart failure, cardiac index, central venous or pulmonary wedge pressure.

OVERDOSE
Supportive: Fluid therapy and vasopressors may be used in severe hypotension for circulatory support.

PATIENT INFORMATION
Milrinone is used to treat heart failure.

AVAILABILITY
Vials—10 mg/10 mL, 20 mg/20 mL
Syringes—5 mg/5 mL
Pre-Mix—20 mg/100 mL D5W

Inotropic and Vasopressor Agents: Adrenergic Receptor Agonists

Drugs that belong to this group (eg, **dobutamine** and **dopamine**) have a common feature: they stimulate cardiac or peripheral tissues at specific adrenergic or dopaminergic receptors to produce a combination of either peripheral vasodilatation or constriction with a positive inotropic support to the heart. They differ in their receptor selectivities and this is reflected in different hemodynamic responses. Because of their pharmacokinetic or pharmacodynamic properties, most are used for short-term hemodynamic support only. Recently the first orally active alpha$_1$-adrenergic agonist was approved for use in patients with orthostatic hypotension (ie, **midodrine**).

Efficacy and Use

These inotropic agents are available for IV, and thus, short-term use. As with the PDE inhibitors, evidence suggests that tachyphylaxis to these drugs may appear with sustained use. To date, there has been no evidence to support their long-term benefit in mortality, and they may even increase the risk of death (Figure 10.1). Nevertheless, these agents are valuable in providing short-term hemodynamic support.

Because these drugs tend to enhance atrioventricular (AV) conduction, they have proarrhythmic potential in patients with atrial arrhythmias. In these cases, pretreatment with **digitalis** may be useful. Because their actions are not identical, they may work synergistically, either together or with other vasodilators. This strategy permits the use of low-dose dopamine when its vasodilatory effects are apparent, rather than risking unwanted vasoconstriction with too high a dose. These drugs have a relatively weak effect on pulmonary wedge pressure. Therefore, when used in combination with preload reducers, such as nitrates or angiotensin converting enzyme (ACE) inhibitors, can produce valuable benefits. Because of the inotropic effects, they can worsen ischemia; it is therefore advisable to use them only with ECG monitoring.

Mode of Action

Dobutamine stimulates beta$_1$-adrenergic receptors and, to a lesser extent, beta$_2$ receptors. It has a very short half-life. When given IV, it raises cardiac output and reduces systemic vascular resistance. Renal blood flow improves and this can result in an improved urine output.

Indications

	Dobutamine	Dopamine
CHF (short-term)	+	+
Cardiogenic shock	+	+
Hypotension	—	+

+—clinically used; —not clinically used (no clear-cut, FDA-approved indications)
CHF—congestive heart failure.

Dopamine is among the oldest known direct inotropic drugs. As a precursor of the catecholamines, it is capable of interacting with a variety of adrenergic receptors. As a result, its hemodynamic actions are, to some extent, dose dependent. Dopamine receptors are found in the renal, mesenteric, coronary, and cerebrovascular beds. Low doses of dopamine stimulate dopamine receptors to produce vasodilatation in these areas. Higher doses release norepinephrine from storage sites. As a result, indirect beta$_1$-adrenergic stimulation is observed producing hemodynamic effects similar to those of dobutamine. At even higher doses, dopamine stimulates alpha-adrenergic receptors, producing vasoconstriction and opposing the dopaminergic vasodilatory action. Hypertension is sometimes observed in this situation. Table 10.2 shows the different pharmacological actions of these inotropic agents.

Isoproterenol is a stimulant of both beta$_1$ and beta$_2$ adrenergic receptors. The drug must be given IV. It causes vasodilatation accompanied by direct and reflex cardiac stimulation. Cardiac output is increased while mean BP falls. It can cause tachycardia and significant arrhythmogenesis, which has limited its clinical use.

Norepinephrine, a naturally-occurring catecholamine, stimulates beta$_1$, alpha$_1$ and alpha$_2$ adrenergic receptors, and to a much less extent, beta$_2$ receptors. Its major hemodynamic effect is to cause vasoconstriction and direct cardiac stimulation leading to increased systolic and diastolic BP. Reflex bradycardia may occur. It has limited clinical use except as a pressor agent in the treatment of shock with hypotension.

Epinephrine, a naturally-occurring catecholamine, stimulates beta-adrenergic receptors, and to a lesser extent, alpha receptors. It causes cardiac stimulation accompanied by venoconstriction. It causes vasoconstriction in certain vascular beds, but dilation in others (eg, skeletal muscle). Cardiac output is increased and systolic BP is elevated, whereas diastolic BP falls, with little change in peripheral vascular resistance. The drug remains an emergency treatment for cardiac arrest, for preserving cerebral blood flow during resuscitation and for treatment of severe allergic reactions. It is used as an adjunctive vasoconstrictor during local anesthesia.

Metaraminol is an IV pressor agent that indirectly causes alpha$_1$ stimulation by causing the release of neuronal norepinephrine.

Methoxamine and **phenylephrine** are both sympathomimetic amines, which act predominantly on post-synaptic alpha-adrenergic receptors to increase arterial BP. In addition, **phenylephrine** has an indirect effect to release **norepinephrine** from its storage sites.

Midodrine is a new orally-active alpha$_1$ receptor agonist that causes both arterial and venous constriction without tachycardia. It is approved for use in patients with symptomatic orthostatic hypotension. It has limited benefit in the management of vasovagal syncope.

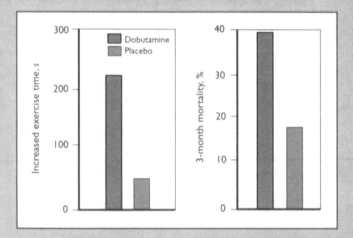

FIGURE 10.1 Effect of intermittent dobutamine infusion on increased exercise capacity and mortality. (*Adapted from* Packer M: Do positive inotropic agents adversely affect the survival of patients with chronic congestive heart failure? II. Protagonist's viewpoint. *J Am Coll Cardiol* 1988; 12:562–566.)

TABLE 10.2 COMPARATIVE AGONIST ACTIVITIES AND ACTIONS OF DOPAMINE AND DOBUTAMINE

Activity	Response to activity	Dopamine	Dobutamine
DA_1	Renal and mesenteric vasodilatation; natriuresis, diuresis	+++	NA
DA_2	Presynaptic sympathetic inhibition of norepinephrine release; generalized reduction of sympathetic tone (excessive stimulation leads to increased risk of nausea and emesis)	++	NA
$Beta_1$	Positive chronotropy or inotropy. Increased AV conduction (leads to increased risk of arrhythmias)	++	+++
$Beta_2$	Peripheral vasodilatation (afterload reduction)	+	++
Alpha	Peripheral and arteriolar vasoconstriction	++	++
Uptake inhibition	Increase in amount of norepinephrine in sympathetic synaptic cleft	++	+

+— mild; ++ —moderate; +++— powerful; Alpha —Alpha-adrenergic receptor; AV—atrioventricular; $Beta_1$ — $Beta_1$-adrenergic receptor; $Beta_2$— $Beta_2$-adrenergic receptor; DA_1— dopamine type 1 receptor; DA_2— dopamine type 2 receptor; NA— not active; uptake inhibition— norepinephrine uptake mechanism.

DOBUTAMINE (Dobutamine, Dobutrex®)

Dobutamine is a selective beta$_1$-adrenergic agonist. In therapeutic doses, dobutamine also exhibits mild beta$_2$- and alpha$_1$-adrenergic activities. Dobutamine does not cause release of endogenous norepinephrine and has no effect on dopaminergic receptors. The major effect of dobutamine is beta$_1$-mediated cardiac stimulation which results in a positive inotropic effect. Dobutamine may reduce peripheral vascular resistance, but BP may remain unchanged or be increased due to increased cardiac output. Heart rate is usually minimally affected, while increased contractility may enhance coronary perfusion and myocardial oxygen consumption. Dobutamine enhances atrioventricular conduction. Thus, in atrial fibrillation with rapid ventricular response, patients should be digitalized prior to dobutamine therapy. Dobutamine may reduce pulmonary vascular resistance, which may benefit patients with elevated pulmonary artery pressure.

SPECIAL GROUPS

Race: no differences in response
Children: safety and effectiveness have not been established
Elderly: no dosage adjustment is required
Renal impairment: no dosage adjustment is required
Hepatic impairment: no dosage adjustment is required
Pregnancy: category B; should only be used if clearly indicated
Breast-feeding: use with caution; not known if the drug is excreted in human milk

DOSAGE

Usual dose range: 2.5–15 µg/kg/min
The infusion rate and the duration of therapy should be adjusted based on clinical response.

IN BRIEF

INDICATIONS
Short-term inotropic support in patients with cardiac decompensation due to depressed contractility.

CONTRAINDICATIONS
Idiopathic hypertrophic subaortic stenosis
Hypersensitivity

DRUG INTERACTIONS
Beta-adrenergic antagonists
General anesthetics: halothene, cyclopropane
Any agents that may affect cardiac/hemodynamic system can potentially interact with dobutamine

ADVERSE EFFECTS
CV: tachycardia, ventricular ectopic beats, hypertension, hypotension, angina
CNS: headache
GI: nausea
Skin: phlebitis, local infiltration/reaction
Other: hypokalemia

PHARMACOKINETICS AND PHARMACODYNAMICS
Duration of action: few minutes
Onset of action: 1–2 min
Peak effect: 10 min
Bioavailability: 100%
Effect of food: not applicable
Clearance: renally excreted as metabolites after methylation and conjugation
Plasma half-life: 2 min
Protein binding: not known

MONITORING
BP, heart rate, ECG, serum electrolytes, urine output, cardiac index, central venous and pulmonary wedge pressure, weight, and improvement in signs and symptoms of heart failure.

OVERDOSE
Supportive: the duration of action is usually short.

PATIENT INFORMATION
Dobutamine is used to increase the contractility of a failing heart.

AVAILABILITY
Vials—250 mg/20 mL (12.5 mg/mL)

DOPAMINE (Dopamine, Intropin®)

Dopamine, an endogenous catecholamine, is the immediate precursor of norepinephrine. Dopamine activates the sympathetic nervous system directly. In addition, dopamine stimulates the release of norepinephrine from storage sites. Dopamine also causes vasodilation by acting on specific dopaminergic receptors in the renal, mesenteric, coronary, and intracerebral vascular beds. The major therapeutic effect of dopamine is dose-dependent. In low doses, up to 10 µg/kg/min, cardiac (beta$_1$) stimulation and renal vascular dilatation (dopaminergic) occur, and in higher doses, > 10 µg/kg/min, vasoconstriction occurs (alpha-adrenergic stimulation). In clinical practice, dopamine may be used to increase cardiac output, BP, and urine output in the management of persistent circulatory failure after adequate fluid resuscitation. Since dopamine may improve cardiac output and stroke volume, it has been used as a short-term, add-on therapy in patients with severe heart failure. The therapy should only be continued if clinical improvement can be achieved without significant adverse effects such as arrhythmias, cardiac ischemia, and signs and symptoms of peripheral tissue ischemia.

SPECIAL GROUPS

Race: no differences in response
Children: safety and effectiveness have not been established
Elderly: no dosage adjustment is required
Renal impairment: no dosage adjustment is required
Hepatic impairment: no dosage adjustment is required
Pregnancy: category C; should only be used if clearly indicated
Breast-feeding: use with caution; not known if the drug is excreted in human milk

DOSAGE

Usual dose range: 1–20 µg/kg/min
Infusion should be started at 1–5 µg/kg/min and increased by 1–4 µg/kg/min, every 10–30 min until the desired response is achieved. Then, the dose should be titrated based on clinical assessment. Infusion rate up to 50 µg/kg/min has been used. As a general rule, lower infusion rate (≤1 µg/kg/min) should be initiated in patients with occlusive vascular disease.

IN BRIEF

INDICATIONS
Hemodynamic imbalances, after adequate fluid resuscitation.

CONTRAINDICATIONS
Pheochromocytoma
Ventricular fibrillation
Uncorrected tachyarrhythmias
Known sulfite allergy (some products)

DRUG INTERACTIONS
Alpha -adrenergic antagonists
Beta-adrenergic antagonists
Monoamine oxidase (MAO) inhibitors
Phenytoin
General anesthetics: halothane, cyclopropane
Diuretics
Any agents that may affect cardiac/hemodynamic system can potentially interact with dopamine

ADVERSE EFFECTS
CV: tachycardia, ventricular ectopic beats, other dysarrhythmias, hypertension, hypotension, angina, polyuria
CNS: headache
GI: nausea, vomiting
Skin: phlebitis, local infiltration/ tissue necrosis
Other: peripheral tissue cyanosis/ gangrene

PHARMACOKINETICS AND PHARMACODYNAMICS
Duration of action: <10 min
Onset of action: <5 min
Peak effect: 5–10 min
Bioavailability: 100%
Effect of food: not applicable
Metabolism: metabolized extensively in plasma, liver, and kidney by MAO and catechol-O-methyltransferase to inactive metabolites; about 25% is metabolized to norepinephrine in the adrenergic nerve terminals
Excretion: in urine mainly as metabolites
Plasma half-life: 2 min
Protein binding: no data

MONITORING
BP, heart rate, ECG , serum electrolytes, urine output, cardiac index, central venous and pulmonary wedge pressure, peripheral tissue perfusion, weight.

OVERDOSE
Supportive: the duration of action is usually short.

PATIENT INFORMATION
Dopamine is used to support cardiac function, blood circulation, and maintain tissue oxygenation.

AVAILABILITY
Vials—
40 mg/mL, in 5, 10, 20 mL
80 mg/mL, in 5, 20 mL
160 mg/mL, in 5 mL
Syringes—
40 mg/mL, in 5, 10 mL
80 mg/mL, in 10 mL
160 mg/mL, in 5 mL
Pre-Mix—
0.8 mg/mL, in 250, 500 mL
1.6 mg/mL, in 250, 500 mL
3.2 mg/mL, in 250, 500 mL

ISOPROTERENOL (Isoproterenol, Isuprel®)

Isoproterenol, a synthetic sympathomimetic agent, acts directly on beta$_1$- and beta$_2$-adrenergic receptors and has negligible effect on alpha-adrenergic receptors. The major therapeutic effects of isoproterenol are bronchodilation, cardiac stimulation and peripheral vasodilation. Isoproterenol also inhibits antigen-induced release of histamine and the slow reacting substance of anaphylaxis.

SPECIAL GROUPS

Race: no differences in response

Children: limited data; dosing based on weight

Elderly: use with caution; no dosage adjustment is required

Renal impairment: use with caution; no dosage adjustment is required

Hepatic impairment: use with caution; dosage adjustment is probably not required

Pregnancy: category C; should only be used if clearly indicated

Breast-feeding: use with caution; not known if the drug is excreted in human milk

DOSAGE

Cardiac arrhythmias (Bradycardia/AV block):

IV—0.02–0.06 mg (1–3 mL of a 1:50,000 dilution); subsequent doses of 0.01–0.2 mg (0.5–10 mL of a 1:50,000 dilution) may be given based on response

IV infusion—The initial rate is 5 µg/min (ie, 2.5 mL/min of a 1:500,000 dilution), and the rate is adjusted based on response (Usual dose range: 2–20 µg/min).

IM/SC—0.2 mg (1 mL of a 1:5,000 dilution); subsequent doses of 0.02–1 mg (0.1–5 mL of a 1:5,000 dilution) may be given based on response

Intracardiac—0.02 mg (0.1 mL of a 1:5,000 dilution)

Shock: Continuous IV infusion (in 1:500,000 dilution, or 2 µg/mL) is initiated at 0.5–5 µg/min and adjusted based on patient's response.

Diagnostic aid: 4 µg/min is administered in the diagnosis of the etiology of mitral valve regurgitation

1–3 µg/min is administered in the diagnosis of coronary artery disease

IN BRIEF

INDICATIONS
Low cardiac output in hypovolemic and septic shock
Bradycardia in cardiopulmonary resuscitation
Heart block and Adams-Stokes attacks
Diagnostic aid for mitral valve regurgitation and coronary artery disease (not FDA-approved)
Bronchospasm

CONTRAINDICATIONS
Known hypersensitivity to isoproterenol or sulfites
History of cardiac arrhythmias
Angina pectoris
Tachycardia and AV block associated with cardiac glycosides intoxication

DRUG INTERACTIONS
Concurrent beta-adrenergic blocking agents
General anesthetics (halogenated hydrocarbons or cyclopropane)
Digitalis
Theophylline derivatives
Other sympathomimetic agents
Ergot alkaloids
Thyroid hormones

ADVERSE EFFECTS
CV: palpitation, tachycardia, arrhythmias, angina, hypertension/hypotension
CNS: headache, dizziness, nervousness, insomnia, tremor, weakness
GI: nausea, vomiting
Skin: flushing, sweating

PHARMACOKINETICS AND PHARMACODYNAMICS
Duration of action: (IV) a few min; (IM/SQ) 2 h
Onset of action: rapid
Peak effect: 15–30 min for bronchodilation
Bioavailability: variable, metabolized in GI mucosa
Effect of food: not known
Metabolism: metabolized in liver, lungs, GI mucosa and other tissue
Clearance: excreted renally (after IV, 40%–50% as unchanged, the rest as metabolites)
Plasma half-life: not known
Protein binding: not known

MONITORING
BP, heart rate, ECG, respiration, urine output, serum electrolytes, and other appropriate monitoring for adequate tissue perfusion (such as blood lactic acid, pH, pO$_2$, and pCO$_2$ levels, and oxygen saturation)

OVERDOSE
Supportive: a beta-adrenergic blocking agent may be used to treat tachycardia if indicated.

PATIENT INFORMATION
Isoproterenol is used to stimulate the heart and maintain cardiac function (or to relieve bronchospasm).

AVAILABILITY
Ampules/Vials—0.2 mg/mL (1:5,000) in 1, 5, 10 mL
Syringes—0.02 mg/mL (1:50,000) in 10 mL
Also available as:
Metered-dose Inhalers—80, 131 mg/metered spray
Solutions for Nebulization—0.5%, 1%
Oral combination preparations for asthma

EPINEPHRINE (Epinephrine, Various Sources)

Epinephrine, a sympathomimetic agent, acts directly on alpha- and beta-adrenergic receptors. At usual doses, it acts predominantly on the beta-receptors of the heart, vasculature, and smooth muscle. At higher doses, alpha-adrenergic stimulation predominates. After rapid intravenous injection, such as in cardiopulmonary resuscitation, epinephrine produces a rapid rise in BP, and increases in heart rate and contractility while it constricts the arterioles in peripheral and splanchnic circulations. These result in improved myocardial and cerebral blood flow during resuscitation. Epinephrine relaxes bronchial smooth muscle by beta$_1$-adrenergic stimulation and constricts bronchial arterioles by alpha -adrenergic stimulation. It has been used in patients with airway obstruction to relieve bronchospasm, congestion and edema. Epinephrine also inhibits histamine release and antagonizes its effect on the end organs. It is useful as an adjunct in the management of anaphylaxis to reverse constriction or obstruction of the airway, vasodilation, and edema associated with mediator release.

SPECIAL GROUPS

Race: no differences in response
Children: dosage should be adjusted based on weight
Elderly: use with caution; no dosage adjustment is required
Renal impairment: use with caution; dosage adjustment is probably not required
Hepatic impairment: use with caution; dosage adjustment is probably not required
Pregnancy: category C; should only be used if clearly indicated
Breast-feeding: use with caution; excreted in human milk

DOSAGE

Cardiac arrest, ventricular fibrillation and pulseless ventricular tachycardia, pulseless electrical activity, or asystole in advanced cardiac life support (ACLS):
Intravenous (IV)—The usual dose is 0.5–1 mg (usually as 5–10 mL of a 1:10,000 injection) administered by IV push. This dose may be repeated every 3–5 minutes if needed.
Other alternative regimens may be considered especially in patients who have failed above regimen:
Epinephrine—3–5 mg IV push every 3–5 minutes
Epinephrine—1 mg, 3 mg and 5 mg IV push, 3 minutes apart
Epinephrine—0.1 mg/kg IV push, every 3–5 min
Or, initial IV administration may be followed by continuous infusion at a rate of 1–4 µg/min.
Intracardiac (into left ventricular chamber) —The usual dose is 0.5–1 mg (usually as 1–10 mL of a 1:10,000 injection). This dose may be repeated every 3–5 minutes if needed.
Endotracheal—1–3 mg diluted in 10 ml of solution before instillation
Symptomatic bradycardia: The usual initial dose is 1 µg/min (1 mg in 500 mL solution) by continuous infusion. The rate is titrated based on clinical response and usually ranges from 2–10 µg/min.

IN BRIEF (Cardiovascular use mainly)

INDICATIONS
Cardiopulmonary resuscitation/cardiac arrest
Syncope and/or bradycardia resulting from AV block

CONTRAINDICATIONS
Known hypersensitivity to sulfites (some products)
Shock other than anaphylactic shock
Dilated cardiomyopathy and coronary insufficiency
Cerebral arteriosclerosis or organic brain damage
General anesthesia with halogenated hydrocarbons or cyclopropane
Narrow-angle glaucoma
Local use in fingers, toes, ears, nose, or genitalia in combination with local anesthetics

DRUG INTERACTIONS
Concurrent alpha- and beta-adrenergic blocking agents
Ergot alkaloids
Diuretics
General anesthetics (halogenated hydrocarbons or cyclopropane)
Digitalis
Phenothiazines
Tricyclic antidepressants
Some antihistamines (especially diphenhydramine, dexchlorpheniramine, tripelennamine)
Guanethidine
Thyroid hormones
Other sympathomimetic agents

ADVERSE EFFECTS
CV: hypertension, palpitation, tachycardia, arrhythmias, angina, MI, hypotension (rare)
CNS: headache, dizziness, weakness, syncope, stroke, anxiety, fear, nervousness, tremor, insomnia, disorientation, assaultive behavior, hallucination, psychosis, memory impairment, exacerbation of Parkinsonian syndrome
Other: metabolic acidosis, hyperglycemia, ↓ urine output, hepatic or renal ischemia/ failure, tissue ischemia, gangrene, or necrosis

PHARMACOKINETICS AND PHARMACODYNAMICS
Duration of action: short, but may persist for a few hours after subcutaneous administration
Onset of action: rapid, within minutes
Peak effect: not known
Bioavailability: (IV) 100%; not known for other routes
Effect of food: not applicable
Metabolism: metabolized in sympathetic nerve endings, liver, and peripheral tissues by catechol-O-methyl-transferase and monoamine oxidase
Clearance: mainly excreted in urine as metabolites
Plasma half-life: not known
Protein binding: not known

MONITORING
BP, heart rate, ECG, mental status, urine output, serum electrolytes, and other appropriate monitoring for adequate tissue perfusion (such as blood lactic acid, pH, pO$_2$, and pCO$_2$ levels, and oxygen saturation).

OVERDOSE
Supportive: an alpha-adrenergic antagonist such as phentolamine may be used for severe hypertension (may be followed by hypotension, which may be treated with a different vasopressor), and a beta-adrenergic antagonist may be used for arrhythmias.

PATIENT INFORMATION
(apply to non-cardiovascular indications only)
Use the medication as directed (for anaphylactic reaction or bronchospasm). If the symptoms persist or get worse, see a physician immediately.

AVAILABILITY
Syringes—1 mg/mL (1:1,000) in 0.3 mL, 1 mL, 2 mL; 0.5 mg/mL (1:2,000) in 0.3 mL; 0.1 mg/mL (1:10,000) in 10 mL
Ampules—5 mg/mL (1:200) in 0.3 mL, suspension; 1 mg/mL (1:1,000) in 1 mL
Vials—5 mg/mL (1:200) in 5 mL, suspension; 1 mg/mL (1:1,000) in 30 mL
Also available as:
Metered-dose Inhalers— 160 and 220 µg/spray
Solutions for Nebulization—1%, 2.25%
Ophthalmic preparations
In various combinations with a local anesthetic agent

The information here is provided as guidance only. Prescribers should always consult the manufacturer's current prescribing information.

203

METARAMINOL (Aramine®)

Metaraminol, a sympathomimetic amine, has similar effects to norepinephrine, but it has a longer duration of action. Metaraminol acts directly on alpha- and beta$_1$-adrenergic receptors. It also acts indirectly by increasing the release of norepinephrine from the storage sites. The major therapeutic effects of metaraminol are vasoconstriction and cardiac stimulation. Tachyphylaxis may occur after prolonged use of metaraminol secondary to depletion of norepinephrine stores in sympathetic nerve endings. Metaraminol may also act as a weak or false neurotransmitter. It may replace norepinephrine in sympathetic nerve endings which may result in vasodilation and hypotension on rare occasions.

SPECIAL GROUPS

Race: no differences in response
Children: safety and effectiveness have not been established
Elderly: no dosage adjustment is required
Renal impairment: use with caution; starting with low dose
Hepatic impairment: use with caution; dosage adjustment is probably not required
Pregnancy: category C; should only be used if clearly indicated
Breast-feeding: use with caution; not known if the drug is excreted in human milk

DOSAGE

Prevention of hypotension:
Usual dose: 2–10 mg IM*. The lowest effective dose should be used for the shortest possible time. At least 10 min should elapse before additional doses are administered.

Severe hypotension or shock:
Usual dose: 0.5–5 mg (direct IV). Direct IV administration may be followed by a continuous infusion (15–200 mg in 500 mL of compatible diluent) if indicated. The rate of infusion should be adjusted to maintain the desired blood pressure.

*Note—Subcutaneous administration of metaraminol has been used. Subcutaneous administration is not recommended because of increased risk of tissue necrosis and abscess formation.

IN BRIEF

INDICATIONS
Hypotension associated with spinal anesthesia (Both prevention and treatment)
Hypotension and shock associated with hemorrhage, reactions to medications, surgical complications, and brain damage due to trauma or tumor

CONTRAINDICATIONS
Known hypersensitivity to sulfites
Suspected peripheral or mesenteric vascular thrombosis
Concurrent halothane or cyclopropane anesthesia

DRUG INTERACTIONS
Concurrent alpha- and beta-adrenergic blocking agents
Other hypotensive agents
General anesthetics (halothane or cyclopropane)
Digitalis
MAO inhibitors
Tricyclic antidepressants
Other sympathomimetic agents

ADVERSE EFFECTS
CV: hypertension, palpitation, tachycardia, bradycardia, arrhythmias, angina, myocardial infarction, hypotension (rare)
CNS: headache, stroke
Skin: local tissue irritation, abscess, necrosis, and sloughing
Other: metabolic acidosis, ↓ urine output, hepatic or renal ischemia/ failure

PHARMACOKINETICS AND PHARMACODYNAMICS
Duration of action: 20–90 min (depends on routes)
Onset of action: (IV) 1–2 min; (IM) <10 min
Peak effect: rapid, < 10 min
Bioavailability: (IV) 100%
Effect of food: not applicable
Metabolism: not clear; partially hepatic
Clearance: excreted in urine and stools mainly as metabolites
Plasma half-life: not known
Protein binding: not known

MONITORING
BP, heart rate, ECG, urine output, serum electrolytes, and other appropriate monitoring for adequate tissue perfusion (such as blood lactic acid, pH, pO$_2$, and pCO$_2$ levels, and oxygen saturation).

OVERDOSE
Supportive: a sympatholytic agent, such as phentolamine may be used for severe hypertension and an appropriate antiarrhythmic agent may be used for symptomatic episodes.

PATIENT INFORMATION
Metaraminol is used to maintain BP or prevent hypotension.

AVAILABILITY
Vials—10 mg/mL in 10 mL (1%)

METHOXAMINE (Vasoxyl®)

Methoxamine, a synthetic sympathomimetic amine, has similar pharmacologic activity to phenylephrine. It acts primarily on alpha-adrenergic receptors and has negligible effect on $beta_1$- or $beta_2$-adrenergic receptors. Methoxamine administration produces a rapid and sustained rise in BP. It is used to maintain BP during anesthesia. Methoxamine is less arrhythmogenic and may be used safely with cyclopropane or halogenated hydrocarbons during anesthesia. Similar to phenylephrine, methoxamine can cause reflex bradycardia and ventricular ectopic beats. Bradycardia may be prevented by administration of atropine. Methoxamine may be useful in terminating paroxysmal atrial or nodal tachycardia, especially in patients with profound hypotension.

SPECIAL GROUPS

Race: no differences in response

Children: safety and effectiveness have not been established

Elderly: use with cautions; no dosage adjustment is required

Renal impairment: use with caution; dosage adjustment is probably not required

Hepatic impairment: use with caution; dosage adjustment is probably not required

Pregnancy: category C; should only be used if clearly indicated

Breast-feeding: use with caution; not known if the drug is excreted in human milk

DOSAGE

Hypotension: Moderate—5–10 mg IM; Severe—3–5 mg IV slowly
This dose may be repeated after 15 min, or supplemented by IM injection of 10–15 mg to provide more prolonged effect.

Prevention of hypotension during anesthesia—The usual dose is 10–15 mg given IM shortly before or with spinal anesthesia (up to 20 mg may be required at high levels of anesthesia).

Supraventricular tachycardia: 10 mg given IV over 3–5 min, or 10–20 mg given IM; systolic BP should not be raised above 160 mmHg

IN BRIEF

INDICATIONS
Hypotension associated with anesthesia
(Both prevention and treatment)
Paroxysmal supraventricular tachycardia associated with hypotension or shock

CONTRAINDICATIONS
Severe hypertension
Known hypersensitivity to methoxamine or sulfites

DRUG INTERACTIONS
Alpha-adrenergic blocking agents and agents with alpha-adrenergic blocking activity (phenothiazines)
Other sympathomimetic agents
MAO inhibitors
Tricyclic antidepressants
Ergot alkaloids
Thyroid hormones
Diuretics
Atropine

ADVERSE EFFECTS
CV: hypertension, reflex bradycardia, heart failure, chest pain, arrhythmias, myocardial infarction
CNS: headache, dizziness, anxiety, nervousness, restlessness, stroke
GI: nausea, vomiting
Skin: cold, piloerection
Other: paresthesia, metabolic acidosis, ↓ urine output, hepatic or renal ischemia/ failure

PHARMACOKINETICS AND PHARMACODYNAMICS
Duration of action: (IV) 10-15 min; (IM) 60–90 min
Onset of action: rapid
Peak effect: (IV) 0.5–2 min; (IM) 15–20 min
Bioavailability: (IV) 100%
Effect of food: not applicable
Metabolism: not known
Clearance: not known
Plasma half-life: not known
Protein binding: not known

MONITORING
BP, heart rate, ECG, mental status, urine output, serum electrolytes, and other appropriate monitoring for adequate tissue perfusion (such as blood lactic acid, pH, pO_2, and pCO_2 levels, and oxygen saturation).

OVERDOSE
Supportive: an alpha-adrenergic antagonist such as phentolamine may be used for severe hypertension, and atropine may be used for severe bradycardia.

PATIENT INFORMATION
Methoxamine is used to maintain BP (or to treat abnormal cardiac rhythm).

AVAILABILITY
Ampules—20 mg/mL, 1 mL

The information here is provided as guidance only. Prescribers should always consult the manufacturer's current prescribing information.

205

VASOPRESSOR WITH SYMPATHOMIMETIC ACTIVITY

MIDODRINE HYDROCHLORIDE (Proamatine®)

Midodrine HCl, an inactive prodrug, is converted to desglymidodrine, a peripheral alpha-agonist, by enzymatic hydrolysis in the body. Desglymidodrine causes vasoconstriction of both arteries and veins. In patients with severe orthostatic hypotension, it can increase both supine and standing BP, and help relieve disabling symptoms. Desglymidodrine also acts on alpha-receptors located within the urinary bladder, which accounts for the dysuria problems observed in certain patient groups. Support stockings, used alone or in combination with fludrocortisone, and/or beta-blockers remain the preferred first-line treatment for patients with orthostatic hypotension. Patient medication profile should also be evaluated to identify and possibly remove any offending agents that may exacerbate the problem. Midodrine should be reserved in patients who remain symptomatic despite standard clinical care. Midodrine may also have a role in the management of hypotension secondary to hemodialysis, anesthesia, or spinal cord lesions, neurocardiogenic syncope, and stress-induced urinary incontinence in females.

SPECIAL GROUPS

Race: no differences in response

Children: safety and effectiveness have not been established

Elderly: no dosage adjustment is required

Renal impairment: use with caution; starting with 2.5 mg doses

Hepatic impairment: use with caution; dosage adjustment is probably not required

Pregnancy: category C; should only be used if clearly indicated

Breast-feeding: use with caution; not known if the drug is excreted in human milk

DOSAGE

10 mg orally three times daily at approximately 3–4 h intervals with first dose administered shortly before or upon arising in the morning; no dose should be administered after dinner or within 3–4 h before bedtime; the dose should be skipped if the patient remains bed-bound

IN BRIEF

INDICATIONS
Symptomatic orthostatic hypotension unresponsive to non-pharmacologic treatment.

CONTRAINDICATIONS
Severe organic heart disease
Urinary retention
Pheochromocytoma
Thyrotoxicosis
Acute renal disease
Supine hypertension, systolic > 180 mmHg
Known hypersensitivity to midodrine

DRUG INTERACTIONS
Cardiac glycosides
Mineralocorticoids
Alpha-adrenergic blocking agents (prazosin, terazosin, etc.)
Vasopressors (phenylephrine, pseudoephedrine, ephedrine, phenylpropanolamine, dihydroergotamine)

ADVERSE EFFECTS
CV: supine and sitting hypertension, bradycardia
GU: urinary retention, frequency and urgency
Skin: pruritus, piloerection, rash
Other: paresthesia, chills

PHARMACOKINETICS AND PHARMACODYNAMICS
Duration of action: 2–6 h
Onset of action: 45–90 min
Peak effect: 1–2 h
Bioavailability: 93%
Effect of food: no effect
Metabolism: metabolized in various tissue and liver to desglymidodrine (active)
Excretion: renal; mainly as desglymidodrine
Plasma half-life: 25 min (midodrine); 3–4 h (desglymidodrine)
Protein binding: insignificant

MONITORING
Supine and standing BP.

OVERDOSE
Supportive: limited data indicate phentolamine may be used to reverse severe hypertension.

PATIENT INFORMATION
To avoid hypertension occurring during sleep, midodrine should not be taken after dinner or within 3–4 h before bedtime. Certain cold remedies and weight control medications may cause hypertension and should be used cautiously with midodrine.

AVAILABILITY
Tablets—2.5 mg, 5 mg

NOREPINEPHRINE (Levophed®)

Norepinephrine, an endogenous catecholamine, acts directly on alpha- and beta$_1$-adrenergic receptors. It does not have beta$_2$-adrenergic activity. The major therapeutic effects of norepinephrine are vasoconstriction and cardiac stimulation. It constricts both arterial and venous blood vessels resulting in an increase in systolic and diastolic BP. This effect may redirect blood flow from peripheral (such as skin and skeletal muscle) and splanchnic circulations to vital organs (such as brain and myocardium). Renal blood flow and urine output may be reduced initially from constriction of renal blood vessels. However, if adequate intravascular volume is maintained, renal perfusion and urine output will increase as the systemic BP is normalized and cardiac output is increased through the positive inotropic effect on the myocardium. Direct coronary artery constriction is usually overcome by increased systemic BP and enhanced cardiac output.

Norepinephrine may be proarrhythmic, especially at higher doses in patients with cardiovascular diseases, concurrent proarrhythmic medications, or metabolic and electrolyte imbalances. Norepinephrine also causes pulmonary vessel constriction resulting in an increase in pulmonary arterial pressure. Norepinephrine is administered IV to provide hemodynamic support via vasoconstriction and cardiac stimulation in patients with profound hypotension after adequate intravascular volume replacement. It has also been used in combination with some local anesthetics to enhance and prolong the duration of local anesthesia.

SPECIAL GROUPS

Race: no differences in response

Children: safety and effectiveness have not been established

Elderly: use with caution; no dosage adjustment is required

Renal impairment: use with caution; no dosage adjustment is required

Hepatic impairment: use with caution; no dosage adjustment is required

Pregnancy: category C; should only be used if clearly indicated

Breast-feeding: use with caution; not known if the drug is excreted in human milk

DOSAGE

Norepinephrine is administered by continuous IV infusion (ie, 4–8 mg in 500–1000 mL solution). The dose should be initiated at a rate of 0.5–1 µg/min and titrated to maintain a desired BP response.

IN BRIEF

INDICATIONS
Hypotensive state
Cardiac arrest (as an adjunct for severe hypotension)

CONTRAINDICATIONS
Known hypersensitivity to sulfites
General anesthesia (halogenated hydrocarbons or cyclopropane)
Suspected peripheral or mesenteric vascular thrombosis
Local use in fingers, toes, ears, nose, or genitalia in combination with local anesthetics

DRUG INTERACTIONS
Concurrent alpha-adrenergic blocking agents
Concurrent beta-adrenergic blocking agents
Diuretics
General anesthetics (halogenated hydrocarbons or cyclopropane)
Digitalis
Atropine
Tricyclic antidepressants
Some antihistamines (especially diphenhydramine, dexchlorpheniramine, tripelennamine)
Thyroid hormones
Guanethidine
Methyldopa
Ergot alkaloids
MAO inhibitors
Other sympathomimetic agents

ADVERSE EFFECTS
CV: hypertension, palpitation, tachycardia, bradycardia, arrhythmias, angina, MI, hypotension (rare)
CNS: headache, dizziness, weakness, syncope, stroke, anxiety, restlessness, tremor, insomnia
Skin: local tissue irritation, extravasation, necrosis, and sloughing
Other: metabolic acidosis, hyperglycemia, ↓ urine output, hepatic or renal ischemia or failure, tissue ischemia, gangrene, or necrosis

PHARMACOKINETICS AND PHARMACODYNAMICS
Duration of action: 1–2 min
Onset of action: rapid
Peak effect: rapid
Bioavailability: (IV) 100%; not absorbed from GI tract
Effect of food: not applicable
Metabolism: metabolized in sympathetic nerve endings, liver, and peripheral tissues by catechol-O-methyltransferase and monoamine oxidase
Clearance: mainly excreted in urine as metabolites
Plasma half-life: not known
Protein binding: not known

MONITORING
BP, heart rate, ECG, mental status, urine output, serum electrolytes, and other appropriate monitoring for adequate tissue perfusion (such as blood lactic acid, pH, pO$_2$, and pCO$_2$ levels, and oxygen saturation).

OVERDOSE
Supportive: the effect should subside within a few minutes, and a beta-adrenergic antagonist such as propranolol may be used for arrhythmias if indicated.

PATIENT INFORMATION
Norepinephrine is used to maintain BP and prevent severe consequences associated with profound hypotension.

AVAILABILITY
Ampules—1 mg/mL, 4 mL

PHENYLEPHRINE

(Phenylephrine, Neo-Synephrine®)

Phenylephrine, a sympathomimetic amine, acts predominantly on postsynaptic α-adrenergic receptors with little effect on the beta$_1$-adrenergic receptors of the heart. It has no effect on the beta$_2$-adrenergic receptors of the bronchi or peripheral blood vessels. Phenylephrine also has an indirect effect by releasing norepinephrine from its storage sites. The major effect of phenylephrine is vasoconstriction. Increased arterial BP may cause an increase in vagal activity and bradycardia. This effect can be blocked by atropine. Phenylephrine is used as an adjunct to provide hemodynamic support in patients with profound hypotension after adequate intravascular volume replacement. Phenylephrine may be used to terminate paroxysmal supraventricular tachycardia, especially in patients with concurrent hypotension or shock. Phenylephrine has also been used in spinal anesthesia to localize and prolong anesthetic activity, as a topical nasal decongestant, and in combination with an inhaled bronchodilator to prolong the effect of bronchodilation while alleviating airway edema and congestion.

SPECIAL GROUPS

Race: no differences in response
Children: dosage should be adjusted based on weight
Elderly: use with caution; no dosage adjustment is required
Renal impairment: use with caution; dosage adjustment is probably not required
Hepatic impairment: use with caution; dosage adjustment is probably not required
Pregnancy: category C; should only be used if clearly indicated
Breast-feeding: probably safe due to limited absorption in the gastrointestinal tract; not known if the drug is excreted in human milk

DOSAGE

Mild or moderate hypotension: The usual dose is 2–5 mg (range: 1–10 mg) administered subcutaneously (SQ) or IM, or 0.2 mg (range: 0.1–0.5 mg) administered IV. The dose may be repeated after 10–15 min if indicated.

Severe hypotension: Continuous IV infusion (ie, 10–20 mg in 500 ml solution) at 100–180 µg/min should be initiated and titrated based on the response. Once the BP is stablized, a maintenance rate of 40–60 µg/min is usually sufficient.

Hypotension associated with spinal anesthesia:
Prophylaxis—2–3 mg administered IM or SQ 3–4 min before administration of the anesthetic agent
Treatment—0.2 mg administered IV; any subsequent doses should be given in increments of 0.1–0.2 mg if indicated and should never exceed 0.5 mg in a single dose

Paroxysmal supraventricular tachycardia: up to 0.5 mg may be given IV over 20–30 sec; subsequent doses may be given in increments of 0.1–0.2 mg if indicated and should never exceed 1 mg in a single dose

IN BRIEF

INDICATIONS
Hypotensive state associated with shock, drug use, or hypersensitivity reactions
Paroxysmal supraventricular tachycardia associated with hypotension or shock
Maintenance of adequate BP during spinal and inhalation anesthesia

CONTRAINDICATIONS
Known hypersensitivity to phenylephrine or sulfites
Severe coronary artery or cardiovascular disease
Pre-existing severe hypertension
Ventricular tachycardia
Hyperthyroidism
Suspected peripheral or mesenteric vascular thrombosis
Local use in fingers, toes, ears, nose, or genitalia in combination with local anesthetics

DRUG INTERACTIONS
Concurrent alpha-adrenergic blocking agents and agents with alpha-adrenergic blocking activity (phenothiazines)
Other sympathomimetic agents
MAO inhibitors
Tricyclic antidepressants
Guanethidine
Thyroid hormones
Diuretics
Atropine
Digitalis
General anesthetics (halogenated hydrocarbons or cyclopropane)

ADVERSE EFFECTS
CV: hypertension, reflex bradycardia, arrhythmias, chest pain, heart failure
CNS: headache, restlessness, excitability, weakness, dizziness, tremor, stroke
Skin: blanching, piloerection, extravasation, necrosis, and sloughing
Other: paresthesia, metabolic acidosis, ↓ urine output, hepatic or renal ischemia or failure

PHARMACOKINETICS AND PHARMACODYNAMICS
Duration of action: (IV) 15-20 min; (IM/SQ) 1–2 hrs
Onset of action: immediate (IV); 10-15 min (IM/SQ)
Peak effect:
Bioavailability: (IV) 100%; (po) 38%
Effect of food: not known
Metabolism: metabolized in liver and intestine by catechol-O-methyltransferase
Clearance: renally excreted, mainly as metabolites
Plasma half-life: 2–3 h
Protein binding: not known

MONITORING
BP, heart rate, ECG, mental status, urine output, serum electrolytes, and other appropriate monitoring for adequate tissue perfusion (such as blood lactic acid, pH, pO$_2$, and pCO$_2$ levels, and oxygen saturation).

OVERDOSE
Supportive: an alpha-adrenergic antagonist, such as phentolamine may be used for severe hypertension, and a beta-adrenergic antagonist, such as propranolol, may be used for arrhythmias if indicated.

PATIENT INFORMATION
Phenylephrine is used to maintain BP (or to treat abnormal cardiac rhythm).

AVAILABILITY
Ampules or Syringes—10 mg/mL (1%), 1 mL
Vials—10 mg/mL (1%), 1 mL and 5 mL
Also available (for non-cardiovascular indications) as:
Metered-dose Inhalers—240 µg/spray + isoproterenol 160 µg/spray
Ophthalmic Preparations
Otic Preparations
Or, in combination with antihistamines, analgesics, antitussives, bronchodilators, decongestants, and expectorants for oral administration (remedies for cold and allergy)

Digitalis differs from other inotropic agents in that it has the pedigree of some 200 years use. It is interesting that despite such a long period of time, the effectiveness of long-term digitalis therapy is repeatedly questioned. However, studies that have compared digoxin with other inotropic and vasodilating drugs in heart failure have demonstrated that the efficacy of many of the newer inotropic agents appears no better than that of this well-tried and inexpensive drug.

EFFICACY AND USE

Cardiac glycosides of the digitalis family are effective inotropic agents for most patients with moderate to severe heart failure and sinus rhythm, particularly those with an S_3 gallop. The beneficial effects of digitalis are additive to those of ACE inhibitors, diuretics, and the inotropic agents. Although cardiogenic shock is a recognized indication for digitalis, the established effective-ness of these drugs is limited to cardiogenic shock with atrial fibrillation or flutter and an increased ventricular rate. In other cases, digitalis benefits only the noninfarcted areas of the ventricle and has little effect on cardiac output. When treating acute atrial fibrillation, the standard digitalizing dose should not be exceeded. Its antiarrhythmic activity is advantageous (see chapter on antiarrhythmic agents) when used in combination with other inotropic agents, such as beta-adrenergic stimulants, that enhance AV conduction. In patients with atrial fibrillation, the use of beta-adrenergic agonists may promote ventricular arrhythmia; correction of atrial function with digitalis may promote safer use of these other agents, but not during exercise. Retrospective analyses suggest that the use of digitalis in the setting of cardiac ischemia, such as after MI, may be associated with increased mortality, particularly in patients with ventricular arrhythmias.

Digitalis drugs are also used in the prevention and treatment of recurrent episodes of paroxysmal atrial tachycardia or paroxysmal AV junctional rhythm in conjunction with measures to increase vagal tone.

MODE OF ACTION

It is now generally accepted that the digitalis glycosides act by binding to and inhibiting the cell membrane-bound sodium-potassium ATPase, the enzyme controlling the cellular sodium pump. This inhibition permits sodium to enter the cardiac cell, which is then expelled using a sodium-calcium exchange process. This, in turn, results in a higher level of intracellular calcium and an increased force of myocardial contraction. This increase in intracellular calcium concentration is accompanied by a fall in intracellular pH, further enhancing sodium movement by a sodium-hydrogen exchange, and further enhancing the inotropic response. Cardiac glycosides slow conduction and increase the refractory period (see chapter on anti-arrhythmic agents) in specialized cardiac conducting tissue. Characteristically, the dominant effect is an increase in vagal tone, which manifests itself as a reduced ventricular rate due to slowing of conduction, and increased refractoriness of AV nodal and functional tissues.

INDICATIONS

	Digoxin
Supraventricular arrhythmias	+
CHF	+
Cardiogenic shock	+

+—FDA approved; CHF—congestive heart failure.

DIGOXIN

(Digoxin, Lanoxicaps®, Lanoxin®)

Digoxin is the most commonly used digitalis glycoside. As a group, digitalis glycosides are the only inotropic agents that have been shown to provide some benefits in the management of chronic heart failure. In patients with heart failure, digoxin increases myocardial contractility and cardiac output, which results in a reflex reduction in sympathetic tone, thus slowing down the heart rate and promoting diuresis in patients with fluid overload. Digoxin also decreases conduction velocity through the AV node and prolongs the effective refractory period of the AV node by increasing vagal activity, by a direct effect on the AV node and by a sympatholytic effect. These effects are useful in patients with supraventricular tachycardia, such as atrial fibrillation or atrial flutter, to reduce the conduction reaching the ventricles and thus the rate of ventricular contractions.

Serum digoxin concentrations should be monitored during therapy. Serum electrolyte disturbances, such as hypokalemia, hypomagnesemia, and hypercalcemia, may predispose the patients to digoxin toxicity and should be monitored routinely for chronic therapy. Since digoxin is mainly excreted in the kidney unchanged, it is important to monitor renal function during chronic digoxin therapy. In patients with acute renal failure, depending on the severity, the dose of digoxin should be adjusted or even be held temporarily.

SPECIAL GROUPS

Race: no differences in response
Children: safety and effectiveness have been established; dosage adjustment is recommended based on age, weight, renal function, and serum levels
Elderly: dosage should be adjusted based on renal function, desired effect, and serum levels
Renal impairment: dosage should be adjusted based on renal function, desired effect, and serum levels
Hepatic impairment: use with caution; dosage adjustment is probably not required
Pregnancy: category C; should only be used if clearly indicated
Breast-feeding: use with caution; the amount excreted in human milk is low and should have no pharmacological effect on a nursing infant

IN BRIEF

INDICATIONS
CHF
Atrial fibrillation
Atrial flutter
Paroxysmal atrial tachycardia

CONTRAINDICATIONS
Ventricular fibrillation
Known hypersensitivity to any digitalis glycosides

DRUG INTERACTIONS
Potassium-depleting agents (corticosteroids, dietetics)

Calcium salts	Propofenone
Sympathomimetics	Indomethacin
Quinidine	Beta-blockers
Verapamil	Calcium-channel blockers
Amiodarone	Antacids
Erythromycin	Kaolin-pectin
Clarithromycin	Cholestyramine
Itraconazole	

Agents that may slow down GI transit (anticholinergics, diphenoxylate, propantheline)

ADVERSE EFFECTS
CV: arrhythmias (ventricular premature contraction or tachycardia, AV dissociation, accelerated junctional rhythm, atrial tachycardia, and AV block
GI: anorexia, nausea, vomiting
CNS: visual disturbance, headache, weakness, dizziness, apathy, psychosis
Other: rash, hypersensitivity reaction, gynecomastia

PHARMACOKINETICS AND PHARMACODYNAMICS
Duration of action: 3–4 d or longer
Onset of action: (po) 0.5–2 h; (IV) 5–30 min
Peak effect: (po) 2–6 h; (IV) 1–4 h
Bioavailability: Tablets/ Elixir—60%–85%
Capsules—90%–100%
IV—100%
Effect of food: slows the rate but not the extent of absorption
Metabolism: small amounts are metabolized in liver or by bacteria in GI tract
Excretion: mainly in urine as unchanged drug (50%–70% as unchanged after IV)
Plasma half-life: 1.5–2 d, normal renal function
≥ 4.5 d, anephric patients
Protein binding: 20%–30%

MONITORING
BP, heart rate, ECG, serum electrolytes, renal function, serum digoxin levels*, and pertinent signs and symptoms for response or toxicity.

OVERDOSE
Supportive: Correction of serum electrolyte and acid-base disturbances is essential. Potassium should not be administered in heart block, unless primarily related to supraventricular tachycardia. In advanced heart block, atropine and/or temporary pacing may be used. Ventricular arrhythmias may be treated with lidocaine, procainamide, propranolol, and phenytoin.
Digoxin is not dialyzable. In life-threatening digoxin overdose, digoxin immune Fab (opine) may be used at a dose equimolar to digoxin in the body to reverse the toxicity . Please see the following Appendix for digoxin immune Fab (opine) dosing guidelines.

PATIENT INFORMATION
Digoxin is used to treat heart rhythm problems or heart failure. Many other medications can interact with digoxin. Do not take any new medications, including over-the-counter products, without consulting a physician or a pharmacist. Check pulse rate routinely as directed. Inform the physician if you experience any unusual palpitation, dizziness, gastrointestinal problems or visual disturbances.

DOSAGE

(*see* Note 1)

Rapid digitalization in adult patients who have not received digoxin in previous 2 wk:

8–12 µg/kg in patients with heart failure and normal sinus rhythm (see Note 2)

10–15 µg/kg in patients with atrial fibrillation or flutter for adequate control of ventricular rate (see Note 2)

This loading dose is usually administered IV in three divided doses, with 50% given as the first dose and two additional doses (25% each) given at 4–8 h intervals after assessing clinical response. The loading dose may also be given orally in similar divided doses every 6–8 h.

Slow digitalization or chronic maintenance therapy in adult patients: Usual dose—100–375 µg/d given orally as a single dose This is the preferred regimen in patients with heart failure and the dose should be administered orally whenever possible. Dosage requirement for each individual should be adjusted based on clinical response and renal function. It may take 1–3 wk for a patient to reach steady state serum digoxin concentrations depending on the renal function (see Notes 3 and 4). In patients with severe renal dysfunction, a maintenance dose administered every 2–3 d may be adequate to maintain desired serum digoxin concentrations.

NOTES

1. The bioavailability of digoxin may vary significantly depending on the products and different dosage forms selected. Although the difference in bioavailability may not be clinically significant for an individual patient, it may be necessary to adjust the dose when switching a patient between different formulations or products.
2. Lower loading doses should be used in patients with severe renal impairment.
3. Serum digoxin levels should be monitored and kept in the range of 0.8–2 ng/mL based on clinical assessment. Sampling of blood should be at least 6–8 h after the dose or ideally just before the next dose.
4. The value of obtaining regular serum digoxin levels, especially in patients with stable renal function is unclear. It is probably reasonable to check digoxin levels every 6–12 mo for chronic therapy. More frequent monitoring is recommended if:
   - heart failure worsens or new onset of arrhythmias
   - renal function deteriorates
   - new medication(s) is(are) initiated that may affect digoxin levels
   - digoxin toxicity is suspected based on clinical symptoms

AVAILABILITY

Tablets—0.125, 0.25 mg
Capsules—0.05, 0.1, 0.2 mg
Elixir—0.05 mg/mL
Injection—0.1 mg/mL, 0.25 mg/mL

The information here is provided as guidance only. Prescribers should always consult the manufacturer's current prescribing information.

211

KEY: Each vial of Digibind contains 38 mg of digoxin-specific Fab fragments, which can bind approximately 0.5 mg of digoxin.

1. For *acute* overdose with *known* amount ingested: Total body load=amount of digoxin liquid or capsules ingested in mg, or 0.8 x (amount of digoxin tablets ingested in mg)
   Dose (# of vials*) = Total body load (mg) ÷ 0.5 (mg/vial)

2. For *acute* overdose with known steady-state serum digoxin concentrations:
   Dose (# of vials*) = digoxin level (ng/mL) x weight (kg) ÷ 100

3. For *acute* overdose with *unknown* amount ingested, 20 vials of digoxin immune Fab is recommended.

4. For *life-threatening* toxicity during *chronic* therapy, six vials of digoxin immune Fab are recommended.

*Dose of digoxin immune Fab (opine) should be rounded up to the next whole vial in calculations. The total dose should be administered IV through a 0.22 micron membrane filter over 30 min. If cardiac arrest is imminent, the dose may be given as an IV bolus.

SELECTED BIBLIOGRAPHY

Alousi AA, Johnson DC: Pharmacology of the bipyridines: amrinone and milrinone. *Circulation* 1986; 70 (Suppl II): II–110–23.

Anversa P, Sonnenblick EH: Ischemic cardiomyopathy: pathophysiological mechanisms. Prog *Cardiovasc Dis* 1990; 33: 49–70.

Braunwald E, Ross J Jr., Sonnenblick EH: Mechanisms of Contraction of the Normal and Failing Heart, 2nd ed. Boston: Little, Brown & Co., 1976.

Captopril-Digoxin Multicenter Research Group: Comparative effects of therapy with captopril and digoxin in patients with mild to moderate heart failure. *JAMA* 1988; 259: 539–44.

Cavusoglu E, Frishman WH, Klapholz M: Vesnarinone: A new inotropic agent for treating congestive heart failure. *J Cardiac Fail* 1995; 1: 249–57.

Cheng W, Li B, Kajstura J, *et al.*: Stretch-induced programmed myocyte cell death. *J Clin Invest* 1995; 96: 2247–59.

Cohn JN, Goldstein SO, Greenberg BH, *et al.*: A dose-dependent increase in mortality with vesnarinone among patients with severe heart failure. *N Engl J Med* 1998, 339:1810–1816.

Dei Cas L, Metrar M, Visioli O: Clinical pharmacology of inolators. *J Cardiovasc Pharmacol* 1989; 14(8): S60–71.

Garofalo F, Lalanne GM, Nanni G: Midodrine for female incontinence: a preliminary report. *Clin Ther* 1986; 9: 44–46.

Goldberg LI: The role of dopamine receptors in the treatment of congestive heart failure. *J Cardiovasc Pharmacol* 1989; 14(5): S19–27.

Goldberg LI, Rajfer SI: Dopamine receptors: Applications in clinical cardiology. *Circulation* 1985; 72: 245–48.

Grose R, Strain J, Greenberg M, LeJemtel TH: Systemic and coronary effects of intravenous milrinone and dobutamine in congestive heart failure. *J Am Coll Cardiol* 1986; 7:1107–13.

Grossman W: Diastolic dysfunction in congestive heart failure. *New Engl J Med* 1991; 325: 1557–64.

Haikala H, Linden I: Mechanisms of action of calcium-sensitizing drugs. *J Cardiovasc Pharm* 1995; 26 (Suppl. 1): S10–19.

Insel PA: Adrenergic receptors - evolving concepts and clinical implications. *N Engl J Med* 1996; 334: 580–85.

Jakovic J, Gilden JL, Hiner BC, *et al.*: Neurogenic orthostatic hypotension: a double-blind, placebo-controlled study with midodrine. *Am J Med* 1993; 95: 38–48.

Kelley RA, Smith TW: Recognition and treatment of digitalis toxicity. *Am J Cardiol* 1992; 69: 108G–119G.

LeJemtel TH, Sonnenblick EH, Frishman WH: Diagnosis and management of heart failure. In Alexander RW, Schlant RC, Fuster V, (eds): *Hurst's the Handbook*, 9th ed. New York: McGraw Hill, 1998: 745–81.

Lewis RP: Clinical use of serum digoxin concentrations. *Am J Cardiol* 1992; 69: 97G–107G.

Lilleberg J, Sundberg S, Nieminen MS: Dose-range study of a new calcium sensitizer, levosimendan, in patients with left ventricular dysfunction. *J Cardiovasc Pharmacol* 1995; 26 (Suppl 1): S63–69.

Low PA, Gilden JL, Freeman R, *et al.*: Efficacy of midodrine vs placebo in neurogenic orthostatic hypotension: a randomized, double-blind multicenter study. Midodrine Study Group. *JAMA* 1997; 227: 1046–1051.

McTavish D, Goa KL: Midodrine: a review of its pharmacological properties and therapeutic use in orthostatic hypotension and secondary hypotensive disorders. *Drugs* 1989; 38: 757–777.

Majerus TC, Dasta JF, Bauman JL, *et al*: Dobutamine: ten years later. *Pharmacotherapy* 1989; 9: 245–59.

Newton GE, Tong JH, Schofield AM, *et al*: Digoxin reduces cardiac sympathetic activity in severe congestive heart failure. *J Am Coll Cardiol* 1996; 28: 155–61.

Packer M: Do positive inotropic agents adversely affect the survival of patients with chronic congestive heart failure? II. Protagonist's viewpoint. *J Am Coll Cardiol* 1988; 12:562–66.

Packer M, Carver JR, Rodeheffer RJ, *et al*: Effect of oral milrinone on mortality in severe chronic heart failure. *N Engl J Med* 1991; 325: 1468–75.

Packer M, Gheorghiade M, Young JB, *et al*: Withdrawal of digoxin from patients with chronic heart failure treated with angiotensin-converting-enzyme inhibitors. *N Engl J Med* 1993; 329: 1–7.

Rector TW, Cohn JN: Assessment of patient outcome with the Minnesota Living with Heart Failure questionnaire: reliability and validity during a randomized, double-blind, placebo-controlled trial of pimobendan. *Am Heart J* 1992; 124: 1017–25.

Ruffolo RR Jr.: Review: The pharmacology of dobutamine. *Am J Med Sci* 1987; 294: 244–48.

Scholz H: Inotropic drugs and their mechanisms of action. *J Am Coll Cardiol* 1984; 4: 389–97.

Smith TW: Digitalis: mechanisms of action and clinical use. *N Engl J Med* 1988; 31: 358–65.

Sonnenblick EH, Frishman WH, LeJemtel TH: Dobutamine: A new synthetic cardioactive sympathetic amine. *N Engl J Med* 1979; 300: 17–22.

Sonnenblick EH, LeJemtel TH: Heart Failure: Its progression and its therapy. *Hosp Pract* 1993; 28: 121–30.

Sonnenblick EH, LeJemtel TH, Frishman WH: Digitalis preparations and other inotropic agents. In Frishman WH, Sonnenblick EH (eds): *Cardiovascular Pharmacotherapeutics*. New York: McGraw Hill, 1997: 237–51.

Tauke J, Goldstein S, Gheorghiade M: Digoxin for chronic heart failure: A review of the randomized controlled trials with special attention to the PROVED and RADIANCE Trials. Prog *Cardiovasc Dis* 1994; 37: 49–58.

The Digitalis Investigation Group: The effect of digoxin on mortality and morbidity in patients with heart failure. *N Engl J Med* 1997; 336: 525–33.

Tisdale JE, Patel R, Webb CR, *et al*: Electrophysiologic and proarrhythmic effects of intravenous inotropic agents. *Prog Cardiovasc Dis* 1995; 38: 167–80.

Uretsky BF, Young JB, Shahidi FE, *et al*.: Randomized study assessing the effect of digoxin withdrawal in patients with mild to moderate chronic congestive heart failure: Results of the PROVED Trial. *J Am Coll Cardiol* 1995; 22: 955–62.

Wright RA, Kaufmann HC, Perera R, *et al*.: A double-blind, dose-response study of midodrine in neurogenic orthostatic hypotension. *Neurology* 1998; 51: 120–124.

The links between coronary artery disease (CAD), diet, and hyperlipidemia (excess serum cholesterol and/or triglycerides) are well established, and the biological factors contributing to hyperlipidemia are now well understood. The hyperlipoproteinemias are defined and treated broadly along the lines of the Fredrickson-Levy classification (Table 11-1).

Cholesterol is an important component of cell membranes but high serum levels are a major risk factor for CAD. Cholesterol is both synthesized in the liver and derived from diet. Dietary cholesterol and triglycerides are carried into the circulation by chylomicrons, the largest and least dense of the lipoproteins. Chylomicrons consist largely of triglycerides (85%), which are hydrolysed at sites in the body that store or use these lipids. The chylomicron remnants are then removed from the circulation by the liver.

The liver secretes very low-density lipoproteins (VLDLs), which are triglyceride-rich but also carry some cholesterol synthesized by the liver. The VLDLs are degraded by lipoprotein lipase into VLDL remnants (or intermediate-density lipoproteins). The VLDL remnants are either removed from the circulation by the liver, where excess cholesterol is converted into bile acids, or degraded further into low-density lipoprotiens (LDLs), the major cholesterol-carrying lipoproteins in

the body, transporting cholesterol to peripheral cells. LDLs, like the VLDL remnants, are removed from the circulation via receptors on the liver cells. Smaller LDL particles tend to penetrate subendothelial tissue and thereby contribute to the development of atherosclerosis more than larger LDL particles. Very small LDL particles surrounded by apolipoprotein[a], a plasmogen-like glycoprotein, are believed to be an independent risk factor for the development of CAD. These small LDL particles are often referred to as lipoprotein[a]. High-density lipoproteins (HDLs) appear to have a protective effect by collecting cholesterol from peripheral cells and transferring it back to VLDL and LDL, so that it can then be removed from the circulation. HDL can be further subdivided into HDL2 and HDL3 fractions, both of which are protective components against CAD. Specific apoproteins carried on the surface of LDL and HDL can also be measured and are independently associated with CAD. Nonetheless, current data suggest that quantification of HDL subfractions and apoproteins adds no predictive value to more conventional lipoproteins. The LDL-HDL ratio is also a convenient method of assessing the atherogenic potential of an individual's plasma lipoproteins.

Because LDLs are the main cholesterol transporters, pharmacological manipulation has focused on decreasing the serum levels of

TABLE 11-1 CLASSIFICATION OF HYPERLIPOPROTEINEMIAS		
Type	**Lipoprotein**	**Elevated Lipid Level**
I (rare)	Chylomicron	Triglyceride ± cholesterol
IIa	LDL	Cholesterol
IIb	LDL plus VLDL	Triglyceride + cholesterol
III (rare)	IDL	Triglyceride + cholesterol
IV	VLDL	Triglyceride ± cholesterol
V	VLDL plus chylomicron	Triglyceride ± cholesterol

IDL —intermediate-density lipoprotein; LDL —low-density lipoprotein; VLDL —very-low-density lipoprotein.

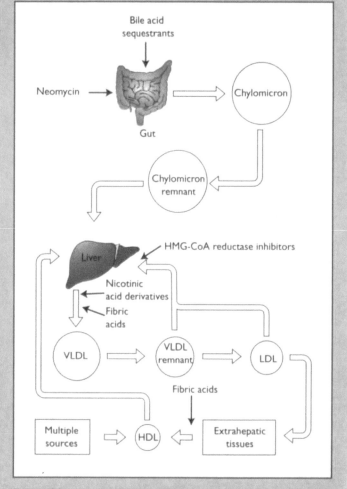

FIGURE 11.1 Interrelationships of the plasma lipoproteins and the sites of action of the lipid-lowering drugs.

The information here is provided as guidance only. Prescribers should always consult the manufacturer's current prescribing information.

215

LDL (by inhibiting VLDL synthesis or increasing the number of LDL receptors on the liver) as well as on reducing cholesterol synthesis and increasing its excretion as bile acids (Figure 11-1).

Most epidemiological studies have shown that high plasma triglyceride levels are also a risk factor for CAD. The recommended approach to the problems of hypertriglyceridemia is described in the report of the NIH Consensus Development Conference on Treatment of Hypertriglyceridemia. Despite the epidemiologic evidence supporting elevated triglyceride concentrations as an independent risk factor for CAD, the absence of pathophysiological or animal evidence that triglycerides are atherogenic or that lowering the plasma level lowers the risk for CAD, intervention specifically directed at this lipid (except rarely in patients with very high concentrations that may cause pancreatitis) is generally not recommended at present. It is noteworthy, however, that the guidelines stating this are several years old and much new data has surfaced since the introduction of these recommendations. On the other hand, many individuals with elevated triglyceride concentrations have associated low concentrations of HDL-cholesterol or high concentrations of LDL-cholesterol, or both, which may influence decisions about intervention to reduce the risk of CAD.

Other factors, such as the presence of lipoprotein A and specific polymorphisms of apolipoprotein E, are also reported to have effects on cardiovascular risk.

Drugs currently used for the treatment of dyslipidemias may be classified into four main groups: bile-acid sequestrants, fibric-acid derivatives, nicotinic acid, and hydroxymethylglutaryl coenzyme A (HMG-CoA) reductase inhibitors. Because of their varying sites and modes of action, these drugs differ in their effects on lipoprotein fractions (Table 11-2).

The link between successful reduction in total cholesterol or triglyceride levels, or both, and increased HDL-cholesterol, as well as morbidity and mortality have been examined in several drug intervention studies. An overview of diet and drug trials indicates that every 1% decrease in serum cholesterol produces a 2% fall in risk of CAD. A more recent analysis found that for every 10% lowering of cholesterol, CAD mortality risk decreased by 15%, and total mortality risk decreased by 11%. Any additional benefit that might be derived from falls in triglyceride levels and rises in HDL-cholesterol remains to be quantified, although there is data from the Helsinki Heart and VA-HIT studies to suggest a 3% decrease in cardiac events with each 1% increase in HDL concentration. The benefit of reducing cholesterol appears as a reduction in the incidence of death, providing cholesterol levels are reduced by more than 9% to 10%; reduction of cholesterol seems also to be associated with a reduction in the progression and promotion in the regression of atheromatous lesions.

TABLE 11-2 SUMMARY OF THE EFFECTS OF THE COMMONLY USED GROUPS OF LIPID-LOWERING AGENTS

| Group | Primarily lower | | Mechanism of action | Lipoprotein effect | | |
	Cholesterol	Triglycerides		VLDL	LDL	HDL
BAS	+		Increased excretion of bile acid in stool; biosynthesis of cholesterol is increased slightly and LDL receptors in liver are increased, resulting in increased disposal of circulating LDL cholesterol	0 or ↑	↓	0 or ↑
FAD		+	Activate lipoprotein lipase; promote lipolysis of VLDL; may also reduce formation of triglycerides	↓	↓↑0	0 or ↑
NA and derivatives	+	+	Inhibit VLDL secretion by liver by decreasing plasma free fatty acids	↓	↓	↑
HMG-CoA reductase inhibitors	+		Inhibit cholesterol synthesis and stimulate suppression of LDL receptors	0 or ↓	↓	0 or ↑

BAS—bile acid sequestrants; FAD—fibric acid derivatives; HDL—high density lipoprotein; HMG-CoA—hydroxymethylglutaryl coenzyme A; NA—nicotinic acid; LDL—low-density lipoprotein; VLDL—very low-density lipoprotein; ↑—increase; ↓—decrease; 0—no change.

LIPID-LOWERING DRUGS: BILE ACID SEQUESTRANTS

The bile acid sequestrants, cholestyramine and colestipol, are safe and effective agents for the treatment of hyperlipidemia. Since they are not absorbed into the circulation, they have the advantages of no systemic drug-drug interactions and few systemic side effects. However, these drugs are not well tolerated due to gastrointestinal side effects and poor palatability. For these reasons, they are now mainly second-line drugs for treating high cholesterol concentrations.

EFFICACY AND USE

The cholesterol-lowering effects of 4 g of **cholestyramine** appear to be equivalent to those obtained with 5 g of **colestipol**. Decreases in LDL concentrations of 12% to 20% may be seen with 5 g **colestipol** or 4 g **cholestyramine** twice daily. The response to therapy varies, but daily dosages of **cholestyramine** of 16 to 24 g and **colestipol** 15 to 30 g can lower concentrations of LDL by 20% to 25%, making these drugs acceptable first-line agents when modest reductions in LDL cholesterol are desired. Concentrations of HDL may increase from 0% to 8% and triglycerides may *increase* (0% to 33%). The benefits of dosages exceeding four packets per day (16 g **cholestyramine**, 20 g **colestipol**) are controversial considering the marginal additional reduction in LDL and the increase in gastrointestinal side effects and poor adherence seen with dosages exceeding this amount.

Bile acid sequestrants have no place in the treatment of lipid disorders other than the reduction of elevated cholesterol levels. They are generally reserved for the treatment of type II hyperlipidemia. These drugs are commonly used for additive or synergistic effects when given in combination with **niacin** or an HMG-CoA reductase inhibitor. Studies have shown **colestipol-niacin** combinations to result in 30% to 55% reductions in LDL and 20% to 45% increases in HDL. **Lovastatin** and **colestipol** have also been used in combination, resulting in a 46% reduction in LDL and a 15% increase in HDL concentrations.

The Lipid Research Clinics Coronary Primary Prevention Trial compared **cholestyramine** (mean daily dose of 16.8 g at 1-year follow-up) to placebo in 3806 men without CAD and with type II hypercholesterolemia receiving a moderate cholesterol lowering diet. After 7 to10 years of follow-up, total and LDL cholesterol concentrations were reduced by 13.4% and 20.3%, respectively, in patients receiving **cholestyramine**. This corresponded to a 19% reduction in risk of the combined primary end point of definite coronary heart disease (CHD) death (24% reduction) and/or definite nonfatal myocardial infarction (19% reduction) compared to placebo (Figure 11.2). A nonsignificant 7% reduction in all cause mortality was seen in the **cholestyramine** group, due primarily to a greater number of violent and accidental deaths in patients taking **cholestyramine**.

Both **cholestyramine** and **colestipol** have been shown to slow the progression of atherosclerosis and promote the regression of atherosclerotic plaques.

Pruritis associated with bile-acid retention is believed to be a result of bile-acid deposition in the skin. By encouraging the loss of bile acids through the intestine, these drugs bring relief of pruritis within 1 to 3 weeks. Diarrhea caused by an excess of fecal bile acids (as in radiation therapy, ileal resection, Crohn's disease, etc.) may also be relieved by bile acid resins. The main problems with these agents, however, are their bulk and gastrointestinal side effects. A report of the 6-year follow-up of the Lipid Research Clinics Program showed that there was an increased incidence of cholecystectomies and gastrointestinal malignancies in subjects receiving **cholestyramine** compared to placebo. Although this association was not statistically significant, it cautions practitioners to pay particular attention to the gastrointestinal complaints of patients receiving bile acid resins.

Cholestyramine and **colestipol** have also been used to treat digoxin toxicity.

The bile acid resins may interfere with normal fat digestion and absorption and consequently prevent the absorption of fat-soluble vitamins (A, D, E, and K), necessitating supplementation of these vitamins with long-term resin therapy. Malabsorption of vitamin K may lead to hypoprothrombinemia and increased bleeding; folic acid malabsorption may lead to decreased serum or red cell folate concentrations.

MODE OF ACTION

Bile acid sequestrants are anion-exchange resins, which exchange a chloride anion for other anions that have a greater affinity for the resin. The mechanism of drug action is to bind bile acids in the intestinal lumen, thereby preventing their absorption. During normal digestion, bile acids are secreted from the liver and gall bladder into the bile, and are then

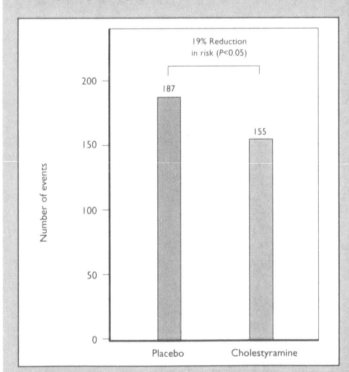

FIGURE 11.2 The effect of cholestyramine treatment on nonfatal myocardial infarction and/or coronary heart disease death in asymptomatic men with type II hyperlipoproteinemia in the LRC-CPPT study. (*Adopted from* Cashin-Hemphill *et al*: Beneficial effects of colestipol-niacin on coronary atherosclerosis: a 4-year follow-up. *JAMA* 1990, 264:3013–3017.)

transported into the intestines. Most of the secreted bile acids are enterohepatically recycled back to the liver through the portal circulation. Bile acids serve to emulsify fats and lipids into a more easily-digestible form. Bile-acid sequestrants, as their name implies, bind bile acids in the intestines to form a complex that is excreted in the feces. Bile acids are therefore removed from enterohepatic recycling.

This process stimulates an increased synthesis of bile acids from endogenous cholesterol, resulting in depletion of the hepatic cholesterol pool. This depletion in turn results in compensatory mechanisms: an increase in the biosynthesis of cholesterol and an increase in the number of specific high-affinity LDL receptors on the liver cell membrane. The increased number of high-affinity LDL receptors expressed on hepatocytes from patients treated with bile acid sequestrants stimulates an enhanced rate of LDL catabolism from plasma and thereby lowers the concentration of this lipoprotein. Despite increased cholesterol production, the net effect of these drugs is a reduction in plasma cholesterol and LDL concentrations in patients with type II hyperlipidemia, possibly because of an increased rate of clearance of LDL from the plasma.

INDICATIONS

	Cholestyramine	Colestipol
Type I hyperlipoproteinemia	–	–
Type IIa hyperlipoproteinemia	+	+
Type IIb hyperlipoproteinemia	+	+
Type III hyperlipoproteinemia	–	–
Type IV hyperlipoproteinemia	–	–
Type V hyperlipoproteinemia	–	–

+—FDA approved; – —not FDA approved

CHOLESTYRAMINE
(Cholestyramine, Questran®, Questran Light®, Prevalite®)

Cholestyramine is an insoluble basic anion-exchange resin containing quaternary ammonium groups that exchange their chloride ions and bind negatively-charged bile acids. The complex is then excreted in the feces along with unchanged resin. This excretion results in partial removal of bile acids from the enterohepatic circulation, which are replaced by the oxidation of endogenous cholesterol. Cholestyramine is as effective as the other bile-acid sequestrant, colestipol.

The Lipid Research Clinics Coronary Primary Prevention Trial compared the efficacy of cholestyramine to placebo in reducing the risk of CHD in 3806 men with primary (type II) hypercholesterolemia and no history of heart disease. In addition to reducing total and LDL cholesterol, the cholestyramine group experienced a 19% reduction in risk of the combined primary end point of definite CHD death (24% reduction) and definite nonfatal myocardial infarction (MI) (19% reduction) compared to placebo. A nonsignificant 7% reduction in all cause mortality was seen in the cholestyramine group. This neutralization of the cardiovascular benefits of cholestyramine was due primarily to a greater number of violent and accidental deaths in patients taking cholestyramine.

Cholestyramine has been shown to retard the progression of atherosclerosis and promote atherosclerotic plaque regression in patients with CAD. Cholestyramine may also help relieve pruritis due to the deposition of bile acids in dermal tissue in patients with partial biliary obstruction.

SPECIAL GROUPS

Race: not evaluated
Children: optimal dosing has not been established; long-term effects are not known in this population; children are at increased risk for hyperchloremic acidosis
Elderly: no dosage adjustment is required unless constipated (see below); more prone to constipation as a side effect; monitor closely
Renal impairment: the possibility of hyperchloremic acidosis is increased in patients with renal insufficiency and cholestyramine should therefore be used cautiously in this group
Hepatic impairment: contraindicated with total biliary obstruction
Pregnancy: category C; not evaluated
Breast-feeding: not evaluated; use cautiously due to potential malabsorption of fat-soluble vitamins; supplementation may be necessary

DOSAGE

Usual adult initial dosage is one packet or scoopful once or twice daily. Usual maintenance dosage is two to four packets or scoopfuls (8–16 g of resin) daily divided into two doses. Dosage increases of 4 g should occur at intervals of no less than 4 wk up to a maximum of 24 g of resin (six packets or scoopfuls) daily. Twice-daily dosing is recommended, but can range from one to six doses per day. Pediatric dose is 240 mg/kg/d in two to three divided doses, normally not exceeding 8 g/d. Since cholestyramine may worsen constipation, patients who are constipated should be started on dosages of one packet or scoop once daily for 5–7 d, increasing by one dose per day every month up to a maximum of 6 doses per day. Consider dosage reductions, combination therapy, or discontinuation or alteration of therapy if triglyceride concentrations increase while on cholestyramine.

IN BRIEF

INDICATIONS
As adjunctive therapy to diet in patients with elevated LDL concentrations (type II hyperlipidemia)
Relief of pruritis associated with partial biliary obstruction

CONTRAINDICATIONS
Complete biliary obstruction; hypersensitivity to product components.

DRUG INTERACTIONS
Phenylbutazone
Warfarin
Thiazide diuretics
Propranolol
Tetracycline
Penicillin G
Phenobarbital
Thyroid and thyroxine preparations
Estrogens and progestins
Digitalis
Drugs that undergo enterohepatic circulation
Fat-soluble vitamins (A, D, E, K)
Spironolactone
Troglitazone

ADVERSE EFFECTS
Adverse effects tend to be gastrointestinal and transient in nature
GI:constipation (8%–39%), gas (12%–32%), heartburn (12%–27%), belching/bloating (9%–27%), abdominal pain (7%–15%), diarrhea (4%–10%), nausea (3%–16%), vomiting (2%–6%)

PHARMACOKINETICS AND PHARMACODYNAMICS
Since cholestyramine is not systemically absorbed, many pharmacokinetic parameters are not applicable (9 g of Questran, 5 g of Questran Light, and 5.5 g of Prevalite or generic cholestyramine all contain 4 g of cholestyramine resin)
Duration of action: 12–24 h (2–4 wk after stopping therapy)
Onset of action: 24–48 h
Peak effect: within 1 mo
Bioavailability: not applicable
Effect of food: none
Metabolism: not applicable
Elimination: 100% fecal
Elimination half-life: not applicable
Protein binding: not applicable

MONITORING
Plasma lipid profile, bowel function, prothrombin time.

OVERDOSE
With an overdose of cholestyramine, the primary potential problem would be intestinal obstruction, best treated by a specialist in that area.

PATIENT INFORMATION
Mix each packetful or scoopful with 2-6 ounces of water or other noncarbonated beverage, soup, or pulpy fruit with a high moisture content (applesauce, crushed pineapple, etc.). Do not consume the powder in its dry form. Sipping or retaining the resin in the mouth may cause teeth discoloration or decay. If you miss a dose take it as soon as you remember. If it is about time for the next dose, take that dose only. Do not take two doses at once. Do not discontinue therapy without your clinician's advice. Take other medications at least 1 h before or 4 h after cholestyramine. Notify your clinician as soon as possible if you become pregnant or intend to become pregnant or breastfeed while taking this medication. Take with plenty of fluid and fiber to minimize constipation. If persistent constipation occurs, notify your clinician. Phenylketonurics: Questran Light contains phenylalanine.

AVAILABILITY
Powder for oral solution: 4 g anhydrous resin per packet or scoopful. Each packet or scoopful contains 9 g (Questran), 5 g (Questran Light), and 5.5 g (Prevalite, generic) powder.

COLESTIPOL

(Colestid®, Flavored Colestid®)

Colestipol is an insoluble high molecular weight basic anion-exchange resin containing secondary and tertiary amine groups. The resin forms complexes with bile acids, which are then excreted in the feces. This excretion results in partial removal of bile acids from the enterohepatic circulation, which are replaced by the oxidation of endogenous cholesterol. Colestipol is as effective as the other bile-acid sequestrant, cholestyramine.

Several studies have demonstrated colestipol, in combination with niacin and/or lovastatin, to slow the progression of atherosclerosis and promote atherosclerotic plaque regression in patients with CAD.

SPECIAL GROUPS

Race: not evaluated

Children: not evaluated

Elderly: no dosage adjustment is required unless constipated (see below); more prone to constipation as a side effect; monitor closely

Renal impairment: the possibility of hyperchloremic acidosis is increased in patients with renal insufficiency and colestipol should therefore be used cautiously in this group

Hepatic impairment: ineffective with total biliary obstruction

Pregnancy: not evaluated; use cautiously due to impaired absorption of fat-soluble vitamins

Breast-feeding: not evaluated; use cautiously due to impaired absorption of fat-soluble vitamins

DOSAGE

Usual adult initial dosage is 1 packet or scoopful once or twice daily. Usual maintenance dosage ranges from 1–6 packets or scoopfuls (5–30 g of resin) daily in single or divided doses. Dosage increases of 5 g should occur at intervals of no less than 4 wk up to a maximum of 30 g of colestipol (6 packets or scoopfuls) daily. Since colestipol may worsen constipation, patients who are constipated should be started on dosages of 1 packet or scoop once daily for 5–7 d, increasing by one dose per day every month up to a maximum of 6 doses / d. Consider dosage reductions, combination therapy, or discontinuation or alteration of therapy if triglyceride concentrations increase while on colestipol.

IN BRIEF

INDICATIONS
As adjunctive therapy to diet in patients with elevated LDL concentrations (type II hyperlipidemia).

CONTRAINDICATIONS
Hypersensitivity to product components.

DRUG INTERACTIONS
Furosemide
Thiazide diuretics
Propranolol
Tetracycline
Penicillin G
Fat-soluble vitamins (A, D, E, K)
Gemfibrozil
Digitalis
Oral phosphate supplements
Hydrocortisone
Drugs that undergo enterohepatic circulation
Spironolactone

ADVERSE EFFECTS
Adverse effects tend to be gastrointestinal and transient in nature. The GI effects reported below are event rates with colestipol-niacin combination therapy:
GI: constipation (31%), stomach discomfort (23%), heartburn (20%), sore throat (14%), abdominal pain (15%), nausea (23%), vomiting (6%)
Hepatic: elevated serum transaminases (<1%)

PHARMACOKINETICS AND PHARMACODYNAMICS
Since colestipol is not systemically absorbed, many pharmacokinetic parameters are not applicable

Duration of action: 12–24 h (2–4 wk after stopping therapy)
Onset of action: 24–48 h
Peak effect: within 1 mo
Bioavailability: not applicable
Effect of food: none
Metabolism: not applicable
Elimination: 100% fecal
Elimination half-life: not applicable
Protein binding: not applicable

MONITORING
Plasma lipid profile, bowel function, prothrombin time, serum transaminases.

OVERDOSE
With an overdose of colestipol, the primary potential problem would be intestinal obstruction, best treated by a specialist in that area.

PATIENT INFORMATION
Mix each packetful or scoopful with ≥3 ounces of water or other noncarbonated beverage, soup, or pulpy fruit with a high moisture content (applesauce, crushed pineapple, etc.). Do not consume the powder in its dry form. Sipping or retaining the resin in the mouth may cause teeth discoloration or decay. If you miss a dose take it as soon as you remember. If it is about time for the next dose, take that dose only. Do not take two doses at once. Do not discontinue therapy without your clinician's advice. Take other medications at least 1 h before or 4 h after colestipol. Notify your clinician as soon as possible if you become pregnant or intend to become pregnant or breast-feed while taking this medication. Take with plenty of fluid and fiber to minimize constipation. If persistent constipation occurs, notify your clinician. Phenylketonurics: Flavored Colestid contains phenylalanine.

AVAILABILITY
Granules for oral suspension: 5 g colestipol per packet or teaspoonful. Each packet or teaspoonful of Flavored Colestid (orange-flavored) contains 5 g colestipol in 7.5 g of product
Tablets—1 g micronized colestipol

LIPID-LOWERING DRUGS: FIBRIC ACID DERIVATIVES

The fibric acid derivatives, **clofibrate**, **gemfibrozil**, and **fenofibrate**, are primarily used for reducing elevated triglyceride concentrations. **Clofibrate** is rarely used due to an increase in mortality in patients taking this drug. **Fenofibrate** has been available outside of the United States for several years, but has just recently been reformulated into a micronized capsule preparation which may be given once daily and has greater bioavailability than the standard fenofibrate preparations. This new formulation has recently been approved for use by the United States Food and Drug Administration (FDA). A long-acting form of **gemfibrozil** (not available in the United States) has also recently been shown to reduce cardiac events in men with a history of CAD.

EFFICACY AND USE

Preliminary data suggests **clofibrate** and **gemfibrozil** to have similar efficacy in reducing total and LDL cholesterol and triglyceride concentrations; however, **gemfibrozil** may be more efficacious at increasing HDL concentrations. **Gemfibrozil** 800 to 1600 mg/day and **clofibrate** 1500 to 2000 mg/day may be expected to reduce triglycerides by about 40% to 60%. **Fenofibrate** has been shown to decrease triglyceride concentrations by 15% to 43% in patients with type IIa hyperlipidemia and by 32% to 53% in patients with type IIb or IV hyperlipidemia. HDL concentrations may be increased anywhere from 1% to 34% with these drugs. LDL concentrations, as mentioned earlier, typically decrease in patients with type II hyperlipidemia and may increase in patients with type IV hyperlipidemia.

A 44% increase in total mortality compared to placebo seen in a World Health Organization study has severely limited the use of **clofibrate**. The excess mortality with **clofibrate** was due primarily to malignancies and complications involving the liver, gallbladder, and pancreas. This study and another, the Coronary Drug Project, also showed higher rates of cholelithiasis, cholecystitis, and cholecystectomy in patients receiving **clofibrate** versus placebo.

Nonmicronized fenofibrate has been shown to reduce total and LDL-cholesterol to a greater extent than **gemfibrozil** with comparable decreases in triglycerides in a small study involving patients with type IIb hyperlipidemia.

The Helsinki Heart Study demonstrated a 34% reduction in the risk of developing a serious cardiac event (MI or sudden cardiac death) in patients receiving **gemfibrozil** versus placebo. This was due mainly to a 37% reduction in the risk of nonfatal MI in patients in the **gemfibrozil** group compared to patients receiving placebo. However, all cause mortality did not differ between the two groups.

Gemfibrozil has also been shown to retard the progression of coronary and vein graft atherosclerosis and the development of new lesions in post-coronary bypass graft patients and to reduce the need for invasive treatment for milder forms of CAD.

The Veterans Administration-HDL Intervention Trial (VA-HIT) studied the effects of a long-acting **gemfibrozil** preparation in patients with a history of CAD and a mean HDL, LDL, and triglyceride concentration of 32, 111, and 161 mg/dL, respectively. In this study, **gemfibrozil** reduced the risk of experiencing another cardiac event (MI or cardiac death) by 22% compared to placebo and also reduced the incidence of cerebrovascular disease.

Fibric acid derivatives are generally well-tolerated, with most side effects being gastrointestinal in nature. Caution should be exercised when combining these drugs with HMG-CoA reductase inhibitors due to the increased risk of rhabdomyolysis. **Clofibrate** increases the incidence of cholesterol gallstones; this adverse effect does not seem as pronounced with other fibric acid derivatives. These drugs may also potentiate the anticoagulant effect of **warfarin**, necessitating close monitoring of prothrombin times in patients on concurrent therapy.

MODE OF ACTION

Fibric acid derivatives increase the activity of the enzyme lipoprotein lipase, thus enhancing the catabolism of triglycerides from VLDL and IDL particles and promoting the transfer of cholesterol to HDL. VLDL production also appears to be decreased. High concentrations of triglyceride-rich VLDL particles may cause a rapid conversion to smaller IDL and LDL particles by lipoprotein lipase, resulting in an increase in LDL concentrations. Patients with normal or only slightly elevated triglyceride concentrations may experience a modest reduction in LDL concentrations.

INDICATIONS

	Clofibrate	Fenofibrate	Gemfibrozil
Type I hyperlipoproteinemia	–	–	–
Type IIa hyperlipoproteinemia	–	–	–
Type IIb hyperlipoproteinemia	–	–	+
Type III hyperlipoproteinemia	+	–	–
Type IV hyperlipoproteinemia	+	+	+
Type V hyperlipoproteinemia	+	+	+

+—FDA approved; – —not FDA approved

CLOFIBRATE
(Clofibrate, Atromid-S ®)

Clofibrate is the protoype fibric acid used in the treatment of hyper-cholesterolemia. Clofibrate is most useful in treating patients with elevated triglyceride concentrations (types IV and V hyperlipidemias). Preliminary data suggests clofibrate and gemfibrozil to have similar efficacy in reducing triglyceride concentrations; however, gemfibrozil may be more efficacious at increasing HDL concentrations. Clofibrate generally has only mild effects on decreasing total and LDL cholesterol concentrations and, in fact, may paradoxically increase LDL concentrations in patients with elevated triglycerides and normal cholesterol concentrations.

Clofibrate is rarely used now due to a 44% increase in total mortality seen in patients receiving clofibrate versus placebo in a World Health Organization study. This excess mortality with clofibrate was due primarily to malignancies and complications involving the liver, gall-bladder, and pancreas. This study and another, the Coronary Drug Project, also showed higher rates of cholelithiasis, cholecystitis, and cholecystectomy in patients receiving clofibrate versus placebo. One study, however, demonstrated combination clofibrate-niacin therapy to reduce total mortality and mortality due to ischemic heart disease in patients with a history of MI.

Clofibrate may also increase the risk of peripheral vascular disease, pulmonary embolism, thrombophlebitis, angina pectoris, arrhythmias, and intermittent claudication.

SPECIAL GROUPS

Race: not evaluated
Children: safety and effectiveness have not been established
Elderly: no dosage adjustment is required
Renal impairment: the risk of rhabdomyolysis and severe hyperkalemia is increased in patients with severe renal insufficiency and clofibrate is therefore contraindicated in this group
Hepatic impairment: contraindicated in patients with clinically-significant hepatic dysfunction
Pregnancy: category C; contraindicated
Breast-feeding: contraindicated

DOSAGE

Usual dosage is 1g twice daily. Some patients may respond to lower dosages.

IN BRIEF

INDICATIONS
As adjunctive therapy to diet in adult patients with type III hyperlipidemia
As adjunctive therapy to diet in adult patients with elevated triglyceride concentrations (types IV and V hyperlipidemias) at risk for pancreatitis

CONTRAINDICATIONS
Clinically-significant hepatic or renal dysfunction, including primary biliary cirrhosis; pregnancy and lactation; hypersensitivity to clofibrate.

DRUG INTERACTIONS
Warfarin
HMG-CoA reductase inhibitors
Phenytoin
Tolbutamide

ADVERSE EFFECTS
Cardiac: rapid or irregular heartbeat (4%), angina (5%)
GI: abdominal pain (9%), epigastric pain (2%), diarrhea (4%), nausea (8%), vomiting (2%)
Skin: rash (7%), pruritis (1%), itching (7%), flushing (5%)
Eyes: blurred vision (2%)
Hepatic: increased serum transaminases (<1%)
Gentiourinary: decreased libido (14%)
Musculoskeletal: myalgia, myositis, myopathy, rhabdomyolysis (<1%)
Hematologic: anemia, leukopenia (<1%)
Other: dizziness (1%), chest pain (1%), headache (3%)

PHARMACOKINETICS AND PHARMACODYNAMICS
Duration of action:	6–12 h (3 wk after stopping therapy)
Onset of action:	2–5 d
Peak effect:	3–4 wk
Bioavailability:	about 100%
Effect of food:	none
Metabolism:	metabolized by CYP3A4; hydrolyzed to the active compound, p-chlorophenoxyisobutyric acid (CPIB)
Elimination:	95%–99% excreted in the urine as free and conjugated clofibric acid
Elimination half-life:	18–22 h
Protein binding:	95%–97%

MONITORING
Plasma lipid profile, serum transaminases, complete blood count (CBC).

OVERDOSE
Treatment should be symptomatic and supportive.
Clofibrate is not removed by hemodialysis.

PATIENT INFORMATION
If you miss a dose take it as soon as you remember. If it is about time for the next dose, take that dose only. Do not take two doses at once. If irregular heartbeats, abdominal pain, or muscle pain, tenderness or weakness occurs, notify your clinician. Do not discontinue therapy without your clinician's advice. This medication should not be taken during pregnancy due to possible harm to the fetus. Notify your clinician as soon as possible if you become pregnant or intend to become pregnant while taking this medication.

AVAILABILITY
Capsule—500 mg

FENOFIBRATE (Tricor™)

Approved in February 1998, fenofibrate is the latest fibric acid derivative to become available in the United States. Fenofibrate is manufactured in micronized form (drug particle diameter <50 μm), which results in more rapid drug dissolution and approximately 30% greater bioavailability compared to the standard formulation . Micronized fenofibrate also has the advantage of single-daily dosing.

Like clofibrate and gemfibrozil, fenofibrate is believed to increase lipoprotein lipase activity and thereby the clearance of triglycerides from the body. Triglyceride concentrations may be decreased by 15% to 43% in patients with type IIa hyperlipidemia and by 32% to 53% in patients with type IIb or IV hyperlipidemia. Studies in patients with type II hyperlipidemia demonstrated fenofibrate, 200 mg/day, to be generally more effective than 20 mg simvastatin or 20 mg pravastatin daily in reducing triglycerides and increasing HDL, although LDL tended to be reduced more with the HMG-CoA reductase inhibitors. Combination therapy of fenofibrate with an HMG-CoA reductase inhibitor has been shown to be safe and effective in reducing both LDL and triglyceride and increasing HDL concentrations.

Nonmicronized fenofibrate, 100 mg three times daily, has been shown to reduce total and LDL-cholesterol to a greater extent than gemfibrozil 600 mg twice daily with comparable decreases in triglycerides in a small study involving patients with type IIb hyperlipidemia. The effects of fenofibrate on morbidity and mortality from CHD have not been evaluated.

SPECIAL GROUPS

Race: not evaluated
Children: safety and effectiveness have not been established
Elderly: no dosage adjustment is required
Renal impairment: dosage may need to be reduced with creatinine clearance <50 mL/min due to a reduction in clearance of the active metabolite
Hepatic impairment: not evaluated
Pregnancy: category C
Breast-feeding: nursing mothers should not use fenofibrate due to the potential for tumorgenicity seen in animal studies

DOSAGE

Usual initial dosage is 67 mg once daily. Dosage may be titrated every 4–8 wk up to 201 mg once daily.

IN BRIEF

INDICATIONS
As adjunctive therapy to diet in adult patients with elevated triglyceride concentrations (type IV and V hyperlipidemia) at risk for pancreatitis.

CONTRAINDICATIONS
Hepatic or severe renal dysfunction; preexisting gallbladder disease; hypersensitivity to fenofibrate.

DRUG INTERACTIONS
Warfarin
HMG-CoA reductase inhibitors
Bile acid sequestrants
Cyclosporine

ADVERSE EFFECTS
CNS: dizziness (2%), decreased libido (2%)
GI: flatulence (3%), nausea/vomiting (4%), constipation (3%), dyspepsia (5%), diarrhea (3%)
Skin: pruritus (3%), rash (6%)
Hepatic: serum transaminases >three times upper limit of normal (8%–10%), hepatitis (<1%)
Pancreatic: pancreatitis (<1%)
Musculoskeletal: rhabdomyolysis (<1%)
Hematologic: decreases in hemoglobin/ hematocrit (<1%), thrombocytopenia (<1%)
Other: infections (18%), localized/misc. pain (8%), flu syndrome (5%), headache (5%)

PHARMACOKINETICS AND PHARMACODYNAMICS
(67 mg micronized = 100 mg nonmicronized fenofibrate)
Duration of action: not evaluated
Onset of action: 2–5 d
Peak effect: ≥12 wk
Bioavailability: cannot be determined due to the unavailability of a parenteral product for comparison
Effect of food: 35% increase in absorption
Metabolism: completely hydrolyzed to the active metabolite fenofibric acid
Elimination: mainly renal; 60% recovered in urine, 25% recovered in feces
Elimination half-life: 20 h
Protein binding: 99%

MONITORING
Plasma lipid profile, serum transaminases, CBC.

OVERDOSE
Treatment should be symptomatic and supportive. Fenofibrate is not removed by hemodialysis.

PATIENT INFORMATION
Take with food to increase drug absorption. If you miss a dose take it as soon as you remember. If it is about time for the next dose, take that dose only. Do not take two doses at once. Notify physician if persistent or unusual side effects occur. Do not discontinue therapy without your physician's advice.

AVAILABILITY
Capsules—67 mg

GEMFIBROZIL (Gemfibrozil, Lopid ®)

Gemfibrozil is currently the most widely used fibric acid derivative in the United States. Gemfibrozil is most useful in treating patients with elevated triglyceride concentrations (types IV and V hyperlipidemias) with the added ability to increase HDL concentrations. Gemfibrozil generally has only mild effects on decreasing total and LDL cholesterol concentrations and, in fact, may paradoxically increase LDL concentrations in patients with elevated triglycerides and normal cholesterol concentrations.

The Helsinki Heart Study evaluated the effects of gemfibrozil in patients with a non-HDL cholesterol of ≥200 mg/dL and no history of CAD. Over a 5-year period, patients receiving gemfibrozil experienced a 34% reduction in the risk of developing a serious cardiac event (sudden cardiac death and/or MI) due mainly to a 37% reduction in the risk of developing nonfatal MI compared to patients receiving placebo. However, all cause mortality did not differ between the two groups. Patients with type IIb hyperlipidemia benefitted the most in this particular study. A subgroup of patients excluded from the Helsinki Heart Study due to CHD or electrocardiographic abnormalities demonstrated no benefit of gemfibrozil in reducing cardiac events or cardiac deaths.

The Lopid Coronary Angiography Trial showed gemfibrozil to retard the progression of coronary and vein graft atherosclerosis and the development of new lesions in post-coronary bypass graft patients with a mean total cholesterol, triglyceride, and HDL concentration of 199, 146, and 31 mg/dL, respectively.

The recently published Veterans Administration-HDL Intervention Trial (VA-HIT) studied the effects of a long-acting gemfibrozil preparation (not currently available in the United States) in patients with a history of CAD and a mean HDL, LDL, and triglyceride concentration of 32, 111, and 161 mg/dL, respectively. In this study, gemfibrozil reduced the risk of experiencing a cardiac event (MI or cardiac death) by 22% compared to placebo and also reduced the incidence of cerebrovascular disease. In this trial, the first study demonstrating the benefit of increasing HDL without lowering LDL concentrations, gemfibrozil increased HDL concentrations by 7.5%, had negligible effects an LDL concentrations, and decreased triglycerides by 24.5%.

Due to the chemical, pharmacological, and clinical similarities between gemfibrozil and clofibrate, many of the adverse effects seen with clofibrate are possible with gemfibrozil, most notably gallstones.

SPECIAL GROUPS

Race: not evaluated
Children: safety and effectiveness have not been established
Elderly: no dosage adjustment is required
Renal impairment: gemfibrozil may worsen renal insufficiency in patients with serum creatinine concentrations >2.0 mg/dL and should therefore be used cautiously in this group
Hepatic impairment: not evaluated
Pregnancy: category C
Breast-feeding: gemfibrozil should not be used in nursing mothers due to the potential for tumorgenicity seen in animal studies

DOSAGE

Usual dosage is 600 mg twice daily 30 min before the morning and evening meal.

IN BRIEF

INDICATIONS
As adjunctive therapy to diet in adult patients with elevated triglyceride concentrations (types IV and V hyperlipidemias) at risk for pancreatitis
Reducing the risk of developing CHD in patients with type IIb hypercholesterolemia with low HDL and no history or symptoms of CHD after other treatments have failed

CONTRAINDICATIONS
Hepatic or severe renal dysfunction, including primary biliary cirrhosis; preexisting gallbladder disease; hypersensitivity to gemfibrozil.

DRUG INTERACTIONS
Warfarin
HMG-CoA reductase inhibitors

ADVERSE EFFECTS
Cardiac: atrial fibrillation (0.7%)
CNS: paresthesias (1%)
GI: dyspepsia (20%), abdominal pain (10%), acute appendicitis (1%) diarrhea (7%), nausea/vomiting (3%), constipation (1%)
Skin: Eczema (2%), rash (2%), pruritis (1%)
Eyes: blurred vision (1%)
Hepatic: increased serum transaminases (<1%)
Endocrine: gout (1%)
Musculoskeletal: extremity pain (1%), myositis (<1%)
Hematologic: decreases in hemoglobin/ hematocrit (<1%), thrombocytopenia, leukopenia (<1%)
Other: dizziness (2%), chest pain (2%), headache (1%), fatigue (4%)

PHARMACOKINETICS AND PHARMACODYNAMICS
Duration of action: 6–8 wk (after stopping therapy)
Onset of action: 2–5 d
Peak effect: 3–4 wk
Bioavailability: 98%
Effect of food: none
Metabolism: hepatic metabolism partially by CYP3A4
Elimination: mainly renal: 70% recovered in urine, mostly as the glucuronide conjugate; 6% recovered in feces
Elimination half-life: 1.5 h
Protein binding: >97%

MONITORING
Plasma lipid profile, serum transaminases, CBC

OVERDOSE
Treatment should be symptomatic and supportive. Gemfibrozil is not removed by hemodialysis.

PATIENT INFORMATION
If you miss a dose take it as soon as you remember. If it is about time for the next dose, take that dose only. Do not take two doses at once. If abdominal pain, muscle pain, tenderness or weakness occurs, notify your clinician. Do not discontinue therapy without your clinician's advice.

AVAILABILITY
Tablet, scored, film-coated—600 mg

LIPID-LOWERING DRUGS: NICOTINIC ACID

Nicotinic acid (**niacin; vitamin B$_3$**) is a water-soluble vitamin that, at doses much larger than those used as a vitamin supplement, lowers total and LDL cholesterol and triglyceride concentrations and increases HDL concentrations. Unlike other available lipid-lowering drugs, niacin has been shown to lower lipoprotein (a) concentrations by as much as 38%.

EFFICACY AND USE

Nicotinic acid, while an effective and inexpensive agent for treating dyslipidemias, is oftentimes overlooked as a first-line drug due to its side effect profile and the availability of the well-tolerated (and more expensive) HMG-CoA reductase inhibitors. Nonetheless, **nicotinic acid** retains a very prominent role in the treatment of dyslipidemias.

In daily doses of 1.5 to 3 g, **nicotinic acid** is effective in most patients with a variety of dyslipidemias. A daily dose of less than or equal to 2 g may lower LDL cholesterol by 20% to 30% and raise HDL cholesterol by as much as 32%. Compared to placebo, patients receiving 3 g daily of **niacin** in the Coronary Drug Project experienced an average reduction in triglyceride concentrations of 26%. When used in combination with **colestipol**, HDL concentrations have been shown to increase and LDL concentrations have been shown to decrease, both by 43%. Adding either an HMG-CoA reductase inhibitor or a bile acid sequestrant to **nicotinic acid** has yielded greater LDL lowering than niacin alone. The combination of **niacin, lovastatin**, and **colestipol** had been shown to produce LDL reductions of almost 70%. Nicotinic acid is effective in the treatment of types II, III, IV, and V hyperlipidemias.

The Coronary Drug Project studied the effect of **nicotinic acid** (3 g daily) on reducing total mortality in 1119 men with a previous MI. After 5 years of treatment, there was no difference in total mortality between the **nicotinic acid** and placebo groups. However, **nicotinic acid** significantly reduced the incidence of definite nonfatal MI by 27% compared to placebo. At an average follow-up of 15 years (about 9 years after the drug was stopped), mortality in the **nicotinic acid** group was 11% less than in the placebo group, a statistically significant difference.

Several studies have demonstrated **nicotinic acid**, in combination with **colestipol** with or without **lovastatin**, to slow the progression of atherosclerosis and promote atherosclerotic plaque regression in patients with CAD. Combination **nicotinic acid-clofibrate** therapy has also been shown to significantly reduce total mortality by 26% and mortality due to ischemic heart disease by 36% in patients with a history of MI.

As mentioned earlier, the more widespread clinical use of **nicotinic acid** has been limited by its side effect profile. The most common side effects are related to the vasodilatory action of the drug: flushing, headache, tingling, itching, and rash. It is believed that slow, gradual upward titration of **nicotinic acid** helps minimize these adverse effects.

Hepatotoxicity is another worrisome side effect of **nicotinic acid**, predominantly with the sustained-release preparations. It is incompletely defined as to why the sustained-release preparations have a greater tendency to damage the liver, but it may relate to the difference in metabolic handling between immediate-release and sustained-release preparations. Some clinicians even advocate avoidance of sustained-release preparations for this reason. A recently released once-daily formulation of **nicotinic acid** is reported to cause transaminase elevations at an incidence similar to HMG-CoA reductase inhibitors and immediate-release niacin.

MODE OF ACTION

The mechanism of action of **nicotinic acid** in treating hyperlipidemia remains largely unknown, but appears to be independent of its role as a vitamin. **Nicotinic acid** appears to act, at least in part, by reducing the synthesis of lipoprotein (a) and the hepatic synthesis and secretion of of apolipoprotein B-containing particles, by reducing free fatty acid release from adipose tissue, and by changing the metabolism of HDL particles with a resultant shift in HDL subtype distribution. Nicotinic acid may also increase the rate of removal of chylomicron triglycerides from the plasma secondary to increased lipoprotein lipase activity. **Nicotinic acid** has no effect on the fecal excretion of fats, sterols, or bile acids.

In addition to its effects on plasma lipid concentrations, **nicotinic acid** produces peripheral vasodilation, thought to be mediated through prostaglandins. **Nicotinic acid** reportedly releases histamine, causing increased gastric motility and acid secretion. It also activates the fibrinolytic system. Large doses of **nicotinic acid** have been reported to decrease uric acid excretion and impair glucose tolerance.

INDICATIONS

	Nicotinic Acid
Type I hyperlipoproteinemia	–
Type IIa hyperlipoproteinemia	+
Type IIb hyperlipoproteinemia	+
Type III hyperlipoproteinemia	–
Type IV hyperlipoproteinemia	+
Type V hyperlipoproteinemia	+

+—FDA approved; —not FDA approved

NICOTINIC ACID (NIACIN)

(Nicotinic Acid, Niacor®, Nicolar®, Slo-Niacin®, Nicobid Tempules®, Niac®, Nia-Bid®, Niacels®, Nico-400®, Nicotinex®, Niaspan®)

Nicotinic acid (niacin; vitamin B₃) is a very effective and inexpensive agent for the treatment of hyperlipidemias. Niacin therapy, however, is usually accompanied by several troublesome side effects necessitating very slow and deliberate dosage titration. Most side effects are secondary to vasodilation (flushing, headaches, etc.) thought to be induced by prostaglandin release. Sustained-release preparations may blunt these side effects somewhat, but in turn may increase the risk of hepatotoxicity.

Niacin decreases total cholesterol, LDL cholesterol, lipoprotein (a), and triglycerides and, more than any other drug, increases HDL cholesterol. The Coronary Drug Project studied the effect of niacin on reducing total mortality in 1119 men with a previous MI. After 5 years, there was no difference in total mortality between the niacin and placebo groups. However, niacin significantly reduced the incidence of definite nonfatal MI compared to placebo. At an average follow-up of 15 years (about 9 years after drug was stopped), mortality in the niacin group was 11% less than in the placebo group, a statistically significant difference.

Several studies have demonstrated niacin, in combination with colestipol with or without lovastatin, to slow the progression of atherosclerosis and promote atherosclerotic plaque regression in patients with CAD. Combination niacin-clofibrate therapy has also been shown to reduce total mortality and mortality due to ischemic heart disease in patients with a history of MI.

SPECIAL GROUPS

Race: not evaluated

Children: not evaluated

Elderly: no dosage adjustment is required

Renal impairment: not evaluated; use cautiously

Hepatic impairment: not extensively studied; use with caution in patients with a history of liver disease, who consume substantial quantities of alcohol, or who have unexplained transaminase elevations; contraindicated with active liver disease

Pregnancy: category C; use cautiously

Breast-feeding: not evaluated; use cautiously

DOSAGE

Note: Immediate and sustained release products are not interchangeable. For patients switching from immediate-release to sustained release preparations, reduce the dosage by 1/2 or more. Therapy should be instituted with the lowest possible dose and gradually titrated upward.

Immediate-release preparations: usual initial dosage is 200–250 mg in single or divided doses. Dosage is increased as tolerated at 4–7d intervals to a normal maintenance dosage of 1.5-6 g/d in three divided doses with meals. Maximum dosage is 8 g/d.

Sustained-release preparations: usual initial dosage is 125–375 mg in single (Niaspan) or two to three divided doses (other sustained release preparations). Usual maintenance dosage is 1–2 g/d. Maximum dosage is 3 g/d.

IN BRIEF

INDICATIONS

As adjunctive therapy to diet for reducing total cholesterol, LDL cholesterol, apolipoprotein B, and triglyceride concentrations in patients with type II hyperlipidemia

As adjunctive therapy in adult patients with elevated triglyceride concentrations (types IV and V hyperlipidemias) at risk for pancreatitis

To reduce the risk of recurrent nonfatal MI in patients with a history of MI and hypercholesterolemia

To slow the progression or promote the regression of atherosclerotic disease in patients with a history of CAD when used with a bile acid sequestrant

CONTRAINDICATIONS

Significant or unexplained hepatic dysfunction; active peptic ulcer disease; arterial bleeding; hypersensitivity to product components.

DRUG INTERACTIONS

HMG-CoA reductase inhibitors

Ganglionic blocking antihypertensives

Vasoactive drugs

Bile acid sequestrants

Niacin-containing vitamins

ADVERSE EFFECTS

Where applicable, the first number represents immediate release niacin (IR), the second, Niaspan®

Skin: flushing (92%, 88%), itching of skin (49% with IR), rash (20%, ≤5%)

GI: abdominal pain (14%, ≤5%), diarrhea (5%, ≤11%), nausea (9%, ≤10%), vomiting (2%, ≤8%)

Hepatic: elevated transaminases (5%, 5%, ≤52% with other sustained-release preparations)

Endocrine: elevated uric acid concentrations (<1%), reduced phosphorous concentrations (<1%)

Hematologic: decreased platelet count (<1%), elevated prothrombin time (<1%)

Other: headache (4%–11% with Niaspan®)

PHARMACOKINETICS AND PHARMACODYNAMICS

Duration of action: 2–6 wk after stopping therapy

Onset of action: 2 wk for cholesterol reduction; several hours for triglyceride reduction

Peak effect: 3–5 wk

Bioavailability: 60%–88%

Effect of food: food may increase bioavailability

Metabolism: rapid, extensive, and saturable first-pass metabolism via two major pathways to form nicotinamide adenine dinucleotide and nicotinuric acid

Elimination: renal, as unchanged drug and metabolites

Elimination half-life: 20–48 min

Protein binding: <20%

MONITORING

Plasma lipid profile, serum transaminases, blood glucose, uric acid, platelet count, prothrombin time, plasma phosphorous concentrations.

OVERDOSE

Treatment is symptomatic and supportive.

PATIENT INFORMATION

Take with food. Do not crush or chew sustained-release preparations. Follow your dosage regimen closely to minimize side effects. Flushing is a common side effect of niacin therapy and usually subsides with repeated dosing. Flushing may last for several hours after dosing and may be minimized by taking aspirin or a NSAID (eg, ibuprofen) about 30–60 min before niacin. Hot beverages or alcohol may worsen flushing. If you miss a dose take it as soon as you remember. If it is about time for the next dose, take that dose only. Do not take two doses at once. Do not discontinue therapy without your clinician's advice. Notify your clinician as soon as possible if you become pregnant or intend to become pregnant or breast-feed while taking this medication.

AVAILABILITY

Tablets, immediate-release—25, 50, 100, 250, 500 mg

Tablets, timed-release—250, 375, 500, 750, 1000 mg

Capsules, timed-release—125, 250, 300, 400, 500 mg

Elixir—50 mg/5 mL

LIPID-LOWERING DRUGS: HMG-CoA REDUCTASE INHIBITORS

Inhibitors of HMG-CoA reductase competitively inhibit the conversion of hydroxymethyl-glutaryl to mevalonic acid, a rate limiting step in the synthesis of cholesterol in the liver and intestines, the main sites for the production of cholesterol in the body. These drugs are highly effective in reducing LDL cholesterol and are very well tolerated. HMG-CoA reductase inhibitors have repeatedly been shown to reduce cardiovascular mortality and morbidity in patients with and without high cholesterol and CAD.

EFFICACY AND USE

The HMG-CoA reductase inhibitors are the most potent drugs available for reducing LDL cholesterol and apolipoprotein B concentrations. In addition, they reduce triglyceride and increase HDL concentrations. Table 11-3 shows the relative efficacy of each of the drugs in this class. These drugs may also be used in combination with bile acid sequestrants or niacin to produce additional decreases in LDL cholesterol, or in combination with a fibric acid derivative for additional reductions in triglyceride concentrations. Combination therapy with niacin or a fibric acid derivative should be approached cautiously, however, due to an increase in the risk of rhabdomyolysis.

Five large, randomized, placebo-controlled studies have proven the efficacy of the HMG-CoA reductase inhibitors in reducing cardiovascular mortality and morbidity. These studies are summarized in Table 11-4.

Additional beneficial effects of these drugs are in slowing atherosclerosis progression and in promoting the regression of atherosclerotic plaques and in reducing the incidence of stroke.

HMG-CoA reductase inhibitors are generally the best tolerated lipid-lowering drugs available. Side effects typically occur in less than 10% of patients and are most commonly abdominal pain, flatulence, headache, constipation, diarrhea, nausea, and vomiting. More serious adverse effects such as rhabdomyolysis, thrombocytopenia, and liver dysfunction are rare but necessitate prospective monitoring and withdrawal of drug therapy if necessary. Persistent serum transaminase elevations more than three times the upper limit of normal, severe myalgias, and precipitous drops in platelet counts are all reasons for considering discontinuation of these medications.

MODE OF ACTION

Most of the cholesterol formed in the body is synthesized in the liver. HMG-CoA reductase inhibitors interrupt an early

TABLE 11-3 RELATIVE LIPID EFFECTS OF THE HGM-CoA REDUCTASE INHIBITORS

Drug	Daily dosage, mg	Usual total cholesterol reduction, %	Usual LDL reduction, %	Usual HDL increase, %	Usual TG reduction, %
Atorvastatin	10.0	25–29	35–39	6–7	17–23
	80.0	45	60	5	37
Cerivastatin	0.3	19	28	10	13
Fluvastatin	20.0	16	20–25	5	10
	80.0	22	30–35	8	15
Lovastatin	20.0	17–19	24–27	6–7	10
	80.0	29–34	40–42	8–10	19–27
Pravastatin	20.0	19–24	26–32	2–6	11
	40.0	21–25	27–34	5–12	11–24
Simvastatin	20.0	25–28	34–38	6–8	15
	80.0	36	47	8	24

HDL—high-density lipoprotein; LDL—low-density lipoprotein; TG—triglyceride.

Adapted from Kong SX, Crawford SY, Gandhi SK, et al.: Efficacy of 3-hydroxy-3methylglutaryl coenzyme A reductase inhibitors in the treatment of patients with hypercholesterolemia: a meta-analysis of clinical trials. Clin Ther 1997; 19:778–97.

rate limiting step in cholesterol synthesis: the conversion of HMG-CoA to mevalonic acid. Rates of synthesis of LDL receptors are inversely related to the amount of cholesterol in cells; thus, the action of HMG-CoA reductase inhibitors reduces cholesterol synthesis, reduces cellular concentrations of cholesterol, and increases the expression of LDL receptors in the liver. Because LDL receptors are responsible for clearing two thirds to three fourths of plasma LDL (and the associated cholesterol), HMG-CoA reductase inhibitors may promote the clearance of LDL as well as VLDL and VLDL remnants. They may also, by reducing cholesterol synthesis, interfere with the hepatic formation of lipoproteins. Because cholesterol synthesis peaks at night, the HMG-CoA reductase inhibitors should be given before the patient goes to bed. HMG-CoA reductase inhibitors may also act by inhibiting platelet aggregation, macrophage foam cell formation, and LDL oxidation, major contributors to atherogenesis.

INDICATIONS

	Atorvastatin	Cerivastatin	Fluvastatin	Lovastatin	Pravastatin	Simvastatin
Type I hyperlipoproteinemia	–	–	–	–	–	–
Type IIa hyperlipoproteinemia	+	+	+	+	+	+
Type IIb hyperlipoproteinemia	+	+	+	+	+	+
Type III hyperlipoproteinemia	+	–	–	–	–	–
Type IV hyperlipoproteinemia	+	–	–	–	–	–
Type V hyperlipoproteinemia	–	–	–	–	–	–

TABLE 11-4 LARGE-SCALE PLACEBO-CONTROLLED STUDIES ASSESSING THE EFFECT OF HMG-CoA REDUCTASE INHIBITORS ON CARDIOVASCULAR MORBIDITY AND MORTALITY

Study	Sample size	Mean or median follow-up, y	CAD?	Drug regimen, mg/d	Mean or median baseline total (LDL) cholesterol concentration, mg/dL*	Mean or median post-treatment total (LDL) cholesterol concentration, mg/dL*	Result of primary endpoint compared to placebo*
4S	4444	5.4	Yes	S 20–40	261 (188)	196 (122)	30% reduction in total mortality
WOSCOPS	6595	4.9	No	P 40	272 (192)	218 (142)	31% reduction in definite nonfatal MI and death from CHD
CARE	4159	5.0	Yes	P 40	209 (139)	NR (97–98)	24% reduction in fatal CHD or nonfatal MI
AFCAPS/TexCAPS	6605	5.2	No	L 20–40	221 (150)†	184 (115)‡	37% reduction in fatal or nonfatal MI, unstable angina, or sudden cardiac death
LIPID	9014	6.1	Yes	P40	218 (150)	179 (NR)	24% reduction in death from CHD

* For the group receiving drug unless stated otherwise.

† For placebo and drug groups combined

‡ At 1-year follow up.

4S — Scandinavian Simvastatin Survival Study; AFCAPS/TexCAPS—Air Force Coronary/Texas Atherosclerosis Prevention Study; CAD—coronary artery disease; CARE—Cholesterol and Recurrent Events Trial; CHD —coronary heart disease; L — lovastatin; LDL—low density lipoprotein; LIPID — Long-Term Intervention with Pravastatin in Ischaemic Diseases; MI—myocardial infarction; NR—not reported; P — pravastatin; S—simvastatin; WOSCOPS — West of Scotland Coronary Prevention Study.

ATORVASTATIN (Lipitor®)

Atorvastatin is a synthetic, reversible HMG-CoA reductase inhibitor indicated for types II, III, and IV hyperlipidemias. Maximum dosages of 80 mg per day have been shown to decrease LDL cholesterol concentrations by 60% in patients with type II hyperlipidemia . This is in comparison to the maximum dosages of other HMG-CoA reductase inhibitors, which yield 30% to 50% reductions in LDL. Atorvastatin (80 mg/day) has also been shown to decrease triglyceride concentrations by 37% in patients with type II hyperlipidemia, compared to 13% to 27% reductions with other HMG-CoA reductase inhibitors. Reductions in triglyceride concentrations of 26% to 46% have been demonstrated with atorvastatin in patients with hypertriglyceridemia, comparable to the 35% to 44% reductions seen with other HMG-CoA reductase inhibitors. Increases in HDL concentrations produced by atorvastatin range from about 5% to 13%, similar to that seen with other HMG-CoA reductase inhibitors.

Atorvastatin has also been shown to lower LDL concentrations to NCEP target levels faster than other HMG-CoA reductase inhibitors. The MIRACL study is currently investigating whether or not aggressive lipid-lowering therapy with atorvastatin, given within 1 to 4 days of hospitalization for unstable angina or acute non–Q-wave MI, will reduce early ischemic events in this patient population. The AVERT study recently demonstrated atorvastatin to be at least as good as coronary angioplasty in reducing cardiovascular events in patients with CAD. The effects of atorvastatin on mortality from CHD have not been evaluated. Two additional trials are currently being conducted: Treat to New Targets (TNT) and Stroke Prevention by Aggressive Reduction of Cholesterol Levels (SPARCL). TNT is investigating the impact of lowering LDL with atorvastatin to target levels of around 75 mg/dL compared with current treatment target levels of 100 mg/dL on cardiovascular endpoints in patients with CAD. SPARCL is investigating whether aggressive lipid lowering will reduce the reoccurrence of cerebrovascular events in patients with a history of stroke and no CAD.

SPECIAL GROUPS

Race: not evaluated
Children: safety and efficacy not established
Elderly: no dosage adjustment is required
Renal impairment: no dosage adjustment is required
Hepatic impairment: liver disease may increase plasma concentrations of atorvastatin
Pregnancy: category X; if the woman becomes pregnant while on atorvastatin, the drug should be discontinued
Breast-feeding: contraindicated

DOSAGE

Usual initial dosage is 10 mg once daily. Dosage may be titrated every 2–4 wk up to 80 mg once daily.

IN BRIEF

INDICATIONS
As adjunctive therapy to diet in adult patients with elevated cholesterol and/or triglyceride concentrations (types II, III, and IV hyperlipidemias).

CONTRAINDICATIONS
Acute liver disease or persistent elevations of serum transaminases; pregnancy; hypersensitivity to product components.

DRUG INTERACTIONS
Cyclosporine
Fibric acid derivatives
Niacin
Erythromycin
Azole antifungals
Antacids
Colestipol
Digoxin (unknown clinical significance)
Norethindrone (unknown clinical significance)
Ethinyl estradiol (unknown clinical significance)

ADVERSE EFFECTS
CNS: dizziness (≥2%), insomnia (≥2%)
Respiratory: bronchitis (≥2%), rhinitis (≥2%)
GI: diarrhea (3%–5%), nausea (≥2%), constipation (1%–2%)
Skin: rash (1%–4%)
Urogenital: urinary tract infection (≥2%)
Extremities: peripheral edema (≥2%)
Hepatic: serum transaminases >three times upper limit of normal (0.7%)
Musculoskeletal: myalgia (1%–6%), arthritis (≥2%), rhabdomyolysis (<1%)
Hematologic: thrombocytopenia (<1%)
Other: infections (3%–10%), chest pain (≥2%), abdominal pain (2%–4%), headache (3%–17%)

PHARMACOKINETICS AND PHARMACODYNAMICS
Duration of action: 4–6 wk after discontinuation
Onset of action: within 2 wk
Peak effect: within 4 wk
Bioavailability: 14%; systemic availability of HMG-CoA reductase inhibition: 30%
Effect of food: food decreases rate and extent of absorption, but does not impair efficacy
Metabolism: extensive hepatic metabolism (most likely by CYP3A4) to active metabolites, which account for 70% of the clinical effect
Elimination: primarily in bile
Elimination half-life: 14 h; 20–30 h half-life for HMG-CoA reductase inhibition
Protein binding: ≥98%

MONITORING
Plasma lipid profile, serum transaminases, signs and symptoms of muscle pain, tenderness, or weakness.

OVERDOSE
Treatment should be symptomatic and supportive. Atorvastatin is not removed by hemodialysis.

PATIENT INFORMATION
If you miss a dose, take it as soon as you remember. If it is about time for the next dose, take that dose only. Do not take two doses at once. If blurred vision, muscle pain, tenderness or weakness occurs, notify your clinician. Follow your prescribed diet. This medication should not be taken during pregnancy due to possible harm to the fetus. Notify your clinician as soon as possible if you become pregnant or intend to become pregnant while taking this medication.

AVAILABILITY
Tablets, film-coated—10, 20, and 40 mg

The information here is provided as guidance only. Prescribers should always consult the manufacturer's current prescribing information.

229

CERIVASTATIN
(Baycol®)

On a milligram per milligram basis, cerivastatin is the most pharmacologically potent HMG-CoA reductase inhibitor, with an approved recommended dosage of 0.4 mg and lower dosages for patients with renal dysfunction. Cerivastatin is effective in reducing LDL-C and helps the majority of patients reach NCEP goals. Cerivastatin is a synthetic, water-soluble HMG-CoA reductase inhibitor which undergoes significant first-pass metabolism and exhibits dose-dependent pharmacokinetics. Cerivastatin has high affinity for hepatic tissue, is extensively (99%) bound to plasma proteins, and is metabolized in the liver via two cytochrome P450 isoenzymes, CYP2C8 and CYP3A4. Cerivastatin is excreted primarily as metabolites in the feces and to a lesser extent in the urine.

Studies with cerivastatin 0.4 mg have shown a 34% mean reduction in LDL-C, a 24% mean reduction in Total-C, a 26% mean reduction in apo B, and a 16% median reduction in TG. Cerivastatin 0.4 mg also increased HDL-C by 7% and, in patients with baseline triglycerides 250–500 mg/dL, cerivastatin 0.4 mg reduced triglycerides by a median of 30%. The effects upon these and other lipid parameters were demonstrated in two pivotal and other supportive clinical trials. Mean reduction in LDL-C at 8 weeks in these studies ranged from 33%–39%. The LDL-C lowering action of cerivastatin 0.4 mg is significantly greater than that seen with cerivastatin 0.3 mg.

Studies completed comparing cerivastatin 0.4 mg with other statins have demonstrated that cerivastatin 0.4 mg is more effective in lowering LDL-C than fluvastatin 40 mg and pravastatin 40 mg. In addition, cerivastatin 0.4 mg is equally effective in lowering LDL-C as lovastatin 40 mg.

Cerivastatin possesses a favorable drug interaction profile as a result of uncomplicated pharmacokinetic properties, a dual metabolic pathway, and the lack of clinically relevant interactions as demonstrated in pharmacokinetic studies with cimetidine, antacids, digoxin, nifedipine, omeprazole, or warfarin. The combined use of cerivastatin and gemfibrozil should be avoided.

Although the effect of cerivastatin upon cardiovascular morbidity and mortality has not been determined, studies have begun enrolling patients to determine the effect of cerivastatin upon the reduction of risk for cardiovascular events in patients with diabetes, the effect upon the reduction of risk of first stroke in elderly patients, and the effect of treatment in postmenopausal women. Additional comparative trials and trials with higher doses are currently being conducted.

SPECIAL GROUPS

Race: no significant differences in pharmacokinetics

Children: safety and efficacy not established

Elderly: no dosage adjustment is required

Renal impairment: plasma cerivastatin concentrations may be elevated in patients with a creatinine clearance ≤ 60 mL/min/1.73 m^2

Hepatic impairment: not evaluated, but contraindicated with acute liver disease or persistent elevations in serum transaminases

Pregnancy: category X; if the woman becomes pregnant while on cerivastatin, the drug should be discontinued

Breast-feeding: contraindicated

DOSAGE

Recommended dosage is 0.4 mg once daily in the evening. Starting dosages of 0.3 or 0.2 mg once daily are recommended in patients with moderate to severe renal dysfunction.

IN BRIEF

INDICATIONS
As adjunctive therapy to diet for the reduction of elevated total and LDL cholesterol levels in patients with primary hypercholesterolemia and mixed dyslipidemia (types IIa and IIb hyperlipidemias)

As an adjunct to diet in the reduction of elevated triglyceride and ApoB levels in patients with primary hypercholesterolemia and mixed dyslipidemia

CONTRAINDICATIONS
Acute liver disease or unexplained persistent elevations of serum transaminases; pregnancy; hypersensitivity to product components.

DRUG INTERACTIONS
Cyclosporine
Fibric acid derivatives
Bile acid sequestrants
Niacin
Erythromycin
Azole antifungals

ADVERSE EFFECTS
CNS: dizziness (2%), insomnia (2%)
Respiratory: rhinitis (11%), pharyngitis (13%), sinusitis (6%)
GI: dyspepsia (4%), diarrhea (3%)
Skin: rash (3%)
Hepatic: serum transaminases >three times upper limit of normal (<0.5%)
Musculoskeletal: arthralgia (7%), myalgia (3%), rhabdomyolysis (<1%)
Other: headache (10%), flu syndrome (5%), asthenia (3%), chest pain (2%)

PHARMACODYNAMICS AND PHARMACOKINETICS
Duration of action: 4–6 wk after discontinuation
Onset of action: within 1 wk
Peak effect: 3–4 wk
Bioavailability: 60% (range 39%–100%)
Effect of food: no effect
Metabolism: hepatic metabolism by CYP2C8 and CYP3A4 with greater affinity for CYP2C8. Two active metabolites, which are 50% and 100% as active as the parent compound; parent compound responsible for most of the clinical activity.
Elimination: active metabolites: 24% recovered in the urine, 70% in the feces
Elimination half-life: 2–3 h
Protein binding: >99%

MONITORING
Plasma lipid profile, serum transaminases, signs and symptoms of muscle pain, tenderness, or weakness, especially if accompanied by malaise or fever.

OVERDOSE
Treatment should be symptomatic and supportive. Cerivastatin is not removed by hemodialysis.

PATIENT INFORMATION
If you miss a dose, take it as soon as you remember. If it is about time for the next dose, take that dose only. Do not take two doses at once. If any unexplained muscle pain, tenderness, or weakness occurs, especially if accompanied by malaise or fever, notify your clinician. Follow your prescribed diet. This medication should not be taken during pregnancy due to possible harm to the fetus. Notify your clinician as soon as possible if you become pregnant or intend to become pregnant while taking this medication.

AVAILABILITY
Tablets—0.2, 0.3, 0.4 mg

FLUVASTATIN (Lescol®)

In 1993, fluvastatin became the first entirely synthetic HMG-CoA reductase approved for use in the United States. At initial dosages, fluvastatin is generally believed to produce the most modest reduction in cholesterol concentrations compared to other available HMG-CoA reductase inhibitors. However, one study showed the maximum dosage of 80 mg per day to decrease LDL cholesterol concentrations more than the maximum dosage of pravastatin (40 mg/day) in patients with type II hyperlipidemia. The least expensive HMG-CoA reductase inhibitor, fluvastatin, may be the most cost-effective drug in this class for lowering cholesterol in patients with mild-to-moderate hypercholesterolemia. Since maximum dosages of fluvastatin would be expected to yield a 30%–35% reduction in LDL cholesterol, patients requiring greater LDL-cholesterol lowering are likely to receive greater benefits from other HMG-CoA reductase inhibitors.

Fluvastatin has also been shown to slow the progression of CAD and may also promote atherosclerotic plaque regression. The efficacy of fluvastatin in reducing cardiovascular mortality and morbidity is currently being investigated. The Lipoprotein and Coronary Atherosclerosis Study showed a nonstatistically significant reduction in clinical events (cardiac morbidity or any fatal event) and need for revascularization in hypercholesterolemic patients receiving fluvastatin compared to placebo. The recently reported Lescol in Severe Atherosclerosis Study demonstrated a 71% reduction in cardiac events (death from cardiovascular causes, MI, occurrence of unstable angina or coronary artery bypass surgery) with fluvastatin compared to placebo in 365 patients with elevated cholesterol and CAD.

Fluvastatin also appears to have unique antifungal activity (mechanism unknown), which may be clinically beneficial when combined with azole antifungal drugs.

SPECIAL GROUPS

Race: not evaluated
Children: safety and efficacy not established
Elderly: no dosage adjustment is required
Renal impairment: no dosage adjustment is required; use cautiously with severe renal impairment
Hepatic impairment: use cautiously since liver disease may increase plasma concentrations of fluvastatin
Pregnancy: category X; if the woman becomes pregnant while on fluvastatin, the drug should be discontinued
Breast-feeding: contraindicated

DOSAGE

Usual initial dosage is 20–40 mg once daily at bedtime. Dosage may be titrated every 4 wk up to 80 mg daily in two divided doses.

IN BRIEF

INDICATIONS
As adjunctive therapy to diet for the treatment of elevated total and LDL cholesterol in patients with type II hyperlipidemia
To slow the progression of coronary atherosclerosis in patients with CHD
As an adjunct to diet in the treatment of elevated triglyceride and ApoB levels in patients with primary hypercholesterolemia and mixed dyslipidemia

CONTRAINDICATIONS
Acute liver disease or persistent elevations of serum transaminases; pregnancy; hypersensitivity to product components.

DRUG INTERACTIONS
Cyclosporine
Gemfibrozil
Cholestyramine
Niacin
Erythromycin
Cimetidine
Ranitidine
Omeprazole
Rifampicin
Digoxin (unknown clinical significance)
Warfarin (unknown clinical significance)

ADVERSE EFFECTS
CNS: dizziness (2%), insomnia (3%)
Respiratory: upper respiratory infections (16%) sinusitis (3%), rhinitis (5%)
GI: diarrhea (5%), nausea (3%), constipation (3%), dyspepsia (8%), flatulence (3%)
Skin: rash (2%)
Hepatic: serum transaminases > three times upper limit of normal (0.2%–2.7%)
Musculoskeletal: myalgia (5%), arthritis (2%), myopathy, rhabdomyolysis (<1%)
Other: flu-like symptoms (5%), abdominal pain (5%), headache (9%), fatigue (3%)

PHARMACOKINETICS AND PHARMACODYNAMICS
Duration of action: 4–6 wk after discontinuation
Onset of action: within 2 wk
Peak effect: 4 wk
Bioavailability: 24%
Effect of food: food decreases rate but not extent of absorption
Metabolism: extensive hepatic metabolism, primarily via CYP2C9; no active metabolites are present systemically
Elimination: about 90% eliminated in the feces as metabolites, <2% as unchanged drug
Elimination half-life: 2–3 h
Protein binding: 98%

MONITORING
Plasma lipid profile, serum transaminases, signs and symptoms of muscle pain, tenderness, or weakness.

OVERDOSE
Treatment should be symptomatic and supportive.
The dialyzability of fluvastatin is not known at present.

PATIENT INFORMATION
If you miss a dose, take it as soon as you remember. If it is about time for the next dose, take that dose only. Do not take two doses at once. If blurred vision, muscle pain, tenderness or weakness occurs, notify your clinician. Follow your prescribed diet. This medication should not be taken during pregnancy due to possible harm to the fetus. Notify your clinician as soon as possible if you become pregnant or intend to become pregnant while taking this medication.

AVAILABILITY
Capsules—20 and 40 mg

LOVASTATIN
(Mevacor®)

Lovastatin is an HMG-CoA reductase inhibitor derived from a strain of the fungus *Aspergillus terreus*. In 1987, lovastatin became the first HMG CoA reductase inhibitor approved for use in the United States. Lovastatin itself is inactive, but is hydrolyzed in vivo to the active beta hydroxyacid metabolite. Starting dosages of 20 mg/day have been shown to decrease total cholesterol by a mean of 17%, decrease LDL by 24%, and increase HDL by 7%. Maximum dosages of 80 mg/day decrease total cholesterol by a mean of 29%, decrease LDL by 40%, and increase HDL by 10%. Triglycerides are decreased by a median of 10% and 19% at daily doses of 20 and 80 mg, respectively. Lovastatin has been shown to slow the progression of atherosclerosis in several trials as well as promote the regression of atherosclerotic plaques. Combining lovastatin with cholestyramine results in additive cholesterol-lowering effects.

The AFCAPS/TexCAPS Study demonstrated the benefit of lovastatin in preventing coronary events in men and women with no prior history of atherosclerotic cardiovascular disease and a mean total cholesterol concentration of 221 mg/dL, LDL concentration of 150 mg/dL and HDL concentration of 36 mg/dL for men and 40 mg/dL for women. After a mean follow-up of 5.2 years, the risk of MI, unstable angina, or sudden cardiac death was reduced by 37% with lovastatin treatment compared to placebo.

SPECIAL GROUPS

Race: not evaluated

Children: not recommended; safety and efficacy not established

Elderly: no dosage adjustment is required

Renal impairment: dosages above 20 mg/d should be used cautiously in patients with creatinine clearances <30 mL/min

Hepatic impairment: use cautiously in patients who consume substantial quantities of alcohol or have a past history of liver disease; contraindicated with acute liver disease

Pregnancy: category X; if the woman becomes pregnant while on lovastatin, the drug should be discontinued

Breast-feeding: contraindicated

DOSAGE

Usual initial dosage is 20 mg once daily for patients requiring ≥ 20% reductions in LDL and 10 mg once daily for patients requiring LDL reductions of <20%, administered with the evening meal. Dosage may be titrated every 4 wk or more up to 80 mg once daily or in divided doses. If used in combination with fibrates or niacin, the dose of lovastatin should not exceed 20 mg.

IN BRIEF

INDICATIONS
As adjunctive therapy to diet for reducing elevated total and LDL cholesterol concentrations in patients with type IIa or IIb hyperlipidemia

Slowing coronary atherosclerosis progression in patients with CHD

Primary prevention of CHD in individuals without symptomatic cardiovascular disease who have average to moderately elevated total cholesterol and LDL cholesterol, and below average HDL cholesterol

CONTRAINDICATIONS
Acute liver disease or persistent elevations of serum transaminases; pregnancy; breast-feeding; hypersensitivity to product components.

DRUG INTERACTIONS
Cyclosporine
Fibric acid derivatives
Niacin
Macrolide antibiotics
Nefazodone
Azole antifungals
Diltiazem
Warfarin (unknown clinical significance)

ADVERSE EFFECTS
CNS: dizziness (1%–2%), headache (2%–10%)
GI: dyspepsia (1%–4%), diarrhea (2%–6%), nausea (2%–5%), constipation (2%–5%), flatulence (3%–6%), abdominal pain (2%–6%)
Skin: rash (1%–5%)
Hepatic: serum transaminases >three times upper limit of normal (1.9%)
Musculoskeletal: myalgia (1%–3%), muscle cramps (1%), rhabdomyolysis (<1%)
Special senses: blurred vision (1%)
Other: asthenia (1% –2%)

PHARMACOKINETICS AND PHARMACODYNAMICS
Duration of action: 4–6 wk after discontinuation
Onset of action: within 2 wk
Peak effect: 4–6 wk
Bioavailability: <5% due to extensive hepatic extraction
Effect of food: food increases bioavailability by 50%
Metabolism: extensive hepatic metabolism predominantly by CYP3A4 to active metabolites, most notably the beta hydroxyacid metabolite
Elimination: 10% of a dose is excreted in the urine; 83% in the feces (biliary excretion and unabsorbed drug)
Elimination half-life: 1.1–1.7 h
Protein binding: >95%

MONITORING
Plasma lipid profile, serum transaminases, signs and symptoms of muscle pain, tenderness, or weakness.

OVERDOSE
Treatment should be symptomatic and supportive.
The dialyzability of lovastatin is presently unknown.

PATIENT INFORMATION
Take with food, preferably in the evening. If you miss a dose, take it as soon as you remember. If it is about time for the next dose, take that dose only. Do not take two doses at once. If blurred vision, muscle pain, tenderness or weakness occurs, notify your clinician. Follow your prescribed diet. This medication should not be taken during pregnancy due to possible harm to the fetus. Notify your clinician as soon as possible if you become pregnant or intend to become pregnant while taking this medication.

AVAILABILITY
Tablets, film-coated—10, 20, and 40 mg

PRAVASTATIN (Pravachol®)

Approved in 1991, pravastatin was the second HMG-CoA reductase inhibitor available for use in the United States. Unlike lovastatin and simvastatin, pravastatin is administered in the active form. Average reductions in LDL of 34% may be seen with pravastatin 40 mg once daily, and reductions of greater than or equal to 50% may be achieved by combining pravastatin with cholestyramine. Pravastatin has been shown to slow the progression of atherosclerosis in several trials as well as reduce the risk of MI and death.

Pravastatin, in a dosage of 40 mg once daily, has been shown to decrease mortality in placebo-controlled studies in patients with a wide range of plasma cholesterol concentrations. The WOSCOP study demonstrated pravastatin to reduce the rate of MI or death by 31% in men with no prior history of MI and a mean total cholesterol concentration of 272 mg/dL. In patients with a history of MI and a mean total cholesterol concentration of 209 mg/dL, pravastatin yielded a 24% risk reduction for the same endpoint in the CARE trial. The LIPID study showed pravastatin to reduce the risk of death from CHD by 24% in patients with a history of MI or unstable angina and a total cholesterol concentration ranging between 155 and 271 mg/dL. The effect of pravastatin on specific subgroups, such as women and the elderly, in these three studies is being examined by the ongoing Prospective Pravastatin Pooling Project .

SPECIAL GROUPS

Race: not evaluated
Children: not recommended; safety and efficacy not established
Elderly: no dosage adjustment is required
Renal impairment: no dosage adjustment is required; patients with renal impairment should be closely monitored
Hepatic impairment: use cautiously in patients who consume substantial quantities of alcohol or have a past history of liver disease; contraindicated with acute liver disease
Pregnancy: category X; if the woman becomes pregnant while on pravastatin, the drug should be discontinued.
Breast-feeding: contraindicated

DOSAGE

Usual initial dosage is 20 mg once daily at bedtime; 10 mg once daily for elderly patients, patients with hepatic or renal impairment, or patients taking drugs that increase the risk of myopathy. Dosage may be titrated every 4 wk up to a maximum dosage of 40 mg once daily; daily dosages > 20 mg should be used cautiously in elderly patients or patients taking drugs which increase the risk of myopathy.

IN BRIEF

INDICATIONS
As adjunctive therapy to diet for reducing elevated total and LDL cholesterol and triglyceride concentrations in patients with type IIa or IIb hyperlipidemia

Slowing coronary atherosclerosis progression and reducing the risk of acute coronary events in patients with clinically evident CAD

Primary prevention of coronary events in hypercholesterolemic patients without clinically evident CHD

Secondary prevention of cardiovascular events and cerebrovascular events in patients with normal (below the 75th percentile of the general population) cholesterol levels

CONTRAINDICATIONS
Acute liver disease or persistent elevations of serum transaminases; pregnancy; breast-feeding; hypersensitivity to product components.

DRUG INTERACTIONS
Immunosuppressive drugs
Gemfibrozil
Niacin
Cholestyramine
Colestipol
Erythromycin

ADVERSE EFFECTS
Cardiac: cardiac chest pain (4%)
CNS: dizziness (3.3%), headache (6.2%)
GI: heartburn (2.9%), diarrhea (6.2%), nausea/vomiting (7.3%), constipation (4%), flatulence (3.3%), abdominal pain (5.4%)
Skin: rash (4%)
Hepatic: serum transaminases > three times upper limit of normal (1.3%)
Musculoskeletal: myalgia (2.7%), localized pain (10%)
Respiratory: cough (2.6%), common cold (7%), rhinitis (4%)
Other: influenza (2.4%), chest pain (3.7%), fatigue (3.8%)

PHARMACOKINETICS AND PHARMACODYNAMICS
Duration of action: 4–6 wk after discontinuation
Onset of action: within 2 wk
Peak effect: 4–6 wk
Bioavailability: 17% due to extensive hepatic extraction
Effect of food: food may decrease bioavailability somewhat, but does not diminish clinical efficacy
Metabolism: hepatic metabolism to inactive or weakly active metabolites. Pravastatin is not metabolized to a clinically significant extent by CYP450 3A4
Elimination: 20% of a dose is excreted in the urine; 70% in the feces (biliary excretion and unabsorbed drug)
Elimination half-life: 1.8 h
Protein binding: 50%

MONITORING
Plasma lipid profile, serum transaminases, signs and symptoms of muscle pain, tenderness, or weakness.

OVERDOSE
Treatment should be symptomatic and supportive.

PATIENT INFORMATION
Take 1 h before or 4 h after cholestyramine or colestipol. Take at bedtime for maximum effect. If you miss a dose, take it as soon as you remember. If it is about time for the next dose, take that dose only. Do not take two doses at once. If blurred vision, muscle pain, tenderness or weakness occurs, notify your clinician. Follow your prescribed diet. This medication should not be taken during pregnancy due to possible harm to the fetus. Notify your clinician as soon as possible if you become pregnant or intend to become pregnant while taking this medication.

AVAILABILITY
Tablets—10, 20 , and 40 mg

The information here is provided as guidance only. Prescribers should always consult the manufacturer's current prescribing information.

233

SIMVASTATIN (Zocor®)

Simvastatin was the third HMG-CoA reductase inhibitor available for use in the United States, receiving approval from the FDA in 1991 immediately after pravastatin. Simvastatin, like lovastatin, is derived from the fungus *Aspergillus terreus* and is itself inactive, requiring in vivo hydrolysis to the active beta hydroxyacid form for clinical effect. Lovastatin and simvastatin differ chemically by only a single methyl group.

Simvastatin has shown efficacy at reducing LDL cholesterol concentrations in patients with homozygous familial hypercholesterolemia, in which LDL-receptor activity is absent or severely diminished. The Multicenter Anti-Atheroma Study showed simvastatin 20 mg daily to slow the progression of atherosclerosis, reduce the proportion of patients with new atherosclerotic lesions, and promote the regression of atherosclerotic plaques in hypercholesterolemic patients with CHD.

Data supporting the use of simvastatin for the treatment of patients with CHD originated from the Scandinavian Simvastatin Survival Study (4S). This trial utilized 20 to 40 mg daily of simvastatin to reduce the risk of mortality by 30%, hospital verified nonfatal MI by 37%, and myocardial revascularization by 37% compared to placebo in patients with a mean baseline total cholesterol concentration of 261 mg/dL, a mean LDL concentration of 188 mg/dL, and a history of angina or acute MI. Simvastatin also reduced the risk of fatal plus nonfatal cerebrovascular events (strokes and transient ischemic attacks [TIAs]) by 28%.

SPECIAL GROUPS

Race: not evaluated

Children: not recommended; safety and efficacy not established

Elderly: dosages ≤20 mg daily are usually sufficient for maximum LDL reduction

Renal impairment: no dosage adjustment is required for patients with mild to moderate renal insufficiency. Patients with severe renal insufficiency should be started at 5 mg daily and closely monitored

Hepatic impairment: use cautiously in patients who consume substantial quantities of alcohol and/or have a past history of liver disease; contraindicated with acute liver disease

Pregnancy: category X; if the woman becomes pregnant while on simvastatin, the drug should be discontinued

Breast-feeding: contraindicated

DOSAGE

Usual initial dosage is 20 mg once daily in the evening, 10 mg once daily for patients requiring only a moderate reduction in LDL cholesterol. Patients taking cyclosporine or who have severe renal insufficiency should be started on 5 mg daily. The recommended dosage for patients with homozygous familial hypercholesterolemia is 40 mg every evening or 80 mg daily in three divided doses (20 mg, 20 mg, and an evening dose of 40 mg). Dosage may be titrated every 4 wk or more up to a maximum dosage of 80 mg every evening. Daily dosages > 20 mg are usually not required in elderly patients. If used in combination with cyclosporine, fibrates or niacin, the daily dosage of simvastatin should not exceed 10 mg.

IN BRIEF

INDICATIONS

As adjunctive therapy to diet for reducing elevated total and LDL cholesterol and triglyceride concentrations in patients with type IIa or IIb hyperlipidemia

Reducing total and LDL cholesterol in patients with homozygous familial hypercholesterolemia

Reducing the risk of death, MI, stroke or TIA, and undergoing myocardial revascularization procedures in patients with CHD and hypercholesterolemia

Increasing HDL cholesterol levels

CONTRAINDICATIONS

Acute liver disease or persistent elevations of serum transaminases; pregnancy; breast-feeding; hypersensitivity to product components.

DRUG INTERACTIONS

Cyclosporine
Fibric acid derivatives
Niacin
Macrolide antibiotics
Nefazadone
Azole antifungals
Warfarin (unknown clinical significance)
Digoxin (unknown clinical significance)

ADVERSE EFFECTS

CNS: headache (3.5%)
GI: dyspepsia (1%), diarrhea (0.5%–2%), nausea (1%), constipation (2.3%), flatulence (1%–2%), abdominal pain (3.2%)
Skin: rash (0.6%), eczema (0.8%), pruritis (0.5%)
Hepatic: serum transaminases >three times upper limit of normal (≈1%)
Musculoskeletal: myalgia, muscle cramps, rhabdomyolysis (<1%)
Respiratory: upper respiratory infection (2.1%)
Special senses: cataract (0.5%)
Other: asthenia (1.6%)

PHARMACOKINETICS AND PHARMACODYNAMICS

Duration of action: 4–6 wk after discontinuation
Onset of action: within 2 wk
Peak effect: 4–6 wk
Bioavailability: <5% due to extensive hepatic extraction
Effect of food: none
Metabolism: extensive hepatic metabolism, in part by CYP3A4, to active metabolites, most notably the beta hydroxyacid metabolite
Elimination: 13% of a dose is excreted in the urine; 60% in the feces (biliary excretion and unabsorbed drug)
Elimination half-life: 1.9 h
Protein binding: ≈95%

MONITORING

Plasma lipid profile, serum transaminases, signs and symptoms of muscle pain, tenderness, or weakness.

OVERDOSE

Treatment should be symptomatic and supportive. The dialyzability of simvastatin is presently unknown.

PATIENT INFORMATION

Take in the evening for maximum benefit. If you miss a dose, take it as soon as you remember. If it is about time for the next dose, take that dose only. Do not take two doses at once. If blurred vision, muscle pain, tenderness or weakness occurs, notify your clinician. Follow your prescribed diet. This medication should not be taken during pregnancy due to possible harm to the fetus. Notify your clinician as soon as possible if you become pregnant or intend to become pregnant while taking this medication.

AVAILABILITY

Tablets, film-coated—5, 10, 20, 40, and 80 mg

Adkins JC, Faulds D: Micronised fenofibrate. A review of its pharmacodynamic properties and clinical efficacy in the management of dyslipidaemia. *Drugs* 1997, 54:615–633.

Anonymous:Cerivastatin for hypercholesterolemia. *Med Lett Drugs Ther* 1998, 40:13–14.

Anonymous: Choice of lipid-lowering drugs. *Med Lett Drugs Ther* 1998, 40:117–122.

Anonymous: Fenofibrate for hypertriglyceridemia. *Med Lett Drugs Ther* 1998, 40:68–69.

Ascah KJ, Rock GA, Wells PS: Interaction between fenofibrate and warfarin. *Ann Pharmacother* 1998, 32:765–768.

Austin MA, Hokanson JE, Edwards KL: Hypertriglyceridemia as a cardiovascular risk factor. *Am J Cardiol* 1998, 81 (suppl.):7B–12B.

Aviram M, Hussein O, Rosenblat M, *et al.*:Interactions of platelets, macrophages, and lipoproteins in hypercholesterolemia: antiatherogenic effects of HMG-CoA reductase inhibitor therapy. *J Cardiovasc Pharmacol* 1998, 31:39–45.

Betteridge DJ, Bhatnager D, Bing RF, *et al.*: Treatment of familial hypercholesterolaemia. United Kingdom lipid clinics study of pravastatin and cholestyramine. *Br Med J* 1992, 304:1335–1338.

Blankenhorn DH, Azen SP, Dramsch DM, *et al.*: Coronary angiographic changes with lovastatin therapy. The Monitored Atherosclerosis Regression Study (MARS). *An Intern Med* 1993, 119:969–976.

Blankenhorn DH, Nessim SA, Johnson RL, *et al.*:Beneficial effects of combined colestipol-niacin therapy on coronary atherosclerosis and coronary venous bypass grafts. *JAMA* 1987, 257:3233–3240.

Bradford RH, Shear CL, Chremos AN, *et al.*: Expanded Clinical Evaluation of Lovastatin (EXCEL) study results. I. Efficacy in modifying plasma lipoproteins and adverse event profile in 8245 patients with moderate hypercholesterolemia. *Arch Intern Med* 1991, 151:43–49.

Brensike JF, Levy RI, Kelsey SF, *et al.*: Effects of therapy with cholestyramine on progression of coronary arteriosclerosis: results of the NHLBI Type II Coronary Intervention Study. *Circulation* 1984, 69:313–324.

Brown WV: Niacin for lipid disorders. Indications, effectiveness, and safety. *Postgrad Med* 1995, 98:185–193.

Brown G, Albers JJ, Fisher LD, *et al.*: Regression of coronary artery disease as a result of intensive lipid-lowering theapy in men with high levels of apolipoprotein B. *N Engl J Med* 1990, 323:1289–1298.

Brown AS, Bakker-Arkema RG, Yellen L, *et al*: Treating patients with documented atherosclerosis to National Cholesterol Education Program-recommended low-density-lipoprotein cholesterol goals with atorvastatin, fluvastatin, lovastatin, and simvastatin. *J Am Coll Cardiol* 1998, 32:665–673.

Bucher HC, Griffith LE, Guyatt GH: Effect of HMGCoA reductase inhibitors on stroke. A meta-analysis of randomized, controlled trials. *Arch Intern Med* 1998, 128:89–95.

Byington RP, Furberg CD, Crouse JR III, *et al.*: Pravastatin, Lipids, and Atherosclerosis in the Carotid Arteries (PLAC-II). *Am J Cardiol* 1995, 76 (suppl. C):54C–59C.

Canner PI, Berge KG, Wenger NK, *et al.*: Fifteen year mortality in Coronary Drug Project patients: long-term benefit with niacin. *J Am Coll Cardiol* 1986, 8:1245–1255.

Carlson LA, Hamsten A, Asplund A: Pronounced lowering of serum levels of lipoprotein Lp(a) in hyperlipidaemic subjects treated with nicotinic acid. *J Intern Med* 1989, 226:271–276.

Carlson LA, Rosenhamer G: Reduction of mortality in the Stockholm Ischaemic Heart Disease Secondary Prevention Study by combined treatment with clofibrate and nicotinic acid *Acta Med Scand* 1988, 223:405–418.

Cashin-Hemphill L, Mack WJ, Pogoda JM, *et al.*: Beneficial effects of colestipol-niacin on coronary atherosclerosis: a 4-year follow-up. *JAMA* 1990, 264:3013–3017.

Castelli WP, Garrison RJ, Wilson PWF, *et al.*: Incidence of coronary heart disease and lipoprotein cholesterol levels. *JAMA* 1986, 256:2835–2838.

Chin NX, Weitzman I, Della-Latta P: In vitro activity of fluvastatin, a cholesterol-lowering agent, and synergy with fluconazole and itraconazole against *Candida* species and *Cryptococcus neoformans*. *Antimicrob Agents Chemother* 1997, 41:850–852.

Committee of Principal Investigators: A co-operative trial in the primary prevention of ischaemic heart disease using clofibrate. *Br Heart J* 1978, 40:1069–1118.

Committee of Principal Investigators: WHO cooperative trail on primary prevention of ischaemic heart disease with clofibrate to lower serum cholesterol: final mortality follow-up. *Lancet* 1984, 2:600–604.

Consensus Development Conference: Treatment of hypertriglyceridemia. *JAMA* 1984, 251:1196–1200.

Coronary Drug Project Research Group: Clofibrate and niacin in coronary heart disease. *JAMA* 1975, 231:360–381.

Dart A, Jerums G, Nicholson G, *et al.*: A multicenter, double-blind, one-year study comparing safety and efficacy of atorvastatin versus simvastatin in patients with hypercholesterolemia. *Am J Cardiol* 1997, 80:39–44.

Downs JR, Clearfield M, Weis S, *et al.*: Primary prevention of acute coronary events with lovastatin in men and women with average cholesterol levels. Results of AFCAPS/TexCAPS. *JAMA* 1998, 279:1615–1622.

Dujovne C, Kwiterovich P, Hunninghake D, Poland M: Comparison of cerivastatin 0.3 mg to pravastatin 20 mg, and cerivastatin 40 mg in 1030 hypercholesterolemic patients (abstract). *Pharmacotherapy* 1999, 19:1193.

Ellen RLB, McPherson R: Long-term efficacy and safety of fenofibrate and a statin in the treatment of combined hyperlipidemia. *Am J Cardiol* 1998, 81 (suppl. 4A):60B–65B.

Farmer JA: Economic implications of lipid-lowering trials: current considerations in selecting a statin. *Am J Cardiol* 1998, 82 (suppl.):26M–31M.

Figge HL, Figge J, Sonney PF, *et al.*: Nicotinic acid: a review of its clinical use in the treatment of lipid disorders. *Pharmacotherapy* 1988, 8:287–294.

Frick MH, Elo O, Haapa K, *et al.*: Helsinki Heart Study: Primary prevention trial with gemfibrozil in middle-aged men with dyslipidemia. *N Engl J Med* 1987, 317:1237–1245.

Frick MH, Heinonen OP, Huttunen JK, *et al.*: Efficacy of gemfibrozil in dyslipidaemic subjects with suspected heart disease. An ancillary study in the Helsinki Heart Study frame population. *Ann Med* 1993, 25:41–45.

Frick MH, Syvänne M, Nieminen MS, *et al.*: Prevention of the angiographic progression of coronary and vein-graft atherosclerosis by gemfibrozil after coronary bypass surgery in men with low levels of HDL cholesterol. *Circulation* 1997, 96:2137–2143.

Frishman WH (ed): Medical Management of Lipid Disorders. New York: Futura Publishing Co., 1992.

Frishman WH, Rapier RC: Lovastatin: an HMG-CoA reductase inhibitor for lowering cholesterol. *Med Clinics N Amer* 1989, 73:437–448.

Frishman WH, Zimetbaum P: Lipid-lowering drugs. In Frishman WH, Sonnenblick EH (eds): *Cardiovascular Pharmacotherapeutics*. New York: McGraw Hill; 1997:399–479.

Furberg CD, Pitt B, Byington RP, *et al.*: Reduction in coronary events during treatment with pravastatin. *Am J Cardiol* 1995, 76 (suppl. C):60C–63C.

Gould AL, Rossouw JE, Santanello NC, *et al.*: Cholesterol reduction yields clinical benefit: impact of statin trials. *Circulation* 1998, 97:946–952.

Grundy SM, Vega GL: Fibric acids: effects on lipids and lipoprotein metabolism. *Am J Med* 1987, 83 (Suppl 5B): 9–20.

Guyton JR, Goldberg AC, Kreisberg RA, *et al.*: Effectiveness of once-nightly dosing of extended-release niacin alone and in combination for hypercholesterolemia. *Am J Cardiol* 1998, 82:737–743.

Hanefield M, Deslypere J-P, Ose L, *et al.*: Efficacy and safety of 300 µg and 400 µg cerivastatin once daily in patients with primary hypercholesterolemia: a multicentre, randomized, double-blind, placebo-controlled study. *J Int Med Res* 1999, 27:115–129.

Henderson RP, Solomon CP: Use of cholestyramine in the treatment of digoxin intoxication. *Arch Intern Med* 1988, 148:745–746.

Herd JA, Ballantyne CM, Farmer JA: Effects of fluvastatin on coronary atherosclerosis in patients with mild to moderate cholesterol elevations (Lipoprotein and Coronary Atherosclerosis Study [LCAS]). *Am J Cardiol* 1997, 80:278–286.

Hjermann I, Holme I, Velve Byre K, Leren P: Effect of diet and smoking intervention on the incidence of coronary heart disease. Report from the Oslo Study Group of a randomised trial in healthy men. *Lancet* 1981, ii:1303–1310.

Holme I: An analysis of randomized trials evaluating the effects of cholesterol reduction on total mortality and CHD incidence. *Circulation* 1990, 82:1916–1924.

Hunninghake D, Bakker-Arkema RG, Wigand JP, *et al.*: Treating to meet NCEP-recommended LDL cholesterol concentrations with atorvastatin, fluvastatin, lovastatin, or simvastatin in patients with risk factors for coronary heart disease. *J Fam Pract* 1998, 47:349–356.

Hunninghake D, Dujovne C, Stein E, *et al.*: The 0.4 mg dose of cerivastatin: comparative safety and efficacy of cerivastatin 0.3 mg versus fluvastatin 40 mg (abstract). *Pharmacotherapy* 1999, 19:1194.

Hunninghake DB, Peters JB: Effect of fibric acid derivatives on blood lipid and lipoprotein levels. *Am J Med* 1987, 83 (Suppl 5B):44–49.

Illingworth DR, Rapp JH, Phillipson BE, Connor WE: Colestipol plus nicotinic acid in treatment of heterozygous familial hypercholesterolemia. *Lancet* 1981, 1:296–298.

Israel MK, Sisson EM: Hyperlipidemias. In: *Pharmcotherapy Self-Assessment Program, 3rd ed.* Kansas City, MO: American College of Clinical Pharmacy, 1998.

Jacotot B, Benghozi R, Pfister P, Holmes D: Comparison of fluvastatin versus pravastatin treatment of primary hypercholesterolemia. *Am J Cardiol* 1995, 76 (suppl.):54A–56A.

Jen SL, Chen JW, Lee WL, Wang SP: Efficacy and safety of fenofibrate or gemfibrozil on serum lipid profiles in Chinese patients with type IIb hyperlipidemia: a single-blind, randomized, and cross-over study. *Chin Med J* 1997, 59:217–224.

Jeppesen J, Hein HO, Suadicani P, Gyntelberg F: Triglyceride concentration and ischemic heart disease. An eight-year follow-up in the Copenhagen Male Study. *Circulation* 1998, 97:1029–1036.

Jukema JW, Bruschke AVG, van Boven AJ, *et al.*: Effects of lipid lowering by pravastatin on progression and regression of coronary artery disease in symptomatic men with normal to moderately elevated serum cholesterol levels. The Regression Growth Evaluation Statin Study (REGRESS). *Circulation* 1995, 91:2528–2540.

Kane JP, Malloy MJ, Tun P, *et al.*: Normalization of low-density-lipoprotein levels in heterozygous familial hypercholesterolemia with a combined drug regimen. *N Engl J Med* 1981, 304:251–258.

Kane JP, Malloy MJ, Ports TA, Phillips NR, *et al.*: Regression of coronary atherosclerosis during treatment of familial hypercholesterolemia with combined drug regimens. *JAMA* 1990, 264:3007–3012.

Knopp RH, Alagona P, Davidson M, *et al.*: Equivalent efficacy of a time-release form of niacin (Niaspan) given once-a-night versus plain niacin in the management of hyperlipidemia. *Metabolism* 1998, 47:1097–1104.

Kong SX, Crawford SY, Gandhi SK, *et al.*: Efficacy of 3-hydroxy-3-methylglutaryl coenzyme A reductase inhibitors in the treatment of patients with hypercholesterolemia: a meta-analysis of clinical trials. *Clin Ther* 1997, 19:778–797.

Kuo PT, Kostis JB, Moreyra AE, Hayes JA: Familial type II hyperlipoproteinemia with coronary heart disease. Effect of diet-colestipol-nicotinic acid treatment. *Chest* 1981, 79:286–291.

LaRosa J: Review of clinical studies of bile acid sequestrants for lowering plasma lipid levels. *Cardiology* 1989, 76 (Suppl 1):55–64.

Lea AP, McTavish D: Atorvastatin. A review of its pharmacology and therapeutic potential in the management of hyperlipidaemias. *Drugs* 1997, 53:828–847.

Lipid Research Clinics Program: The Lipid Research Clinics Coronary Primary Prevention Trial results. I. Reduction in incidence of coronary heart disease. *JAMA* 1984, 251:351–364.

Lipid Research Clinics Program: The Lipid Rearch Clinics Coronary Primary Prevention Trials results. II. The relationship of reduction in incidence of coronary heart disease to cholesterol lowering. *JAMA* 1984, 251:365–374.

Lipid Research Clinics Investigators: The Lipid Research Clinics Coronary Primary Prevention Trial. Results of 6 years of post-trial follow-up. *Arch Intern Med* 1992, 152:1399–1410.

Long-Term Intervention with Pravastatin in Ischaemic Disease (LIPID) Study Group: Prevention of cardiovascular events and death with pravastatin in patients with coronary heart disease and a broad range of initial cholesterol levels. *N Engl J Med* 1998, 339:1349–1357.

MAAS Investigators: Effect of simvastatin on coronary atheroma: the Multicentre Anti-Atheroma Study (MAAS). *Lancet* 1994, 334:633–638.

Malloy MJ, Kane JP, Kunitake ST, *et al.*: Complimentarity of colestipol, niacin, and lovastatin in treatment of severe familial hypercholesterolemia. *Ann Intern Med* 1987, 107:616–623.

McClellan KJ, Wiseman LR, McTavish D: Cerivastatin. *Drugs* 1998, 55:415–420.

McKenney JM, Proctor JD, Harris S, Chinchili VM: A comparison of the efficacy and toxic effects of sustained- vs immediate-release niacin in hypercholesterolemic patients. *JAMA* 1994, 271:672–677.

Muck W: Rational assessment of the interaction profile of cerivastatin supports its low propensity for drug interactions. *Drugs* 1998, 56 (Suppl 1):15–23.

Ose L, Luurila O, Eriksson J, *et al.*: Efficacy and safety of cerivastatin, 0.2 mg and 0.4 mg, in patients with primary hypercholesterolemia: a multinational, randomised, double-blind study. *Curr Med Res Opin* 1999, 15:228–240.

Payne VW, Secter RA, Noback RK: Use of colestipol in a patient with digoxin intoxication. *Drug Intell Clin Pharm* 1981, 15:902–903.

Pitt B, Mancini GBJ, Ellis SG, Rosman HS, *et al.*: Pravastatin limitation of atherosclerosis in the coronary arteries (PLAC I): reduction in atherosclerosis progression and clinical events. *J Am Coll Cardiol* 1995, 26:1133–1139.

Pitt B, Waters D, Brown WV, *et al.*: Aggressive lipid-lowering therapy compared with angioplasty in stable coronary artery disease. *N Engl J Med* 1999, 341:70–76.

Prevention of cardiovascular events and death with pravastatin in patients with coronary heart disease and a broad range of initial cholesterol levels: the long-term intervention with pravastatin in Ischaemic Disease (LIPID) Study Group. *N Engl J Med* 1998, 339:1349–1357.

Probstfield JL, Margitic SE, Byington RP, *et al.*: Results of the primary outcome measure and clinical events from the asymptomatic carotid artery progression study. *Am J Cardiol* 1995, 76 (suppl.):47C–53C.

PPP Project Investigators: Design, rationale, and baseline characteristics of the Prospective Pravastatin Pooling (PPP) Project: a combined analysis of three large-scale randomized trials: Long-term Intervention with Pravastatin in Ischemic Disease (LIPID), Cholesterol and Recurrent Events (CARE), and West of Scotland Coronary Prevention Study (WOSCOPS). *Am J Cardiol* 1995, 76:899–905.

Report from the Committee of Principal Investigators: A cooperative trial in the primary prevention of ischaemic heart disease using clofibrate. *Br Heart J* 1978, 40:1069–1118.

Rubins HB, Robins SJ, Collins D, *et al.*: Gemfibrozil for the secondary prevention of coronary heart disease in men with low levels of high-density lipoprotein cholesterol. *N Engl J Med* 1999, 341:410–418.

Sacks FM, Pfeffer MA, Moye LA, *et al.*: The effect of pravastatin on coronary events after myocardial infarction in patients with average cholesterol levels. *N Engl J Med* 1996, 335:1001–1009.

Salonen R, Nyyssönen K, Porkkala E, *et al.*: Kuopio Atherosclerosis Prevention Study (KAPS). *Circulation* 1995, 92:1758–1764.

Scandinavian Simvastatin Survival Study Group: Randomised trial of cholesterol lowering in 4444 patients with coronary heart disease: the Scandinavian Simvastatin Survival Study (4S). *Lancet* 1994, 344:1383–1389.

Schwartz GG, Oliver MF, Ezekowitz MD, *et al.*: Rationale and design of the myocardial ischemia reduction with aggressive cholesterol lowering (MIRACL) study that evaluates atorvastatin in unstable angina pectoris and in non-Q-wave acute myocardial infarction. *Am J Cardiol* 1998, 81:578–581.

Shepherd J, Cobbe SM, Ford I, *et al.*: Prevention of coronary heart disease with pravastatin in men with hypercholesterolemia. *N Engl J Med* 1995, 333:1301–1307.

Slater EE, MacDonald JS: Mechanism of action and biological profile of HMG-CoA reductase inhibitors. A new therapeutic alternative. *Drugs* 1988, 36:72–82.

Stein EA: Cerivastatin in primary hyperlipidemia: a multicenter analysis of efficacy and safety. *Am J Cardiol* 1998, 82(4B):40J–46J.

Stein EA: Extending therapy options in treating lipid disorders. A clinical review of cerivastatin, a novel HMG-CoA reductase inhibitor. *Drugs* 1998, 56 (suppl. 1):25–31.

Stein EA, Lane M, Laskarzewski P: Comparison of statins in hypertriglyceridemia. *Am J Cardiol* 1998, 81 (suppl. 4A):66B–69B.

The Expert Panel: Report of the National Cholesterol Education Program Expert Panel on Detection, Evaluation, and Treatment of High Blood Cholesterol in Adults. *Arch Intern Med* 1988, 148:36–39.

Tyroler HA: Total serum cholesterol and ischaemic heart disease risk in clinical trials and observational studies. *Am J Prev Med* 1985, 1:18–24.

Todd PA, Ward A: Gemfibrozil: a review of its pharmacodynamic and pharmacokinetic properties and therapeutic use in dyslipidaemia. *Drugs* 1988, 36:314–339.

Vega GL, Grundy SM: Mechanisms of primary hypercholesterolemia in humans. *Am Heart J* 1987, 112:493–502.

Walker JF: HMG-CoA reductase inhibitors: current clinical experience. *Drugs* 1988, 36 (Suppl 3):83–86.

Warshafsky S, Frishman WH: Efficacy of the HMG-CoA reductase inhibitors for prevention of fatal and nonfatal stroke: a meta-analysis. *J Gen Intern Med* 1999, in press.

Waters D, Higginson L, Gladstone P, *et al.*: Effects of monotherapy with an HMG-CoA reductase inhibitor on the progression of coronary atherosclerosis as assessed by serial quantitative ateriography. The Canadian Coronary Atherosclerosis Intervention Trial. *Circulation* 1994, 89:959–968.

Watts GF, Lewis B, Brunt JNH, *et al.*: Effects on coronary artery disease of lipid-lowering diet, or diet plus cholestyramine, in the St Thomas' Atherosclerosis Regression Study (STARS). *Lancet* 1992, 339:563–569.

Wild SH, Fortmann SP, Marcovina SM: A prospective case-control study of lipoprotein (a) levels and Apo (a) size and risk of coronary heart disease in Stanford Five-city Project participants. *Arterioscler Thromb Vasc Biol* 1997, 17:239–245.

XIII International Symposium on Drugs Affecting Lipid Metabolism, Florence, Italy, June 2, 1998.

NEURONAL AND GANGLIONIC BLOCKERS

Some of the earliest antihypertensive treatments involved the use of neuronal and ganglionic blockers, but they proved to have numerous unpleasant side effects. As a result, these blockers are now used as third- or fourth-line agents in the management of severe hypertension when the combination of better-tolerated agents has failed to achieve adequate blood pressure (BP) control. **Trimethaphan** is used for the reduction of BP during surgery and the treatment of hypertensive emergencies.

EFFICACY AND USE

Guanethidine is an adrenergic neural blocking drug that is effective for the treatment of high BP, but it is rarely used today. Because of its ability to reduce BP by decreasing the degree of vasoconstriction that accompanies increased sympathetic activity on moving to an upright posture, it tends to cause orthostatic hypotension. Because postural hypotension is more common in the morning, a low dose may be given then, with the balance of the daily dose given later in the day. Thus, the diurnal 24-hour BP pattern reverses, with relative hypotension during the waking hours and relative hypertension at night. Because prolonged standing, excessive heat, alcohol, or exercise can increase the risk for orthostatic hypotension, its use is now restricted.

Reserpine, a rauwolfia alkaloid, is one of the oldest drugs used to treat hypertension, and has been available for almost 50 years. Recently it was shown to be effective as an adjunct therapy in older patients with isolated systolic hypertension in relatively low dosages. It is commonly used as a second- or third-line agent to treat refractory mild-to-moderate hypertension. It is fairly well tolerated, especially when used in low doses and concomitantly with a diuretic agent. Its use is limited primarily by its side effect profile; depression and other central nervous system (CNS) effects in particular can be a significant problem.

Trimethaphan has a special place in this small group of drugs. As a short-acting drug given only intravenously, it is used for the rapid reduction of BP in hypertensive emergencies or to produce elective hypotension during surgery.

Although systemic vascular resistance is depressed in patients undergoing treatment with ganglionic blockers, the response of individual organ beds is variable. Splanchnic and cerebral blood flow may be reduced slightly, while the blood flow of skin may increase. Attempting to exploit these differential effects, **reserpine** has been used with mixed success in the treatment of Raynaud's phenomenon and migraine headaches; **guanethidine** has been used in the treatment of reflex sympathetic dystrophy. The renal effects of ganglionic blockade are of particular importance because of the association of severe hypertension with renal disease. In normotensive and some hypertensive subjects, ganglionic blockade may lead to a fall in glomerular filtration rate (GFR) and renal blood flow (RBF) and an increase in renal vascular resistance (RVR). These effects occur acutely but may also persist. In some hypertensive patients, RBF is unchanged or may increase, while RVR is reduced. Apart from the peripheral effects of ganglionic blockers (Table 12.1), those that penetrate the CNS can produce prominent unwanted effects such as mental confusion.

MODE OF ACTION

Guanethidine and **guanadrel** interfere with the release of norepinephrine from postganglionic adrenergic nerve endings. They are taken up and stored in the neuron via the same mechanisms by which norepinephrine is handled. Reduced catecholamine release results in reduced arteriolar vasoconstriction and reduction in the reflex increase in sympathetic activity that accompanies a change in position. **Guanethidine** also causes depletion of norepinephrine from nerve endings and structural changes that are slow to reverse. **Guanethidine** has a long duration of action; its effects are observable for 1 to 3 weeks after discontinuation of treatment. Peak effect occurs within 8 hours after a single oral dose. However, full therapeutic effects are not observed until 1 to 3 weeks after initiation of therapy. By contrast, **guanadrel** has a rapid onset of action, reaching its peak effect in 4 to 6 hours.

Reserpine acts by depleting catecholamines and serotonin in the brain and in many other organs. It exerts its antihypertensive effect by reducing sympathetic peripheral vasoconstriction and by reducing cardiac output with chronic administration. Depletion of biogenic amines may be inhibited by the action of monoamine oxidase inhibitor (MAOI) agents, which in turn would limit the effectiveness of reserpine to reduce BP. **Reserpine** has a long duration of action, and when

TABLE 12.1 SITE OF ACTION AND PREDOMINANT NEURAL TONE WITH CONSEQUENT EFFECTS OF AUTONOMIC GANGLIONIC BLOCKADE

Site	Predominant tone	Effect of ganglionic blockade
Arterioles	Sympathetic (adrenergic)	Vasodilatation, increased peripheral flow, hypotension
Veins	Sympathetic (adrenergic)	Dilatation, pooling of blood, decreased venous return, decreased cardiac output
Heart	Parasympathetic (cholinergic)	Tachycardia
Iris	Parasympathetic (cholinergic)	Mydriasis
Ciliary muscle	Parasympathetic (cholinergic)	Cycloplegia
Gastrointestinal tract	Parasympathetic (cholinergic)	Reduced tone and motility, constipation
Urinary bladder	Parasympathetic (cholinergic)	Urinary retention
Salivary glands	Parasympathetic (cholinergic)	Xerostomia
Sweat glands	Sympathetic (cholinergic)	Anhidrosis

Adapted from Taylor P: Agents acting at the neuromuscular junction and autonomic ganglia. In Goodman and Gilman's The Pharmacological Basis of Therapeutics, edn 8. London: MacMillan; 1990: 183.

The information here is provided as guidance only. Prescribers should always consult the manufacturer's current prescribing information.

239

taken chronically, exerts additive effects through progressive catecholamine depletion. This depletion has been implicated in the unwanted occurrence of mental depression and the deregulation of pituitary hormone synthesis and secretion, yielding increased serum prolactin levels.

Trimethaphan is a ganglion-blocking agent that competitively inhibits adrenergic transmission in autonomic ganglia. It is short acting, blocking transmission in both sympathetic and parasympathetic ganglia. It does not impair nerve conduction in the pre- or postganglionic neurons, but it blocks the action of acetylcholine liberated from the presynaptic nerve endings and has a peripheral vasodilating effect.

Mecamylamine is a very potent oral ganglionic blocker, its effect being predominantly orthostatic.

The ganglionic blockers produce widespread effects in the body (Table 12.1). Changes in cardiac rate following ganglionic blockade depend primarily upon the concurrent vagal tone: mild tachycardia usually accompanies the fall in BP. In patients with normal cardiac function, ganglionic blockers often reduce cardiac output because venous dilatation diminishes venous return. In patients with congestive heart failure (CHF), ganglionic blockers frequently increase cardiac output because peripheral resistance is reduced, thus decreasing afterload.

INDICATIONS

	Guanadrel	Guanethidine	Reserpine	Mecamylamine	Trimethaphan
Unresponsive moderate to severe hypertension	+	+	+	+	—
Hypertensive emergencies	—	—	—	—	+
Malignant hypertension	—	—	—	+	+
Controlled hypotension (in surgery)	—	—	—	—	+
Renal hypertension	—	+	—	—	—
Psychosis	—	—	+	—	—
Pulmonary edema	—	—	—	—	+
Dissecting aortic aneurysm	—	—	—	—	+

+—FDA approved; — —not FDA approved.

GUANADREL

(Hylorel®)

Guanadrel sulfate blocks the efferent peripheral sympathetic pathways selectively. It suppresses sympathetic vasoconstriction by inhibiting norepinephrine release from neuronal storage sites in response to stimulation of the nerve. Guanadrel also causes depletion of norepinephrine from the nerve ending, resulting in relaxation of vascular smooth muscle. This in turn decreases total peripheral vascular resistance and decreases venous return, both of which decrease the ability to maintain BP in the upright position.

Guanadrel reduces systolic BP more than diastolic BP. Since this agent can reduce or eliminate cardiovascular reflexes, greater reductions of BP are observed when patients are upright than when they are supine. Renal blood flow and glomerular filtration usually are unchanged when patients are in the supine position, but may be reduced by 30%–40% when they are in the upright position.

Given the equal antihypertensive effectiveness of guanethidine and guanadrel, guanadrel's shorter duration of action may make it preferable to limit the duration of possible unwanted side effects. Postural and postexercise hypotension is common in patients receiving this drug. Heat-induced vasodilation may also increase the hypotensive effect of guanadrel. However, tolerance to the hypotensive effect of guanadrel may also result during prolonged therapy due to sodium and water retention induced by this agent. For this reason, the concurrent use of a diuretic with this agent is recommended.

SPECIAL GROUPS

Race: no differences in response

Children: not recommended; safety and effectiveness have not been established

Elderly: lower dosages are recommended; elderly are more susceptible to hypotensive effects of the drug

Renal impairment: may increase plasma half-life and diminish clearance; recommend dose reduction or use prolonged dosing intervals, especially with a creatinine clearance of < 60 mL/min

Hepatic impairment: not known

Pregnancy: category B; no adequate and well controlled studies in pregnant women have been performed

Breast-feeding: not recommended; may be excreted in breast milk

DOSAGE

Initially, give 5mg twice daily. Adjust dosage weekly, or monthly until BP is controlled.

Maintenance dose is usually 20–75 mg/d in two to four divided doses. For patients with creatinine clearance of 30–60 ml/min, initiate therapy with 5 mg every 24 h. For patients with creatinine clearance of < 30 mL/min, increase dosage interval to 48 h. Dosage increments should be made cautiously at intervals ≥ 7 d for patients with moderate renal insufficiency and ≥ 14 d for patients with severe renal insufficiency.

IN BRIEF

INDICATIONS
Hypertension

CONTRAINDICATIONS
Hypersensitivity; Pheochromocytoma; Concurrent treatment or within one week of treatment with monoamine oxidase inhibitors (MAOIs); Frank CHF.

DRUG INTERACTIONS
Anesthetic agents
Sympathomimetic agents
Beta blockers
Tricyclic antidepressants
Hypotension-producing medications
Vasodilators
MAOIs
Vasopressors
Phenothiazines

ADVERSE EFFECTS
Cardiovascular: chest pain; orthostatic hypotension; peripheral edema
CNS: fatigue; headache; drowsiness
GI/GU: increased bowel movements; dry mouth; dry throat; nocturia; ejaculation disturbances
Respiratory: shortness of breath
Others: excessive weight gain/loss

PHARMACOKINETICS AND PHARMACODYNAMICS
Duration of action: 9 h (range, 4–14 h) after single dose
Onset of action: 2 h
Peak effect: 4–6 h
Bioavailability: rapidly and almost completely absorbed from the gastrointestinal tract
Effect of food: not known
Metabolism: hepatic
Elimination: 85% renal (≈ 40% as unchanged drug)
Plasma half-life: 10 h; increased in renal impairment
Protein binding: ≈ 20%

MONITORING
Since guanadrel may cause orthostatic hypotension, monitor both supine and standing pressures, especially during dosage adjustments. In addition to the contraindications listed above, use with extreme caution in patients with diabetes mellitus, regional vascular disease, asthma, recent MI, angina pectoris, history of peptic ulcer, sinus bradycardia, cerebrovascular insufficiency, diarrhea, fever, salt, depletion, anemia, or Addison's disease.

OVERDOSE
Usually produces dizziness and blurred vision; patient should lie down until symptoms subside. Treatment should be supportive. Persistent, excessive hypotension may require intensive therapy to support vital functions. Vasoconstrictors will counteract guanadrel's effects; use with caution.

PATIENT INFORMATION
Postural hypotension is greatest in morning and on standing up. Avoid getting up suddenly from a lying or sitting position. This may be heightened by fever, heat, exercise, prolonged standing, and alcohol use. Patient should sit or lie down at first sign of dizziness. Notify physician if persistent or unusual side effects occur. Consult physician before taking nonprescription remedies for colds, allergies, or asthma. Take medication as prescribed; do not discontinue therapy without physician's advice.

AVAILABILITY
Tablets—10 mg, 25 mg

GUANETHIDINE (Ismelin®)

Guanethidine is a postganglionic adrenergic-blocking agent which is structurally and pharmacologically related to guanadrel. Guanethidine acts by displacing norepinephrine from terminal vesicle storage sites and by inhibiting norepinephrine release and re-uptake. Consequently, guanethidine exerts its antihypertensive effects by reducing peripheral sympathetic vasoconstriction. Although rarely used, it is indicated for the treatment of moderate to severe hypertension in addition to other better-tolerated drugs when those, in combination, have failed to achieve adequate BP control. Absorption of guanethidine varies considerably among patients, necessitating individualization of dosage.

Due to its long duration of action, guanethidine may be taken on a once daily regimen, which may be considered an advantage over guanadrel if patient compliance is a significant concern. Similar to guanadrel, guanethidine decreases systolic BP more than diastolic BP. Since guanethidine reduces or eliminates cardiovascular reflexes, further lowering of BP is observed when patients are upright than when they are supine.

Postural and postexercise hypotension are common in patients receiving guanethidine. Guanethidine is most effective in treating hypertension when used in conjunction with a diuretic to avoid tolerance from salt and fluid retention.

Guanethidine also has been used in the treatment of reflex sympathetic dystrophy by intravenous infusion to produce a regional intravascular sympathetic block. This type of administration may be longer acting and technically simpler than other regional neural blocks. Intravenous guanethidine injection has been used with limited success in the treatment of Raynaud's phenomenon. Further studies are required to support guanethidine use with these indications.

Other uses of guanethidine include effective treatment of refractory variant angina that has failed to be controlled by nitrates and calcium channel blockers. Guanethidine has also been used successfully to control hyperreflexic bladders in spinal cord trauma patients.

SPECIAL GROUPS

Race: no differences in response
Children: use with caution; safety and effectiveness have not been established
Elderly: may be more sensitive to hypotensive effect
Renal impairment: since decreased BP may further compromise renal function, use with extreme caution in hypertensive patients with renal dysfunction
Hepatic impairment: reduced metabolism and excessive accumulation of guanethidine may occur; lower doses or increased dosage interval may be required
Pregnancy: category C; safety for use during pregnancy has not been established
Breast-feeding: not recommended; guanethidine is excreted in breast milk

DOSAGE

Adult: Initially, give 10 or 12.5 mg/d orally; increased gradually according to response (10–12.5 mg increments at weekly intervals). Usual maintenance dose is 25–50 mg/d. Dosage may be increased more rapidly and with larger dosage increments under careful hospital supervision.
Elderly: Use lower dose.
Children: Initially, give 0.2 mg/kg body weight orally once a day. Daily dose can be increased by 0.2 mg/kg body weight at 7–10 d intervals, up to five to eight times the initial daily dose.

IN BRIEF

INDICATIONS
Moderate to severe hypertension
Renal hypertension

CONTRAINDICATIONS
Hypersensitivity; Pheochromocytoma; Concurrent treatment or recent treatment with MAOIs; Frank CHF.

DRUG INTERACTIONS
Anesthetic agents
Anorexiants
Antidiabetic agents
Haloperidol
Loxapine
Methylphenidate
Minoxidil
MAOIs
Phenothiazines
Sympathomimetics
Trimeprazine
Thioxanthenes
Tricyclic antidepressants

ADVERSE EFFECTS
Cardiovascular: bradycardia; orthostatic hypotension; peripheral edema; angina
CNS: fatigue; weakness; syncope; headache; mental depression; blurred vision
GI/GU: nausea; vomiting; dry mouth; diarrhea; increase in bowel movements; inhibition of ejaculation
Respiratory: dyspnea; nasal congestion
Others: myalgia; weight gain; dermatitis; alopecia

PHARMACOKINETICS AND PHARMACODYNAMICS
Duration of action: 24–48 h (BP returns gradually to pretreatment levels within 1–3 wk after discontinuing therapy)
Onset of action: 0.5–2 h
Peak effect: within 8 h after single dose. The full effect may not be noticed until 1–3 wk after initiation of therapy
Bioavailability: 3%–30% (varies tenfold)
Effect of food: not known
Metabolism: partially metabolized by the liver to three metabolites that are less active than the parent drug
Elimination: 25%–60% of a dose excreted in urine as unchanged drug
Plasma half-life: 1.5 d (alpha), 4–8 d (beta)
Protein binding: not known

MONITORING
Monitor BP and other vital signs. In addition to the contraindications listed above, use guanethidine with extreme caution in patients with cerebrovascular insufficiency, cardiac ischemia, and peptic ulcers.

OVERDOSE
Gastric lavage may be useful for very recent ingestion. Treatment should be symptomatic and supportive.

PATIENT INFORMATION
This medication may cause gastrointestinal side effects (particularly diarrhea), headache, blurred vision, fatigue, and dizziness. If severe, do not drive or operate machinery. Notify physician if persistent or unusual side effects occur. Consult physician before taking nonprescription remedies for colds, allergies, or asthma. Avoid alcohol use. Take medication as prescribed; do not discontinue therapy without physician's advice.

AVAILABILITY
Tablets—10 mg, 25 mg

MECAMYLAMINE (Inversine®)

Mecamylamine is a very potent oral ganglionic blocker used in the treatment of moderately severe or severe hypertension and uncomplicated malignant hypertension. It is rarely used now except as additional therapy when better tolerated agents have failed to achieve the desired level of BP control. The use of mecamylamine is limited by its numerous side effects; other drugs may produce rapid falls in BP and be better tolerated. Other uses for mecamylamine include the treatment of hyperreflexia in patients with spinal cord injuries and the promotion of smoking cessation. The latter effect occurs by mecamylamine inhibiting central nicotinic cholinergic receptors. Despite an initial increase in the number of cigarettes smoked, continued use of this medication may lead to conditioning that suppresses the nicotine craving. Adequate studies to exclude the contribution of a placebo effect must be performed to clarify this issue.

SPECIAL GROUPS

Race: no differences in response

Children: not recommended; safety and effectiveness have not been established

Elderly: may be more sensitive to hypotensive effect

Renal impairment: excretion may be reduced; reduce dose

Hepatic impairment: little, if any, impact on elimination; dose reduction unnecessary

Pregnancy: category C; not recommended; may decrease intestinal motility in fetus, resulting in meconium or paralytic ileus

Breast-feeding: not recommended; may be excreted in breast milk

DOSAGE

Initially, give 2.5 mg twice daily; increase in increments of 2.5 mg at intervals of at least every 2 d according to response. Smallest dose should be taken in the mornings to limit the orthostatic adverse effects of the drug. Maintenance dose is usually 25 mg/d in three divided doses.

Note: It is recommended that mecamylamine be administered at consistent times in relationship to meals because hypotension may occur after a meal. Mecamylamine ingestion with meals may slow the drug's absorption and thereby produce desired gradual correction of severe hypertension. Discontinuation of mecamylamine in an abrupt manner may result in severe rebound hypertension, especially in patients being treated for malignant hypertension. Gradual withdrawal is recommended when mecamylamine therapy is discontinued, and the substitution of other antihypertensive therapy may be necessary.

IN BRIEF

INDICATIONS
Essential hypertension, moderately severe
Esssential hypertension, severe
Malignant hypertension, uncomplicated

CONTRAINDICATIONS
Hypersensitivity
Patients with chronic pyelonephritis who are receiving antibiotics and sulfonamides
Recent MI
Recent cardiac ischemia
Recent cerebrovascular insufficiency
Glaucoma
Organic pyloric stenosis
Uremia

DRUG INTERACTIONS

Alcohol	Drugs that increase urinary pH (eg, sodium bicarbonate, acetazolamide)	Hypotensive agents
Antibiotics		Sulfonamides
Bethanechol		

ADVERSE EFFECTS
Cardiovascular: orthostatic hypotension; syncope
CNS: fatigue; weakness; blurred vision; paresthesia; tremor; choreiform movements; mental changes (confusion, excitement, depression); convulsions
GI/GU: anorexia; dry mouth; nausea; vomiting; constipation; ileus; impotence; urinary retention
Respiratory: nasal congestion; interstitial pulmonary edema; fibrosis

PHARMACOKINETICS AND PHARMACODYNAMICS
Duration of action: 6–12 h
Onset of action: 0.5–2 h
Peak effect: 3–5 h
Bioavailability: not known
Effect of food: administration of mecamylamine after meals may provide more gradual control of BP than that produced when the drug is given on an empty stomach
Metabolism: little hepatic metabolism
Elimination: renal, largely unchanged (clearance is decreased in alkaline urine and is increased in acidic urine.)
Plasma half-life: not known
Protein binding: not known

MONITORING
Monitor BP and observe for tolerance. Additional diuretic treatment may be required. In addition to the contraindications listed above, use mecamylamine with caution in patients with prostatic hypertrophy, bladder neck obstruction, and urethral stricture because urinary retention may occur.

OVERDOSE
Treatment should be symptomatic and supportive. Pressor agents may be required, but sensitivity to their effects may be exaggerated.

PATIENT INFORMATION
Take mecamylamine after meals. This medication may cause gastrointestinal side effects, urinary retention, CNS effects, weakness, vision problems, drowsiness, and dizziness. If affected, do not drive or operate machinery. You may experience dizziness when getting up from a sitting or lying position; do this slowly. Do not take antacids, especially those containing sodium bicarbonate. Do not take other medications without consulting your physician. If any unusual effects appear, consult your physician immediately. Avoid alcohol use. Take medication as prescribed; do not discontinue therapy without physician's advice.

AVAILABILITY
Tablets—2.5 mg

RESERPINE

(Reserpine, Serpalan®)

Reserpine, a rauwolfia alkaloid, is one of the earliest drugs that was used effectively for the treatment of systemic hypertension. It acts at post-ganglionic sympathetic nerve endings and causes a depletion of CNS stores of catecholamines and serotonin. With repeated administration, depletion of catecholamine stores happens slowly, causing a gradual decrease in peripheral vascular resistance and BP, which is usually associated with bradycardia. With prolonged therapy, venous dilation decreases venous return to the heart and cause a reduction of cardiac output. Reserpine is the least expensive nondiuretic, antihypertensive agent available and is fairly well tolerated when used in low doses (0. 1 to 0. 2 mg daily) in combination with a diuretic agent. Depression and other CNS effects were very common when high doses of reserpine were used. The drug is found in many combination products, which include diuretics and hydralazine. Reserpine was one of the drugs used in the National Institutes of Health- sponsored Systolic Hypertension in the Elderly program to treat isolated systolic hypertension.

By depleting catecholamine stores in sympathetic nerve terminals, reserpine diminishes adrenergic vasoconstriction in cutaneous blood vessels. Consequently, reserpine may be useful in the Raynaud's syndrome by reducing both the severity and frequency of vasospastic episodes. A placebo effect may account for the limited success noted in using reserpine for this indication. Similarly, reserpine has been used with variable success in the treatment of migraine headaches by reducing cerebral vasoconstriction. Reserpine may also be used as a second-line agent to control the cardiovascular and neurologic symptoms associated with hyperthyroidism in patients who are resistant to propranolol or in whom beta blockade is contraindicated.

SPECIAL GROUPS

Race:	no differences in response
Children:	safety and effectiveness have not been established; however, there is experience with the use of reserpine in children
Elderly:	more sensitive to the hypotensive and CNS effects
Renal impairment:	no dosage adjustment is necessary; avoid use with severe impairment
Hepatic impairment:	reduce dose in severe impairment
Pregnancy:	category C; not recommended
Breast-feeding:	not recommended; possible adverse reactions in infants from reserpine in breast milk

IN BRIEF

INDICATIONS
Hypertension
Psychotic disorders

CONTRAINDICATIONS
Hypersensitivity
Active peptic ulcer disease
Ulcerative colitis
Gallstones
Electroconvulsive therapy
Mental depression

DRUG INTERACTIONS
Alcohol
Anticholinergics
Beta blockers
Bromocriptine
Digitalis glycosides
Hypotension-producing agents
Levodopa
MAOIs
Nonsteroidal anti-inflammatory drugs (NSAIDs)
Sympathomimetics
Quinidine
Tricyclic antidepressants

ADVERSE EFFECTS
Cardiovascular: bradycardia; arrhythmias; hypotension;syncope; edema
CNS: drowsiness; fatigue; lethargy; mental depression; headache; dizziness; nervousness; anxiety; nightmares; Parkinsonian syndrome and other extrapyramidal tract symptoms (rare)
GI/GU: abdominal cramps; diarrhea; nausea; vomiting; anorexia; dryness of mouth; hypersecretion; pseudolactation; impotence; dysuria
Respiratory: dyspnea; epistaxis; nasal congestion
Others: purpura; rash; pruritus; weight gain; muscular aches; deafness (rare); optic atrophy (rare); glaucoma (rare)

PHARMACOKINETICS AND PHARMACODYNAMICS
Duration of action: 1–6 wk
Onset of action: several days–3 wk
Peak effect: 3–6 wk
Bioavailability: ≈ 50%
Effect of food: not known
Metabolism: hepatic; inactive metabolites
Elimination: renal; fecal, 60% unchanged
Plasma half-life: 4.5 h, initial; 45–168 h, terminal
Protein binding: 96%

MONITORING
Monitor BP. In addition to the contraindications listed above, reserpine should be used with extreme caution in patients with cardiac arrhythmias, epilepsy, CHF, Parkinson's disease, or pheochromocytoma.

OVERDOSE
Treat with immediate evacuation of stomach and installation of an activated charcoal slurry. Use vasopressors if necessary to support BP (norepinephrine, phenylephrine). Observe for at least 72 h.

PATIENT INFORMATION
Take reserpine with food or milk. This medication may cause gastrointestinal side effects (dry mouth, stomach pains), mental depression, drowsiness, or dizziness. If severe, do not drive or operate machinery. Avoid alcohol use. Take medication as prescribed; do not discontinue therapy without physician's advice.

DOSAGE

Adults: Usual maintenance dose is 0.1–0.25 mg/d, taken with meals to avoid gastric irritation.

Children: 0.005–0.02 mg/kg (5–20 ug/kg) or 0.15–0.60 mg/m² (150–600 ug/m²) of body surface area a day in one or two divided daily doses

AVAILABILITY

Tablets—0.1 mg, 0.25 mg
Combination formulations:
Diupres—Reserpine/chlorothiazide combination tablets
  0. 125 mg/250 mg
  0. 125 mg/500 mg
Regroton—Reserpine/chlorthalidone combination tablets
  0.25 mg/50 mg
Demi-Regroton—Reserpine/chlorthalidone combination tablets
  0.125 mg/25 mg
Hydropres—Reserpine/hydrochlorothiazide combination tablets
  0. 125 mg/25 mg
  0.125 mg/50 mg
Salutensin—Reserpine/hydroflumethiazide combination tablets
  0. 125 mg/50 mg
Diutensen-R—Reserpine/methyclothiazide combination tablets
  0. 1 mg/2.5 mg
Metatensin—Reserpine/trichlormethiazide combination tablets
  0.1 mg/2 mg
  0.1 mg/4 mg
Renese-R—Reserpine/trichlormethiazide combination tablets
  0.25 mg/2 mg
Hydrap-ES
Marpres
Ser-Ap-Es
Tri-Hydroserpine
Unipres—Reserpine/hydrochlorothiazide/hydralazine HCl combination
  tablets
  0.1 mg/15 mg/25 mg

TRIMETHAPHAN (Arfonad®)

Trimethaphan camsylate is a short-acting ganglionic blocking agent that is generally used for the acute and short-term reduction of BP during surgery or during a hypertensive crisis. In general, it is best given diluted as an intravenous infusion. Pseudotolerance to trimethaphan may develop very rapidly mainly as a result of water retention; this may be alleviated with a diuretic agent. As with all the neuronal and ganglionic blockers, side effects limit the usefulness of this drug. Although useful clinically, experimental studies suggest that trimethaphan may reduce spinal cord blood flow during surgery, increasing the risk for spinal cord injury.

Trimethaphan and nitroprusside have similar indications, but they have certain notable differences. Trimethaphan may exhibit reduced cardiac output, whereas nitroprusside may render no change or a slight increase in cardiac output. Early pseudotolerance secondary to fluid retention seen with trimethaphan may not be noted with nitroprusside. Recovery of BP following discontinuation of these medications is more rapid with nitroprusside. Effective combined use of both drugs has been associated with lower doses of nitroprusside required and diminished risk of cyanide toxicity. Trimethaphan may be particularly useful in treating hypertensive crises involving acute dissecting aneurysm, and in the emergency treatment of pulmonary edema in patients with pulmonary hypertension associated with systemic hypertension.

SPECIAL GROUPS

Race: no differences in response

Children: dosage based on body weight; use with caution

Elderly: may be more sensitive to hypotensive effect

Renal impairment: reduced excretion results in enhanced effects; reduce dosage

Hepatic impairment: metabolism may be reduced; reduce dosage

Pregnancy: category D; not recommended; may decrease intestinal motility in fetus resulting in meconium ileus or neonatal paralytic ileus

Breast-feeding: not recommended; may be excreted in breast milk

DOSAGE

Adult: For controlled hypotension during surgery, give 3–4 mg/min by intravenous infusion initially. Adjust according to response to a maintenance infusion dose ranging from 0.2–6 mg/min. Trimethaphan should be administered after the patient is anesthetized and this drug should be discontinued prior to wound closure to allow BP to return toward normal.

For hypertensive emergency, initially give 0.5–1 mg/min; adjust according to response. Maintain BP at a dose of 1–5 mg/min by intravenous infusion.

Elderly: Use lower dose.

Children: Initially, administer 0.05 mg/kg/min to 0.15 mg/kg/min as an intravenous infusion; adjust according to response.

IN BRIEF

INDICATIONS
Controlled hypotension during surgical procedures
Hypertensive emergencies
Pulmonary edema
Dissecting aortic aneurysm

CONTRAINDICATIONS
Hypersensitivity
Anemia
Asphyxia
Uncorrected respiratory insufficiency
Hypovolemia
Shock
Glaucoma
Severe cardiac disease

DRUG INTERACTIONS
Anesthetics
Hypotension-producing medication
NSAIDs
Neostigmine
Neuromuscular blocking agents
Procainamide
Pyridostigmine
Sympathomimetics

ADVERSE EFFECTS
Cardiovascular: orthostatic hypotension; tachycardia; precipitation of angina
GI/GU: anorexia; nausea; vomiting; constipation; dryness of mouth; urinary retention; paralytic ileus
Respiratory: respiratory depression
Others: mydriasis; cycloplegia; urticaria; itching; hyperglycemia; hypokalemia

PHARMACOKINETICS AND PHARMACODYNAMICS
Duration of action: 10–15 min
Onset of action: immediate (intravenous)
Peak effect: very rapid
Bioavailability: not known
Metabolism: hepatic, possibly by pseudocholinesterase
Elimination: renal, mostly unchanged
Plasma half-life: very short
Protein binding: not known

MONITORING
Not intended for prolonged use. Monitor BP and respiratory function. In addition to the contraindications listed above, trimethaphan should be used with extreme caution in patients who are debilitated, in those receiving steroids, in those with a history of allergy, Addison's disease, cardiac ischemia, cerebrovascular insufficiency, diabetes, or degenerative disease of the CNS.

OVERDOSE
Withdraw treatment. Correct hypotension, if necessary. Severe hypotension or respiratory arrest are possible treatment complications. Treatment should be symptomatic and supportive. Vasopressor agents may be used to correct undesirable hypotension during surgery.

PATIENT INFORMATION
Trimethaphan is intended to produce a short-term reduction in BP. It may cause gastrointestinal side effects, dizziness, urinary retention, or chest pain.

AVAILABILITY
Injection—50 mg/mL in 10 mL ampules

Applebaum SM: Pharmacologic agents in micturitional disorders. *Urology* 1980, 16:555–568.

Bennett WM, Aronoff GR, Golper TA, *et al.*: Drugs Prescribing in Renal Failure. Philadelphia: American College of Physicians, 1987.

Bonelli S, Conoscente F, Movilia PG, *et al.*: Regional intravenous guanethidine versus stellate ganglion blocker in reflex sympathetic dystrophies. A randomized trial. *Pain* 1983, 16:297–307.

Braddom RL, Johnson EW: Mecamylamine in control of hyperreflexia. *Arch Phys Med Rehab* 1969, 50:448–456.

Cheah JS: A double blind trial of reserpine in small doses as an adjunct in the treatment of hyperthyroidism. *Med J Aus* 1972, 1:322.

Driessen JJ, van der Werken C, Nicolai JPA, *et al.*: Clinical effects of regional intraveinous guanethidine (Ismelin) in reflex sympathetic dystrophy. *Acta Anaesthesiol Scand* 1983, 27:505–509.

Eriksen S: Duration of sympathetic blockade: stellate ganglion versus intravenous regional guanethidine block. *Anaesthesia* 1981, 36:768–771.

Frenneaux M, Kaski JC, Brown M, *et al.*: Refractory variant angina relieved by guanethidine and clonidine. *Am J Cardiol* 1988, 62:832–833.

Glynn CJ, Basedow RW, Walsh JA: Pain relief following post-ganglionic sympathetic blockade with IV guanethidine. *Br J Anaesth* 1981, 53:1297–1302.

Halstenson CE, Opsahl JA, Abraham PA, *et al.*: Disposition of guanadrel in subjects with normal and impaired renal function. *J Clin Pharmacol* 1989, 29:128–32.

Keller S, Frishman WH, Epstein J: Neuropsychiatric manifestations of cardiovascular drug therapy. *Heart Dis* 1999, 1:241–254.

Krakoff L: Antiadrenergic drugs with central action, ganglionic blockers and neuron depletors. In *Cardiovascular Pharmacotherapeutics*. Edited by Frishman WL, Sonnenblick EH. New York: McGraw Hill 1997:267–273.

Krakoff L: Antiadrenergic drugs with central action, ganglionic blockers and neuron depletors. In *Cardiovascular Pharmacotherapeutics Companion Handbook*. Edited by Frishman WH, Sonnenblick EH. New York: McGraw Hill 1998:220–227.

Martin BR, Onaivi ES, Martin TJ: What is the nature of mecamylamine's antagonism of the central effects of nicotine? *Biochem Pharmacol* 1989, 38:3391–3397.

Miller R, Toth C, Silva DA, *et al.*: Nitroprusside versus a nitroprusside-trimethaphan mixture: a comparison of dosage requirements and hemodynamic effects during induced hypotension for neurosurgery. *Mt. Sinai J Med* 1987, 54:308–312.

Murphy JM, Sage JI: Trimethaphan or nitroprusside in the setting of intracranial hypertension. *Clin Neuropharmacol* 1988, 11:436–442.

Nattero G, Lisino F, Brandi G, *et al.*: Reserpine for migraine prophylaxis. *Headache* 1976, 15:279–281.

Nunn-Thompson CL, Simon PA: Pharmacotherapy for smoking cessation. *Clin Pharm* 1989, 8:710–720.

Phillips WA, Hensinger RN: Control of blood loss during scoliosis surgery. *Clin Orthopaed & Related Res* 1988, 229:88–93.

Pomerleau CS, Pomerleau OF, Majchrzak MJ: Mecamylamine pretreatment increases subsequent nicotine self-administration as indicated by changes in plasma nicotine level. *Psycho-Pharmacol* 1987, 91:391–393.

Rose JE, Sampson A, Levin ED, *et al.*: Mecamylamine increases nicotine preference and attenuates nicotine discrimination. *Pharmacol Biochem Behav* 1989, 32:933–938.

Samuels AH, Taylor AJ: Reserpine withdrawal psychosis. *Aust NZ J Psych* 1989, 23:129–130.

SHEP Cooperative Research Group: Prevention of stroke by antihyperintensive drug treatment in older persons with isolated systolic hypertension: Final results of the Systolic Hypertension in the Elderly Program (SHEP). *JAMA* 1991, 265:3255–3264.

Siegel RC, Fried JF: Intraaterially administered reserpine and saline in scleroderma. *Arch Intern Med* 1974, 134:515–518.

Stolerman IP. Could nicotine antagonists be used in smoking cessation? *Br J Addict* 1986, 81:47–53.

Stumph JL: Drug therapy of hypertensive crises. *Clin Pharmacol* 1988, 7:582–591.

Taylor P: Agents acting at the neuromuscular junction and autonomic ganglia. In *Goodman & Gilman's The Pharmacological Basis of Therapeutics*, 9th ed. Edited by Hardman JG, Gilman AG, Limbird LE. New York: McGraw Hill 1995:177–197.

Tindall JP, Whalen RE, Burton EE Jr.: Medical uses of intraarterial injections of reserpine. Treatment of Raynaud's syndrome and of some vascular insufficiencies of the lower extremities. *Arch Dermatol* 1974, 110:233–237.

The information here is provided as guidance only. Prescribers should always consult the manufacturer's current prescribing information.

247

In addition to the angiotensin II receptor blockers, the angiotensin converting enzyme inhibitors, and the calcium channel blockers, which are discussed in other chapters, there are other peripheral vasodilators that include a wide variety of compounds with highly disparate mechanisms of action. These drugs also differ enormously in their effects on small and large arteries and in their differential vasodilatory actions on arterial and venous vessels. Several drugs have poorly defined pharmacologic profiles and many nonspecific agents have little clinical usefulness despite having been available for many years, but some drugs in this broad group have a valuable place in cardiovascular therapy.

EFFICACY AND USE

Hydralazine and **minoxidil** are two potent and effective arterial vasodilators. Because of the oncogenic potential of **hydralazine** and the antihypertensive efficacy of **minoxidil**, which is associated with fluid retention, edema and pericardial effusion, they are used as second-, third- and fourth-line drugs in complicated or resistant hypertension. They are frequently used as adjunctive therapy in patients with uremia and complicated hypertension. They have been shown to be ineffective in reversing left ventricular hypertrophy, possibly because of volume overload and the stimulation of growth factors such as angiotensin II and catecholamines.

Nitrates have, for many years, been the mainstay of treatment of angina, as well as other cardiovascular problems. They are useful in the acute reduction of blood pressure (BP) and for the relief of heart failure. They have an adjunctive role in percutaneous coronary angioplasty and in maintaining cardiac function after thrombolytic therapy. However, recent work indicates that the chronic application of nitrates results in tolerance and that this may develop within 24 hours of transdermal delivery devices. Combination vasodilator therapy is particularly valuable. A useful combination is that of **hydralazine** and **isosorbide dinitrate**, as used in the Veteran's Administration Heart Failure Trial (VHeFT-1). This demonstrated a decrease in mortality in patients with NYHA Class II-III congestive heart failure (CHF) receiving **isosorbide-hydralazine** compared with those given **prazosin**. Mortality reduction, however, was lower in patients on the combination than in patients on **enalapril**. **Diazoxide** is a powerful and fast-acting vasodilator used, like **nitroprusside**, for situations in which rapid reduction in BP is desired; that is, hypertensive crises or hypotensive anesthesia. **Nitroprusside** is also useful when swift unloading of the heart is required, as in acute heart failure.

Fenoldopam is a selective dopamine1 agonist that is available in intravenous form and approved for the short-term management of hypertension and for patients with malignant hypertension having end-organ dysfunction. The drug has hemodynamic effects similar to **nitroprusside**, but unlike **nitroprusside**, it can also induce both a diuresis and natriuresis and does not cause cyanide toxicity. **Epoprostenol** is a naturally occurring prostaglandin approved for intravenous use in patients having advanced primary pulmonary hypertension. The drug can be used long term as a continuous chronic infusion therapy.

Pentoxifylline and **cilostazol** are both active drugs that are approved for use in patients with intermittent claudication. **Papaverine** is a vasodilator approved for use as a treatment for vascular spasm. **Tolazoline**, which produces vasodilation by means of histamine-like effect, is used to treat persistent pulmonary hypertension of the newborn. **Isoxsuprine**, an oral vasodilator that now has limited use, is indicated for relieving symptoms associated with cerebral vascular insufficiency and peripheral vascular disease. Vasodilator agents now used to treat vascular causes of impotence in men include **papaverine** and the prostaglandin agent **alprostadil**, which are administered by injection, and the orally active, selective phosphodiesterase inhibitor, **sildenafil**.

MODE OF ACTION

Hydralazine exerts a peripheral vasodilating effect through a direct relaxant action on arterial smooth muscle. Its main activity appears to be via interference with the cellular calcium movements responsible for initiating or maintaining a contractile state. **Minoxidil** appears to interfere with calcium uptake by the smooth muscle cell membrane. Some of its actions may be the result of enhanced opening of a potassium channel in smooth muscle. The observation that endogenously formed nitric oxide is a natural vasodilator (endothelium-derived relaxing factors, [EDRF]) suggests that the organic nitrates may mimic this action. **Diazoxide** has a direct action on smooth muscle by opening potassium channels. It exerts its effects on all circulatory beds.

Cilostazol is a selective phosphodiesterase III inhibitor that suppresses cyclic AMP degradation with a resultant elevation of cyclic adenosine monophosphate (AMP) in blood platelets and blood vessels, thus leading to an inhibition of platelet aggregation and vasodilation. **Pentoxifylline** appears to improve microcirculatory flow by improving erythrocyte flexibility. **Sildenafil** is a selective inhibitor of cyclic guanosine monophosphate (cGMP) specific phosphodiesterase V that improves vascular flow to the penis by activating the nitric oxide cyclic monophosphate cGMP pathway during sexual stimulation, to cause vascular engorgement and an improved erection.

INDICATIONS

	Alpros	Cilos	Diaz	Epo	Fenold	Hydral	Minox	Nitrates	Nitrop	Pentox	Silden	Tolaz
Angina pectoris	—	—	—	—	—	—	—	+	—	—	—	—
Adjunctive therapy for MI	—	—	—	—	—	—	—	+	—	—	—	—
Cerebrovascular insufficiency	—	—	—	—	—	—	—	—	—	(+)	—	—
Congestive heart failure	—	—	—	—	—	(+)	—	(+)	+	—	—	—
Controlled hypotension during surgery	—	—	—	—	—	—	—	+	+	—	—	—
Severe hypertension/hypertensive crises	—	—	+	—	+	+	+	(+)	+	—	—	—
Peripheral vascular disease	—	+	—	—	—	—	—	—	—	+	—	—
Pulmonary hypertension	—	—	—	+	—	—	—	—	—	—	—	+
Vascular impotence	+	—	—	—	—	—	—	—	—	—	+	—

+—FDA approved; — —not FDA approved; (+)—clinical use not FDA approved.

Alpros—alprostadil; Cilos—cilostazol; CHF—congestive heart failure; Diaz—diazoxide; Epo—epoprostenol; Fenold—fenoldopam; Hydral—hydralazine; MI—myocardial infarction; Minox—minoxidil; Nitrop—nitroprusside; Pentox—pentoxifylline; Silden —sildenafil; Tolaz—tolazoline .

ALPROSTADIL

(Caverject® Injection, Edex®Injection, Muse® Pellet, Prostin VR Pediatric® Injection)

Alprostadil is a naturally occurring prostaglandin E_1. It is a vasodilator and a platelet-aggregation inhibitor. Alprostadil has been used for the treatment of erectile dysfunction in adult males, and for temporary maintenance of patency of the ductus arteriosus in neonates. Alprostadil causes erection by relaxing trabecular smooth muscle and dilating cavernosal arteries. This leads to a process referred to as the corporal veno-occlusive mechanism, where lacunar spaces expand and blood becomes entrapped due to compression of venules against the tunica albuginea. When alprostadil is given by intracavernosal injection, there is no significant rise in levels of prostaglandin E_1 in the systemic circulation. Alprostadil is metabolized by the lungs with a short half-life of 30 seconds to 10 minutes, which may explain the low rate of priapism associated with intracavernosal injection with this agent.

In neonates with a closing ductus arteriosus, alprostadil relaxes and therefore may reopen the ductus. By maintaining ductal patency, alprostadil may improve blood flow and oxygenation in neonates with congenital heart defects and who depend upon the patent ductus for survival until corrective or palliative surgery can be performed.

SPECIAL GROUPS

Race: no differences in response
Children: has been used as palliative therapy to temporarily maintain the patency of the ductus arteriosus until corrective or palliative surgery can be performed in neonates who have congenital heart defects
Elderly: initiate with low dose; individualize dose according to response
Renal impairment: initiate with low dose; individualize dose according to response
Hepatic impairment: initiate with low dose; individualize dose according to response
Pregnancy: category X; not indicated for use in women

DOSAGE

Adults: For erectile dysfunction, initiate with low dose and individualize dose by careful titration. Refer to package literature for details on dosage and administration.

Neonates: The preferred administration route is continuous intravenous infusion into a large vein. Alternatively, alprostadil may be given through an umbilical artery catheter placed at the ductal opening. Alprostadil must be diluted in the appropriate amount of sodium chloride injection or dextrose injection prior to infusion. Initiate infusion with 0.05 to 0.1 µg/kg/minute. After a therapeutic response is achieved (increased pO2 in infants with restricted pulmonary blood flow or increased systemic blood pressure and blood pH in infants with restricted systemic blood flow), reduce the infusion rate to the lowest dosage that maintains the response. This may be achieved by lowering the dosage from 0.1 to 0.05 to 0.025 to 0.01 µg/kg/minute. If response to 0.05 µg/kg/minute is inadequate, dosage can be increased gradually up to 0.4 µg/kg/minute. However, infusion rates higher than 0.1 µg/kg/minute generally do not produce greater response.

IN BRIEF

INDICATIONS
Erectile dysfunction (Caverject injection, Edex Injection, Muse Pellet)
Temporary maintenance of patency of ductus arteriosus in neonates who have congenital heart defects and who depend upon the patent ductus for survival until corrective or palliative surgery can be performed (Prostin VR Pediatric Injection)

CONTRAINDICATIONS
Hypersensitivity
Conditions that might predispose patients to priapism
Patients with anatomical deformation of the penis
Patients with penile implants
Use in women
For sexual intercourse with a pregnant woman unless the couple uses a condom barrier
Respiratory distress syndrome (hyaline membrane disease)

DRUG INTERACTIONS
Anticoagulants
Cyclosporine

ADVERSE EFFECTS
Cardiovascular: flushing, bradycardia, hypotension, tachycardia, cardiac arrest, edema
CNS: fever, headache, dizziness, seizures
GI: diarrhea
Respiratory: apnea, upper respiratory infection, flu syndrome, sinusitis, bronchial wheezing, nasal congestion, respiratory depression, cough
GU: penile pain, prolonged erection, penile fibrosis, injection site hematoma, penile disorder

PHARMACOKINETICS AND PHARMACODYNAMICS
Duration of action: the dose of alprostadil that is selected for self-injection treatment should provide patient with an erection that is sufficient for sexual intercourse and that is maintained for no longer than one hour (adults). Closure of the ductus arteriosus usually begins within 1 to 2 hours after the discontinuation of infusion (neonates)
Metabolism: pulmonary. In patients with normal respiratory function, up to 80% of a dose may be metabolized in one pass through the lungs
Elimination: metabolites excreted in urine (90% within 24 hours)
Half-life: 30 seconds to 10 minutes
Protein binding: ≈ 80% to albumin

MONITORING
For adults: degree of penile pain, length of erection, signs of infection.
For neonates: arterial blood gases, arterial blood pH, blood pressure, heart rate, respiratory rate, temperature, respiratory status, renal output.

OVERDOSE
If intracavernous overdose occurs, monitor patient until any systemic effects have resolved or until penile detumescence has occurred. Symptomatic treatment of any systemic symptoms would be appropriate. Symptoms of overdose when treating patent ductus arteriosus include apnea, bradycardia, pyrexia, hypotension and flushing. If apnea or bradycardia occurs, discontinue alprostadil infusion and provide appropriate medical therapy. Use caution in restarting the infusion. If pyrexia or hypotension occurs, decrease the infusion rate until symptoms subside. Flushing is usually a result of incorrect intra-arterial catheter placement; repositioning the catheter may help.

PATIENT INFORMATION
For adult patients using alprostadil for erectile dysfunction, refer to patient package literature for proper administration and storage of alprostadil. Do not change the dose of alprostadil established in the physician's office without consulting the physician. Erection may be expected within 5 to 20 minutes after administration of medication. Do not use alprostadil if the female partner is pregnant, unless a condom barrier is used. Inform physician as soon as possible if any new penile pain, nodules, hard tissue or signs of infection develop.

AVAILABILITY
Caverject Injection (powder for injection, lyopholized): 6.15 µg (5 µg/mL), 11.9 µg (10 µg/mL), 23.2 µg (20 µg/mL)
Edex Injection—5 µg, 10 µg, 20 µg, 40 µg
Muse (pellet)—125 µg, 250 µg, 500 µg, 1000 µg
Prostin VR Pediatric (injection)—500 µg/mL (1 mL ampule)

The information here is provided as guidance only. Prescribers should always consult the manufacturer's current prescribing information.

CILOSTAZOL (Pletal®)

Cilostazol is a phosphodiesterase III inhibitor demonstrated to be effective for the management of intermittent claudication. It suppresses cAMP degradation with a resultant elevation of cAMP in blood platelets and blood vessels, thus leading to an inhibition of platelet aggregation and vasodilation. Cilostazol's vasodilatory effect, however, is not homogeneous. A greater degree of dilation seems to be demonstrated by the femoral artery than the vertebral, carotid, and superior mesenteric arteries. The renal arteries are not responsive to cilostazol.

Money *et al.*, studied the effects of cilostazol on walking distance in 239 patients with intermittent claudication. Compared with patients treated with placebo, patients treated with cilostazol 100 mg twice daily demonstrated significant improvements in absolute claudication distance at weeks 8, 12, and 16. Improvements in walking distances for cilostazol-treated patients were also demonstrated in another study conducted by Dawson et. al., where 81 patients with intermittent claudication were randomized to either 12 weeks of treatment with cilostazol or placebo. At present, there are no studies on the effects of cilostazol on long-term outcome in patients with intermittent claudication. Additional studies on the efficacy and safety of chronic cilostazol use are required to establish the long-term utility of this agent.

SPECIAL GROUPS

Race: no differences in response
Children: safety and efficacy have not been established
Elderly: dosage adjustment is usually not required
Renal impairment: dosage adjustment is usually not required in patients with mild to moderate renal impairment
Hepatic impairment: dosage adjustment is usually not required in patients with mild to moderate hepatic impairment
Smokers: smoking reduces cilostazol exposure by approximately 20%
Pregnancy: category C; use only if the potential benefit justifies the potential risk to the fetus
Breast-feeding: not recommended; cilostazol may be excreted in breast milk

DOSAGE

The recommended dose is 100 mg twice daily, taken at least 30 min before or 2 h after breakfast and dinner. Clinical response may be observed after 2–4 wk from initiation of therapy. However, treatment for up to 12 wk may be needed before a beneficial effect is experienced. The dose should be reduced to 50 mg twice daily when cilostazol is coadministered with cytochrome P450 3A4 or 2C19 inhibitors such as ketoconazole, itraconazole, erythromycin, diltiazem, and omeprazole. Since cytochrome P450 3A4 is also inhibited by grapefruit juice, this beverage should also be avoided in patients receiving cilostazol.

IN BRIEF

INDICATIONS
Intermittent claudication (reduction of symptoms of intermittent claudication as indicated by an increased walking distance)

CONTRAINDICATIONS
Hypersensitivity
CHF

DRUG INTERACTIONS
Aspirin (may not be clinically significant)
Cytochrome P450 3A4 inhibitors (eg, erythromycin, ketoconazole, itraconazole, diltiazem, and grapefruit juice.)
Cytochrome P450 2C19 inhibitors (eg, omeprazole)
Warfarin (possible interaction)

ADVERSE EFFECTS
Cardiovascular: palpitation, tachycardia, peripheral edema
CNS: headache (1%–4%), dizziness, vertigo
GI: diarrhea, abnormal stool, dyspepsia, flatulence, nausea
Respiratory: cough, pharyngitis, rhinitis
Others: infection, back pain, myalgia

PHARMACOKINETICS AND PHARMACODYNAMICS
Time to peak plasma
concentration: 3–4 hours
Bioavailability: not known
Effect of food: administration of cilostazol with a high fat meal increases its absorption as indicated by an approximately 90% increase in the maximum plasma concentration
Metabolism: extensively metabolized by hepatic cytochrome P450 3A4 isoenzyme, and to a lesser extent by the 2C19 isoenzyme. Two active metabolites are formed. The more active metabolite, 3,4-dehydrocilostazol, accounts for approximately 50% of the total phosphodiesterase III inhibition
Elimination: urine (74%), feces (20%)
Half-life: 11–13 h
Protein binding: 95%–98%

MONITORING
BP, heart rate, complete blood count (CBC), maximal walking distance.

OVERDOSE
Signs and symptoms of cilostazol overdosage include severe headache, diarrhea, hypotension, tachycardia, and possibly cardiac arrhythmias. Observe the patient carefully and give supportive treatment as needed. Since cilostazol is highly protein-bound, it is unlikely to be removed by hemodialysis.

PATIENT INFORMATION
Take cilostazol at least 30 min before or 2 h after breakfast and dinner. Beneficial effects of this medication may not be immediate. Although improvements may be observed at 2–4 wk after initiation of therapy, treatment for up to 12 wk may be required before a beneficial effect is experienced.
This medication may cause headache, palpitations, and diarrhea. Notify physician if persistent or unusual side effects occur. Do not discontinue therapy without your physician's advice.

AVAILABILITY
Tablets—50 mg, 100 mg

DIAZOXIDE

(Diazoxide, Hyperstat® I.V., Proglycem®)

Diazoxide is a benzothiadiazine derivative that is structurally related to the thiazides. It is used orally for the treatment of intractable hypoglycemia and intravenously for the acute management of hypertensive crisis associated with renal disease. In contrast to the thiazide diuretics, diazoxide causes sodium and water retention. This can result in expansion of plasma and extracellular fluid volume, edema, and CHF, especially during prolonged therapy. The sodium- and water-retaining effects may be prevented by concurrent administration of diazoxide with a diuretic. The hyperglycemic effect is primarily a result of the inhibition of insulin release from the pancreas, as well as an extrapancreatic (catecholamine-induced) effect.

Diazoxide is an extremely useful drug for the emergency management of high BP, as in patients with hypertensive encephalopathy. It offers the advantage of rapidly and consistently lowering the arterial pressure toward normal values, but rarely achieves values below normal. In comparison with nitroprusside, diazoxide has the advantage that constant patient monitoring is not necessary, but it lacks nitroprusside's advantage of immediate dose adjustability. Its diabetogenic effect limits its usefulness, and enthusiasm for its use has declined because of occasional episodes of profound BP reduction.

SPECIAL GROUPS

Race: no differences in response

Children: diazoxide-induced edema occurs most frequently in infants given the oral form; may lead to CHF; no problems seen with parenteral diazoxide in children

Elderly: may require reduction in dose or lengthening of dosage interval

Renal impairment: reduced dose may be necessary, especially with repeated administration

Hepatic impairment: administer with caution; lower doses may be needed

Pregnancy: category C; only to be used when condition may put the mother's life at risk; crosses placenta; may cause harm to fetus; safety is not established

Breast-feeding: not recommended; diazoxide may be excreted in breast milk

DOSAGE

Hypertension: Adults—Intravenously, give 1–3 mg/kg body weight or up to 150 mg every 5–15 min if necessary to obtain desired response. Further doses may be administered every 4–24 h as needed to maintain desired BP until oral antihypertensive medication is effective, usually within 4–5 d. Limit to 1.2 g/d. Do not use for more than 10 d.

Note: Intravenous injection should be administered only into a peripheral vein. Because the alkalinity of the solution is irritating to tissue, avoid extravascular injection or leakage. Treatment is most effective if intravenous administration is completed within 10–30 s. Patient should remain recumbent during and for 15–30 min after administration.

Children—Intravenous 1–3 mg/kg body weight or 30–90 mg/m² body surface area, every 5–15 min as necessary to obtain desired response. Further doses may be given every 4–24 h, as needed to maintain desired BP until oral antihypertensive medication is effective. Injection should be rapid and not exceed 30 s.

IN BRIEF

INDICATIONS
Hypertensive emergencies (intravenous)
Hypoglycemia (oral)

CONTRAINDICATIONS
Hypersensitivity to diazoxide, other thiazides, or other sulfonamide-derived drugs
Compensatory hypertension, such as that associated with aortic coarctation or arteriovenous shunt
Hypertension caused by pheochromocytoma
Dissecting aortic aneurysm
Coronary or cerebral insufficiency
Diabetes mellitus
Inadequate cardiac reserve (*ie*, uncompensated CHF)

DRUG INTERACTIONS
Hydantoins
Hypotension-producing medications
Sulfonylureas
Thiazide diuretics
Warfarin

ADVERSE EFFECTS
Cardiovascular: hypotension (7%), sodium and water retention, myocardial ischemia, atrial and ventricular arrhythmias, electrocardiogram (ECG) changes
CNS: dizziness/weakness (2%), cerebral ischemia, convulsions, confusion, headache
GI: nausea, vomiting (4%), abdominal discomfort, anorexia, alterations in taste, dry mouth, constipation, diarrhea
Others: hyperglycemia, dyspnea, cough, choking sensation, hirsutism, tinnitus, neutropenia, leukopenia, thrombocytopenia, hyperuricemia, decreased libido

PHARMACOKINETICS AND PHARMACODYNAMICS
Duration of action: 2–12 h (intravenous)
Onset of action: 1 min (intravenous)
Time to peak effect: 2–5 min (after intravenous push)
Bioavailability: oral formulation is readily absorbed
Effect of food: not known
Metabolism: hepatic
Elimination: approximately 50% excreted unchanged in the urine
Half-life: 9–24 h (children), 20–36 h (adults), >30 h (end stage renal disease)
Protein binding: >90%

MONITORING
BP, blood glucose, serum uric acid.
Cardiac and BP monitoring are required for intravenous administration.

OVERDOSE
Can result in hyperglycemia (which responds to insulin); monitor patient for up to 7 d while blood sugar concentration stabilizes. Severe hypotension responds to vasopressor treatment.

PATIENT INFORMATION
If the suspension has been prescribed, shake well before using. Check blood glucose carefully. This medication may cause dizziness, headache, edema, weakness, nausea, and vomiting. Notify physician if persistent or unusual side effects occur. Do not discontinue therapy without your physician's advice.

DOSAGE (CONTINUED)

Elderly—May require reduction in dose or lengthening of dosage interval.

Hypoglycemia: Adults and Adolescents—Oral, initially 1 mg/kg of body weight every 8 h, adjusted according to clinical response. For maintenance, 3–8 mg/kg of body weight a day, divided into two or three equal doses every 12 or 8 h, respectively.

Neonates and Infants—Oral, 3.3 mg/kg body weight every 8 h, adjusted according to clinical response. For maintenance, 8–15 mg/kg of body weight a day divided into two or three equal doses every 12 or 8 h, respectively.

Elderly—More likely to have age-related renal function impairment, which may require a reduction in dosage and/or longer dosing interval.

AVAILABILITY
Injection (Hyperstat I.V.)—15 mg/mL (20 mL)
Capsules (Proglycem)—50 mg
Suspension, oral (Proglycem)—50 mg/mL (30 mL)

EPOPROSTENOL (Flolan®)

Epoprostenol, a metabolite of arachidonic acid, is a naturally occurring prostaglandin. It causes direct vasodilation of pulmonary and systemic arterial vascular beds, inhibits platelet aggregation, and has antiproliferative effects. Epoprostenol is rapidly hydrolyzed in the blood, with a half-life of approximately six minutes. A 12 week controlled trial in 81 patients with severe primary pulmonary hypertension showed that the addition of epoprostenol to conventional treatment was associated with better exercise capacity, fewer symptoms and no deaths among 40 patients, compared to eight deaths among 41 patients treated with conventional therapy alone. In a recent study involving 27 patients with advanced primary pulmonary hypertension, McLaughlin et al., found that long-term (>1 year) therapy with epoprostenol lowered pulmonary vascular resistance beyond the level achieved in the short term with intravenous adenosine.

The use of epoprostenol in patients with CHF, however, has not been very successful as demonstrated by the FIRST trial in which the combination of epoprostenol infusion and standard therapy was compared to standard therapy alone in 471 patients with class IIIB/IV CHF and decreased left ventricular ejection fraction. Although epoprostenol infusion was associated with a significant increase in cardiac index, a decrease in pulmonary capillary wedge pressure, and a decrease in systemic vascular resistance, this trial was terminated early because of a strong trend toward decreased survival in the patients treated with epoprostenol. Hence, the manufacturer of epoprostenol states that this medication should not be used on a chronic basis in patients with CHF due to severe left ventricular systolic dysfunction.

SPECIAL GROUPS

Race: not studied
Children: safety and effectiveness have not been established
Elderly: use with caution; reduced doses may be needed
Renal impairment: use with caution; the metabolites of epoprostenol are excreted in the urine
Hepatic impairment: use with caution
Pregnancy: category B; this drug should be used during pregnancy only if clearly indicated
Breast-feeding: not recommended; epoprostenol may be excreted in breast milk

IN BRIEF

INDICATIONS
Primary pulmonary hypertension (epoprostenol is indicated for the long-term intravenous treatment of primary pulmonary hypertension in NYHA Class III and Class IV patients)

CONTRAINDICATIONS
Hypersensitivity
CHF due to severe left ventricular systolic dysfunction

DRUG INTERACTIONS
Antiplatelet agents (may not be clinically significant)
Anticoagulants (may not be clinically significant)
Diuretics
Other vasodilators

ADVERSE EFFECTS
Cardiovascular: flushing, tachycardia, hypotension, chest pain, bradycardia
CNS: dizziness, headache, anxiety, nervousness, tremor, hyperesthesia, paresthesia
GI: nausea, vomiting, diarrhea, abdominal pain
Musculoskeletal: jaw pain, myalgia, nonspecific musculoskeletal pain
Others: chills, fever, catheter-associated sepsis, flu-like symptoms, hemorrhage, dyspnea

PHARMACOKINETICS AND PHARMACODYNAMICS
Duration of action: 5 min (cardiovascular effects), 2 h (platelet aggregation inhibition)
Time to steady state concentration: 15 min (continuous infusion)
Metabolism: rapidly hydrolyzed at neutral pH in blood and is also subjected to enzymatic degradation. Epoprostenol is metabolized to two primary metabolites, both of which have pharmacological activity orders of magnitude less than the parent drug in animal test systems.
Elimination: metabolites of epoprostenol are found mainly in the urine.
Half-life: ≤6 min

MONITORING
Monitor for improvements in pulmonary function and dose-related adverse effects. Adjust infusion rate accordingly. Pump device and catheters should be checked frequently to avoid system related failure.

OVERDOSE
Signs and symptoms of excessive doses of epoprostenol during clinical trials are the expected dose-limiting pharmacologic effects of epoprostenol, including flushing, headache, hypotension, tachycardia, nausea, vomiting, and diarrhea. Treatment will ordinarily require dose reduction of epoprostenol. One patient with secondary pulmonary hypertension accidentally received 50 ml of an unknown concentration of epoprostenol. The patient vomited and became unconscious with an initially unrecordable BP. Epoprostenol was discontinued and the patient regained consciousness within seconds. No fatal events have been reported following overdosage of epoprostenol.

DOSAGE

Acute Dose-Ranging: The infusion rate is initiated at 2 ng/kg/min and increased in increments of 2 ng/kg/min every 15 min or longer until dose-limiting pharmacologic effects occur. The most common dose-limiting pharmacologic effects are nausea, vomiting, headache, hypotension, and flushing. During acute dose-ranging in clinical trials, the mean maximum dose which did not result in dose-limiting pharmacologic effects was 8.6 ± 0.3 ng/kg/min

Note: Epoprostenol must be reconstituted only with sterile diluent for epoprostenol. Reconstituted solutions of epoprostenol must not be diluted or administered with other parenteral solutions or medications.

Continuous Chronic Infusion: Chronic infusions of epoprostenol should be initiated at 4 ng/kg/min less than the maximum-tolerated infusion rate determined during acute dose-ranging. If the maximum-tolerated infusion rate is less than 5 ng/kg/min, the chronic infusion should be started at one half the maximum-tolerated infusion rate. During clinical trials, the mean initial chronic infusion rate was 5 ng/kg/min

Note: Chronic continuous infusion of epoprostenol should be administered through a central venous catheter. Temporary peripheral intravenous infusions may be used until central access is established.

Dosage Adjustments: Alterations in the chronic infusion rate should be based on persistence, recurrence, or worsening of the patient's symptoms of primary pulmonary hypertension and the occurrence of adverse events due to excessive doses of epoprostenol. In general, increases in dose from the initial chronic dose should be expected. Increments in dose should be considered if symptoms of primary pulmonary hypertension persist or recur after improving. The infusion should be increased by 1–2 ng/kg/min increments at intervals sufficient to allow assessment of clinical response; these intervals should be at least 15 min. In contrast, decreased dosage of epoprostenol should be considered when dose-related pharmacological events occur. Dosage decreases should be made gradually in 2 ng/kg/min decrements every 15 min or longer until the dose-limiting adverse effects resolve.

Note: Abrupt withdrawal of epoprostenol or sudden large reductions in infusion rates should be avoided with the exception of life-threatening situations such as unconsciousness or collapse. Consult epoprostenol package literature for detailed information on administration and reconstitution of epoprostenol.

PATIENT INFORMATION

Epoprostenol must be reconstituted only with sterile diluent for epoprostenol. Epoprostenol is infused continuously through a permanent indwelling central venous catheter via a small, portable infusion pump. Therefore, therapy with epoprostenol requires commitment by the patient to drug reconstitution, drug administration, and care of the permanent central venous catheter. Sterile technique must be followed in preparing the drug and in the care of the catheter. Even brief interruptions in the delivery of epoprostenol may result in rapid symptomatic deterioration. Base the decision to receive epoprostenol for primary pulmonary hypertension on the understanding that there is a high likelihood that therapy with this medication will be needed for prolonged periods, possibly years. Infusion rates of epoprostenol should be adjusted only under the direction of a physician.

AVAILABILITY

Powder for reconstitution—0.5 mg, 1.5 mg (mannitol, NaCl. In 17 mL flint glass vials)

FENOLDOPAM (Corlopam® I.V.)

Fenoldopam mesylate is a dopamine agonist that induces peripheral vasodilation through stimulation of dopamine$_1$ receptors. Fenoldopam also causes renal vasculature vasodilation, which leads to an increase in renal blood flow. Fenoldopam has been compared with sodium nitroprusside in the management of patients with hypertensive urgencies and emergencies.

Treatment with fenoldopam was demonstrated to be as effective as treatment with sodium nitroprusside in a randomized, open-label, multi-center trial involving 153 severely hypertensive patients with diastolic BP of 120 mmHg or higher. A dose-dependent reduction in arterial pressure for up to 24 hours without evidence of tolerance, rebound on withdrawal or significant changes in heart rate was observed with intravenous infusion of fenoldopam.

Fenoldopam has also been shown to be an appropriate alternative to sodium nitroprusside for patients who develop hypertension after coronary artery bypass graft surgery. Additional evidence has demonstrated fenoldopam to be effective in treating hypertension after noncardiac surgery. The adverse event profiles of fenoldopam and sodium nitroprusside were generally comparable in comparative trials. In contrast to sodium nitroprusside, fenoldopam produces a dose-related modest increase in intraocular pressure and may be associated with a lower incidence of hypotension. In addition, intravenous fenoldopam may offer advantages over sodium nitroprusside because it can induce both a diuresis and natriuresis, is not light sensitive, and is not associated with cyanide toxicity.

SPECIAL GROUPS

Race: no differences in response
Children: safety and effectiveness have not been established
Elderly: dosage adjustments are generally not necessary
Renal impairment: dosage adjustments are generally not necessary
Hepatic impairment: dosage adjustments are generally not necessary
Pregnancy: category B; fenoldopam should be used in pregnancy only if clearly indicated
Breast-feeding: not recommended; fenoldopam may be excreted in breast milk

DOSAGE

The initial dose of fenoldopam is chosen according to the desired magnitude and rate of BP reduction in a given clinical situation. In general, there is a greater and more rapid BP reduction as the initial dose is increased. Lower initial doses (0.03–0.1 µg/kg/min) titrated slowly have been associated with less reflex tachycardia than have higher initial doses (≥0.3 µg/kg/min). The recommended increments for titration are 0.05–0.1 µg/kg/min at intervals of ≥15 min. Doses below 0.1 µg/kg/min have very modest effects and appear only marginally useful in patients with severe hypertension. Fenoldopam infusion can be abruptly discontinued or gradually tapered prior to discontinuation. Oral antihypertensive agents can be added during fenoldopam infusion (after BP is stable) or following its discontinuation. Patients in clinical trials have received intravenous fenoldopam for a maximum of 48 h.

Note: Fenoldopam should be administered by continuous intravenous infusion only. A bolus dose should not be used. The fenoldopam injection ampule concentrate must be diluted with the appropriate amount of 0.9% sodium chloride or 5% dextrose before infusion. See fenoldopam package insert for details on proper dilution.

IN BRIEF

INDICATIONS
Short term management of severe hypertension
Malignant hypertension associated with deteriorating end-organ function

CONTRAINDICATIONS
Hypersensitivity to fenoldopam and sodium metabisulfite

DRUG INTERACTIONS
Formal drug-drug interaction studies using intravenous fenoldopam have not been performed
Concomitant use of a beta blocker should be avoided

ADVERSE EFFECTS
Cardiovascular: hypotension (>5%), palpitation, tachycardia, bradycardia, edema, heart failure, ischemic heart disease, myocardial infarction (MI), angina pectoris
CNS: headache (>5%), dizziness
GI: nausea (>5%), vomiting, diarrhea
Others: flushing (>5%), hypokalemia, increased intraocular pressure, dyspnea, elevated blood urea nitrogen (BUN), elevated serum glucose, elevated transaminase, leukocytosis, bleeding, limb cramp, oliguria, pyrexia

PHARMACOKINETICS AND PHARMACODYNAMICS
Duration of action: ≈ 1 h (intravenous)
Onset of action: ≈ 5 min (intravenous)
Time to steady state plasma concentration: ≈ 20 min
Metabolism: hepatic to inactive metabolites
Elimination: renal (90%), fecal (10%); only 4% of a dose is eliminated as unchanged drug
Half-life: ≈ 5 min

MONITORING
Monitor BP and heart rate at frequent intervals (ie, every 15 min) to avoid hypotension and rapid reductions of BP. Electrolytes should also be monitored frequently (electrolytes were monitored at intervals of 6 h during clinical trials).
Fenoldopam may increase intraocular pressure; administer with caution in patients with glaucoma or intraocular hypertension.

OVERDOSE
Intentional fenoldopam overdosage has not been reported. The most likely reaction would be excessive hypotension, which should be managed with drug discontinuation and appropriate supportive measures.

PATIENT INFORMATION
This drug is used for short-term management of severe hypertension. Adverse effects such as headache, flushing, nausea, and dizziness may occur.

AVAILABILITY
Injection, concentrate—10 mg/mL (5 mL ampules)

HYDRALAZINE (Hydralazine, Apresoline®)

The predominant effect of hydralazine is direct vasodilatation of arterioles, with only slight effect on veins. Hydralazine reduces peripheral resistance, an action probably important in its antihypertensive effect, although the exact mechanism by which this action is accomplished is unknown. The increase in cardiac output, decrease in systemic resistance, and reduction in afterload may explain its efficacy in treating CHF, where, in combination with nitrates it has been shown to reduce mortality more than prazosin. This combination, however, has since been shown to be less effective in reducing mortality than an angiotensin converting enzyme (ACE) inhibitor.

Apparent tolerance to the antihypertensive effects of hydralazine may develop with chronic administration. Concurrent diuretic therapy may decrease this tendency and enhance the antihypertensive effects. Hydralazine does not appear to reverse left ventricular hypertrophy. Lupus erythematosus is a recognized adverse effect that is apparently more frequent in those who are slow to form acetyl derivatives. Despite this effect, the drug is well tolerated when used as a third drug after the concomitant use of a diuretic agent and a beta-blocker.

SPECIAL GROUPS

Race: no differences in response

Children: safety and efficacy have not been established; however, there is experience with the use of hydralazine in children

Elderly: may require reduction in dose or lengthening of dosage interval

Renal impairment: in severe renal impairment, interval between doses should be prolonged to avoid accumulation

Hepatic impairment: may require reduction in dose or lengthening of dosage interval

Pregnancy: category C; use only when potential benefits outweigh potential hazards to the fetus. However, intravenous hydralazine has been used effectively and generally is considered the parenteral hypotensive agent of choice for the management of hypertensive emergencies associated with pregnancy (eg, preeclampsia, eclampsia)

Breast-feeding: not recommended; hydralazine is excreted in breast milk

IN BRIEF

INDICATIONS
Essential hypertension (oral formulation)

Severe essential hypertension when the drug cannot be given orally or when the need to lower BP is urgent (parenteral formulation)

CONTRAINDICATIONS
Hypersensitivity to hydralazine or any of its components such as tartrazine and sulfites

Mitral valve rheumatic heart disease

DRUG INTERACTIONS
Beta blockers (metoprolol, propranolol)

Indomethacin

Monoamine oxidase (MAO) inhibitors

ADVERSE EFFECTS
Cardiovascular: palpitation, tachycardia, hypotension, angina pectoris

CNS: headache, peripheral neuritis, numbness and tingling, dizziness, tremors, depression, anxiety

GI: nausea, vomiting, anorexia, diarrhea, constipation, paralytic ileus

Hematologic: blood dyscrasias, leukopenia, agranulocytosis and purpura, lymphadenopathy, splenomegaly

Others: nasal congestion, flushing, edema, muscle cramps, dyspnea, urination difficulty, lupus-like syndrome, rash, urticaria, fever, arthralgia, eosinophilia, hepatitis (rare)

PHARMACOKINETICS AND PHARMACODYNAMICS
Duration of action: 6–12 h (oral), 2–4 h (intravenous)

Onset of action: 45 min (oral), 10–20 min (intravenous)

Time to peak effect: 1 h (oral), 15–30 min (intravenous)

Bioavailability: 30%–50%

Effect of food: administration with food results in higher plasma hydralazine concentrations

Metabolism: hepatic, extensive

Elimination: in urine as active drug (12%–14%) and metabolites

Half-life: 3–7 h

Protein binding: 87%

MONITORING
BP, heart rate, antinuclear antibody (ANA) titer determinations, complete blood counts. In addition to the contraindications listed above, hydralazine should be used with extreme caution in patients with cerebrovascular accidents, pulmonary hypertension, severe renal damage, or coronary artery disease (CAD).

OVERDOSE
Symptoms of overdose include hypotension, tachycardia, headache, and generalized skin flushing. Complications can include myocardial ischemia and subsequent MI, cardiac arrhythmias and shock. Treatment is primarily supportive and symptomatic. In acute overdose, perform gastric lavage as soon as possible. Supportive measures include the administration of intravenous fluids. In hypotension, raise pressure without increasing or aggravating tachycardia. Avoid adrenaline use. Tachycardia responds to beta blockers. Digitalization may be necessary.

PATIENT INFORMATION
Take hydralazine with meals. Since this medication may cause dizziness, use caution when driving or performing other activities that require alertness. Notify physician if persistent or unusual side effects such as tiredness, fever, muscle or joint aches, or chest pain occur. Do not discontinue therapy without your physician's advice.

The information here is provided as guidance only. Prescribers should always consult the manufacturer's current prescribing information.

257

HYDRALAZINE (CONTINUED)

DOSAGE

Oral: Adults—For hypertension, give 40 mg/d for the first 2–4 d, 100 mg/d for the balance of week one, and 200 mg/d for week 2 and subsequent weeks in four divided daily doses. Maintain dose at lowest effective level. Maximum dose is 300 mg/d. Higher doses have been used in the treatment of CHF.

Children—For hypertension, give 750 µg (0.75 mg)/kg body weight or 25 mg/m^2 body surface area per day divided into four doses; increase gradually over 3–4 wk as needed. Maximum dose is 7.5 mg/kg of body weight or 200 mg/d.

Parenteral: Adults—For hypertension, give 10–40 mg intravenously or intramuscularly; repeat as needed.

Note: Hydralazine should not be diluted with solutions containing dextrose or other sugars, because it can form potentially toxic hydrazones.

Children—For hypertension, give 0.1–0.2 mg/kg/dose intravenously or intramuscularly every 4–6 h as needed.

AVAILABILITY

Tablets—10 mg, 25 mg, 50 mg, 100 mg.
Injection—20 mg/mL (1 mL)
Combination formulations:
Apresazide—Hydralazine hydrochloride/ hydrochlorothiazide combination capsules
  25 mg/ 25 mg
  50 mg/ 50 mg
  100 mg/ 50 mg
Hydra-Zide—Hydralazine hydrochloride/ hydrochlorothiazide combination capsules
  25 mg/ 25 mg
  50 mg/ 50 mg
  100 mg/ 50 mg
Hydrap-ES
Marpres
Ser-Ap-Es
Tri-Hydroserpine
Unipres—Reserpine/ hydrochlorothiazide/hydralazine HCl combination tablets
  0.1 mg/ 15 mg/ 25 mg

ISOSORBIDE DINITRATE

(Isosorbide dinitrate, Isordil®, Sorbitrate®, Dilatrate®-SR)

Isosorbide dinitrate is an important member of the organic nitrate ester family. Although the exact mechanism of action of the nitrates is not fully known, the principal pharmacologic action of these agents is relaxation of vascular smooth muscle, resulting in generalized vasodilation. Nitrates are well established in the treatment of various cardiovascular disorders, most notably angina pectoris and CHF. Attenuation of hemodynamic effects may occur with all long-acting nitrates. Continuous administration tends to promote this tolerance, whereas intermittent administration appears to maintain efficacy.

Isosorbide dinitrate reduces left ventricular preload and afterload because of venous (predominantly) and arterial dilatation, with a more efficient redistribution of blood flow within the myocardium. Because of its venodilatory action, it has been advantageously combined with hydralazine, an arterial vasodilator, to produce a balanced effect leading to a greater reduction in mortality in heart failure than has been seen with prazosin but less of an effect than that seen with ACE inhibitors. Isosorbide dinitrate is available in various formulations. Slow-release formulations are available for prophylaxis, and chewable forms are available to provide rapid absorption and relief of symptoms. Isosorbide dinitrate is indicated for the prophylaxis and treatment of angina. Low-dose nitrate treatment has been regarded as well tolerated in the treatment of acute MI. It improves left ventricular performance, possibly limiting infarct size and reducing complications. However, nitrates should be used under close clinical observation and with hemodynamic monitoring in acute MI. A short-acting form should be used in this setting because its effects can be terminated rapidly should excessive hypotension or tachycardia develop.

SPECIAL GROUPS

Race: no differences in response

Children: safety and effectiveness have not been established

Elderly: lower doses may be required

Renal impairment: no dosage adjustment is usually necessary Use with caution in severe renal impairment

Hepatic impairment: lower doses may be advisable; avoid use in severe hepatic impairment

Pregnancy: category C; use only when clearly needed and when potential benefits outweigh potential hazards to the fetus

Breast-feeding: not recommended; nitrates may be excreted in breast milk

IN BRIEF

INDICATIONS
Angina pectoris (treatment and prevention of angina pectoris)

CONTRAINDICATIONS
Hypersensitivity or idiosyncrasy to nitrates
Severe anemia
Closed angle glaucoma
Postural hypotension
Head trauma or cerebral hemorrhage

DRUG INTERACTIONS
Alcohol
Aspirin
Calcium channel blockers
Dihydroergotamine

ADVERSE EFFECTS
Cardiovascular: hypotension, tachycardia, retrosternal discomfort, palpitation, syncope, arrhythmias, edema
CNS: headache, lightheadedness, dizziness, weakness, anxiety, confusion, insomnia
GI: nausea, vomiting, diarrhea, dyspepsia, dry mouth
Dermatologic: drug rash, pruritus, exfoliative dermatitis, cutaneous vasodilation with flushing
Others: flushing, arthralgia, dysuria, impotence, urinary frequency, hemolytic anemia, asthenia, blurred vision, methemoglobinemia (rare, usually with overdose)

PHARMACOKINETICS AND PHARMACODYNAMICS
Duration of action: oral, 4–6 h; sublingual, 1–2 h; chewable, 1–2 h; sustained-release, 6–8 h
Onset of action: oral, 20–40 min; sublingual, 2–5 min; chewable, 2–5 min; sustained-release, 30 min–4 h
Bioavailability: sublingual, 59%; oral, 22%
Effect of food: for faster absorption, administer oral nitrates on an empty stomach with a glass of water.
Metabolism: hepatic (very rapid and nearly complete) and in blood (enzymatically). Two active metabolites are isosorbide 5-mononitrate and isosorbide-2-mononitrate
Elimination: renal, as metabolites
Half-life: oral, 4 h; sublingual, 1 h
Protein binding: minimal

MONITORING
BP, heart rate.

OVERDOSE
Gastric lavage may be useful if the medication has only recently been swallowed. If excessive hypotension occurs, elevate legs to aid venous return. Administer oxygen and artificial ventilation if needed. Monitor methemoglobin concentrations as indicated.

PATIENT INFORMATION
Take oral nitrates on an empty stomach with a glass of water. Do not chew or crush sublingual or sustained release dosage form. Do not change from one brand of this drug to another without consulting your physician or pharmacist. Avoid alcohol. This medication may cause headache, dizziness, flushing, blurred vision, or dry mouth. Notify physician if persistent or unusual side effects occur. Do not discontinue therapy without your physician's advice.

DOSAGE

Oral tablets, short acting (Isosorbide dinitrate, Isordil Titradose, Sorbitrate): As an antianginal agent, give 5–20 mg in tablet form three times daily; adjust as needed and tolerated. Usual dosage range is 10–40 mg three times daily. Elderly may be more sensitive to hypotensive effect. Use with caution in those with impaired hepatic and renal functions; a reduction in dosage may be required.

Note: A daily nitrate-free interval of at least 14 h is advisable to minimize tolerance. The optimal interval will vary with the individual patient, dose, and regimen.

Oral tablets and capsules, sustained-release (Isosorbide dinitrate, Isordil Tembids, Dilatrate-SR, Isordil Tembids): Administer sustained-release preparations once daily or twice daily in doses given 6 h apart (*ie*, 8 am and 2 pm). Do not exceed 160 mg/d.

Sublingual and chewable tablets (Isosorbide dinitrate, Isordil, Sorbitrate): For angina pectoris, the usual starting dose is 2.5 –5 mg for sublingual tablets and 5 mg for chewable tablets. Titrate upward until angina is relieved or when dose-related adverse effects occur. For acute prophylaxis, administer 5–10 mg sublingual or chewable tablets every 2–3 h.

Note: Limit use of sublingual or chewable isosorbide dinitrate for terminating an acute anginal attack in patients intolerant of or unresponsive to sublingual nitroglycerin.

AVAILABILITY

Oral tablets (Isosorbide dinitrate)—5 mg, 10 mg, 20 mg, 30 mg
Oral tablets (Isordil Titradose, Sorbitrate)—5 mg, 10 mg, 20 mg, 30 mg, 40 mg
Tablets, sublingual (Isosorbide dinitrate, Isordil)—2.5 mg, 5 mg, 10 mg
Tablets, sublingual (Sorbitrate)—2.5 mg, 5 mg
Tablets, chewable (Sorbitrate)—5 mg, 10 mg
Tablets, sustained release (Isosorbide dinitrate, Isordil Tembids)—40 mg
Capsules, sustained release (Dilatrate-SR, Isordil Tembids)—40 mg

ISOSORBIDE MONONITRATE

(Ismo®, Monoket®, Imdur®)

The active metabolite of isosorbide dinitrate, isosorbide-5-mononitrate, is available for the prophylaxis of angina pectoris. Since it is not subjected to first-pass metabolism in the liver, its bioavailability is almost complete. With an eccentric dosing regimen, the tolerance problem with nitrates may be less prominent, and rebound (early morning worsening of angina) is less of a problem. Regular formulations for twice daily dosing and a once daily extended-release formulation are available. In a placebo-controlled outcomes study, ISIS-4, there was no demonstrable effect of mononitrates on survival in patients with acute MI. The effects of isosorbide mononitrate are difficult to terminate rapidly. Therefore, the use of these agents should be avoided in patients with acute MI or CHF.

SPECIAL GROUPS

Race: no differences in response
Children: safety and effectiveness have not been established
Elderly: lower doses are not usually required. However, older patients may be more susceptible to risks for hypotension
Renal impairment: no dosage adjustment is usually necessary; use with caution in severe renal impairment
Hepatic impairment: no dosage adjustment is usually necessary; use with caution in severe hepatic impairment
Pregnancy: category C; use only when clearly needed and when potential benefits outweigh potential hazards to the fetus
Breast-feeding: not recommended; nitrates may be excreted in breast milk

DOSAGE

For angina prophylaxis, tablets should be swallowed whole. Administer 20 mg (Ismo, Monoket) twice daily with doses given 7 h apart. An initial dose of 5 mg twice daily may be appropriate for persons of small stature. Imdur may be initiated at 30 or 60 mg once daily. Dosage of Imdur may be increased to 120 mg once daily after several days if necessary.

IN BRIEF

INDICATIONS
Angina pectoris (prevention of angina pectoris)

CONTRAINDICATIONS
Hypersensitivity or idiosyncrasy to nitrates
Acute MI with low-filling pressures
Severe anemia
Closed angle glaucoma
Postural hypotension
Head trauma or cerebral hemorrhage

DRUG INTERACTIONS
Alcohol
Aspirin
Calcium channel blockers
Dihydroergotamine

ADVERSE EFFECTS
Cardiovascular: hypotension, tachycardia, retrosternal discomfort, palpitation, syncope, arrhythmias, edema
CNS: headache, lightheadedness, dizziness, weakness, anxiety, confusion, insomnia
GI: nausea, vomiting, diarrhea, dyspepsia
Dermatologic: drug rash, pruritus, exfoliative dermatitis, cutaneous vasodilation with flushing
Others: flushing, arthralgia, dysuria, impotence, urinary frequency, hemolytic anemia, asthenia, blurred vision, methemoglobinemia (rare, usually with overdose)

PHARMACOKINETICS AND PHARMACODYNAMICS
Duration of action: 1–10 h (Ismo, Monoket), ≈ 12 h (Imdur) Duration of action may vary due to development of tolerance
Onset of action: 30–60 min
Time to peak plasma concentration: 30–60 min (Ismo, Monoket), 3–4 h (Imdur)
Bioavailability: ≈ 100%
Effect of food: concomitant food intake may decrease the rate but not the extent of absorption of isosorbide mononitrate
Metabolism: hepatic
Elimination: renal, mainly as inactive metabolites.
Half-life: ≈ 5 h (Ismo, Monoket), ≈ 6 h (Imdur)
Protein binding: minimal, <5%

MONITORING
BP, heart rate.

OVERDOSE
Gastric lavage may be useful if the medication has only recently been swallowed. If excessive hypotension occurs, elevate legs to aid venous return. Administer oxygen and artificial ventilation if needed. Monitor methemoglobin concentrations as indicated.

PATIENT INFORMATION
Extended-release tablets (Imdur) should not be chewed or crushed and should be swallowed together with a half-glassful of fluid. Avoid alcohol. This medication may cause headache, dizziness, flushing, blurred vision, or dry mouth. Notify physician if persistent or unusual side effects occur. Do not discontinue therapy without your physician's advice.

AVAILABILITY
Tablets (Ismo)—20 mg
Tablets (Monoket)—10, 20 mg
Extended-release tablets (Imdur)—30 mg, 60 mg, 120 mg

The information here is provided as guidance only. Prescribers should always consult the manufacturer's current prescribing information.

261

ISOXSUPRINE

(Isoxsuprine, Vasodilan®, Voxsuprine®)

Isoxsuprine is a vasorelaxant that stimulates beta receptors in the vascular wall. Isoxsuprine produces peripheral vasodilatation through a direct effect on vascular smooth muscle, primarily within skeletal muscle, with a smaller effect on cutaneous blood flow. It decreases peripheral resistance, administration of large oral doses may decrease BP. Isoxsuprine also lowers blood viscosity and relaxes the myometrium, thereby inhibiting uterine contractions. This agent may have positive inotropic and chronotropic effects on the heart and may increase cardiac output. Isoxsuprine has been recommended for the treatment of cerebrovascular insufficiency or peripheral vascular disease, but data supporting these claims are very weak. Isoxsuprine has also been used in the management of dysmenorrhea, threatened abortion, and premature labor. However, the efficacy of this agent in the treatment of these conditions has not been established.

SPECIAL GROUPS

Race: no differences in response
Children: safety and efficacy have not been established
Elderly: risk for hypotension may be increased with isoxsuprine; initiate with lower doses
Renal impairment: lower doses may be needed
Hepatic impairment: lower doses may be needed
Pregnancy: category C; use only if the potential benefit justifies the potential risk to the fetus
Breast-feeding: not recommended; isoxsuprine may be excreted in breast milk.

DOSAGE

The usual adult dose is 10–20 mg three to four times daily. Medication may be given with meals to reduce gastrointestinal irritation.

IN BRIEF

INDICATIONS
Relief of symptoms associated with cerebral vascular insufficiency (possibly effective)
Peripheral vascular disease (possibly effective)
Raynaud's disease (possibly effective)

CONTRAINDICATIONS
Hypersensitivity
Immediately postpartum
Arterial bleeding

DRUG INTERACTIONS
Hypotensive agents

ADVERSE EFFECTS
Cardiovascular: hypotension, tachycardia, chest pain
CNS: dizziness, weakness
GI: nausea, vomiting, abdominal distress
Others: rash

PHARMACOKINETICS AND PHARMACODYNAMICS
Time to peak
plasma concentration: within 1 h
Bioavailability: ≈ 100%
Effect of food: not known
Metabolism: partially conjugated in the liver
Elimination: primarily in urine
Half-life: 1.25 h
Protein binding: not known

MONITORING
BP, heart rate.

OVERDOSE
Symptoms of overdose include hypotension, flushing, and vasodilation. Treat with intravenous fluids. Alpha-adrenergic pressors may be required.

PATIENT INFORMATION
This medication may cause dizziness, use caution when driving or performing other activities that require alertness. Notify physician if persistent or unusual side effects occur.

AVAILABILITY
Tablets—10 mg, 20 mg

MINOXIDIL (Minoxidil, Loniten®, Rogaine®)

Minoxidil is a direct-acting peripheral vasodilator. Although minoxidil is indicated for the treatment of hypertension, it has serious side effects and is, therefore, not considered a primary agent in treating essential hypertension. It is recommended for use only in patients with symptomatic or organ-damaging hypertension not responsive to other treatment. Its exact mechanism of action is unknown, but some of its action may be the result of the opening of potassium channels in smooth muscle cells. Its predominant effect is direct vasodilatation of arterioles, with marginal effects on veins. Minoxidil reduces peripheral resistance and causes a reflex increase in heart rate and cardiac output. It should not be used as the sole agent to initiate therapy. Rather, it should be given in conjunction with both a diuretic, to control salt and water retention, and a beta blocker, to control reflex tachycardia.

SPECIAL GROUPS

Race: no differences in response

Children: safety and efficacy have not been established; however, there is experience with the use of minoxidil in children

Elderly: may be more sensitive to hypotensive effects; lower doses may be required

Renal impairment: lower doses may be required

Hepatic impairment: dosage adjustment is usually not necessary

Pregnancy: category C; use only when clearly needed and when potential benefits outweigh potential hazards to the fetus

Breast-feeding: not recommended; minoxidil is excreted in breast milk

DOSAGE

Oral: Adults—Usual initial dose is 5 mg/d as a single dose; may be increased by 10 mg every 3 d (seldom necessary to exceed 50 mg/d). Usual maintenance dose is 10–40 mg/day in one–two divided doses. Maximum dose is 100 mg/d.

Children—For children under 12 y, the usual initial dose is 0.1–0.2 mg/kg once daily; maximum initial dose is 5 mg/d. Increase gradually every 3 d as needed and tolerated. Usual maintenance dose is 0.25–1 mg/kg/d in one to two divided doses. Maximum dose is 50 mg/d.

Topical: Apply 1 mL to affected areas of the scalp twice daily (morning and night). Wash hands after applying.

IN BRIEF

INDICATIONS
Severe hypertension (oral formulation)
Resistant or refractory hypertension (oral formulation)
Male-pattern baldness of the vertex of the scalp (topical formulations)

CONTRAINDICATIONS
Hypersensitivity
Pheochromocytoma
Acute MI
Dissecting aortic aneurysm

DRUG INTERACTIONS
Guanethidine
Other hypotensive agents (additive hypotensive effects)

ADVERSE EFFECTS
Cardiovascular: ECG changes, tachycardia, CHF, hypotension, edema, pericardial effusion and tamponade (<1%)
CNS: headache, fatigue
GI: nausea, vomiting
Hematologic: transient hematocrit and hemoglobin decrease, thrombocytopenia (<1%), leukopenia (rare)
Others: rash, breast tenderness, darkening of skin, hypertrichosis, fluid and electrolyte imbalance

PHARMACOKINETICS AND PHARMACODYNAMICS
Duration of action: up to 100 h (oral)
Onset of action: 30 min (oral)
Time to peak effect: within 2–8 h (oral)
Bioavailability: 90% (oral); 1%–4% (topical)
Effect of food: not known
Metabolism: hepatic, 90%; predominantly by conjugation with glucuronic acid; metabolites exert much less pharmacologic effect than the parent drug (oral)
Elimination: primarily in the urine
Half-life: 4.2 h
Protein binding: not significant

MONITORING
BP, heart rate, CBC, electrolytes.

OVERDOSE
If marked hypotension occurs, give normal saline intravenously.
Avoid epinephrine and norepinephrine because of their stimulant effects on the heart.
Use vasopressors such as phenylephrine, vasopressin, and dopamine only if a vital organ is underperfused.

PATIENT INFORMATION
If the topical formulation of this product is prescribed, apply to affected areas of the scalp twice daily. Wash hands after applying. Hair growth usually takes 4 mo. The oral formulation of this medication may cause dizziness, use caution when performing tasks that require alertness. Get up slowly from a sitting or lying position. Notify physician if persistent or unusual side effects occur (ie, increased heart rate; rapid weight gain; unusual swelling of extremities, face, or abdomen; breathing difficulty, especially when lying down; chest pain). Do not discontinue therapy without your physician's advice.

AVAILABILITY
Tablets—2.5 mg, 10 mg
Topical solution—2% (60 mL), 5% (60 mL)

NITROGLYCERIN

(Nitroglycerin, Tridil®, Nitro-Bid®, Nitrostat®, Nitrolingual®, Nitrogard®, Nitrong®, Nitrocine® Timecaps, Nitroglyn®, Minitran®, Nitro-Dur®, Transderm-Nitro®, Nitrodisc®, Deponit®, Nitro-Derm®, Nitrol®)

Nitroglycerin has been the mainstay in the acute management of angina pectoris for many years. It reduces left ventricular preload and afterload because of venous (predominantly) and arterial dilatation, with a beneficial redistribution of blood flow within the myocardium. It may be successfully combined with other vasodilators and is available as parenteral, capsule, tablet, topical, sublingual, buccal, aerosol, ointment, and transdermal formulations. As with all other nitrate formulations, nitroglycerin is associated with pharmacologic tolerance and with continued use must be administered intermittently. Low-dose treatment with intravenous nitroglycerin has been regarded as safe and effective for use after MI. Its use results in reduced infarct size and improved left ventricular performance.

SPECIAL GROUPS

Race: no differences in response
Children: safety and effectiveness have not been established
Elderly: lower doses may be required
Renal impairment: no dosage adjustment is usually necessary; use with caution in severe renal impairment
Hepatic impairment: lower doses may be advisable; avoid use in severe hepatic impairment
Pregnancy: category C; use only when clearly needed and when potential benefits outweigh potential hazards to the fetus
Breast-feeding: not recommended; nitrates may be excreted in breast milk

DOSAGE

Sublingual tablets (Nitrostat): Dissolve one tablet under tongue or in buccal pouch at first sign of an acute anginal attack. Repeat approximately every 5 min until relief is obtained. No more than three tablets should be taken in 15 min. If pain persists, notify physician or get to emergency room immediately. May be used prophylactically 5–10 min prior to activities which might trigger an acute attack.

Translingual spray (Nitrolingual): At the onset of an attack, spray one to two metered doses onto or under the tongue. No more than three metered doses should be administered within 15 min. If chest pain continues, seek immediate medical attention. May use prophylactically 5–10 min before engaging in activities which might trigger an acute attack. Do not inhale spray.

Transmucosal, buccal tablets (Nitrogard): Administer 1 mg every 3–5 h during waking hours. Place tablet between lip and gum above incisors, or between cheek and gum. Do not chew or swallow tablet.

Sustained-release capsules (Nitroglycerin, Nitro-Bid Plateau Caps, Nitrocine Timecaps, Nitroglyn): Initiate with 2.5 mg three times daily. Titrate upward to an effective dose or until dose-related adverse effects occur.

Note: Tolerance may develop when nitroglycerin is administered without a nitrate-free interval. Consider administering on a reduced schedule (once or twice daily).

IN BRIEF

INDICATIONS

Prevention of angina pectoris (oral sustained-release tablets and capsules, transdermal system)

Prevention and treatment of angina pectoris (sublingual tablets, translingual spray, transmucosal tablets, topical ointment)

Control of BP in perioperative hypertension (intravenous)

CHF associated with acute MI (intravenous)

Angina pectoris unresponsive to recommended doses of organic nitrates or beta blockers (intravenous)

Controlled hypotension during surgical procedures (intravenous)

CONTRAINDICATIONS

Hypersensitivity or idiosyncrasy to nitrates
Severe anemia
Closed angle glaucoma
Postural hypotension
Head trauma or cerebral hemorrhage
Increased intracranial pressure
Hypotension or uncorrected hypovolemia (intravenous)
Cerebral ischemia (intravenous)
Restrictive cardiomyopathy (intravenous)
Constrictive pericarditis (intravenous)
Pericardial tamponade (intravenous)

DRUG INTERACTIONS

Alcohol
Aspirin
Calcium channel blockers
Dihydroergotamine
Heparin

ADVERSE EFFECTS

Cardiovascular: hypotension, tachycardia, retrosternal discomfort, palpitation, syncope, arrhythmias, edema
CNS: headache, lightheadedness, dizziness, weakness, anxiety, confusion, insomnia
GI: nausea, vomiting, diarrhea, dyspepsia
Dermatologic: drug rash, pruritus, exfoliative dermatitis, contact dermatitis (transdermal systems), cutaneous vasodilation with flushing
Others: flushing, arthralgia, dysuria, impotence, urinary frequency, hemolytic anemia, asthenia, blurred vision, methemoglobinemia (rare, usually with overdose)

PHARMACOKINETICS AND PHARMACODYNAMICS

Dosage form	Onset of action	Duration
Sublingual tablet	1–3 min	30–60 min
Translingual spray	2 min	30–60 min
Transmucosal tablet	1–2 min	3–5 h
Sustained release	20–45 min	3–8 h
Topical ointment	≤30 min	2–12 h
Transdermal system	30–60 min	8–24 h
Intravenous	Immediate	3–5 min

Note: The duration of action of nitroglycerin may vary due to development of tolerance.

Bioavailability: variable
Effect of food: not known
Metabolism: hepatic (very rapid and nearly complete) and in blood (enzymatically). Oral dosage forms undergo extensive first-pass metabolism
Elimination: renal, as metabolites
Half-life: 1–4 min
Protein binding: 60%

MONITORING

BP, heart rate.

DOSAGE (CONTINUED)

Sustained-release tablets (Nitrong): Initiate with 2.6 mg three times daily. Titrate upward to an effective dose or until dose-related adverse effects occur.

Note: Tolerance may develop when nitroglycerin is administered without a nitrate-free interval. Consider administering on a reduced schedule (once or twice daily).

Topical ointment (Nitroglycerin, Nitro-Bid, Nitrol): Initiate at 15–30 mg (1–2 in) every 8 h, increasing by one-half inch per application every 6 h to a maximum of 75 mg (5 in) per application every 4 h.

Note: Any regimen of nitroglycerin ointment administration should include a daily nitrate-free interval of about 10–12 h to avoid tolerance. To apply the ointment using the dose-measuring paper applicator, place the applicator on a flat surface, printed side down. Squeeze the necessary amount of ointment from the tube onto the applicator, place the applicator (ointment side down) on the desired area of skin (usually on nonhairy skin of chest or back), and tape the applicator into place. Do not rub in.

Transdermal Systems (Nitroglycerin Transdermal, Minitran, Nitro-Dur, Nitro-Derm, Transderm-Nitro, Nitrodisc, Deponit): Initiate with a 0.1 or 0.2 mg/h patch. Apply patch for 12–14 h; remove for 10–12 h before applying a new patch. Patch should be applied on to clean, dry, hairless skin of chest, inner upper arm, or shoulder. Avoid placing below knee or elbow. Vary site of placement to decrease skin irritation. Apply a new patch if the first patch loosens or falls off.

Intravenous (Nitroglycerin I.V., Tridil I.V., Nitro-Bid I.V., Nitroglycerin in 5% Dextrose): Initiate intravenous infusion at 5 μg/min (0.005 mg); increase by increments of 5 μg/min at 3–5 min intervals until desired effect is obtained or to 20 μg/min. Dosage may be increased beyond 20 μg/min by 10 μg/min increments at 3–5 min intervals, then by 20 μg/min increments until desired effect is reached. Reduce dosage increments and frequency of dosage increments as partial effect are noted. There is no fixed optimum dose. Continuously monitor physiologic parameters such as BP and heart rate and other measurements, such as pulmonary capillary wedge pressure (PCWP), to achieve accurate dose. Maintain adequate blood and coronary perfusion pressures.

Note: Intravenous infusion is not direct, but must be given through a special nonpolyvinylchloride (non-PVC) intravenous infusion set or infusion pump. Refer to manufacturers' package literature for dilution and administration recommendations. Do not administer with other medications.

OVERDOSE

Gastric lavage may be useful if the medication has only recently been swallowed. Treat severe hypotension and reflex tachycardia by elevating the legs and administering intravenous fluids. The rapid metabolism of nitroglycerin usually makes additional measures unnecessary. However, if additional correction of severe hypotension is needed, administration of an intravenous alpha-adrenergic agonist such as methoxamine or phenylephrine may be considered. Epinephrine should be avoided since it aggravates the shock-like reaction. Methemoglobin concentrations in blood should be monitored and methemoglobinemia be treated with high-flow oxygen and intravenous methylene blue.

PATIENT INFORMATION

Do not chew or crush sustained release dosage form.

Do not swallow or chew sublingual form; contact physician or go to emergency room if no relief after three sublingual doses. To avoid falling, use sublingual tablets or translingual spray only when sitting or lying down. Keep tablets and capsules in original container; keep tightly closed. Do not change from one brand of this drug to another without consulting your physician or pharmacist. Avoid alcohol. This medication may cause headache, dizziness, flushing, blurred vision, or dry mouth. Notify physician if persistent or unusual side effects occur. Do not discontinue therapy without your physician's advice.

(In addition, please look under the dosage section for administration instructions for various nitroglycerin dosage forms.)

AVAILABILITY

Sublingual tablets (Nitrostat)—0.15 mg, 0.3 mg, 0.4 mg, 0.6 mg

Translingual spray (Nitrolingual)—0.4 mg per metered dose

Transmucosal tablets, controlled release—1 mg, 2 mg, 3 mg

Capsules, sustained-release (Nitroglycerin, Nitro-Bid Plateau Caps, Nitrocine Timecaps, Nitroglyn)—2.5 mg, 6.5 mg, 9 mg

Capsules, sustained-release (Nitroglyn)—13 mg

Tablets, sustained-release (Nitrong)—2.6 mg, 6.5 mg, 9 mg

Topical ointment (Nitroglycerin, Nitro-Bid, Nitrol)—2% in a lanolin petrolatum base

Transdermal systems (Nitroglycerin)—0.2mg/hour, 0.4 mg/hour, 0.6 mg/hour

Transdermal system (Deponit)—0.2 mg/hour, 0.4 mg/hour

Transdermal system (Nitrodisc, Nitro-Dur)—0.3 mg/hour

Transdermal systems (Minitran, Nitro-Dur, Transderm-Nitro)— 0.1 mg/hour, 0.2 mg/hour, 0.4 mg/hour, 0.6 mg/hour

Transdermal systems (Nitro-Dur, Transderm-Nitro, Nitro-Derm)— 0.8 mg/hour

Intravenous (nitroglycerin I.V., Nitro-Bid I.V., Tridil I.V.)—5 mg/mL (1,5, and 10 mL vials)

Intravenous (Tridil I.V.)—0.5 mg/mL, 10 mL ampules

Intravenous (Nitroglycerin in 5% dextrose)—25 mg in 250 mL, 50 mg in 250 and 500 mL, 100 mg in 250 mL, 200 mg in 500 mL)

PAPAVERINE

(Genabid®, Pavagen®, Pavabid®Plateau CAPS®)

Papaverine hydrochloride is a benzylisoquinoline alkaloid. It can be prepared synthetically or derived from opium. In contrast to morphine, the principal opium alkaloid, papaverine usually does not lead to tolerance or addiction. Papaverine has little effect on the CNS, although large doses may cause sedation and sleepiness in some patients. The major therapeutic action of papaverine is its spasmolytic effect on smooth muscles, which is most pronounced on blood vessels including the coronary, cerebral, pulmonary, and peripheral arteries. By depressing cardiac conduction, prolonging the refractory period, and depressing the excitability of the myocardium, papaverine induces relaxation of the cardiac muscle. Papaverine also relaxes smooth muscles of the bronchi, gastrointestinal tract, ureters, and biliary system. At present, the oral formulation of papaverine is indicated for the relief of cerebral and peripheral ischemia associated with arterial spasm and myocardial ischemia complicated by arrhythmias.

SPECIAL GROUPS

Race: no differences in response
Children: safety and efficacy have not been established
Elderly: lower doses may be required
Renal impairment: lower doses may be required
Hepatic impairment: lower doses may be required
Pregnancy: category C; use only when clearly needed and when the potential benefits outweigh the potential harm to the fetus
Breast-feeding: not recommended; papaverine may be excreted in breast milk

DOSAGE

Oral, sustained release: 150 mg every 12 h. 150 mg every 8 h or 300 mg every 12 h may be given in difficult cases.
Note: It is uncertain if effective plasma concentrations are maintained for 12 h with sustained-release preparations. In the past, the Food and Drug Administration has recommended that papaverine products be withdrawn from the market.

IN BRIEF

INDICATIONS
Oral formulations:
Relief of peripheral and cerebral ischemia associated with arterial spasm
Myocardial ischemia complicated by arrhythmias

CONTRAINDICATIONS
Hypersensitivity to papaverine or its components
Complete atrioventricular heart block

DRUG INTERACTIONS
CNS depressants
Levodopa

ADVERSE EFFECTS
Cardiovascular: tachycardia, arrhythmia, mild hypertension
CNS: vertigo, drowsiness, sedation, headache
GI: nausea, abdominal discomfort, anorexia, constipation, diarrhea
Others: flushing, sweating, skin rash, malaise, hepatic hypersensitivity, chronic hepatitis

PHARMACOKINETICS AND PHARMACODYNAMICS
Duration of action: up to 12 h (sustained-release)
Onset of action: rapid
Time to peak
plasma concentration: 1–2 h
Bioavailability: 30%–54%
Effect of food: not known
Metabolism: hepatic
Elimination: papaverine is excreted in the urine primarily as inactive metabolites
Half-life: estimates of papaverine's biologic half-life vary widely; however, reasonably constant plasma concentrations can be maintained after 4 d with regular administration at 6 h intervals
Protein binding: 90%

MONITORING
BP, heart rate, ECG, liver function test. Use with caution in patients with glaucoma.

OVERDOSE
In case of papaverine overdose, the patient's airway should be protected and ventilation and perfusion supported. Carefully monitor vital signs, blood gases, and blood chemistry values. If seizures occur, they may be managed with diazepam, phenytoin, or phenobarbital. Administration of intravenous fluids and/or a vasopressor and elevation of the patient's legs may be used to treat hypotension. Calcium gluconate may be useful for the treatment of papaverine-induced adverse cardiac effects. Plasma calcium concentrations and ECG should be monitored. It is not known if papaverine is removed by hemodialysis.

PATIENT INFORMATION
The sustained-release capsules must be swallowed whole, without crushing, dividing, or chewing. This medication may cause dizziness, drowsiness, nausea, flushing, and headache. Use caution when driving or performing other tasks that require alertness. Avoid alcohol intake. Notify physician if persistent or unusual side effects occur.

AVAILABILITY
Capsules, sustained-release—150 mg

PENTOXIFYLLINE (Pentoxifylline, Trental®)

Pentoxifylline is thought to decrease blood viscosity and improve erythrocyte flexibility, microcirculatory flow, and tissue oxygen concentrations. Improvement in erythrocyte flexibility appears to be caused by inhibition of phosphodiesterase and a resultant increase in cyclic AMP in red blood cells. Reduction in blood viscosity may be the result of decreased plasma fibrinogen concentrations and inhibition of red blood cells and platelet aggregation. Pentoxifylline has modest efficacy in improving treadmill exercise performance in patients with intermittent claudication. Before the approval of cilostazol, this agent was the only approved claudication drug in the United States.

SPECIAL GROUPS

Race: no differences in response
Children: safety and efficacy have not been established
Elderly: lower doses may be required
Renal impairment: lower doses may be required
Hepatic impairment: dosage adjustment is usually not necessary
Pregnancy: category C; use only when clearly needed and when potential benefits outweigh potential hazards to the fetus
Breast-feeding: not recommended; pentoxifylline and its metabolites are excreted in breast milk

DOSAGE

Usual initial dose is 400 mg three times daily with meals, reduced to 400 mg twice daily if GI or CNS side effects occur. While therapeutic effects may be observed within 2–4 wk, continue treatment for ≥8 wk.

IN BRIEF

INDICATIONS
Intermittent claudication

CONTRAINDICATIONS
Hypersensitivity, intolerance to pentoxifylline or methylxanthines (eg, caffeine, theophylline)
Recent cerebral or retinal hemorrhage

DRUG INTERACTIONS
Antihypertensive agents
Cimetidine
Theophylline
Warfarin

ADVERSE EFFECTS
Cardiovascular: angina/chest pain, edema, hypotension, arrhythmia (rare)
CNS: dizziness, headache, seizures (<1%)
GI: dyspepsia, nausea, vomiting

PHARMACOKINETICS AND PHARMACODYNAMICS
Duration of action: not known
Onset of action: multiple doses, 2–4 wk
Bioavailability: 20%
Effect of food: food intake delays absorption, but does not affect total absorption
Metabolism: liver, extensive; erythrocytes, minor
Elimination: primarily in urine
Half-life: 24–48 min, parent drug; 60–96 min, metabolites
Protein binding: bound to erythrocyte membrane, 45%

MONITORING
BP, heart rate, maximal walking distance.

OVERDOSE
Symptoms of overdose include hypotension, flushing, seizures, somnolence, loss of consciousness, agitation, bradycardia, and atrioventricular block. Treatment is supportive and symptomatic.

PATIENT INFORMATION
Take this medication with food or meals. If gastrointestinal or central nervous system side effects (ie, dizziness, headache, indigestion, nausea, and vomiting) continue, contact physician. While improvement may be experienced in 2–4 wk, continue treatment for at least 8 wk. Do not discontinue therapy without your physician's advice.

AVAILABILITY
Tablets, controlled release—400 mg

The information here is provided as guidance only. Prescribers should always consult the manufacturer's current prescribing information.

267

SILDENAFIL CITRATE (Viagra®)

Sildenafil, a specific inhibitor of type 5 cyclic guanosine monophosphate (cGMP) phosphodiesterase, is used as oral therapy for erectile dysfunction. The physiologic mechanism of penile erection consist of nitric oxide release in the corpus cavernosum during sexual stimulation. Nitric oxide then activates guanylate cyclase, which causes elevation in cGMP levels, leading to relaxation of smooth muscle in the corpus cavernosum. This in turn increases blood flow into the corpus cavernosum, an essential phase in the erectile process. Sildenafil has no direct relaxant effect on isolated human corpus cavernosum but enhances the effect of nitric oxide by inhibiting phosphodiesterase type 5, which is responsible for the degradation of cGMP in the corpus cavernosum. At usual recommended doses, sildenafil has no effect in the absence of sexual stimulation.

Since the potential for cardiac risk is associated with sexual activity, treatments of erectile dysfunction generally should be avoided in men for whom sexual activity is inadvisable due to their underlying cardiovascular status. Patients who experience symptoms such as angina pectoris or dizziness upon initiation of sexual activity should be advised to refrain from further activity. In addition, sildenafil was shown to potentiate the hypotensive effects of nitrates. Therefore, sildenafil is contraindicated in patients who are concurrently using organic nitrates in any form.

SPECIAL GROUPS

Race: no differences in response
Children: sildenafil is not indicated for use in children
Elderly: initiate with lower dose
Renal impairment: initiate with lower dose in patients with severe renal impairment (CrCl < 30 mL/min)
Hepatic impairment: initiate with lower dose
Pregnancy: category B; sildenafil is not indicated for use in women
Breast-feeding: sildenafil is not indicated for use in women

DOSAGE

The usual recommended dose is 50 mg taken as needed approximately one hour before sexual activity. However, sildenafil may be taken anywhere from 4 hours to 30 minutes prior to sexual activity. The dose may be increased to 100 mg or decreased to 25 mg based on effectiveness and tolerance. The maximum recommended dosing frequency is once daily. For patients who are older than 65 years, patients with hepatic impairment or severe renal impairment, or patients who are taking potent cytochrome P450 3A4 inhibitors (eg, erythromycin, ketoconazole, itraconazole), consider initiating with a lower dose of 25 mg.

IN BRIEF

INDICATIONS
Erectile dysfunction

CONTRAINDICATIONS
Hypersensitivity
Patients concurrently or intermittently using organic nitrates in any form

DRUG INTERACTIONS
Amlodipine   Ketoconazole
Cimetidine   Nitrates
Erythromycin   Rifampin
Itraconazole

ADVERSE EFFECTS
Cardiovascular: flushing, angina pectoris, syncope, tachycardia, hypotension, myocardial ischemia, cerebral thrombosis, cardiac arrest, heart failure, abnormal electrocardiogram
CNS: headache, ataxia, hypertonia, neuralgia, tremor, vertigo, insomnia, decreased reflexes, hypesthesia, seizure, anxiety
GI: dyspepsia, diarrhea, vomiting, glossitis, colitis, dysphagia
Dermatologic: rash, urticaria, herpes simplex, pruritus
Genitourinary: urinary tract infection, cystitis, nocturia, urinary frequency, abnormal ejaculation, prolonged erection, priapism, hematuria
Others: nasal congestion, abnormal vision, anemia, leukopenia, thirst, hyperglycemia, edema, arthritis, dyspnea

PHARMACOKINETICS AND PHARMACODYNAMICS
Onset of action: 30 minutes to 1 hour
Time to maximum plasma concentration: 30–120 min
Bioavailability: ≈ 40%
Effect of food: the rate of absorption is decreased when sildenafil is taken with a high-fat meal
Metabolism: predominantly cleared by the CYP3A4 (major route) and CYP2C9 (minor route) hepatic microsomal isoenzymes. Sildenafil is converted into an active metabolite by N-desmethylation and is further metabolized. Active metabolite accounts for about 20% of sildenafil's pharmacologic effects
Elimination: predominantly in the feces as metabolites (≈ 80%), and to a lesser extent in the urine (≈ 13%)
Half-life: ≈ 4 hours
Protein binding: ≈ 96%

MONITORING
Blood pressure, length of erection, signs of infection.

OVERDOSE
Standard supportive measures should be employed as required. Hemodialysis is not expected to accelerate clearance as sildenafil is highly protein bound and is not predominantly eliminated in the urine.

PATIENT INFORMATION
Sildenafil is contraindicated in patients who are taking organic nitrates concurrently. If symptoms such as angina pectoris, dizziness, and nausea are experienced upon initiation of sexual activity, refrain from further activity and discuss the episode with physician. Sildenafil offers no protection against sexually transmitted diseases, consider counseling regarding protective measures necessary to guard against sexually transmitted diseases. Sildenafil has no effect in the absence of sexual stimulation.

AVAILABILITY
Tablets—25 mg, 50 mg, 100 mg

SODIUM NITROPRUSSIDE
(Sodium Nitroprusside, Nitropress®)

Nitroprusside is a potent and rapidly acting vasodilator. It is effective only when given intravenously and is used for the acute management of hypertensive crises, heart failure, or during surgery when elective hypotension is desirable. It acts on both peripheral arterial and venous vessels. Its effects are dose-related and depend on the preexisting hemodynamic state of the patient. In hypertensive and normotensive patients, a slight increase in heart rate is observed with a slight reduction in cardiac output. In those with heart failure, substantial improvements in left ventricular performance are seen, together with a slight reduction in heart rate and a reduction in arrhythmias.

Because nitroprusside is metabolized rapidly to cyanogen (cyanide radical) and then to thiocyanate in the liver, care must be taken to ensure that the dosage rate does not exceed the capacity of the body to remove the cyanide radical; if this happens, toxicity manifest as coma, dilated pupils, pink coloration of the skin, and weak vital signs may result. For this reason, thiocyanate concentrations should be monitored periodically in patients with renal insufficiency and in those receiving prolonged infusion of sodium nitroprusside (>48–72 h).

SPECIAL GROUPS

Race: no differences in response

Children: appropriate studies have not been performed; however, pediatrics-specific problems that would limit the usefulness of this agent in children are not expected

Elderly: may be more sensitive to hypotensive effects; age-related renal impairment are also more likely to exist; use with caution

Renal impairment: dosage may have to be reduced because excretion of thiocyanate is reduced; use with caution

Hepatic impairment: dosage may have to be reduced because hepatic enzymes are involved in the metabolism of cyanide; use with caution

Pregnancy: category C; administer to a pregnant woman only if clearly needed; use only when potential benefits outweigh potential hazards to the fetus

Breast-feeding: not recommended; nitroprusside and its metabolites may be excreted in breast milk

IN BRIEF

INDICATIONS
Hypertensive crises
Controlled hypotension during surgery to reduce bleeding into the surgical field
Acute CHF

CONTRAINDICATIONS
Hypersensitivity
To produce hypotension during surgery in patients with known inadequate cerebral circulation or in moribund patients coming to emergency surgery
Increased intracranial pressure
Arteriovenous shunt or coarctation of the aorta (ie, compensatory hypertension)
Congenital (Leber's) optic atrophy
Tobacco amblyopia
Acute CHF associated with reduced peripheral vascular resistance such as high-output heart failure that may be seen in endotoxic sepsis

DRUG INTERACTIONS
Dobutamine
Hypotension-producing medications
Sympathomimetics

ADVERSE EFFECTS
Cardiovascular: hypotension, palpitations, substernal distress, ECG changes, bradycardia, tachycardia
CNS: disorientation, headache, dizziness, restlessness
GI: nausea, vomiting, abdominal pain
Hematologic: decreased platelet aggregation, methemoglobinemia
Others: flushing, diaphoresis, irritation at the infusion site, hypothyroidism, increased intracranial pressure, tinnitus, muscle twitching, thiocyanate toxicity

PHARMACOKINETICS AND PHARMACODYNAMICS
Duration of action: 1–10 min after infusion is stopped
Onset of action: almost immediate
Time to peak effect: almost immediate
Metabolism: nitroprusside is metabolized by an enzyme present in red blood cells to cyanide with subsequent metabolism in the liver and the kidney, by the enzyme rhodanase, to thiocyanate
Elimination: thiocyanate is eliminated renally
Half-life: parent drug: 3–4 min
Thiocyanate: 3–4 d with normal renal function; half-life increases as renal function decreases
Protein binding: not known

MONITORING
BP, heart rate, ECG, acid-base status, serum thiocyanate concentrations (during prolonged infusion or in patients with renal impairment), methemoglobin concentrations.

OVERDOSE
Signs of excessive hypotension usually disappear if infusion rate is slowed or temporarily discontinued.
If signs and symptoms of thiocyanate toxicity occur, discontinue drug therapy.
Treat massive overdose and signs and symptoms of cyanide toxicity immediately. Serum cyanide concentrations may be reduced by intravenous infusions of sodium nitrate and sodium thiosulfate.

DOSAGE

Adults: The usual initial dose is 0.3 µg/kg/min (range, 0.1–0.5 µg/kg/min) intravenous infusion; can be adjusted slowly in increments of 0.5 µg/kg/min according to response. Usual dose is 3 µg/kg/min. The maximum recommended infusion rate is 10 µg/kg/min. Infusion at the maximum dose rate (10 µg/kg/min) should never last for more than 10 min. To keep the steady-state thiocyanate concentration below 1 mmol/L, the rate of a prolonged infusion should not exceed 3 µg/kg/min (1 µg/kg/min in anuric patients). When >500 µg/kg of nitroprusside is administered faster than 2 µg/kg/min, cyanide is generated faster than the unaided patient can eliminate it.

Note: After reconstitution with appropriate diluent, sodium nitroprusside injection is not suitable for direct injection. The reconstituted solution must be further diluted in the appropriate amount of sterile 5% dextrose injection before infusion. Protect the diluted solution from light by promptly wrapping with the supplied opaque sleeve, aluminum foil or other opaque material. Sodium nitroprusside should not be infused through an ordinary intravenous apparatus, regulated only by gravity and mechanical clamps. Only an infusion pump, preferably a volumetric pump, should be used. Refer to manufacture's package literature for complete prescribing information.

Children: Appropriate studies have not been performed. Dosage recommendation is same as for adults.

PATIENT INFORMATION

This medication may cause headache, dizziness, drowsiness, confusion, nausea, and abdominal pain. Notify physician if persistent or unusual side effects occur.

AVAILABILITY

Powder for injection—50 mg/vial (2 and 5 mL vials)

TOLAZOLINE (Priscoline®)

Tolazoline produces vasodilatation by means of a direct, histamine-like relaxation of vascular smooth muscle. It also has moderate competitive alpha-adrenergic blocking activity. Tolazoline increases heart rate and cardiac output. Response of BP to this agent depends on the relative contributions of its vasodilating and cardiac stimulating effects. Tolazoline usually reduces pulmonary arterial pressure and pulmonary vascular resistance. Its use is generally restricted to the treatment of pulmonary hypertension in children.

SPECIAL GROUPS

Race: no differences in response
Children: tolazoline is indicated for persistent pulmonary hypertension of the newborn
Elderly: not applicable
Renal impairment: no specific dosing guidelines exist for administering tolazoline in neonates with renal failure; lower doses may be considered; it is recommended to monitor renal function during tolazoline administration; one investigator has recommended that tolazoline be discontinued in the presence of compromised renal function
Hepatic impairment: no information
Pregnancy: category C; use only when clearly needed and when potential benefits outweigh potential hazards to the fetus
Breast-feeding: not recommended; tolazoline may be excreted in breast milk

DOSAGE

Newborns: For pulmonary hypertension, the recommended dose is 1–2 mg/kg body weight via scalp vein over a 10 min period. Maintenance is best with 1–2 mg/kg/h, increased if necessary (in increments of 1–2 mg/kg/h) up to 6–8 mg/kg/h. May be withdrawn gradually when arterial blood gases remain stable. If necessary, the initial bolus dose may be repeated during the maintenance infusion. There is very little experience with infusions lasting more than 36 –48 h. Response can be expected within 30 min after the initial dose if it occurs.
Note: Use of diluents containing benzyl alcohol is not recommended for use in neonates; fatal toxic syndrome may result. See manufacturer's package literature for instructions on administration.

IN BRIEF

INDICATIONS
Persistent pulmonary hypertension of the newborn

CONTRAINDICATIONS
Hypersensitivity
CAD

DRUG INTERACTIONS
Epinephrine
Ethanol

ADVERSE EFFECTS
Cardiovascular: hypotension, tachycardia, arrhythmias, hypertension, edema, pulmonary hemorrhage
GI: GI bleed, abdominal pain, nausea, vomiting, diarrhea
Hematologic: thrombocytopenia, leukopenia
Others: flushing, rash, oliguria, hematuria, increased pilomotor activity

PHARMACOKINETICS AND PHARMACODYNAMICS
Duration of action: continuous upon infusion
Onset of action: within 30 min
Effect of food: not known
Metabolism: little
Elimination: renally as the unchanged drug
Half-life: 3–10 h, in neonates; half-life is increased with decreased renal function
Protein binding: not known

MONITORING
Administer tolazoline in a highly supervised setting where vital signs, oxygenation, acid-base status, and fluid and electrolytes can be monitored and maintained. In addition to the contraindications listed above, tolazoline should be used with extreme caution in patients with severe obliterative vascular disease, cerebrovascular disease, recent MI, stress ulcers, hypotension, and mitral stenosis.

OVERDOSE
Symptoms of overdosage include increased pilomotor activity, peripheral vasodilation, skin flushing, and rarely, hypotension and shock. Hypotension is treated by placing the patient in the Trendelenburg position and administering intravenous fluids. The use of epinephrine or norepinephrine is not recommended because of the risk for a further decrease in BP followed by an exaggerated rebound increase. If fluid expansion fails to maintain BP, an infusion of dopamine or ephedrine may be effective. Dopamine should be used cautiously because severe hypotension has resulted when tolazoline and dopamine were administered together.

PATIENT INFORMATION
Side effects may decrease with continued therapy.

AVAILABILITY
Injection—25 mg/mL (4 mL ampules)

Selected bibliography

Abdelwahab W, Frishman W, Landau A: Management of hypertensive urgencies and emergencies. *J Clin Pharmacol* 1995, 35:747–762.

Barst RJ, Rubin LJ, Long WA, *et al.*: A comparison of continuous intravenous epoprostenol (prostacyclin) with conventional therapy for primary pulmonary hypertension. The Primary Pulmonary Hypertension Study Group. *N Engl J Med* 1996, 334:296–302.

Brogden RN, Markham A: Fenoldopam: a review of its pharmacodynamic and pharmacokinetic properties and intravenous clinical potential in the management of hypertensive urgencies and emergencies. *Drugs* 1997, 54:634–650.

Burns-Cox N, Gingell C: Medical treatment of erectile dysfunction. *Postgrad Med J* 1998, 74:336–342.

Califf RM, Adams KF, McKenna WJ, *et al.*: A randomized controlled trial of epoprostenol therapy for severe congestive heart failure: The Flolan International Randomized Survival Trial (FIRST). *Am Heart J* 1997, 134:44–54.

Campese VM: Minoxidil: A review of its pharmacological properties and therapeutic use. *Drugs* 1981; 22:237–278.

Cheng JWM: The use of cilostazol for the management of intermittent claudication. *Heart Disease* 1999, 1:182–186.

Coffman J: Drug treatment of peripheral vascular disease. In *Cardiovascular Pharmacotherapeutics*. Edited by Frishman WH, Sonnenblick EH. New York: McGraw Hill; 1997;1185–1193.

Cohn JN, Archibald DG, Ziesche S, *et al.*: Effect of vasodilator therapy on mortality in chronic congestive heart failure. Results of a Veterans Administration Cooperative Study. *N Engl J Med* 1986; 314:1547–1552.

Cohn JN, Johnson G, Ziesche S, *et al.*: A comparison of enala-pril with hydralazine-isosorbide dinitrate in the treatment of chronic congestive heart failure. *N Engl J Med* 1991, 325:303–310.

Dawson DL, Cutler BS, Meissner MH, Strandness DE: Cilostazol has beneficial effects in treatment of intermittent claudication: results from a multicenter, randomized, prospective, double-blind trial. *Circulation* 1998; 98:678–686.

Fink AN, Frishman WH, Azizad M, Agarwal Y: Use of prostacyclin and its analogues in the treatment of cardiovascular disease. *Heart Disease* 1999, 1:29–40.

Frishman WH: Tolerance, rebound and time-zero effect of nitrate therapy. *Am J Cardiol* 1992, 70(Suppl 17): 43G–48G.

Frishman WH: Management of hypertensive urgencies and emergencies. In Frishman WH, Sonnenblick EH (eds): *Cardiovascular Pharmacotherapeutics*. New York: McGraw Hill; 1997:1577–1592.

Frishman WH, Fink AN, Ahmad A: Prostacyclin in cardiovascular disease. In Frishman WH, Sonnenblick EH (eds): *Cardiovascular Pharmacotherapeutics Companion Handbook*. New York: McGraw Hill; 1998:419–426.

Frishman WH, Hotchkiss J: Selective and non-selective dopamine receptor agonists: an innovative approach to cardiovascular disease treatment. *Am Heart J* 1996, 132:861–870.

Goldstein I, Lue TF, Padma-Nathan H, *et al.*: Oral sildenafil in the treatment of erectile dysfunction. *N Engl J Med* 1998, 338: 1397–1404.

Hiatt WR: Current and future drug therapies for claudication. *Vasc Med* 1997, 2:257–262.

Koch Weser J: Diazoxide. *N Engl J Med* 1976, 294: 1271–1274.

McLaughlin VV, Genthner DE, Panella MM, Rich S: Reduction in pulmonary vascular resistance with long-term epoprostenol (prostacyclin) therapy in primary pulmonary hypertension. *N Engl J Med* 1998, 338:273–277.

Money SR, Herd JA, Isaacsohn JL, *et al.*: Effect of cilostazol on walking distances in patients with intermittent claudication caused by peripheral vascular disease. *J Vasc Surg* 1998, 27:267–274.

Phillips BB, Gandhi AJ: Epoprostenol in the treatment of congestive heart failure. *Am J Health Sys Pharm* 1997, 54:2613–2615.

Post JB, Frishman WH: Fenoldopam: a new dopamine agonist for the treatment of hypertensive urgencies and emergencies. *J Clin Pharmacol* 1998, 38:2–13.

Price DE, Boolell M, Gepi-Attee S, *et al.*: Sildenafil: study of a novel oral treatment of erectile dysfunction in diabetic men. *Diabet Med* 1998, 15: 821–825.

Thadani U: Nitrate tolerance, rebound, and their clinical relevance in stable angina pectoris, unstable angina, and heart failure. *Cardiovasc Drugs Ther* 1997, 10:735–742.

DRUGS IN DEVELOPMENT: NEW AGENTS, NEW CLASSES, NEW INDICATIONS

Despite the large number of pharmacologic agents available for the treatment of cardiovascular disease, the search for additional drugs and pharmacotherapeutic approaches continues. In this chapter, ongoing investigations of new drugs, drug classes, and the clinical applications of these treatments are discussed.

DRUGS AFFECTING THE RENIN-ANGIOTENSIN-ALDOSTERONE SYSTEM

The renin-angiotensin system is a major contributor to the pathophysiology of various cardiovascular diseases. For this reason attempts to modulate this system have been a pharmacotherapeutic goal for more than 25 years. Blockade of the renin-angiotensin system has been attempted at four pivotal areas: 1) using beta-adrenergic blockers to inhibit release of renin from the juxtaglomerular cells; 2) inhibiting the rate-limiting angiotensinogen-renin step with renin inhibitors; 3) blocking the conversion of angiotensin I to angiotensin II by the angiotensin converting enzyme (ACE) inhibitors; and 4) blocking the active receptor sites for the terminal products of angiotensin II and **aldosterone**.

ACE inhibitors have been studied successfully in patients with systemic hypertension and congestive heart failure (CHF), and in patients with and without diabetes mellitus, to prevent progressive glomerulonephropathy. There are ongoing clinical studies evaluating ACE inhibitors in survivors of acute myocardial infarction (MI) with normal left ventricular ejection fractions. An antithrombotic mechanism has been postulated for the benefit of ACE inhibition against reinfarction. The drugs have also been shown to reduce the risk of sudden cardiac death in post-MI patients.

Five trials have demonstrated a reduction in recurrent MI in patients who received long-term treatment with an ACE inhibitor. The reduction was remarkably consistent from trial to trial, ranging from 7% to 8% per year of treatment, despite the fact that a different ACE inhibitor was used in each trial and the duration of follow up was different.

The ACE Inhibitor Collaborative Group reported findings in 100,000 patients who participated in randomized trials in which ACE inhibitors were given within 24 hours of MI onset. Analysis of the effect of treatment on 30-day mortality showed a statistically significant reduction in deaths during this period in patients who received ACE inhibitors compared with controls. The difference emerged within the first day of treatment and was evident in all groups except those who were hypotensive on admission. The investigators concluded that use of ACE inhibitors in patients with acute MI has the potential to save about five lives in a thousand.

The effects of ACE inhibitors in patients with endothelial dysfunction have been studied in 11 trials. The hypertension trials had mixed results, half showing some improvement and half showing no improvement. In contrast, studies of patients with coronary disease have consistently shown improvement in endothelial function with an ACE inhibitor. The largest of these trials was the Trial on Reversing En-

dothelial Dysfunction (TREND), where 129 patients with coronary artery disease (CAD) but no left ventricular dysfunction were randomized to either the ACE inhibitor **quinapril** 40 mg daily or placebo. After 6 months, acetylcholine-induced vasoconstriction had decreased significantly compared with baseline in the quinapril-treated patients, but not in the placebo group. In a substudy, the investigators evaluated the effect of ACE inhibition on microvascular coronary blood flow, as measured by Doppler ultrasound. The results paralleled those of the larger study. In the placebo group, responses to acetylcholine and adenosine infusion did not change significantly from baseline, but in the **quinapril** group there was a 48% increase in coronary blood flow. It is suggested that the microvasculature, like the epicardium, benefits from ACE inhibitor therapy.

The Quinapril Anti-Ischemia and Symptoms of Angina Reduction (QUASAR) trial, which is currently in the enrollment phase, is based on the premise that adverse outcomes are linked to the presence of ischemic episodes and that endothelial dysfunction is a mechanism underlying these episodes. Thus, it is hypothesized that if **quinapril** reduces tissue angiotensin production and increases bradykinin and endothelial-derived vasodilators like nitric oxide, it will improve endothelial function and reduce ischemia.

There are now 10 oral ACE inhibitors available and one parenteral formulation (enalaprilat). Studies are now in progress evaluating the effects of ACE inhibitors on left ventricular and vascular wall hypertrophy, myocardial aging, and myocardial and vascular apoptosis. The drugs have not been shown to be effective for preventing or inhibiting the development of post-angioplasty restenosis.

RENIN INHIBITION

Inhibition of the action of renin on angiotensinogen was demonstrated with early inhibitory peptides and in studies with specific antibodies. The most currently available renin inhibitors are nonpeptides, which must be given intravenously, such as **enalkiren** and **CGP 38560A**. Orally effective agents include **Ro 42-5892** and **A-74273**, but they appear to have low bioavailability and short pharmacologic half-lives, which could limit their clinical effectiveness. The concept of renin inhibition still remains an attractive one because these drugs not only inhibit the production of angiotensin I and II, but also prevent the reactive rise in renin release that follows the use of ACE inhibitors and angiotensin II receptor blockers.

ANGIOTENSIN II RECEPTOR BLOCKADE

Currently there are five AT_1 receptor blockers available for the treatment of systemic hypertension: **candesartan, irbesartan, losartan, telmisartan**, and **valsartan**. The drugs are being studied in patients with CHF, in comparison to ACE inhibitors and in combination with ACE inhibitors. Their protective action in patients with diabetic glomerulonephropathy and left ventricular hypertrophy, and on myocardial aging are being assessed. Morbidity and mortality studies are also being carried out in hypertensive patients, comparing A-II receptor blockers to other antihypertensive treatments.

ANTI-ALDOSTERONE AGENTS

The results of a recent study (Randomized Aldactone Evaluation Study [RALES]) demonstrated the benefit of using **spironolactone**, an aldosterone-inhibiting diuretic, in addition to triple therapy (ACE inhibition, loop diuretics, and digoxin) in patients with severe CHF. This study in 1600 patients showed the additional efficacy of **spironolactone** compared to placebo on reductions in death, hospitalization, and the need for coronary artery revascularization.

Unlike spironolactone, **triamterene** and **amiloride**, which antagonize the effects of aldosterone at the distal renal tubule site, agents are currently in development that directly bind to aldosterone: the aldosterone antagonists (*eg*, eplerenone). These newer agents might reduce some of the side effects associated with aldosterone (gynecomastia) while providing a diuretic- and potassium-conserving activity similar to that of spironolactone.

ANTIARRHYTHMIC DRUGS

Following publication of the CAST findings, few new drugs were developed and studied for the treatment of ventricular arrhythmias. Most of the new drugs are being studied as therapies for supraventricular arrhythmias, specifically for arrhythmia conversion and prevention, and are shown in Table 14.1.

Amiodarone has significant toxicity with chronic use, and a new orally active class III antiarrhythmic, **azimilide**, which is now being investigated in patients with supraventricular tachycardia, may be approved for use in preserving normal sinus rhythm in patients with atrial fibrillation and paroxysmal atrial tachycardia.

Ibutilide and **dofetilide** are two intravenous type III agents that are approved as converting agents in patients with atrial fibrillation. Studies using these drugs in patients with ventricular arrhythmias are in progress.

Studies are now in progress to assess whether pharmacologic slowing of heart rate in patients with atrial fibrillation is as effective in reducing morbidity and mortality as the conversion of arrhythmia to normal sinus rhythm.

ANTITHROMBOTIC AGENTS

THROMBOLYTIC AGENTS

Multiple studies using available thrombolytic treatments are being carried out. These studies are examining more effective approaches for thrombolysis delivery, adjunctive therapies, and protocols to maximize early patient treatment in larger numbers of patients. Thrombolysis is also being used beyond the treatment of patients with acute MI and pulmonary embolus, such as those with thrombosed prosthetic valves and peripheral and cerebral intra-arterial thromboses.

Single-chain tissue plasminogen activator (tPA) occurs naturally, but is synthesized for commercial use using a recombinant DNA technique and is known as **alteplase**. A double-chain form of tPA, **duteplase**, was also synthesized and appeared to have similar activity when tested in vitro, but this is not commercially available. The tPA molecule has a binding site enabling it to bind specifically to fibrin in thrombus. Thus, it should theoretically be clot specific and not result in activation of generally circulating plasminogen. Plasminogen activator inhibitor-1 (PAI-1) is important, and under natural conditions it can neutralize endogenous tPA, but not with the administration of therapeutic doses of tPA.

Another mutant of native tPA, TNK-tPA, has amino acid substitutions at three different sites which result in reduced plasma clearance, increased fibrin specificity, and resistance to PAI-1. Its prolonged half-life allows it to be given as a single intravenous bolus over 5 to 10 seconds. The results of the TIMI 10B angiographic trial showed that when TNK-tPA was given as a 40 mg intravenous bolus, 90 minute TIMI grade three flow was similar to that achieved with tPA. Investigators also found a trend toward higher minute TIMI three flow with no increase in bleeding risk. TNK-tPA was evaluated in a large (n=16,950) phase III, randomized, double-blind mortality trial (ASSENT-2 [Assessment of the Safety and Efficacy of a New Thrombolytic TNK-tPA Trial]), and was found to be comparable to tPA.

Lanoteplase is a novel synthetic plasminogen activator (nPA), which lacks fibronectin fingerlike and epidermal growth factor domains. It is more potent than **alteplase**, has a much longer plasma clearance, and can be administered as a single bolus. At comparable lytic doses, both **BMS-200980** and **alteplase** have comparable effects on fibrinogen and alpha$_2$-antiplasmin. The drug was compared to alteplase in the inTIME-II study (Intravenous nPA for Treatment of Infarcting Myocardium Early), using a multicenter, double-blind, randomized, angiographic protocol, with 150,000 patients randomized. **Lanoteplase** was equivalent to **alteplase** in reducing 30-day all-cause mortality, however, its use was associated with a higher rate of intracerebral hemorrhage than tPA.

TABLE 14.1 ANTIARRHYTHMIC AGENTS UNDER INVESTIGATION

Drugs	Cardiac myocyte membrane effect	Route of administration	Likely major indication(s)	Approval due
Azimilide	Blocks I_{kr} and I_{ks}	Oral	AF (Fl)/PSVT	2000
Dofetilide	Blocks I_{kr}	Oral	AF (Fl)/PSVT	1999
Dronedarone	Multiple actions	IV and oral	AF (Fl)/PSVT/VAs/SCD Proph	2002
Ersentilide	Blocks I_{kr} and β_1 receptor	IV and ?oral	AF (Fl)/PSVT/VAs/SCD Proph	?
Tedisamil	Blocks I_{kr} and I_{to}	IV and oral	VAs/?PSVT	2002
Trecetilide	Probably similar to ibutilide	IV and oral	AF (Fl)	2001

AF (Fl) — atrial fibrillation (flutter); IV—intravenous; PSVT — paroxysmal supraventricular tachycardia; SCD Proph —prophylaxis against sudden cardiac death; VAs —sustained ventricular arrhythmias; I_{kr} — rapidly activating delayed rectifier potassium channel; I_{ks} —slowly activating delayed rectifier potassium channel; I_{to} — transient outward current.

Recombinant **staphylokinase** (STAR), a profibrinolytic agent of bacterial origin, has shown promise for arterial thrombolysis. Unlike the streptokinase-plasma complex, in the absence of fibrin the staphylokinase-plasmin complex is rapidly inhibited by C-2 antiplasmin. STAR has been shown to recanalize coronary arteries efficiently and rapidly (coronary reperfusion within 20 minutes), and is significantly more fibrin-specific than r-tPA without decreasing circulating fibrinogen and C-2 antiplasmin levels. Also, in the great majority of patients with peripheral arterial occlusion, STAR quickly restored vessel patency and limb viability. STAR can induce neutralizing antibodies, but protein engineering can significantly reduce its antigenicity without functional inactivation.

The fibrin specificity of thrombolytic agents may be improved by targeting the agent to a fibrin clot. This is achieved by conjugating monoclonal antibodies which are fibrin specific and do not cross react with fibrinogen. These conjugates are being developed for clinical use, and in animal experiments they have been found to be more potent than tPA and cause less fibrinogen and alpha-antiplasmin consumption.

Recombinant **prourokinase** (r-ProUK) is the single chain precursor of urokinase. It is the only natural PA which is a zymogen and hence inactive until its conversion to double-chain urokinase. This conversion requires clot-bound plasminogen, which is converted to clot-bound plasmin, which in turn converts other ProUK molecules to active urokinase on the clot surface. ProUK is being developed as a clot-specific treatment for lysing thrombi in acute MI.

Other drugs currently being evaluated in patient trials include **ancrod**, which is a pit viper venom derivative that lowers the level of fibrinogen in the bloodstream, **saruplase** and **difibrotide**.

ANTIPLATELET AGENTS

Studies have shown that GP IIb/IIIa inhibition is beneficial in patients undergoing percutaneous coronary interventions, including endovascular stenting. More recent evidence has shown the benefit of these treatments in patients presenting with non-ST segment elevation acute coronary syndromes. The results of studies with **tirofiban** and **eptifibatide** have shown a 1.5% absolute reduction in 30-day mortality or nonfatal MI when administered to patients with non-ST elevated syndromes who are receiving **aspirin**, with and without **heparin**. Most of this benefit is on non-fatal infarction rather than on mortality.

The nonpeptide agents, **lamifiban** and **lefradafiban**, have also shown promise in treating unstable coronary syndromes, but are not yet available. The orally active GP IIb/IIIa inhibitors, **orbofiban** and **xemilofiban**, were studied in patients with MI and unstable angina, and in patients undergoing coronary angioplasty. The trial with these agents was discontinued because of hemorrhagic complications. Other orally active agents are being studied (*e.g.* **sibrofiban**).

Recently, the antiplatelet agent, **clopidogrel**, was shown to be as effective as **ticlopidine** for reducing the risk of stent thrombosis after coronary stent implantation.

Low Molecular Weight Heparins

Features of low molecular weight heparins (LMWH) that distinguish it from standard **heparin** can result in the following clinical advantages: 1) a more predictable dose response with patient variability to a fixed dose; 2) a long half-life and reduced bleeding for equivalent antithrombotic effects; and 3) enhanced safety and efficacy in the treatment of patients with venous thrombosis.

In a recent study of thrombolytic therapy with **enoxaparin** plus **aspirin** versus unfractionated **heparin** plus **aspirin**, enoxaparin plus aspirin was more effective in reducing the incidence of ischemic events in patients with unstable angina or non-Q wave MI in the early stage. Based on this study, **enoxaparin** was approved for use in unstable coronary syndromes.

Vasoflux is another LMWH derivative under investigation that has been shown to be more effective than heparin and LMWH in activating fibrin-bound thrombin.

Direct Thrombin Inhibitors

Hirudin is a naturally occurring antithrombotic substance found in the saliva of leeches and a recombinant form for diagnostic and therapeutic purposes was developed in 1986. **Hirudin** is a potent and specific thrombin inhibitor. It binds directly to both free and fibrin bound thrombin, forming a 1:1 complex causing blockage of all proteolytic functions of the enzyme, including fibrinogen clotting and activation of clotting factors V, VIII and XIII. By blocking factor V activation, the prothrombinase complex is inhibited, thereby interrupting further production of thrombin. Thrombin-induced platelet aggregation and release reactions are prevented while hirudin has no direct effect on platelet reactions or functions, nor is it inactivated by platelet factors.

Hirulogs are synthetic peptides modeled after **hirudin**. **Hirulog-1** (hirulog) is an amino acid peptide containing two domains joined by a glycine residue linker region. Similar to **hirudin**, **hirulog** binds to thrombin, forming a 1:1 complex causing inhibition of all known functions, including cleavage of fibrinogen, activation of platelets, and clotting factors.

The potential advantages of the selective thrombin inhibitors **hirudin** and **hirulog** over **heparin** include an inhibition of clot-bound thrombin, a lack of immunogenicity, no requirement of AT III as a cofactor (which may lead to a more consistent dose response), and a lack of inactivation by platelet factor. The drugs are being evaluated as treatments for acute coronary syndromes. Other direct antithrombin agents under investigation include **inogatran**, **melagatran**, **efegatran**, and **argatroban**.

Vascular Surfactants

Poloxamer 188 (RheothRx) is a nonionic, block copolymer surfactant. As a surfactant, **Rheoth Rx** reduces surface tension and hydrophobic interactions of cellular elements, which may inhibit free movement of blood in the intravascular space. Its mechanisms of action include a potentiation of the action of thrombolysis with decreased reocclusion and improvement of collateral blood flow, and an alteration of the fibrin structure of clots. It has been used in small clinical trials where it has been shown to decrease infarct size, reduce the rate of reinfarction, and improve ventricular function. It has no known anticoagulant properties and can be used safely with thrombolytic agents, **heparin** or **aspirin** without increasing the risk of bleeding. The drug also has no hemodynamic actions. However, studies with the drug revealed no clinical benefit in patients with CAD. The agent is now being evaluated as a drug to ameliorate vaso-occlusive crises in patients with sickle cell disease.

BETA-ADRENERGIC BLOCKERS

Beta-adrenergic blockers are available for a wide variety of cardiovascular conditions and in recent years a great deal of attention has been given to their use as adjunctive treatments to conventional therapy (ie, ACE inhibitors, diuretics, digoxin) in patients with heart failure secondary to left ventricular systolic dysfunction.

Two large studies have been completed with two beta$_1$ selective blockers, **bisoprolol** and long-acting **metoprolol**. MERIT-HF (Metoprolol CR/SL Randomized Intervention Trial in Congestive Heart Failure) evaluated 4,000 patients with predominantly class II and III CHF who were randomized to receive placebo or **metoprolol** 25–200 mg once daily. The addition of **metoprolol** to standard triple therapy was associated with a 35% reduction in mortality. In the CIBIS-II trial (Cardiac Insufficiency Bisoprolol Study), 2,600 patients with class III-IV CHF on standard therapy were randomized to receive placebo or **bisoprolol** 1.25–10 mg once daily. Adjunctive **bisoprolol** treatment caused a 32% relative reduction in all cause mortality.

Currently, a study is in progress evaluating a new vasodilator beta blocker, **bucindolol**, as an adjunctive therapy in patients with CHF. Preliminary results suggest little efficacy with the agent. The drug is also being evaluated in patients with systemic hypertension. New formulations of beta blockers are also being tested, which include **nevobilol**, a vasodilator beta blocker agent with nitric oxide-enhancing activity, and a sublingual beta blocker, **esprolol**, for patients with angina pectoris.

CALCIUM-CHANNEL BLOCKERS

Despite some initial fears about the dangers of calcium blockers in hypertension, an extensive database supports their overall safety.

A new dihydropyridine, **lercapidipine**, is being evaluated in patients with hypertension and angina pectoris. The dihydropyridine calcium blockers **amlodipine** and **felodipine** are being studied as adjunctive therapies in CHF. Long-acting felodipine is also being evaluated in a low-dose combination formulation with metoprolol-XL in patients with hypertension. **Nicardipine** and **nimodipine** are being evaluated in acute stroke. A new dihydropyridine, **clevidipine**, is being evaluated in perioperative hypertension.

Significant drug drug interactions led to the voluntary removal of the selective T-channel calcium blocker, **mibefradil**, which had been marketed for use in patients with hypertension and angina pectoris.

CENTRALLY ACTING AGENTS

The role of the central nervous system (CNS) in regulating vascular tone and control of blood pressure (BP) has been well documented. **Rilmenidine** and **monoxidine** are representatives of a new class of centrally acting antihypertensive drugs, the imidazoline receptor agonists. There are two subtypes of imidazoline receptors found in the brain, designated as I-1 and I-2. Studies have shown that **rilmenidine** exerts its antihypertensive effects at the same CNS sites as **clonidine**, except that rilmenidine has greater agonist receptor selectivity for the imidazoline receptor and clonidine for the alpha$_2$-adrenergic receptor. Rilmenidine appears to decrease central sympathetic outflow and has been shown to be an effective, orally active, antihypertensive drug, and may have specific neuro-protective actions in the presence of cerebral ischemia through its actions on the I-2 receptor. Used once daily, the drug appears to be comparable to other antihypertensive drugs, and causes less dry mouth and tiredness than clonidine. Rilmenidine appears to work as a vasodilator, and there are significant reductions in both serum norepinephrine and renin levels with drug treatment. The drug causes an increase in sodium excretion and cleared osmoles through central inhibition of renal sympathetic nerve activity. **Monoxidine** is a more selective I-1 receptor agonist. The drug is also an effective antihypertensive drug, which causes less orthostatic hypotension than prazosin. The imidazoline receptor agonists are effective second generation, centrally acting, antihypertensive drugs, associated with fewer CNS side effects compared to clonidine and alpha methyldopa. The antisympathetic effects of the imidazoline receptor agonists make them potential treatments for regression of left ventricular hypertrophy and treatment of CHF. Preliminary results of a study using monoxidine in the treatment of CHF show no benefit from the drug.

DIURETICS

The natriuretic peptides are naturally occurring vasodilator-natriuretic substances produced in the heart and brain.. They are also biologic markers that are elevated in patients with CHF.

When the natriuretic peptide **nesiritide** is infused in patients with CHF, it reduces pulmonary capillary wedge pressure and systemic vascular resistance while increasing stroke volume and cardiac index. It suppresses plasma aldosterone but does not change the plasma renin, norepinephrine or epinephrine. It increases renal plasma flow and glomerular filtration rate, as well as insulin excretion without affecting BP and heart rate. **Nesiritide** was recently approved for clinical use in the treatment of acute heart failure.

The direct aldosterone inhibitor **eplerenone** is also being evaluated as a diuretic agent in CHF and as an antihypertensive.

INOTROPIC AGENTS

Inotropic agents for long-term treatment of CHF have not been associated with favorable mortality outcomes. They provide hemodynamic support when used intravenously in patients with acute MI, and following open heart surgery. There also is experience using these drugs intravenously as a palliative treatment in patients with advanced chronic heart failure (eg, **dobutamine, milrinone**).

One new inotropic agents under investigation is **levosimendan**, which is being developed in an oral form. **Levosimendan** is an inodilatory benzimidazoline phosphodiesterase inhibitor, which acutely increases cardiac output and improves exercise tolerance in heart failure patients, while reducing ventricular filling pressure. **Levosimendan** may also have additional effects to enhance calcium binding to troponin C, a calcium-sensitizing action. Theoretically, this could enhance contractile response for a given amount of cytotoxic calcium, which could lead to less arrhythmogenicity, but this needs to be proven.

Studies with other phosphodiesterase inhibitors, such as **vesnarinone** and **OPC 18790** have suggested an increase in mortality risk, and clinical research programs with these agents have been discontinued.

LIPID LOWERING AGENTS

Drugs that reduce low-density lipoprotein (LDL) cholesterol levels in the blood can prevent the formation of, slow the progression of, and cause regression of atherosclerotic lesions throughout the circulation, thereby reducing the risk of MI and death. These agents also have been shown to improve endothelium-dependent vasodilation, to prevent clot formation by an anticoagulant action, and to stabilize atherosclerotic vascular lesions by possibly reducing inflammatory stimuli. It remains controversial whether elevated serum triglyceride levels appear to be an independent risk factor for cardiovascular disease in human beings. However, there is direct evidence from clinical trials of the benefit of reducing triglycerides with pharmacologic treatment.

Pravastatin and **simvastatin** have also been used to reduce mortality from graft rejection after heart transplantation. **Lovastatin** was shown to decrease saphenous vein atherosclerosis after bypass surgery. In a recent study comparing the use of **atorvastatin** alone to angioplasty in patients with stable CAD, the statin group were shown to have fewer cardiovascular events.

In a primary prevention study of hypercholesterolemic men, **pravastatin** was shown to reduce the risk of major coronary events. In another primary prevention study of normocholesterolemic men and women with below average HDL cholesterol levels, lovastatin reduced the risk of acute coronary events.

Niacin is another agent that lowers LDL cholesterol and triglycerides but can cause flushing, pruritis and gastrointestinal distress. **Niaspan**, a new extended-release niacin formulation, appears to be better tolerated. Hepatic toxicity has been reported to occur with some of the older sustained-release niacin formulations, when used in higher doses.

The fibric acid derivatives (FADs), which include **gemfibrozil, fenofibrate,** and **clofibrate,** are used to reduce triglycerides, lipoprotein(a) and HDL-cholesterol. They can also lower LDL cholesterol, but less than the statins. There are data from a recent study to suggest that individuals having a low HDL cholesterol and normal LDL cholesterol can benefit from treatment with gemfibrozil.

Fenofibrate has been available in tablet form outside the United States, but a new micronized formulation is being marketed, which may have a greater effect on LDL cholesterol than gemfibrozil. The dose of fenofibrate must be adjusted in patients with renal disease. There are also no available data on the effects of fenofibrate in patients with CAD. Other FADs that are marketed overseas include **bezafibrate,** which has been shown in preliminary studies to benefit men who have had a previous MI.

A recent animal study suggested the possible use of an angiogenesis inhibitor drug (*e.g.,* **endostatin**) to arrest the development or progression of atherosclerotic plaque by inhibiting blood vessel growth.

New approaches to cholesterol lowering currently being investigated are the **acyl coenzyme-A transferase (ACAT)** inhibitors, the **squalene synthetase inhibitors,** the cholesterol esterase inhibitors, **the 7-alpha hydroxylase inhibitors,** and **plant sterols.**

The inhibitors of ACAT catalyzed cholesterol esterification are thought to be potent inhibitors of intestinal cholesterol absorption. In addition, they are thought to influence LDL synthesis in the liver and prevent the formation of foam cells in blood vessel walls.

The **squalene synthetase** inhibitors inhibit the conversion of farnesyl pyrophosphate to squalene by inhibiting squalene synthetase. Squalene is the immediate precursor compound to cholesterol. Inhibiting the formation of cholesterol at this level would have a more specific effect rather than at the level of HMG-CoA where the formation of other essential substances, such as **ubiquinone** and **dolichol,** would be inhibited. Whether or not **squalene synthetase** inhibition will provide a safer means than HMG-CoA for blocking cholesterol synthesis must be determined.

The enzyme **7-alpha hydroxylase** is the regulatory substance in the conversion of cholesterol to bile salts. Bile acid biosynthesis represents the major route of catabolism and removal of cholesterol in the body. An enzyme-inhibiting drug could potentially reduce plasma cholesterol levels and have a preventive influence on gallstone production.

The cholesterol lowering activity of **plant sterols and stanols,** in particular their predominant components, **sitosterol and sitostanol,** have been established in clinical trials. The plant sterols lower serum cholesterol by inhibiting the intestinal absorption of cholesterol. Because of their safety and efficacy, they have the potential for use in clinical practice. The use of fatty acid esters of stanols is particularly promising because stanols may easily mix with dietary fats in this form, and their hypocholesterolemic effects are greater than in the free form.

COMBINATION ANTIHYPERTENSIVE PRODUCTS

Most combination formulations include a diuretic as one treatment component, but recently low dose combinations of calcium-channel blockers and ACE inhibitors have been available. A combination of **felodipine** with **ramipril** is in clinical trials. A study is in progress evaluating a calcium blocker-beta blocker combination formulation (extended-release **metoprolol** and **felodipine**) and studies are being planned for using combination formulations of ACE inhibitors and A-II receptor blockers.

NEWER APPROACHES FOR SYSTEMIC HYPERTENSION

New drugs and new classes of drugs are being examined for the treatment of hypertension and include new ACE inhibitors and A-II receptor blockers, the aldosterone antagonists, neutral endopeptidase inhibitors, the neutral endopeptidase-ACE inhibitors, the endothelin receptor blockers, potassium ion channel openers, adenosine receptor agonists, and beta-adrenergic blockers.

The orally acting ACE inhibitor agents, **cilazapril, perindopril** and **spirapril,** have undergone extensive clinical testing and some are already approved for use in hypertension. **Sampatrilat** is currently being studied in patients with hypertension and CHF.

A-II receptor blockers under investigation include **eprosartan**, **forasartan** and **ripisartan**. **Tasosartan**, which had been studied extensively in hypertensive patients, will not be marketed.

The direct aldosterone blocking agent, **eplerenone**, is being studied as an antihypertensive agent. The neutral endopeptidase inhibitors are drugs that structurally resemble the ACE inhibitors. Orally active neutral endopeptidase (NEP) inhibitors have been developed to inhibit the metabolism of naturally occurring atrial natriuretic peptides (Fig. 14.1), which, in turn, act on the kidney to produce increased sodium excretion, on the vasculature to induce vasodilation, and on the adrenal glands to reduce aldosterone secretion. Multiple agents in this class have been tested in patients having chronic systemic hypertension with equivocal benefit observed (**candoxatril**, SCH 42495).

It is believed that the attenuation of responsiveness to endogenous atrial natriuretic peptides (ANPs) with endopeptidase inhibition is due to activation of the renin-angiotensin-aldosterone system (RAAS). This has prompted the development of agents that both augment the action of ANP and block the RAAS, the dual NEP-ACE inhibitor drugs (**omelapril**, **alatriopril**), which are now being examined in patients with systemic hypertension and CHF.

Endothelin, the most potent vasoconstrictor known to date, is a naturally occurring polypeptide produced predominantly by the endothelial cells. Its release is influenced by A-II and other physiologic mediators. The receptors for endothelin have been isolated and their genes cloned. Heightened endothelin release has been identified in many cardiovascular disease states, including systemic hypertension. Active clinical research programs are in place evaluating various endothelin receptor blockers in patients with systemic hypertension. A large study with the endothelin-inhibitor **bosentan** demonstrated its antihypertensive activity in patients, however, further development of the drug has been discontinued because of its hepatotoxicity. Endothelin-converting enzyme inhibitors are also being investigated; they interfere with the biosynthesis of native vasoactive endothelin.

Potassium ion channel openers cause vasodilation by enhancing potassium efflux from vascular smooth muscle.

Pinacidil, **nicorandil**, and **cromakalim** are orally active drugs in this class that have been evaluated in patients with hypertension. Their effects appear to be similar to **minoxidil** and **diazoxide**. Their clinical utility may be limited by the need to dose these drugs thrice daily and the occurrence of tachycardia in some patients.

Adenosine receptor agonists have direct vasodilatory effects and can inhibit neurotransmitter release. They can lower BP while inhibiting renin release and causing a natriuresis. The drugs have been shown to be effective in various animal models, and are being considered for use in clinical trials.

A new beta-adrenergic receptor (beta$_3$) has recently been characterized. This receptor appears to mediate thermogenesis in humans and beta$_3$ stimulation may reduce requirements of insulin needed to maintain glycemic control. Since hyperinsulinemia has been suspected to be a cause of systemic hypertension, drugs in the beta$_3$ agonist class are being developed for the treatment of obesity as well as a potential therapy of high BP. Other classes of insulin sensitizing drugs are being evaluated for the treatment of hypertension.

NEW CLASSES OF DRUGS FOR ANGINA PECTORIS AND MYOCARDIAL ISCHEMIA

Seven new classes of drugs are being evaluated in patients with stable angina pectoris and myocardial ischemia. The first are the potassium channel openers. Potassium ATP channels are located in the cell membranes of various organs, including the myocardium and blood vessels. During myocardial ischemia, there is a reduction in intracellular myocardial ATP that causes opening of KATP channels. This results in an efflux of intracellular potassium, hyperpolarization of the cell membrane, shortening of action potential duration, and both myocardial and vaso-relaxation. The potassium efflux that occurs during ischemia has been shown to be protective and prevents further myocardial damage, thereby preserving myocardial function. There are currently large scale trials in progress assessing the antianginal efficacy and safety profile of these drugs, which includes **nicorandil**. **Nicorandil** is a coronary and peripheral vasodilator that has a complex mechanism of action and appears to be a short duration of action, requiring frequent dosing. Its potential advantage is that, unlike nitrates, it is not associated with tolerance. The drug is available for clinical use outside the United States. Other orally active adenosine triphosphate (ATP) potassium channel openers have been developed for use in angina.

The second class of drugs are the nitric oxide donors, which include **molsidomine** and **persidomine**. Nitric oxide has been shown to be an important biological substance involved in normal physiologic functioning. It appears to be an endogenous vasodilator. Endothelial cell dysfunction often leads to diminished nitric oxide production, which may be an etiological factor in atherosclerotic vascular diseases. **Persidomine** is a nitric oxide donor of the sydnonimine class . The drug is not associated with pharmacologic tolerance, and ongoing clinical trials using this compound in patients with angina pectoris are now in progress.

The third class of drugs is composed of the sinus node inhibitors. These drugs reduce heart rate by a nonbeta-adrenoceptor mediated mechanism, and produce no direct negative

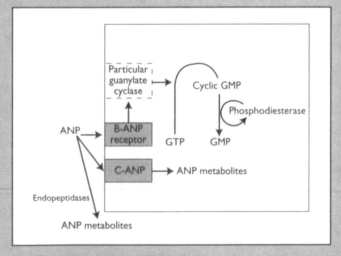

FIGURE 14.1 Mechanisms of action for atrial natriuretic peptide. (*Adapted from* Achilihu G, Frishman WH, Landau A: Neutral endopeptidase inhibitors and atrial natriuretic peptide. *J Clin Pharmacol* 1991;31:758–762.)

inotropic effects. The prototype agent, **zatebradine**, decreases the rate of spontaneous depolarization of pacemaker cells in the sinoatrial node, thereby producing a sinus node inhibition. **Zatebradine** has no effect on calcium channels, it has no effect on the peripheral vasculature or the myocardium. The drug can antagonize an isoproterenol-mediated increase in heart rate in a noncompetitive fashion, without affecting contractility. However, preliminary findings suggest that **zatebradine** may not be effective in angina pectoris despite their heart rate lowering effects. **Tedisaril**, another sinus node inhibitor, is now being evaluated in clinical trials.

The fourth class is composed of agents that have favorable effects on myocardial metabolism. **Ranolazine** is a drug without hemodynamic effects, however, it appears to improve myocardial ischemia by altering myocardial substrate metabolism. The drug has been evaluated in patients with angina, and has shown benefit in improving exercise tolerance.

Similar to **ranolazine**, **trimetazidine** demonstrates a number of potentially useful cytoprotective actions, which include a limitation of mitochondrial and membrane damage caused by oxygen free radicals, a reduction of intracellular acidosis, and an inhibitory effect of neutrophil infiltration in the perfused myocardium. In multiple clinical studies, **trimetazidine** has demonstrated significant anti-ischemic actions. In patients with chronic stable angina, trimetazidine has reduced angina attack frequency and nitroglycerin consumption, while increasing treadmill exercise time and the time to the development of 1mm ST segment depression on the exercise ECG. The drug is also as effective as **propranolol** and **nifedipine** on both angina and exercise parameters, and can provide additional benefit when added to **diltiazem**, **nifedipine**, or beta blockers. **Trimetazidine** also reduced the number of ischemic episodes in patients with angina pectoris who underwent ambulatory ECG monitoring.

The fifth class of drugs is composed of the aldose reductase inhibitors. They are shown to preserve the tissue redox ratio of nicotinamide adenine dinucleotide to the reduced form of NAD (NAD/NADH), which can be protective in myocardial ischemia. In experimental isolated heart studies using diabetic rats, it has been shown that the aldose reductase inhibitor **zopolrestat** preserved ATP during global ischemia, reduced ischemic injury as indicated by creatine phosphokinase (CPK) release, and improved functional recovery of the myocardium after reperfusion. In addition, aldose reductase inhibition with **zopolrestat** in the isolated diabetic rat heart model was shown to increase Na+/K+-ATPase activity with limitation in the rise of intracellular sodium and hence the intracellular calcium rise during ischemia and reperfusion. Clinical trials with **zopolrestat** in diabetic and nondiabetic patients with angina pectoris are in progress.

The sixth class of drugs is composed of the inhibitors of sodium-hydrogen ion exchanger (NHE), which is markedly active in ischemia and reperfusion. Inhibition of this exchanger definitely decreases intracellular Na+ and subsequently decreases intracellular Ca+ overload. Inhibitors also decrease the rate of ATP depletion during ischemia and reperfusion. Such action reduces the chances of malignant arrhythmias occurring, as well as the development of myocardial necrosis. **Amiloride** and analogues have been proved potent NHE inhibitors. However, **amiloride** alone is nonspecific and for it to be effective it must be taken at excessively high levels. This can prove to be toxic. In contrast, analogues, such as **cariporide**, which is undergoing clinical investigation, are more potent and more selective, accomplishing the same desired results of NHE inhibition, while not requiring excessive doses for effectiveness. Therefore, analogues are preferred as potential treatment for clinical use to prevent reperfusion injury. However, a recent study with **cariporide** showed no clinical benefit in patients with myocardial ischemia.

The seventh class of drugs is composed of the statins and acyl-coA: cholesterol acyltransferase inhibitors (eg, **avasimibe**), which appear to improve endothelial cell functioning and vascular reactivity independent of the cholesterol lowering effects. These drugs are now being evaluated as antianginal drugs.

The eighth class of drugs is composed of biological substances that stimulate angiogenesis. Angiogenesis is a term for the formation of new capillaries from existing blood vessels. Angiogenesis takes place in the following manner. In response to cytokines, endothelial cells degrade their basement membrane; migrate from the parent blood vessel in a directional manner toward a stimulus; and invade the extravascular space. Endothelial cells then proliferate to replace the invading cells; migrate through the connective tissue to a target site where cells assemble to form a new vessel and lumen; and secrete a basement membrane (Fig. 14.2). Angiogenesis stimulators are shown in Table 14.2. Some of these factors are being used in clinical trials to treat patients with CAD and angina pectoris (Table 14.3).

Vascular endothelial growth factor (VEGF) is a secreted homodimeric glycoprotein with 4 different isoforms generated from a single gene, through an alteration splicing mechanism in humans. The 4 isoforms have 121, 165, 189, and 206 amino acids respectively. VEGF binds to specific cell receptors, flt-1 and flk-1. The biologic activity of **VEGF-165** has been studied most extensively since it is the predominant isoform secreted by a variety of cells. **VEGF-165** and **VEGF-121** are being studied in clinical trials of patients with severe angina pectoris, with the substance being injected directly into the coronary circulation and peripherally. In other studies, naked DNA containing the VEGF gene was injected directly into sites in the myocardium identified by angiography. Access was obtained via mini-thoracotomy. Other investigators injected the VEGF gene into cardiac muscle aboard a disarmed adenovirus vector during coronary artery bypass surgery or during a mini-thoracotomy. Some short-term preliminary studies have revealed clinical benefit in patients with severe angina pectoris, with evidence of increased blood flow to the heart. In some studies, the results have been unimpressive.

Another angiogenesis substance under investigation has been **fibroblast growth factor (FGF)**. The FGF gene presently contains nine members. FGF-1 (acidic) and FGF-2 (basic) are single-chain polypeptides. These molecules promote formation of new blood vessels and the proliferation of vascular smooth muscle cells. FGF-1 and FGF-2 have been administered to humans with angina pectoris and severe CAD by direct intracoronary injection and by direct intramyocardial injection. Intramyocardial delivery of naked DNA containing the FGF gene and delivery of the FGF gene by adenovirus have also been utilized. FGF-2 has been implanted in pellet form in the myocardium in patients undergoing incomplete coronary revascularization procedures. Early results with FGF have been favorable, but more long-term data are needed.

Other angiogenesis stimulatory substances under investigation are **hypoxia inducible factor (HIF)** where the gene for HIF is delivered by adenovirus injected into the myocardium. Inflammatory mediators of angiogenesis are also being investigated as potential clinical agents.

DRUGS FOR MYOCARDIAL INFARCTION AND UNSTABLE ANGINA

The direct antithrombin agents, **inogatran**, **melagatran**, **efegatran**, and **argatroban**, are being evaluated as alternative therapies to heparin in patients with heparin-induced thrombocytopenia and as an adjunct to thrombolytic therapy in patients with acute MI. The direct antithrombins have an advantage in preventing rethrombosis, by inhibiting thrombin bound to clot, which is not affected by heparin. The antithrombin agent **hirudin**, which is approved for use in heparin-induced thrombocytopenia, is being evaluated for use in acute coronary syndromes, and **hirulog (bevalirudin)**, another direct thrombin inhibitor, is being evaluated as an adjunctive therapy in patients undergoing transluminal coronary angioplasty.

A recombinant antithrombin III is being developed and evaluated in patients undergoing cardiopulmonary bypass

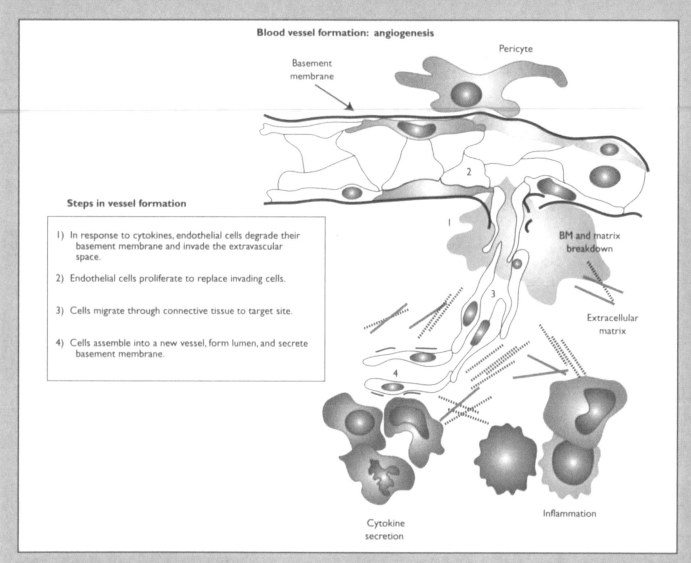

Blood vessel formation: angiogenesis

Pericyte

Basement membrane

Steps in vessel formation

1) In response to cytokines, endothelial cells degrade their basement membrane and invade the extravascular space.

2) Endothelial cells proliferate to replace invading cells.

3) Cells migrate through connective tissue to target site.

4) Cells assemble into a new vessel, form lumen, and secrete basement membrane.

BM and matrix breakdown

Extracellular matrix

Cytokine secretion

Inflammation

FIGURE 14.2 Blood vessel formation: angiogenesis.

who develop heparin resistance. New LMWH are being studied in patients with unstable coronary syndromes.

Newer thrombolytic agents under investigation in acute MI include pro-urokinase, which is the single-chain precursor of urokinase, **lanoteplase** (r-nPA), a novel synthetic plasminogen activator that lacks fibronectin finger-like and epidermal growth factor domains, and TNK-tPA, which appears to be more fibrin specific than tPA.

Newer glycoprotein IIb/IIIa antagonists under investigation in unstable coronary syndromes include oral and intravenous agents such as **fradafiban, lefradifiban, sibrifiban,** and **lamifiban.**

Cariporide (Hoe 642) is an inhibitor of the membrane sodium-hydrogen ion exchanger, and is being evaluated as a cardioprotective agent in acute coronary syndromes. **Lazaroids,** a group of 21-aminosteroids that inhibit lipid peroxidation without glucocorticoid activity, are also being evaluated in myocardial ischemia-reperfusion.

When **adenosine** is combined with thrombolytics to treat MI, the area of infarct may be reduced by as much as an additional 67% over thrombolytics alone. Other adenosine agonists or potentiators (eg, **acadesine**) have been used as myocardial preserving agents in patients undergoing coronary revascularization. Adenosine-regulating agents can theoretically act in any ischemic microcirculatory bed to attenuate reperfusion injury, inflammation or thrombogenesis.

Another innovative approach to preserving myocardial function in acute MI are interventions that interfere with cardiac myocyte apoptosis (programmed cell death), a process that is activated with myocardial ischemia. Utilization of A-II receptor blockers and infusion of insulin-growth factor during myocardial ischemia in rats can inhibit the amount of cardiac myocyte

TABLE 14.2 ANGIOGENIC AGENTS (TYPES OF STIMULATORS)

Extracellular matrix molecule	Growth factors and cytokines		Hormones
Fibronectin	FGF		GM-CSF
Fibrin	VEGF		Estrogen
Collagen	PDGF		Progesterone
Laminin	EGF	HIF	
	Angiogenin	HGF	
	Vasculotropin	TNFα	
	Pleiotropin	PGE$_2$	
	Proliferin	TGFβ	

CSF—granulocyte macrophage-colony stimulating factor; ECG — epidermal growth factor; FGF—fibroblast growth factor; GM- HGF—hepatocyte growth factor; HIF—hypoxia inducible factor; PDGF—platelet-derived growth factor; PGE$_2$—prostaglandin E$_2$; TGFβ—transforming growth factor beta; TNFα—tumor necrosis factor alpha; VEGF—vascular endothelial growth factor.

Adapted from Frishman WH, Greenberg S, Goldschmidt M, Patel K, et al.: Innovative pharmacologic approaches for the treatment of myocardial ischemia. In Frishman WH, Sonnenblick EH (eds): Cardiovascular Pharmacotherapeutics. New York: McGraw Hill, 1997:861.

TABLE 14.3 CLINICAL TRIALS OF THERAPEUTIC MYOCARDIAL ANGIOGENESIS

Growth factor	Delivery	Phase	Patients treated with active agent/placebo
FGF-1	Intramyocardial	I	20/20
FGF-2	Intracoronary	I	
FGF-2	Local(polymer)	I	16/8
FGF-2	Intracoronary	I	52/0
FGF-2	Intravenous	I	14/0
FGF-2	Intracoronary	II	
FGF-4	Intracoronary (adenovirus)	I	
VEGF$_{165}$	Intracoronary	I	15/0
VEGF$_{165}$	Intravenous	I	27/0
VEGF$_{165}$	Intracoronary/intravenous	II	
VEGF$_{165}$	Intramyocardial (plasmid)	I	13/0*
VEGF$_{121}$	Intramyocardial (adenovirus)	I	7/0*
HIF-1α	Intramyocardial (adenovirus)	I	

* Enrollment not completed at this time.

The information here is provided as guidance only. Prescribers should always consult the manufacturer's current prescribing information.

281

apoptosis by 50%, and suggests future therapeutic approaches in human beings. Capsase, an enzyme in the apoptosis process, can be inhibited pharmacologically with evidence of myocardial preservation in experimental infarct models.

Markers of inflammation are elevated in patients with acute coronary syndromes, suggesting that acute inflammation may play a role in plaque destabilization and rupture. Antibiotic regimens against *chlamydia pneumoniae* and *hylobacteria pylori* are being evaluated as possible protective agents in patients with CAD, but the results of clincial trials have not shown benefit.

DRUGS FOR CEREBROVASCULAR DISEASE

Recombinant tissue plasminogen activator (tPA) is approved for use in acute ischemic stroke within 3 hours of symptom onset. An investigational thrombolytic agent, **pro-urokinase**, was shown to have long-term morbidity benefit if used within 6 hours of symptom onset in patients with middle cerebral artery stroke. A fibrinogen-depleting agent, **ancrod**, which is derived from snake venom, was shown to be of benefit in patients if used within 3 hours of stroke onset.

Innovative clinical strategies are being developed to protect neurons from ischemic damage (Table 14.4), and are being utilized with and without thrombolysis in patients with stroke. The final common pathway for ischemic neuronal death appears to be influx of calcium. Calcium enters cells from stimulation of the N-methyl-D-aspartate (NMDA) receptors by the excitatory amino acids glutamate and aspartate, which are released during cerebral ischemia. This influx of calcium is not inhibited by calcium channel blockers and is believed to be the main source of calcium responsible for ischemic neuronal death. Noncompetitive NMDA receptor antagonists (**aptigenel, dextorphan, ramacemide, magnesium**), competitive antagonists (**selfotel**), glycine site inhibitors (**ACEA 1021, ACPC 2D9379, GV150-526A**), and polyamine site inhibitors (**eliprodil**) are currently in clincial trials but are difficult to manage because of their psychotic effects. Inhibition of the initial ischemic releases of glutamate is also being evaluated with the sodium channel blocker **riluzole**, the anticonvulsant **lamotrigine**, and **BW619C89**.

The calcium influx from NMDA receptor stimulation causes delayed neuronal death occurring at about 8 hours after the onset of ischemia. The initiating event for the excitotoxic ischemic cascade induced by glutamate appears to be the influx of sodium induced by stimulation of the AMPA (kainic acid) glutamate receptor site. Siesjo has hypothesized inhibition of the AMPA site by phosphonates such as APV and quinoxaline diones such as NBQX. In animal models, NMDA receptor antagonists have been more effective in reducing infarct volume in models of focal ischemia that are analogous to arterial occlusive disease. AMPA receptor antagonists, on the other hand, have been more effective in reducing infarct volume in models of global ischemia analogous to cardiac arrest or hypovolemic shock.

Free radicals have also been implicated in ischemic neuronal damage, particularly in animal models involving reperfusion. A steroid derivative, **tirilazad mesylate**, with antioxidant properties, has been employed in clinical trials, but no definitive benefits have been demonstrated as yet for ischemic stroke.

Lubeluzole is a novel benzothiazole compound that has emerged as a neuroprotective agent in animal models of focal ischemia. Blockade of sodium channels may be one of the mechanisms contributing to its neuroprotective effect. Lubeluzole also inhibits glutamate release after ischemia and reduces potassium-induced increases in intracellular calcium. Finally it prevents glutamate-mediated increases in nitric oxide production by inhibiting the activity of nitric oxide synthase. A phase II clinical trial of lubeluzole in acute ischemic stroke suggests that lubeluzole lowers mortality and disability in some patients. Lubeluzole is also being evaluated in two studies: a pivotal large phase III trial stratified to treatment between 0 and 6 or 6 and 8 hours from symptom onset (LUB-13), and a trial of lubeluzole versus placebo in combination with intravenous recombinant tPA therapy (LUB-USA-6). The latter study has been interrupted pending analysis of the LUB-13 study, which was reportedly negative.

The anticonvulsants **clomethiazole** and **vigabatrin** are GABA agonists recently shown to be neuroprotective in animal models of focal and global ischemia. The results of a phase III trial of 1,360 patients randomized to receive either placebo or 75 mg/kg of **clomethiazole** intravenously over 24 hours, beginning within 12 hours of stroke onset, were reported. The difference between clomethiazole and placebo on the primary endpoint (percentage of patients scoring greater than 60 on the Barthel Index at 3 months post stroke) was not statistically significant. Prespecific subgroup analysis revealed a positive effect of clomethiazole in patients with larger strokes; confirmation of these results awaits completion of an ongoing phase III trial in North America.

Piracetam, a GABA derivative and nootropic agents, was shown to be neuroprotective in two pilot trials of acute ischemic stroke. Although its mechanism of action is not entirely clear,

TABLE 14.4 NEUROPROTECTIVE AGENTS IN CLINICAL TRIALS
Calcium channel blockers (nimodipine, nicardipine)
NMDA receptor antagonists (selfotel, dextorphan, cerestat, eliprodil, magnesium, lamotrigine, glycine site antagonists)
Lubeluzole
Free radical scavengers (tirilizad)
Anti-ICAM-1 antibody
GM-1 ganglioside
GABA agonists (clomethiazole)
Fosphenytoin
Nootropic agents (piracetam)
Glutamate release inhibitors (BW619C89)
AMPA receptor antagonists
Adenosine agonists
Kappa-selective opioid antagonists (nalmafene)
Calpain inhibitors
Basic fibroblast growth factor
Selective serotonin agonists (BAYx3702)
Combined cytoprotective strategies
Cytoprotection plus thrombolysis
Adapted from Hickenbottom SL, Grotta J: Neuroprotective therapy. *Sem Neurol* 1998; 18: 488.

it is thought that its neuroprotective properties are mediated through restoration of cell membrane fluidity and, thus, maintenance of membrane-bound cell functions. However, a recent randomized, placebo-controlled trial of 927 patients given **piracetam** intravenously within 12 hours of stroke onset demonstrated no difference in mortality or neurologic outcomes at 12 weeks post stroke. Post hoc subgroup analysis of patients treated within 7 hours of symptom onset showed a trend toward better outcome, and a multicenter, randomized, placebo-controlled trial of early use of piracetam may begin.

One innovative treatment under investigation is **citicoline**, an endogenous substance that regulates the rate-limiting step involved in phosphatidylcholine synthesis and reduces production of free fatty acids. Others under investigation include the use of adenosine agonists, growth factor, and **enlimomab**, a murine anti-ICAM-I monoclonal antibody that has been shown to inhibit neutrophil adhesion, migration and cytotoxicity. However, preliminary studies with **enlimomab** have shown considerable toxicity with the drug, and no apparent clinical benefit.

TABLE 14.5 OUTLINE OF PHARMACOLOGICAL APPROACHES FOR PREVENTION OF RESTENOSIS

Antiplatelet agents and antithrombotics

Aspirin

Dipyridamole

TXA_2 receptor antagonists (vapiprost, sulotroban, S-1452)

TXA_2 synthetase inhibitors

TXB_2 synthetase inhibitors (ridogrel)

Prostacyclin and prostacyclin analogs (ciprostene, beraprost)

Fish oils (omega 3 fatty acids, eicosapentaenoic acid, Maxepa)

Ticlopidine

Dextran

Heparin (unfractionated)

Low molecular weight heparin (enoxaparin, reviparin, dalteparin)

Exogenous antithrombin III

Direct thrombin antagonists (hirudin, hirulog, antistasin)

Factor Xa inhibitors (antistasin, tick anticoagulant peptide)

Vitamin K antagonists (warfarin)

Early coagulation cascade inhibitors (rTFPI, DEGR-VIIa)

Thrombolytic agents (tissue plasminogen activator, urokinase)

IIb/IIIa receptor antagonists (c7E3 fab, abciximab, integrelin, tirofiban, xemilofiban, RGD and KCD peptides)

Defibrinogenating agents (ancrod)

cAMP phosphodiesterase inhibitors (cilostazol)

Anti-inflammatory Drugs

Steroids

NSAIDs (ebselen, sulfinpyrazone)

Anti-allergic agents (tranilast)

Growth Factor Antagonists

PDGF antagonists (trapidil, polyclonal α-PDGF antibodies, PDGF-receptor tyrosine kinase inhibitor)

Pituitary growth hormone antagonists (angiopeptin, octreotide)

Serotonin antagonists (ketanserin)

ACE inhibitors (cilazapril, captopril, fosinopril, enalapril, irbesartan)

Estrogen

β-Adrenergic receptor antagonists (prazosin, urapidil)

β_1-adrenergic receptor antagonists (carvedilol)

Nitric oxide donors (L-arginine, nitrosated albumin, linsidomine, molsidomine)

Leucocyte and endothelial adhesion molecule antagonists (α-CD/11 CD18 adhesion complex antibodies)

Endothelial Growth Factors

VEGF

(Human) HGF

Vasodilators

Calcium channel antagonists (diltiazem, nifedipine, nisoldipine, verapamil)

Antiproliferatives and Antineoplastics

Microtubule inhibitors (colchicine, taxol)

Other antineoplastics (etoposide, vincristine, dactinomycin, cyclosporine, azathioprine, methotrexate)

Photodynamic Therapy

8-methoxypsoralen (8MOP)

Phthalocyanine

Photofrin (QLT Phototherapeutics)

Lipid-lowering Agents

LDL apheresis

HMG-CoA reductase inhibitors (lovastatin, pravastatin, fluvastatin)

Probucol

Antioxidants

Vitamins, E, C

Probucol

Radiotherapy

γ-irradiation (192Ir)

β-irradiation (90 Sr/Y)

Delivery methods: wire-delivered, liquid-filled source, external beam radiation

Molecular Strategies

Recombinant chimeric toxins

ASODNs (c-myc, c-myb, PCNA, nonmuscle myosin)

Gene therapy (thymidine kinase, retinoblastoma gene product)

Note: Drugs have been classified according to what is thought to be their principal pharmacodynamic mechanism in reducing restenosis, although there is certainly overlap among the categories, with several antithrombotic agents, for example, having also been found to have direct antiproliferative effects on smooth muscle cells.

ACE—angiotensin converting enzyme; ASODNs—antisense oligodeoxynucleotides; cAMP—cyclic adenosine monophosphate; DEGR-VIIa—active site inactivated factor VIIa; HGF—human growth factor; LDL—low-density lipoprotein; NSAIDs—nonsteroidal anti-inflammatory drugs; PCNA— proliferating cell nuclear antigen; PDGF—platelet derived growth factor; rTFPI—recombinant tissue factor pathway inhibitor; TXA_2—thromboxane A_2; TXB_2—thromboxane B_2; VEGF—vascular endothelial growth factor.

Adapted from Landzberg BR, Frishman WH, Lerrick K: Pathophysiology and pharmacological approaches for prevention of coronary artery restenosis following coronary artery balloon angioplasty and related procedures. Prog Cardiovasc Dis 39: 361–398, 1997.

Drugs for Treating Restenosis in Patients Following PTCA with and without Stenting

Multiple therapeutic approaches have been employed to prevent coronary restenosis following angioplasty (Table 14.5). However, most pharmacologic regimens have shown no beneficial effect.

Angiopeptin (**lamreotide**), a somatostatin analogue, is now under consideration as a possible treatment modality for post angioplasty restenosis. Angiopeptin reduces growth hormone secretion and can prevent an increase in insulin-like growth factor (IGF-1), an important serum and tissue factor responsible for cell proliferation in the vascular wall. Another agent under consideration to prevent post angioplasty restenosis is **hyaluronan**.

New Drugs for Congestive Heart Failure

Various vasodilator drug classes are being evaluated in the treatment of patients with chronic CHF, and include new ACE inhibitors, the A-II receptor blockers, the neutral endopeptidase inhibitors (**candoxatril**), dual neutral endopeptidase inhibitors, calcium-entry blockers (**amlodipine, felodipine**), the endothelin inhibitors, and the vasopressin inhibitors.

Newer diuretic approaches include the direct aldosterone antagonists (**eplerenone**) and the addition of spironolactone to loop diuretics for maximizing cardioprotection. A recent clinical trial demonstrated a benefit of adding aldactone to loop diuretic therapy as part of a heart failure treatment regimen, with reductions in patient morbidity and mortality. Continuous infusions of **torsemide**, a loop diuretic, may be a better treatment approach for chronic and acute congestion than bolus injections of the drug.

Inotropic drugs continue to be investigated and the calcium-sensitizing agent **levosimendan** is now being evaluated in clinical trials.

Drugs interfering with sympathetic nervous activity, such as beta-adrenergic blocking drugs, have been shown to be useful adjunctive therapies in patients with heart failure. Long-acting **metoprolol, bisoprolol**, and the vasodilator-beta blocker **bucindolol** are currently being evaluated for this indication.

The centrally acting antihypertensive agent **moxonidine**, an imidazole receptor agonist, is now undergoing clinical trials in CHF. Moxonidine's actions are similar to clonidine.

Patients with advanced heart failure have considerable skeletal muscle weakness, cachexia and anorexia, and growth hormone is being evaluated as a stimulant for enhancing cardiac and skeletal muscle function.

Patients with heart failure appear to have enhanced cardiac apoptosis. The use of IGF-1 and A-II receptor blockers may reduce the rate of cell death.

Cytokines are a group of small pleiotropic endogenous peptides produced by a variety of cell types in response to different stimuli. Tumor necrosis factor alpha (TNFα), interleukin 1- alpha (IL-1α), interleukin-1 beta (IL-1β), and interleukin-6 (IL-6) are classified as "proinflammatory" cytokines. These substances are responsible for initiating the primary host response to bacterial infections, as well as initiating the repair of injured tissues.

Cytokines are involved in augmenting the expression of adhesion molecules and for enhanced cell-to-cell interactions involved in inflammation. In addition, the proinflammatory cytokines are able to affect cardiovascular functioning by promoting left ventricular remodeling, causing ventricular dysfunction and uncoupling myocardial beta receptors. They are elevated in the serum in various cardiovascular disorders, and are often a marker of disease severity.

Many experimental and clinical studies have shown that there is an association between depressed myocardial function in heart failure patients and elevated levels of TNFα. However, the nature of this association is not clear or agreed upon. There are studies that suggest elevated levels of TNFα play a major role in causing myocardial depression, whereas other studies conclude that TNFα is likely to play a part in the alleviation of this condition. A third school of thought suggests that the elevated levels of TNFα are merely a marker that may indicate the stage of progression of the disease. Thus, although it is clear that there are elevated levels of TNFα in various cardiac diseases, the reasons for these increased levels and the mechanism(s) for their effects are not agreed upon.

Current studies are in progress evaluating the effects of a soluble recombinant human TNF R fusion protein on the clinical course of patients with advanced heart failure. Other inflammatory cytokines may be therapeutic targets in the future.

TABLE 14.6 Beta blocker mortality trials

Trial	Number of patients	Drugs	NYHA class	EF, %	Mean follow-up, mo	Progress
BEST	2708	Bucindolol	III-IV	≤35	36	In follow-up
CIBIS II	2647	Bisoprolol	III-IV	≤35	17	Benefit
MERIT-HF	3991	Metoprolol XL	II-IV	≤40	12	Benefit
COPERNICUS	2000	Carvedilol	IIIb-IV	≤25	36	Recruiting
COMET	3073	Carvedilol/Metoprolol	II-IV	≤35	36	In follow-up
Total 14,349						

BEST—Beta Blocker Evaluation of Survival Trial; CIBIS II—Cardiac Insufficiency Bisoprolol Study; COMET—Carvedilol or Metoprolol Trial. COPERNICUS—Carvedilol Prospective Randomized Cumulative Survival Trial; EF—ejection fraction; MERIT-HF—Metoprolol CR/XL Randomized Intervention Trial in Heart Failure; NYHA—New York Heart Association.

Adapted from Internal Medicine World Report. ACC Symposium Issue April 1999; 14: 4. Medical World Business Press Inc.

The natriuretic peptide **nesiritide** has received clinical approval for use in the treatment of patients with acute heart failure.

DRUGS FOR PERIPHERAL VASCULAR DISEASE

Multiple agents are being evaluated to prevent and treat peripheral venous and arterial thromboses, and these include new low molecular weight heparin (**tinzaperin**), **hirudin**, SR90107/ **pentasaccharide**, and HMR2906.

Poloxamer 188, a nonionic co-polymer surfactant is being evaluated as a treatment for vaso-occlusive crisis in sickle cell disease.

New prostacyclin analogues are being evaluated in patients with peripheral vascular disease and other thrombotic disorders. **Iloprost** is a more stable analogue of **epoprostenol**, and is undergoing clinical investigation in various vascular disorders including primary pulmonary hypertension. An oral agent, **beraprost**, is being evaluated as a treatment for leg pain caused by vascular disease.

Other agents under investigation for intermittent claudication and other vasospastic conditions include the serotonin blockers **ketanserin** and **naftidrofuryl**, and the endothelin inhibitors. Recently the antiplatelet-vasodilator compound **cilostazol**, a phosphosidesterase III inhibitor, was approved for use in intermittent claudication.

Major treatments for male erectile dysfunction secondary to peripheral vascular disease include the use of self-injectible prostaglandins and the phosphodiesterase V inhibitory drug **sildenafil**.

HORMONES, VITAMINS, AND HERBAL REMEDIES

Estrogen replacement with and without progestins has been suggested as a treatment for reducing the rates of morbidity and mortality from CAD in postmenopausal women. Estrogen appears to have favorable effects on plasma lipids and lipoproteins, but its major benefit may stem from a direct vasculoprotective action. However, a recent placebo-controlled study did not show any morbidity and mortality benefit when hormone replacement was given to postmenopausal women with known CAD. In this study, an increased incidence of venoembolic complications with hormone replacement was seen. The Womens Health Initiative Trial is evaluating the utility of hormone replacement as a primary prevention intervention in postmenopausal women aged 50 to 80 years. At this juncture, hormone replacement therapy should not be recommended to prevent CAD in postmenopausal women. Two synthetic estrogen receptor modulators, **tamoxifen** and **raloxifene**, have been shown to have possible activity in reducing CAD morbidity and mortality in postmenopausal women, and are currently being evaluated in clinical trials.

As mentioned previously, growth hormone is being evaluated in patients with advanced heart failure to improve hemodynamic function and musculoskeletal strength.

Vitamin E supplementation does appear to have benefit in reducing the risk of coronary heart disease (CHD). It is recommended that 400 IU/day be used as prophylactic therapy, especially in patients with known CAD. There is also evidence that supplementation of folate, Vitamin B12, and pyridoxine in the diet protects against premature CAD by reducing plasma homocysteine, a substance that may be toxic to the vascular endothelium in high levels. It is now recommended that 400 µg/day (0.4 mg/d) of folate be taken as a prophylactic treatment. Studies with Vitamin C are less conclusive regarding its cardioprotective action.

The results of recent studies have suggested that the use of fish oil supplements containing omega-3 fatty acids can slow the progression of atherosclerosis, as well as reduce the mortality risk in post-MI patients.

Multiple herbal remedies are now being marketed for various cardiovascular conditions. Most of these have no substantive clinical benefit, and some are potentially toxic.

DRUGS FOR CARDIAC ARREST

Pharmacotherapy for patients undergoing cardiac arrest now include the use of intravenous **amiodarone** to help treat refractory life-threatening arrhythmias. A recent study of long-term survival after cardiac arrest was no better with repeated high doses of **epinephrine** than with repeated standard doses. The vasopressor agent, **vasopressin**, is being evaluated as a cardiac stimulator and a potential substitute for epinephrine.

GENE THERAPY

Gene therapy is the newest form of pharmacotherapy and is defined as the introduction of DNA into cells as a means of replacing a congenitally deficient protein or expressing a foreign protein within the cell nucleus and cytoplasm. These proteins can then act within the cell or be secreted into the systemic circulation to exert an effect on remote organ systems.

The technology needed to perform gene therapy has become available because of the ability to isolate individual human genes, to clone and sequence the genes, to synthesize the corresponding complimentary DNA (cDNA) and to insert this cDNA into a plasmid expression vector or recombinant virus. The foreign DNA can then be introduced through the cell membrane using a variety of delivery systems including viruses or chemical delivery systems such as liposomes. Once the DNA enters the cell, it is taken up into the cell nucleus by unknown mechanisms to be transcribed to messenger RNA and translated into therapeutic protein.

Currently, gene therapy is being considered as a means of replacing congenitally absent or defective proteins. Ongoing studies are in progress using hepatic gene therapy as a treatment for homozygous familial hypercholesterolemia, a condition associated with premature CAD.

Gene therapy is also being considered as a means to prevent restenosis after coronary angioplasty and for stimulating angiogenesis in patients with chronic myocardial ischemia.

ACE Inhibitor Myocardial Infarction Collaborative Group: Indications for ACE inhibitors in the early treatment of acute myocardial infarction; systematic overview of individual data from 100,000 patients in randomized trials. *Circulation* 1998; 97: 2202–12.

Alpert JS, Bakx ALM, Braun S, Frishman WH, *et al.*: Antianginal and anti-ischemic effects of mibefradil in the treatment of patients with chronic stable angina pectoris. *Am J Cardiol* 80(4B): 20C–26C, 1997.

Alter M for the SASS Investigators: Ganglioside GM-1 in acute ischemic stroke. The SASS trial. *Stroke* 1994; 25: 1141–48.

Anderson JL, Muhlestein JB, Carlquist J, Allen A, *et al.*: Randomized secondary prevention trial of azithromycin in patients with coronary artery disease and serological evidence for *Chlamydia pneumoniae* infection. The Azithromycin Coronary Artery Disease: Elimination of Myocardial Infarction with Chlamydia (ACADEMIC) Study. *Circulation* 1999; 99: 1540–47.

Barinaga M: Finding new drugs to treat stroke. *Science* 1996; 272: 664–66.

Bialik S, Greenen DL, Bennett MR, Sivapalasingam, *et al.*: Cardiac myocyte apoptosis: a new therapeutic target? In, Frishman WH, Sonnenblick EH (eds): *Cardiovascular Pharmacotherapeutics*. New York: McGraw Hill 1997:955–72.

Biasucci LM, Vitelli A, Liuzzo G, Altamura S, *et al*: Elevated levels of interleukin-6 in unstable angina. *Circulation* 1996; 94: 874–77.

Blum A, Cannon RO III: Effects of oestrogens and selective oestrogen receptor modulators on serum lipoproteins and vascular function. *Curr Opin Lipid* 1998; 9: 575–86.

Bilder G, Wentz T, Leadley R, *et al.*: Restenosis following angioplasty in the swine coronary artery is inhibited by an orally active PDGF-receptor tyrosine kinase inhibitor, RPR101511A. *Circulation* 1999, 99: 3292–99.

Bostom AG, Selhub J: Homocysteine and arteriosclerosis. Subclinical and clinical disease associations. *Circulation* 1999; 99: 2361–63.

Brunner LaRocca HP, Vaddadi G, Esler MD: Recent insight into therapy of congestive heart failure: focus on ACE inhibition of angiotensin II antagonism. *J Am Coll Cardiol* 1999; 33: 1163–73.

Buttrick P: Gene therapy in the cardiovascular system. In, Frishman WH, Sonnenblick EH (eds): *Cardiovascular Pharmacotherapeutics*. New York: McGraw Hill 1997: 945–53.

Cannon CP, Maraganore JM, Loscalzo J, McAllister A, *et al.*: Anticoagulant effects of hirulog, a novel thrombin inhibitor in patients with coronary artery disease. *Am J Cardiol* 1993; 71: 778–782.

Cannon CP, McCabe CH, Gibson MS, Adgey JA, *et al*: TNK-tissue plasminogen activator compared with front-loaded tissue plasminogen activator in acute myocardial infarction: primary results of the TIMI 10B trial. *Circulation* 1997; 96 (Suppl I): I–206 (abstr).

Cannon CP, McCabe CH, Gibson MC, *et al.* and the TIMI 10A Investigators: TNK-tissue plasminogen activator in acute myocardial infarction. Result of the thrombolysis in myocardial infarction (TIMI) 10A Dose-Ranging Trial. *Circulation* 1997; 95: 351–56.

Cardiac Arrhythmia Suppression Trial (CAST) Investigators: Preliminary report: Effect of encainide and flecainide on mortality in a randomized trial of arrhythmia suppression after myocardial infarction. *N Engl J Med* 1989; 321: 406–412.

CIBIS II Investigators and Committees: The Cardiac Insufficiency Bisoprolol Study II (CIBIS-II): a randomized trial. *Lancet* 1999; 353: 9–13.

Clark KWM, Hazel JS, Coull BM: Lazaroids: CNS pharmacology and current research. *Drugs* 1995; 50: 971–83.

Cody RJ: The clinical potential of renin inhibitors and angiotensin antagonists. *Drugs* 1994; 47: 586–598.

Cohen M, Demers C, Gurfinkel E, *et al.* for the Efficacy and Safety of Subcutaneous Enoxaparin vs Non-Q-Wave Coronary Events Study Group: A comparison of low molecular weight heparin with unfractionated heparin for unstable coronary artery disease. *N Engl J Med* 1997; 337: 447–52.

Cohn JN, Goldstein SO, Greenberg BH, *et al*: A dose-dependent increase in mortality with vesnarinone among patients with severe heart failure. *N Engl J Med* 1998; 339: 1810–16.

Collaborative Organization of RheothRx Evaluation (CORE): Effects of RheothRx on mortality, morbidity, left ventricular function and infarct size in patients with acute myocardial infarction. *Circulation* 1997; 96: 192–201.

Collen D: On the regulation and control of fibrinolysis. Thromb Haemost 1980; 43: 77–89.

Collen D, Lijnen H: Staphylokinase, a fibrin specific plasminogen activator with therapeutic potential? *Blood* 1994; 84: 680–86.

Collen D, van de Werf F: Coronary thrombolysis with recombinant staphylokinase in patients with evolving myocardial infarction. *Circulation* 1993; 87: 1850–53.

Dalla Volta S, Maraglino G, Della-Valentina P, Viena P, Desideri A: Comparison of trimetazidine with nifedipine in effort angina: a double-blind crossover study. *Cardiovasc Drug Ther* 1990; 4: 853–59.

Dangas G, Badimon JJ, Smith DA, *et al*: Pravastatin therapy in hyperlipidemia: effects of thrombus formation and the systemic hemostatic profile. *J Am Coll Cardiol* 1999; 33: 1294–1304.

DeClerck PJ, Vanderschueren S, Billiet J, Moreau H, *et al.*: Prevalence and induction of circulating antibodies against recombinant staphylokinase. *Thromb Haemost* 1994; 71: 129–33.

De Deyn PP, Reuck JD, Deberdt W, Vlietinck R, Orgogozo J for the Members of the Piracetam in Acute Stroke Study (PASS) Group: Treatment of acute ischemic stroke with piracetam. *Stroke* 1997; 28: 2347–52.

Demaison L, Fantini E, Sentex E, Grynberg A, *et al.*: Trimetazidine: in vitro influence on heart mitrochondrial function. *Am J Cardiol* 1995; 76: 31B–37B.

den Heijer P, Vermeer F, Ambrosioni E, *et al*: Evaluation of a weight-adjusted, single-bolus plasminogen activator in patients with myocardial infarction. A double-blind, randomized, angiographic trial of lanoteplase versus alteplase. *Circulation* 1998; 98: 2117–25.

Deswal A, Bozkurt B, Seta Y, *et al.*: Safety and efficacy of a soluble P75 tumor necrosis factor receptor (Enbrel, Etanercept) in patients with advanced heart failure. *Circulation* 1999, 99: 3224–26.

Detry J-MR, Leclercq PJ on behalf of the TEMS Steering Committee: Trimetazidine European Multicenter Study versus propranolol in stable angina pectoris: contribution of Holter electrocardiographic ambulatory monitoring. *Am J Cardiol* 1995; 76: 8B–11B.

Diener HC, Hacke W, Hennerici M, Radberg J, *et al.*: Lubeluzole in acute ischemic stroke: a double blind placebo controlled phase II trial. *Stroke* 1996; 27: 76–81.

Domanski M, Exner DV, Borkowf CB, *et al*: Effect of ACE inhibition on sudden cardiac death in patients following acute myocardial infarction. *J Am Coll Cardiol* 1999; 33: 598–604.

Downs JR, Clearfield M, Weis S, Whitney E, *et al*: Primary prevention of acute coronary events with lovastatin in men and women with average cholesterol levels. Results of the AFCAPS/TexCAPS. *JAMA* 1998; 279: 1615-22.

Duff HJ, Brown E, Cragoe EJ, Rahmberg M: Antiarrhythmic activity of amiloride: mechanisms. *J Cardiovasc Pharmacol* 1991; 17: 879-88.

Duty S, Wester AH: Potassium channel openers. Pharmacological effects and future uses. *Drugs* 1990; 40: 785-791.

Edwards PA, Fogelman AM: Cellular enzymes of cholesterol metabolism. *Curr Opin Lipid* 1990; 1: 136-39.

Eitzman DT, Chi L, Saggin L, Schwartz RS, *et al.*: Heparin neutralization by platelet-rich thrombi. *Circulation* 1994 89: 1523-1529.

Enlimomab Acute Stroke Trial Study Group: The enlimomab acute stroke trial final results (abst). *Neurology* 1997; 48: A270.

EPIC Investigators: Use of a monoclonal antibody directed against the platelet glycoprotein IIb/IIIa receptor in high-risk coronary angioplasty. *N Engl J Med* 1994; 330: 956-61.

EPISTENT Investigators: Randomised, placebo-controlled and balloon-angioplasty-controlled trial to assess safety of coronary stenting with use of platelet glycoprotein IIb/IIIa blockade. *Lancet* 1998; 352: 87-92.

Ericsson C-G, Hamsten A, Nilsson J, Grip L, *et al.*: Angiographic assessment of effects of bezafibrate on progression of coronary artery disease in young male postinfarction patients. *Lancet* 1996; 347: 849-53.

Fenton II JW, Villanueva GB, Ofosu FA, Maraganore JM: Thrombin inhibition by hirudin: how hirudin inhibits thrombin. *Haemostasis* 1991; 21 (Suppl 1): 27–31.

Fink AN, Frishman WH, Azizad M, Agarwal Y: Use of prostacyclin and its analogues in the treatment of cardiovascular disease. *Heart Disease* 1999; 1: 29–40.

Flamm ES, Demopoulos HB, Seligman ML, Power RG, *et al.*: Free radicals in cerebral ischemia. *Stroke* 1978; 9:445–447.

Folláth F, Hinkka S, Jäger D, *et al.*: Dose-ranging and safety with intravenous levosimendan in low output heart failure: experience in three pilot studies and outline of the levosimendan infusion versus dobutamine (LIDO) trial. *Am J Cardiol* 1999, 83(12B): 21I–25I.

Forman R, Frishman WH, Strizik B: Thrombolytic agents. In, Frishman WH, Sonnenblick EH (eds): *Cardiovascular Pharmacotherapeutics Companion Handbook*. New York: McGraw Hill, 1998: 324–45.

Francis G: TNF-α and heart failure. The difference between proof of principle and hypothesis testing (editorial). *Circulation* 1999, 99: 3213-14.

Frank D, Haytoglu T, Frishman WH: Cardiovascular effects of raloxifene, a selective estrogen receptor modulator. *J Clin Pharmacol* 1999 in press.

Frick MH, Syvänne M, Nieminen MS, Kauma H, *et al.*: Prevention of the angiographic progression of coronary and vein-graft atherosclerosis by gemfibrozil after coronary bypass surgery in men with low levels of HDL-cholesterol. *Circulation* 1997; 96: 2137–43.

Friedel HA, Brogden RN: Pinacidil. *Drugs* 1990; 39: 929–967.

Frishman WH: Imidazoline receptor agonist drugs (abst). *Am J Hypertens* 1999; 12(4 Pt 2):213A.

Frishman WH, Cheng A: Secondary prevention of myocardial infarction: the role of beta-adrenergic blockers and angiotensin converting enzyme inhibitors. *Am Heart J* 1999; 137: S25–34.

Frishman WH, Chiu R, Landzberg BR, Weiss M: Medical therapies for the prevention of restenosis after percutaneous coronary interventions. *Curr Probl Cardiol* 1998; 23(10): 533–640.

Frishman WH, Fan SC, Boczko J, Hussain J: Fish oils, vitamins and folic acid as cardiovascular protective agents. In, Frishman WH, Sonnenblick EH (eds): *Cardiovascular Pharmacotherapeutics*. New York: McGraw Hill 1997: 511–34.

Frishman WH, Fozailoff A, Lin C, Dike C: Renin inhibition: a new approach to cardiovascular therapy. *J Clin Pharmacol* 1994; 34: 873–80.

Frishman WH, Gabor R, Pepine C, Cavusoglu E: Heart rate reduction in the treatment of chronic stable angina pectoris. Experience with the sinus node inhibitor. *Am Heart J* 1996; 131: 204–10.

Frishman WH, Goldman A: Inhibitors of neutral endopeptidase. In, Frishman WH, Sonnenblick EH (eds): *Cardiovascular Pharmacotherapeutics*. New York: McGraw Hill, 1997: 611–17.

Frishman WH, Klein MD, Blaufarb I, Borge R, *et al.*: Antiplatelet and other antithrombotic drugs. In, Frishman WH, Sonnenblick EH (eds): *Cardiovascular Pharmacotherapeutics*. New York: McGraw Hill 1997: 323–79.

Frishman WH, Lin C: Specific inhibitors of renin in cardiac therapy. In Frishman WH, Sonnenblick EH (eds): *Cardiovascular Pharmacotherapeutics*. New York: McGraw Hill, 1997: 757–68.

Frishman W, Pepine CJ, Weiss R, Baiker WM for the Zatebradine Study Group: Addition of zatebradine, a direct sinus node inhibitor, provides no greater exercise tolerance benefit in patients with angina pectoris taking extended-release nifedipine: results of a multicenter, randomized, double-blind, placebo-controlled, parallel group study. *J Am Coll Cardiol* 1995; 26: 305–12

Frishman WH, Tamirisa P, Kumar A: Endothelin and endothelin antagonism. In, Frishman WH, Sonnenblick EH (eds): *Cardiovascular Pharmacotherapeutics*. New York: McGraw Hill, 1997: 689–701.

Frishman WH, Vahdat S, Bhatta S: Innovative pharmacologic approaches to cardiopulmonary resuscitation. *J Clin Pharmacol* 38: 765–772, 1998.

Frishman WH, Wang S, Gurell D, Yashar P: Potassium channel openers and sodium-hydrogen channel effectors. In, Frishman WH, Sonnenblick EH (eds): *Cardiovascular Pharmacotherapeutics*. New York: McGraw Hill, 1997: 619–37.

Frishman WH, Weisner M, Somer BG, Deutsch A, *et al.*: Natriuretic peptides and other vasoactive peptides: implications for furture drug therapy. In, Frishman WH, Sonnenblick EH (eds): *Cardiovascular Pharmacotherapeutics*. New York: McGraw Hill; 1997: 573–609.

Frishman WH, Yu A: Imidazole receptor agonist drugs for the treatment of systemic hypertension. In, Frishman WH, Sonnenblick EH (eds): *Cardiovascular Pharmacotherapeutics*. New York: McGraw Hill, 1997; 677–87.

Frishman WH, Zimetbaum P, Derman M: HMG-CoA reductase inhibitors. In, Frishman WH (ed): *Medical Management of Lipid Disorders: Focus on Prevention of Coronary Artery Disease*. Mt. Kisco, Futura Publ., 1992: 153–80.

Gokce N, Keaney Jr JF, Frei B, *et al.*: Long-term ascorbic acid administration reverses endothelial vasomotor dysfunction in patients with coronary artery disease. *Circulation* 1999, 99: 3234–40.

Goldberg D, Frishman WH: *Beta$_3$-Adrenergic Agonists: A New Approach to Human Pharmacotherapy*. Mt. Kisco, Futura Publishing: 1995.

Goldschmidt M, Frishman WH: Ranolazine: a new anti-ischemic drug which affects myocardial energetics. *Am J Therap* 1995; 2: 269–74.

Goldschmidt M, Landzberg BR, Frishman WH: Nicorandil: A potassium-channel opening drug for the treatment of ischemic heart disease. *J Clin Pharmacol* 1996; 36: 559–72.

Gomberg-Maitland M, Frishman WH: Recombinant growth hormone: a new cardiovascular drug therapy. *Am Heart J* 1996; 132: 1244–62.

Grayston JT: Controlled trial of azithromycin in patients with coronary artery disease. *Circulation* 1999; 99: 1538–39.

Grossman M, Raper SE, Kozarsky K, Stein EA, *et al.*: Successful ex vivo gene therapy directed to liver in a patient with familial hypercholesterolemia. *Nature Genet* 1994; 6: 335–41.

Gueugniaud P-Y, Mols P, Goldstein P, *et al.*: A comparison of repeated high doses and repeated standard doses of epinephrine for cardiac arrest outside the hospital. *N Engl J Med* 1998; 339: 1595–1601.

Guyton JR, Goldberg AC, Kreisberg RA, Sprecher DL, *et al.*: Effectiveness of once-nightly dosing of extended release niacin alone or in combination for hypercholesterolemia. *Am J Cardiol* 1998; 82: 737–43.

Haber E, Quertermous T, Matsueda GR, Runge MS: Innovative approaches to plasminogen activator therapy. *Science* 1989; 243: 51–56. 145.

Hamroff G, Katz SD, Mancini D, Blaufarb I, *et al.*: Addition of angiotensin II receptor blockade to maximal angiotensin converting enzyme inhibition improves exercise capacity in patients with severe congestive heart failure. *Circulation* 1999; 99: 990–92.

Hansson L, Lindholm LH, Niskanen L, *et al.*: Effect of ACE inhibition compared with conventional therapy on cardiovascular morbidity and mortality in hyeprtension. The Captopril Prevention Project (CAPPP) randomised trial. *Lancet* 1999; 353: 611–16.

Harper IS, Bond JM, Chacon E, Reece JM, *et al.*: Inhibition of N+/H+ exchange preserves viability, restores mechanical function and prevents the pH paradox in reperfusion injury to rat neonatal myocytes. *Basic Res Cardiol* 1993; 88: 430–42.

Hasenfuss G, Pieske B, Castell M, *et al.*: Influence of the novel inotropic agent levosimendan on isometric tension and calcium cycling in failing human myocardium. *Circulation* 1998; 98: 2141–47.

Helisch A, Ware JA: Therapeutic angiogenesis in ischemic heart disease. *J Thromb Hemost* 1999 in press.

Henry TD, Annex BH, Azrin MA, McKendall GR, *et al.*: Double blind, placebo-controlled trial of recombinant human vascular endothelial growth factor - the VIVA trial (abstr). *J Am Coll Cardiol* 1999; 33 (Suppl A): 384A.

Herrera-Garza EH, Stetson SJ, Cubillos-Garzon A, *et al.*: Tumor necrosis factor-α. A mediator of disease progression in the failing human heart. *Chest* 1999; 115: 1170–74.

Hickenbottom SL, Grotta J: Neuroprotective therapy. *Sem Neurol* 1998; 18: 485–92.

Holvoet P, Dewerchin M, Stassen JM, Lijnen HR, *et al.*: Thrombolytic profiles of clot-targeted plasminogen activators: parameters determining potency and initial and maximal rates. *Circulation* 1993; 87: 1007–16.

Hulley S, Grady D, Bush T, Furberg C, *et al.*: Randomized trial of estrogen plus progestin for secondary prevention of coronary heart disease in postmenopausal women. *JAMA* 1998; 280: 605–13.

Ikeda I, Sugano M: Inhibition of cholesterol absorption by plant sterols for mass intervention. *Curr Opin Lipid* 1998; 9: 527–31.

IMPACT II Investigators: Randomised placebo-controlled trial of effect of eptifibatide on complications of percutaneous coronary intervention: IMPACT II. *Lancet* 1997; 349: 1422–28.

Ismail A, Khosvavi H, Olson H: The role of infection in atherosclerosis and coronary artery disease. A new therapeutic target. *Heart Disease* 1999; 1(4):233–240.

Jeppeson J, Hein HO, Suadicani P, Gyntelberg F: Triglyceride concentration and ischemic heart disease. An eight-year follow up in the Copenhagen Male Study. *Circulation* 1998; 97: 1029–36.

Kang PM, Landau AJ, Eberhardt RT, Frishman WH: Angiotensin II receptor antagonists: a new approach to blockade of the renin-angiotensin system. *Am Heart J* 1994; 127: 1388–1401.

Katz SD, Rao R, Berman JW, Schwarz M, *et al.*: Pathophysiological correlates of increased serum tumor necrosis factor in patients with congestive heart failure: relation to nitric oxide dependent vasodilation in the forearm circulation. *Circulation* 1994; 90: 12–16.

Kesäniemi YA: Relevance of the reduction of triglycerides in the prevention of coronary heart disease. *Curr Opin Lipid* 1998; 9: 571–74.

Kobashigawa JA, Katznelson S, Laks H, Johnson JA, *et al.*: Effect of pravastatin on outcomes after cardiac transplantation. *N Engl J Med* 1995; 333: 621–27.

Knopp RH, Alagona P, Davidson M, Goldberg AC, *et al.*: Equivalent efficacy of a time-release form of niacin (Niaspan) given once-a-night versus plain niacin in the management of hyperlipidemia. *Metabolism* 1998; 47: 1097–1104.

Krum H, Viskoper RJ, Lacourciere Y, Budde M, *et al.*: The effect of an endothelin-receptor antagonist, bosentan, on blood pressure in patients with essential hypertension. *N Engl J Med* 1998; 338: 784–90.

Laham RJ, Leimbach M, Chronos NA, Vansant JP, *et al.*: Intracoronary administration of recombinant fibroblast growth factor-2 (rFGF-2) in patients with severe coronary artery disease: results of Phase I (abstr). *J Am Coll Cardiol* 1999; 33 (Suppl A): 383A.

Laham RJ, Sellke FW, Ware JA, Pearlman JD, *et al.*: Results of a randomized, double-blind, placebo-controlled study of local perivascular basic fibroblast growth factor (bFGF) treatment in patients undergoing coronary artery bypass surgery (abstr). *J Am Coll Cardiol* 33 (Suppl A): 383A.

Leri A, Claudio PP, Li Q, Wang X, *et al.*: Stretched-mediated release of angiotensin II induced myocyte apoptosis by activating p53 that enhances the local renin-angiotensin-system and decreases the Bcl-2-to-Bax protein ratio in the cell. *J Clin Invest* 1998; 101: 1326–42.

Lijnen HR, Nelles L, Holmes WE, Collen D: Biochemical and thrombolytic properties of a lower molecular weight form (comprising Leu144 through Leu411) of recombinant single-chain urokinase type plasminogen activator. *J Biol Chem* 1988; 163: 5594–98.

Loskove JA, Frishman WH: Nitric oxide donors in the treatment of cardiovascular and pulmonary diseases. *Am Heart J* 1995; 129: 604–13.

Mahoffey KW, Puma JA, Barbagelata A, Casas CA, *et al.*: Does adenosine in conjunction with thrombolysis reduce infarct size? Results from the Controlled Randomized AMISAD trial (abstr). *Circulation* 1997; 96: I–206.

Mancini GB, Henry GC, Mcacya C, O'Neill BJ, *et al.*: Angiotensin converting enzyme inhibition with quinapril improves endothelial vasomotor dysfunction in patients with coronary artery disease. The TREND (Trial on Reversing Endothelial Dysfunction) Study. *Circulation* 1996; 94: 258–65.

Mangano DT: Effects of acadesine on myocardial infarction, stroke and death following surgery: a meta-analysis of the 5 international randomized trials. The Multicenter Study of Perioperative Ischemia (McSPI) Research Group. *JAMA* 1997; 277: 325–32.

Mann DL, Young JB: Basic mechanisms in congestive heart failure: recognizing the role of proinflammatory cytokines. *Chest* 1994; 105: 897–904.

Maridonneau-Parini I, Harpey C: Effect of trimetazidine of membrane damage induced by oxygen free radicals in human red cells. *Br J Clin Pharmacol* 1985; 20: 148–51.

Markwardt F: Past, present and future of hirudin. *Haemostasis* 1991; 21 (Suppl 1): 11–26.

Mashour NH, Lin GI, Frishman WH: Herbal medicine in the treatment of cardiovascular disease: clinical considerations. *Arch Intern Med* 158: 2225–2234, 1998.

McKenney JM, Proctor JD, Harris S, Chinchili VM: A comparison of the efficacy and toxic effects of sustained-versus immediate-release niacin in hypercholesterolemic patients. *JAMA* 1994; 271: 672–77.

McNeely W, Goat KL: Nebivolol in the management of essential hypertension. A review. *Drugs* 1999; 57: 633–51.

Melman A, Christ GJ: The hemodynamics of erection and the pharmacotherapy of erectile dysfunction. In, Frishman WH, Sonnenblick EH (eds): *Cardiovascular Pharmacotherapeutics*. New York: McGraw Hill 1997: 1221–29.

MERIT-HF Study Group: Effect of metoprolol CR/XL in chronic heart failure (MERIT-HF). *Lancet* 1999; 353: 2001–2007.

Mokrzycki M, Tamirisa P, Frishman WH: Diuretic therapy in cardiovascular disease. In, Frishman WH, Sonnenblick EH (eds); *Cardiovascular Pharmacotherapeutics Companion Handbook*. New York: McGraw Hill, 1998: 152–74.

Moulton KS, Heller E, Konerding MA, Flynn E, *et al.*: Angiogenesis inhibitors endostatin and TNP-470 reduce intimal neovascularization and plaque growth in apolipoprotein E-deficient mice. *Circulation* 1999; 99: 1726–32.

Moussa I, Oetgen M, Roubin G, *et al.*: Effectiveness of clopidogrel and aspirin versus ticlopidine and aspirin in preventing stent thrombosis after coronary stent implantation. *Circulation* 1999; 99: 2364–66.

Muir KW, Lees KR. Clinical experience with excitatory amino acid antagonist drugs. *Stroke* 1995; 26:503–513.

Muller DWM: Gene therapy for the management of cardiovascular disease. *J Noninvas Cardiol* 1994; 6: 89–96.

Opie LH, Sonnenblick EH, Frishman WH, Thadani U: Beta-blocking agents. In, Opie LH (ed): *Drugs for the Heart* 4th ed. Philadelphia: W.B. Saunders Co., 1995: 1–30.

Organisation to Assess Strategies for Ischemic Syndromes (OASIS-2) Investigators: Effects of recombinant hirudin (lepirudin) compared with heparin on death, myocardial infarction, refractory angina, and revascularization procedures in patients with acute myocardial ischaemia without ST elevation: a randomised trial. *Lancet* 1999; 353: 429–38.

Pepine CJ, Wolff AA on behalf of the Ranolazine Study Group: A controlled trial with a novel anti-ischemic agent, ranolazine, in chronic stable angina pectoris that is responsive to conventional antianginal agents. *Am J Cardiol* 1999, 84: 46–50.

Pitt B, Segal R, Martinez FA, *et al.* on behalf of ELITE Study Investigators: Randomised trial of losartan versus captopril in patients over 65 with heart failure (Evaluation of Losartan in the Elderly Study: ELITE) *Lancet* 1997; 349.

Pitt B, Waters D, Brown WV, *et al.* for the Atorvastatin versus Revascularization Treatment Investigators: Aggressive lipid-blocking therapy compared with angioplasty in stable coronary artery disease. *N Engl J Med* 1999, 341: 70–76.

PRISM-PLUS Study Investigators: Inhibition of platelet glycoprotein IIb/IIIa receptor with tirofiban in unstable angina and non-Q-wave myocardial infarction. *N Engl J Med* 1998; 338: 1488–97.

PRISM Study Investigators: A comparison of aspirin plus tirofiban with aspirin plus heparin for unstable angina. *N Engl J Med* 1998; 338: 1498–1505.

Progress in Clinical Trials. *Clin Cardiol* 1999; 22: 369–72.

PURSUIT Trial Investigators: Inhibition of platelet glycoprotein IIb/IIIa with eptifibatide in patients with acute coronary syndromes. *N Engl J Med* 1998; 339: 436–43.

Ramasamy R, Liu H, Schaefer S: Aldose reductase inhibition limits the rise in intracellular sodium and calcium and protets diabetic hearts from ischemic injury. Presented at the 56th Annual Meeting of the American Diabetes Assn, San Francisco, Ca., June 8–11, 1996.

Ramasamy R, Schaefer S, Oates P: Improved ischemic tolerance in diabetic hearts treated with an aldose reductase inhibitor. Presented at 55th Annual Meeting of American Diabetes Assn. Atlanta, Ga., June 10–13, 1995.

Ranolazine Study Group: Double-blind efficacy and safety of a novel anti-ischemic agent, ranolazine, versus placebo in patients with chronic stable angina pectoris. *Circulation* 1994; 90: 726–34.

Renaud JF: Internal pH, Na+ and Ca2+ regulation by trimetazidine during cardiac cell acidosis. *Cardiovasc Drug Ther* 1988; 1: 677–86.

RESTORE Investigators: Effects of platelet glycoprotein IIb/IIIa blockade with tirofiban on adverse cardiac events in patients with unstable angina or acute myocardial infarction undergoing coronary angioplasty. *Circulation* 1997; 96: 1445–53.

Rongen GA, Lenders JWM, Kleinbloessem CH, *et al*: Efficacy and tolerability of the renin inhibitor Ro 42–5892 in patients with hypertension. *Clin Pharmacol Ther* 1993; 54: 567–577.

Rothman S. Synaptic release of excitatory amino acid neurotransmitter mediates anoxic neuronal death. *J Neurosci* 1984;4:1884–1891.

Rubins HB, Robins SJ, Collins D: The Veterans Affairs High-Density Lipoprotein Intervention Trial: baseline characteristics of normocholesterolemic men with coronary artery disease and low levels of high-density lipoprotein cholesterol. Veterans Affairs Cooperative Studies Program High-Density Lipoprotein Intervention Trial Study Group. *Am J Cardiol* 1996; 78: 572–75.

Ruddy MC, Kostis JB, Frishman WH: Drugs that affect the renin-angiotensin system. In, Frishman WH, Sonnenblick EH (eds): *Cardiovascular Pharmacotherapeutics*. New York: McGraw Hill 1997; 131–92.

Ruddy MC, Kostis JB, Frishman WH: Drugs that affect the renin angiotensin system. In, Frishman WH, Sonnenblick EH (eds): *Cardiovascular Pharmacotherapeutics Companion Handbook*. New York: McGraw Hill, 1998: 107–151.

Runge MS, Bode C, Matsueda GR, Haber E: Antibody-enhanced thrombolysis: targeting of tissue plasminogen activator in vivo. *Proc Natl Acad Sci USA* 1987; 84: 7659–62.

Ruotolo G, Ericsson C-G, Tettamanti C, *et al*: Treatment effects on serum lipoprotein lipids, apolipoproteins and low density lipoprotein particle size and relationships of lipoprotein variables to progression of coronary artery disease in the Bezafibrate Coronary Atherosclerosis Intervention Trial (BECAIT). *J Am Coll Cardiol* 1998; 32: 1648–56.

Schlaifer JD, Wargovich TJ, O'Neill B, Mancini GB, *et al.*: Effects of quinapril on coronary blood flow in coronary artery disease patients with endothelial dysfunction. TREND Investigators. *Am J Cardiol* 1997; 80: 1594–97.

Sellier P, Audouin P, Payen B, Corona P, *et al.*: Acute effects of trimetazidine evaluated by exercise testing. *Eur J Clin Pharmacol* 1987; 33: 205–07.

Sellier P: Chronic effects of trimetazidine on ergometric parameters of effort angina. *Cardiovasc Drug Ther* 1990; 4: 822–23.

Shepherd J, Cobbe SM, Ford I, Isles CG, *et al.*: Prevention of coronary heart disease with pravastatin. *N Engl J Med* 1995; 333: 1301–07.

Siesjo BK. Pathophysiology and treatment of focal cerebral ischemia. Part I: Pathophysiology. *J Neurosurg* 1992; 77:169–184.

Siesjo BK. Pathophysiology and treatment of focal cerebral ischemia. Part II: Mechanisms of damage and treatment. *J Neurosurg* 1992; 77:337–354.

Sonnenblick EH, LeJemtel TH, Frishman WH: Digitalis preparations and other inotropic agents. In, Frishman WH, Sonnenblick EH (eds): *Cardiovascular Pharmacotherapeutics Companion Handbook*. New York: McGraw Hill; 1998: 188–202.

Stephens NG, Parsons A, Schofield PM, Kelly F, *et al*: Randomised controlled trial of vitamin E in patients with coronary disease. Cambridge Heart Antioxidant Study (CHAOS). *Lancet* 1996; 347: 781–86.

Szczeklik A, Musial J, Undas A, *et al*: Inhibition of thrombin generation by simvastatin and lack of additive effects of aspirin in patients with marked hypercholesterolemia. *J Am Coll Cardiol* 1999; 33: 1286–93.

Takahashi T, Takeyoshi I, Haegawa Y, *et al*: Lazaroid U-74389G ameliorates ischemia-reperfusion injury in canine hearts: a histologic study. *Transplant Proc* 1998; 30: 3334–36.

Taylor DG, Kaplan HD: New antihypertensive drugs. In, Kaplan NM, Brenner BM, Laragh JH (eds): *New Therapeutic Strategies in Hypertension*. New York: Raven Press, 1989: 125–139.

The Post Coronary Artery Bypass Graft Trial Investigators: The effect of aggressive lowering of low density lipoprotein cholesterol levels and low-dose anticoagulation on obstructive changes in saphenous vein coronary artery bypass grafts. *N Engl J Med* 1997; 336: 153–62.

The STIPAS Investigators: Safety study of tirilazad mesylate in patients with acute ischemic stroke (STIPAS). *Stroke* 1994; 25: 418–23.

The Women's Health Initiative Study Group: Design of the Women's Health Initiative Clinical Trial and observational study. *Controlled Clin Trials* 19: 61–109, 1998.

Torgano G, Cosentini R, Mandelli C, Perondi R, *et al*: Treatment of *Helicobacter pylorii* and *Chlamydia pneumoniae* infections decreases fibrinogen plasma level in patients with ischemic heart disease. *Circulation* 1999; 99: 1555–59.

Vale PR, Losordo DW, Dunnington CH, Lahti K, *et al.*: Direct intramyocardial injection of VEGF results in effective gene transfer for patients with chronic myocardial ischemia (abstr). *J Am Coll Cardiol* 1999; 33 (Suppl A): 384A.

Vanderschuren S, Stockx L, Wilms G, Lacroix H, *et al.*: Thrombolytic therapy of peripheral arterial occlusion with recombinant staphylokinase. *Circulation* 1995; 92: 2050–57.

Vanderschuren SMF, Stassen JM, Collen D: On the immunogenicity of recombinant staphylokinase in patients and in animal models. *Thromb Haemost* 1994; 72: 297–301.

Van de Werf F, Cannon CP, Luyten A, *et al.* for the ASSENT-1 Investigators: Safety assessment of single-bolus administration of TNK tissue-plasminogen activator in acute myocardial infarction: The ASSENT-1 trial. *Am Heart J* 1999, 137: 86–91.

Veitch K, Maisin L, Hue L: Trimetazidine effects on the damage to mitochondrial functions caused by ischemia and reperfusion. *Am J Cardiol* 1995; 76: 25B–30B.

von Schacky C, Angerer P, Kothny W, Theisen K, *et al.*: The effect of dietary omega-3 fatty acids on coronary atherosclerosis: a randomized, double-blind, placebo-controlled trial. *Ann Intern Med* 1999; 130: 554–62.

Ware JA, Simons M: *Angiogenesis and Cardiovascular Disease*. New York: Oxford University Press, 1999.

Weber KT: Aldosterone and spironolactone in heart failure. *N Engl J Med* 1999, 341: 753–54.

Weitz JI, Young E, Johnston M, *et al*: Vasoflux, a new anticoagulant with a novel mechanism of action. *Circulation* 1999; 99: 682–89.

Weitz JI, Hudoba M, Massel D, Maraganore J, *et al*: Clot-bound thrombin is protected from inhibition by heparin-antithrombin III but is susceptible to inactivation by antithrombin III-independent inhibitors. *J Clin Invest* 1990; 86: 385–391.

The information here is provided as guidance only. Prescribers should always consult the manufacturer's current prescribing information.

291

ACRONYMS OF CARDIOVASCULAR DRUG TRIALS

AASK—African American Study of Kidney Disease and Hypertension

AAASPS—African American Antiplatelet Stroke Prevention Study

ABCD—Appropriate Blood Pressure Control in Diabetes Trial

ACAD—Azithromycin in Coronary Artery Disease

ACADEMIC—Azitromycin in Coronary Artery Disease: Elimination of Myocardial Infarction with Chlamydia

ACAPS—Asymptomatic Carotid Artery Plaque Study

ACAPS—Asymptomatic Carotid Artery Progression Study

ACAS—Asymptomatic Carotid Atherosclerosis Study

ACBS—Asymptomatic Cervical Bruit Study

ACCEPT—Accupril Canadian Clinical Evaluation and Patient Teaching

ACCESS—Acute Candesartan Cilexetil Evaluation in Stroke Survival

ACCESS—Atorvastatin Comparative Cholestereol Efficacy and Safety Study

ACCORD — Angioplastie Coronaire, Corvasal Diltiazem

ACCT—Amlodipine Cardiovascular Community Trial

ACE—Aspirin and Carotid Endarterectomy Trial

ACES—Azithromycin and Coronary Events Study

ACET—Azmacort Cost Effetiveness Trial

ACHIEVE—Accupril Congestive Heart Failure Investigation and Economic Variable Evaluation

ACIP—Asymptomatic Cardiac Ischemia Pilot Study

ACIT—Asymptomatic Cardiac Ischemia Trial

ACME—Angioplasty Compared to Medicine

ACP —Asymptomatic Cardiac Ischemia Pilot Study

ACT—Arteriopathic Chronique Ticlopidine

ACT—Attacking Claudication with Ticlopidine

ACTION—A Coronary Disease Trial Investigating Outcome with Nifedipine GITS

ACTS—American Canadian Thrombosis Study

ADEG—Antiarrhythmic Drug Evaluation Group Trial

ADEP—Atherosclerotic Disease Evolution by Picotamide Study

ADMIRAL—Abciximab with Percutaneous Coronary Angioplasty and Stent in Acute Myocardial Infarction

ADMIRE—AMP579 Delivery for Myocardial Infarction Reduction

ADMIT—Arterial Disease Multiple Intervention Trial

ADOPT—Accupril Decision on Pharmacotherapy

ADVENT—Antithrombin for Deep Venous Thrombosis

AFASAK—Atrial Fibrillation, Aspirin, Antikoagulation

AFCAPS/TexCAPS—Air Force Coronary/Texas Atherosclerosis Prevention Study

AFFIRM—Atrial Fibrillation Follow-up Investigation of Rhythm Management

AFI—Atrial Fibrillation Investigators 1993 Pooled Study

AFIB—Atrial Fibrillation Investigation with Bidisomide

AFIRME—Antagonist of the Fibrinogen Receptor after Myocardial Events

AFTER—Anistreplase Following Thrombolysis Effect on Reocclusion

AFTER—Aspirin/Anticoagulant Following Thrombolysis with Eminase in Recurrent Infarction

AIMS—Anisoylated Plasminogen Streptokinase Complex Intervention Mortality Study

AIPRI—Angiotensin Converting Enzyme Inhibition in Progressive Renal Insufficiency

AIRE — Acute Infarction Ramipril Efficacy Study

AIRE—Acute Infarction Reperfusion Efficacy Study

AIREX—Acute Infarction Ramipril Efficacy Extension Study

AITIA—Aspirin in Transient Ischemic Attacks

AITIAIS—Aspirin in Transient Ischemic Attacks Italian Study

ALDUSA—Aspirin Low Dosage in Unstable Angina

ALERT—Amiodarone vs Lidocaine inpatient Emergency Resuscitation Trial

ALIVE—Adenosine Lidocaine Infarct Zone Viability Enhancement Trial

ALIVE—Amiodarone vs Lidocaine in Prehospital Refractory Ventricular Fibrillation

ALIVE—Azimilide Post Infarct Survival Evaluation

ALL—Antihypertensive and Lipid Lowering studies

ALLHAT—Antihypertensive and Lipid Lowering Treatment to Prevent Heart Attack Trial

AMI—Argatroban in Myocardial Infarction Study

AMIABLE—Acute Myocardial Infarction Angioplasty Bolus Lysis Evaluation

AMICUS—Austrian Multicenter Isradipine Cum Spirapril Study

AMIS—Aspirin in Myocardial Infarction Study

AMISTAD—Acute Myocardial Infarction Study of Adenosine

AMP—Adenosine Monophosphate Study

AMPI—APSAC in Acute Myocardial Infarction Placebo Controlled Investigation

AMT—Adenosine-scan Multicenter Trial

ANBP—Australian National Blood Pressure Trial

ANS—American Nimodipine Study

ANZ—Australia and New Zealand Heart Failure Collaborative Study

APASS—Antiphospholipid Antibodies in Stroke Study

APIC—Acenocoumarin vs Pentoxifylline in Intermittent Claudication

APIS—Antihypertensive Patch Italian Study

APLAUSE—Antiplatelet Treatment After Intravascular Ultrasound Guided Optimal Stent Expansion Trial

APPI—Actilyse Persantine in Postischemic Injury

APRAISE—Antisense to Prevent Restenosis after Intervention, Stent Evaluation

APRICOT—Antithrombotics in the Prevention of Reocclusion in Coronary Thrombosis

APRICOT—Aspirin vs Coumadin Trial

APRICOT—Aspirin vs Coumadin in the Prevention of Reocclusion and Recurrent Ischemia after Successful Thrombolysis Trial

APSI—Acebutolol Prevention Secondaire de l'Infarctus

APSIM—APSAC dans l'Infarctus du Myocarde

APSIS—Angina Prognosis Study in Stockholm

APSIS—Angina Prognosis Study with Isoptin and Seloken Trial

APT—Antiplatelet Trials

APTH—Ambulatory Blood Pressure Monitoring and Treatment of Hypertension

ARCH—Amiodarone Reduction Coronary Heart Study

AREVA—Anticoagulation et Remplacement Valvulaire

ARGAMI—Argatroban Compared with Heparin in Myocardial Infarction Treated with rtPA

ARGAMI-2 Direct Antithrombin—Argatroban in Acute Myocardial Infarction

ARIC—Atherosclerosis Risk in Communities

ARIS—Anturan Reinfarction Italian Study

ARMS—APSAC Reocclusion Multicenter Study

ARREST—Amiodarone in Out of Hospital Resuscitation of Refractory Sustained Ventricular Tachyarrhythmias

ART—Anturane Reinfarction Trial

ASAAC—Acetyl Salicylic Acid Aortocoronary Bypass Surgery

ASAAC—Acetyl Salicylic Acid vs Anticoagulants Study

ASAP—Acetyl Salicylic Acid Persantine Study

ASAP—Azimilide Supraventricular Arrhythmia Program

ASCB—Asymptomatic Cervical Bruit Study

ASCOT—Anglo Scandinavian Cardiac Outcomes Trial

ASIS—Angina and Silent Ischemia Study

ASIST—Atenolol Silent Ischemia Trial

ASK—Australian Streptokinase Trial in Stroke

ASPECT—Anticoagulants in Secondary Prevention of Events in Coronary Thrombosis

ASPIRE—Action on Secondary Prevention through Intervention to Reduce Events

ASPS—Australian Swedish Pindolol Study

ASS—Acute Stroke Study

ASS—Auckland Stroke Study

ASSENT—Assessment of the Safety and Efficacy of a New Thrombolytic Agent

ASSENT 2—Assessment of the Safety and Efficacy of a New Thrombolytic Agent: TNK-tPA

ASSET—Anglo–Scandinavian Study of Early Thrombolysis

ASSET—Atorvastatin Simvastatin Safety and Efficacy Trial

ASSIST—American Stop Smoking Intervention Study

AST—Australian Streptokinase Trial

ATACS—Antithrombotic Therapy in Acute Coronary Syndromes

ATBC—Alpha Tocopherol/Beta Carotene Study

ATEST—Atenolol and Streptokinase Trial

ATIAIS—Anturane Transient Ischemic Attack Italian Study

ATIME—Accupril Titration Intervention Management Interval Management Evaluation Trial

ATLANTIS—Alteplase Thrombolysis for Acute Noninterventional Therapy in Ischemic Stroke

ATLAS—Acolysis during Treatment of Lesions Affecting Saphenous Vein Bypass Grafts

ATLAS—Aspirin and Ticlid vs Anticoagulation for Stents Study

ATLAS—Assessment of Treatment with Lisinopril and Survival

ATLAST—Antiplatelet Therapy vs Lovenox plus Antiplatelet Therapy for Patients with Increased Risk of Stent Thrombosis

ATLAST—Aspirin/Ticlopidine vs Low Molecular Weight Heparin/Aspirin/Ticlopidine Stent Trial

ATP—Adult Treatment Panel of the National Cholesterol Education Program

ATTMH—Australian Therapeutic Trial of Mild Hypertension

AUST—Australian Urokinase Stroke Trial

AUS-TASK—Australian Arm of the International TPA/SK Mortality Trial

AVERT—Atorvastatin vs Revascularization Treatments

AVID—Antiarrhythmics vs Implantable Defibrillators Trial

AVID—Angiography vs Intravascular Ultrasound Directed Coronary Stent Placement Trial

BAATAF—Boston Area Anticoagulation Trial for Atrial Fibrillation

BASIS—Basel Antiarrhythmic Study of Infarct Survival

BBPP—Beta Blocker Pooling Project

BCAPS—Beta Blocker Cholesterol-Lowering Asymptomatic Plaque Study

BCIS—British Cardiovascular Intervention Study

BCSP—Bavarian Cholesterol Screening Project

BECAIT—Bezafibrate Coronary Atherosclerosis Intervention Trial

BENEDICT—Bergamo Nephrology Diabetes Complication Trial

BEPS—Belgian Eminase Prehospital Study

BERCI-I—Beraprost et Claudication Intermittenti

BEST—Beta Blocker Evaluation of Survival Trial

BEST—Beta Blocker Stroke Trial

BEST—Bolus Dose-Escalation Study of Tissue-Type Plasminogen Activator

BEST—Bucindolol Evaluation of Survival Trial

BHAT—Beta Blocker Heart Attack Trial

BHFS—Benazepril Heart Failure Study

BIG-MAC—Beaumont Interventional Group–Mevacor, Angiotensin Converting Enzyme Inhibitor, Colchicine Restenosis Trial

BIP—Bezafibrate Infarction Prevention Study

BLASP—Barbados Low-Dose Aspirin Study in Pregnancy

BMRC—British Medical Research Council Trial of the Effect of Aspirin in Postoperative Deep Venous Thrombosis

BMS—Belfast Metoprolol Study

BNS—Belfast Nifedipine Study

BOILER—Balloon Occlusive Intravascular Lysis Enhanced Recanalization Strategy

BRAVO—Blockade of the GP IIb/IIIa Receptor to Avoid Vascular Occlusion

BRCT—Brain Resuscitation Clinical Trial

BRILLIANT—Blood Pressure, Renal Effects, Insulin Control, Lipids, Lisinopril and Nifedipine Trial

BTRS—Belgian Ticlopidine Retinopathy Study

BUFUL—Bumetanide and Furosemide on Lipid Profile

CAASET—Canadian Amlodipine and Atenolol Stress Echo Trial

CABADAS—Prevention of Coronary Artery Bypass Graft Occlusion by Aspirin, Dipyridamole and Acenocoumarol/Phenoprocoumon Study

CABRI—Coronary Artery Bypass Revascularization Investigation

CACHET—Comparison of Abciximab Complications with Hirulog (and Abciximab Backup) for Ischemic Events Trial

CACTIS—Comparison of Aspirin with Clopidogrel or Ticlopidine in Stents

CADILLAC—Controlled Abciximab and Device Investigation to Lower Late Angioplasty Complications

CADS—Captopril and Digoxin Study

CAFA—Canadian Atrial Fibrillation Anticoagulation Study

CAFS—Canadian Atrial Fibrillation Study

CALYPSO—Cylexin as an Adjunct to Lytic Therapy to Prevent Superoxide Reflow Injury

CAMCAT—Canadian Multicenter Clentiazem Angina Trial

CAMIAT—Canadian Amiodarone Myocardial Infarction Arrhythmia Trial

CAMIAT—Canadian Myocardial Infarction Amiodarone Trial

CAPE—Circadian Anti-ischemia Program in Europe

CAPITOL—Captopril Postinfarction Tolerance

CAPP—Captopril Prevention Project

CAPPHY—Captopril Primary Prevention in Hypertension

CAPPP—Captopril Prevention Project

CAPRICORN—Carvedilol Postinfarct Survival Control Evaluation

CAPRIE—Clopidogrel vs Aspirin in Patients at Risk of Ischemic Events

CAPS—Cardiac Arrhythmia Pilot Study

CAPTIN—Captopril before Reperfusion in Acute Myocardial Infarction

CAPTIN—Captopril plus Tissue Plasminogen Activator Following Acute Myocardial Infarction

CAPTISM—Captopril Insulin Sensitivity Multicenter Study

CAPTURE—Chimeric 7E3 Antiplatelet in Unstable Angina Refractory to Standard Treatment

CARE—Calcium Antagonist in Reperfusion

CARE—Carevedilol Atherectomy Restenosis Trial

CARE—Cholesterol and Recurrent Events

CARET—Beta Carotene and Retinol Efficacy Trial

CARMEN—Carvedilol Angiotensin Converting Enzyme Inhibitors Remodeling Mild Heart Failure Evaluation

CARPORT—Coronary Artery Restenosis Prevention on Repeated Thromboxane A_2-Antagonism Study

CARS—Coronary Artery Regression Study

CARS—Coumadin Aspirin Reinfarction Study

CART—Colchicine Angioplasty Restenosis Trial

CASANOVA—Carotid Artery Stenosis with Asymptomatic Narrowing: Operation vs Aspirin

CASCADE—Cardiac Arrest in Seattle: Conventional vs Amiodarone Drug Evaluation

CASCADE—Conventional Antiarrhythmic vs Amiodarone in Survivors of Cardiac Arrest Drug Evaluation

CASCO—Calcium Sensitization in Congestive Heart Failure

CASH—Cardiac Arrest Study Hamburg

CASIS—Canadian Amlodipine/Atenolol in Silent Ischemia Study

CASSIS—Czech and Slovak Spirapril Intervention Study

CAST—Cardiac Arrhythmia Suppression Trial

CAST—Chinese Acute Stroke Trial

CAT—Cardiomyopathy Trial

CAT—Chinese Angiotensin Converting Enyme Inhibitor in Acute Myocardial Infarction Trial

CATS—Canadian American Ticlopidine Study

CATS—Captopril and Thrombolysis Study

CCAIT—Canadian Coronary Atherosclerosis Intervention Trial

CCHAT—Canadian Cozaar Hyzaar Amlodipine Trial

CCSI—Chinese Captopril Study 1

CCT—Chinese Captopril Trial

CDP—Coronary Drug Project

CDPAS—Coronary Disease Prevention with Aspirin Study

CDPAS—Coronary Drug Project Aspirin Study

CEDIM—Carnitina Echocardiografia Digitalizzata Infarto Miocardico

CEI-AMI—Converting Enzyme Inhibitor Treatment of Patients in China with Acute Myocardial Infarction

CEPRIM—Cebutid 50 en Prevention des Reocclusions Coronaires apres Repefusion Myocardique a la phase aigue d'un Infarctus

CESG—Cerebral Embolism Study Group Trial

CESNA—Comparative Efficacy and Safety of Nisoldipine and Amlodipine in the Treatment of Subjects with Mild to Moderate Hypertension

CESNA II—Comparative Efficacy and Safety of Nisoldipine and Amlodipine in Hypertensive Subjects with Ischemic Heart Disease

CHAD—Cholesterol Hypertension and Diabetes Study

CHAMP—Combination Hemotherapy and Mortality Prevention

CHAOS—Cardiovascular Disease, Hypertension and Hyperlipidemia, Adult-Onset Diabetes, Obesity, and Stroke

CHAPS—Carvedilol Heart Attack Pilot Study

CHARM—Candesartan in Heart Failure Assessment in Reduction of Mortality and Morbidity

CHEAPER—Confirmation that Heparin is an Alternative to Promote Early Reperfusion in Acute Myocardial Infarction

CHF-STAT—Congestive Heart Failure–Survival Trial of Antiarrhythmic Therapy

CHOICE—Congestive Heart Failure Mortality Investigation on Carvedilol's Efficacy

CHRISTMAS—Carvedilol Hibernation Reversible Ischemia Trial: Marker of Success

CIAIT—Chinese Infarction Angiotensin Converting Enzyme Inhibitor Trial

CIBIS—Cardiac Insufficiency Bisoprolol Study

CIBIS-II—Cardiac Insufficiency Bisoprolol Study II

CIDS—Canadian Implantable Defibrillator Study

CITO—Collaborazione Italiana per la Trombosi in Ortopedia

CITTS—Central Illinois Thrombolytic Therapy Study

CLAPT—Cholesterol Lowering Atherosclerosis Percutaneous Transluminal Coronary Angioplasty Trial

CLAS—Cholesterol Lowering Atherosclerosis Study

CLASP—Collaborative Low Dose Aspirin Study in Pregnancy

CLASP—Preeclampsia Prevention with Low Dose Aspirin

CLASS—Clomethiazole Acute Stroke Study

CLASS-IHT—Clomethiazole Acute Stroke Study in Ischemic Hemorrhagic and Tissue Plasminogen Activator-Treated Patients

CLASSICS—Clopidogrel Aspirin Stent International Cooperative Study

CLEOPAD—Clopidogrel in Peripheral Arterial Disease

CLIP—Cholesterol Lowering Intervention Program

COBALT—Continuous Infusion vs Bolus Altreplase Trial

COBALT—Continuous Infusion vs Double-Bolus Administration of Altreplase

COLUMBUS—A Study of Low Molecular Weight Heparin in the Treatment of Venous Thromboembolism named after Columbus

COMET—Carvedilol or Metoprolol Evaluation Trial

COMMIT—Comprehensive Multidisciplinary Interventional Trial for Regression of Coronary Artery Disease

COMPASS—Comparative Trial of Saruplase vs Streptokinase

CONSENSUS—Cooperative North Scandinavian Enalapril Survival Study

CONSENSUS II—Cooperative North Scandinavian Enalapril Survival Study II

CONVINCE—Controlled Onset Verapamil Investigation for Cardiovascular Endpoints

COPERNICUS—Carvedilol Prospective Randomized Cumulative Survival Trial

CORE—Collaborative Organization for RheothRx Evaluation

CORTES—Clivarin Assessment of Regression of Thrombus, Efficacy and Safety

COTAIM—Continuation of Trial of Antihypertensive Interventions and Management

CPAS—Canadian Prinivil Atenolol Study

CPEP—Chicago Coronary Prevention Evaluation Program

CPHRP—Coronary Prevention and Hypertension Research Project

CPPT—Coronary Primary Prevention Trial

CPRG—Coronary Prevention Research Group Study with Oxprenolol following Myocardial Infarction

CPSTS—Chinese Post Stroke Treatment Study

CRAFT—Catheterization Rescue Angioplasty Following Thrombolysis

CRAFT—Controlled Randomized Atrial Fibrillation Trial

CREDO—Clopidogrel Reduction of Events During Extended Observation

CREW—Coronary Regression with Estrogen in Women

CRIS—Calcium Antagonist Reinfarction Italian Study

CRISP—Cholesterol Reduction in Seniors Program

CSG—Collaborative Study Group Trial of Irbesartan

CSGTEI—Collaborative Study Group Trial on the Effect of Irbesartan

CTAF—Canadian Trial of Atrial Fibrillation

CURE—Clopidogrel in Unstable Angina to Prevent Recurrent Ischemic Events

CURVES—CURVES of Efficacy for Various Doses of Statins on Low-Density Lipoprotein Cholesterol Reduction in the Study

DAAF—Digoxin in Acute Atrial Fibrillation

DAMAD—Diabetic Microangiopathy Modification with Aspirin vs Dipyridamole

DANAMI—Danish Trial in Acute Myocardial Infarction

DANDERYD—Danderyd-Stockholm Intervention Study

DASS—Dilazep Aspirin Stroke Study

DATA—Diltiazem as Adjunctive Therapy to Activase

DAVIT—Danish Verapamil Infarction Trial

DCAF—Dilated Cardiomyopathy and Atrial Fibrillation Trial

DCCT—Diabetes Control and Complications Trial

DCM—Dilated Cardiomyopathy Study

DEFIANT—Doppler Flow and Echocardiography in Functional Cardiac Insufficiency: Assessment of Nisoldipine Therapy

DES—Danish Enoxaparin Study

DIAB-HYCAR—Diabetes Hypertension Cardiovascular Morbidity and Mortality and Ramipril

DIAMOND—Danish Investigation of Arrhythmia and Mortality on Dofetilide

DIAMOND-CHF—Danish Investigations of Arrhythmia and Mortality on Dofetilide in Congestive Heart Failure

DIAMOND-MI—Danish Investigations of Arrhythmias and Mortality on Dofetilide in Myocardial Infarction

DiDi—Diltiazem in Dilated Cardiomyopthy Trial

DIG—Digitalis Investigation Group Study

DIGAF—Digoxin in Atrial Fibrillation Study

DIGAMI—Diabetic Patients Receiving Insulin Glucose Infusion during Acute Myocardial Infarction

DILCACOMP—Diltiazem Captopril Comparative Study

DILDURANG—Diltiazem Duration in Angina

DILPLACOMP—Diltiazem Placebo Comparative Trial

DIMT—Dutch Ibopamine Multicenter Trial

DIPAP—Dipyridamole in Peripheral Arteriopathy

DOFISK—Dose Finding of Streptokinase Trial

DOUBLE—Double Bolus Lytic Efficacy Trial

DPPS—Duesseldorf Percutaneous Transluminal Coronary Angioplasty Platelet Study

DRS—Diltiazem Reinfarction Study

DUE—Drug Use Evaluation

DUET—Dispatch Urokinase Efficacy Trial

DURAC—Duration of Anticoagulation after Venous Thromboembolism

DUTCH-TIA—DUTCH Transient Ischemic Attack Study

DVT—Danish Verapamil Trial

EAFT—European Atrial Fibrillation Trial

EAGAR—Estrogen and Graft Atherosclerosis Research Trial

EASI—European Antiplatelet Stent Investigation

ECASS-II—European and Australian Cooperative Stroke Study II

ECAT AP—ECAT Angina Pectoris Study

ECCE—Effects of Captopril on Cardiopulmonary Exercise Parameters Post Myocardial Infarction

ECSG—European Cooperative Study Group for rtPA in Acute Myocardial Infarction

EDEN—Estudio in Ventricular Dysfunction of Enalapril after Myocardial Infarction

EDIC—Echocardiography Dobutamine International Cooperative Study

EDIT—Early Diagnosis and Thrombolytic Therapy in Acute Myocardial Infarction without Significant ST Segment Elevation in the Electrocardiogram

EFERF—Enalapril Felodipine Extended Release Factorial Study

EFICAT—Ejection Fraction in Carvedilol-Treated Transplant Candidates

EFS—European Fraxiparin Study

ELITE—Evaluation of Losartan in the Elderly

ELSA—European Lacidipine Study on Atherosclerosis

EMERA—Estudio Multicentrico Estreptoquinasa Republica Argentina

EMERALD—European and Australian Multicenter Evaluation Research on Atrial Dofetilide

EMERAS—Estudio Multicentrico Estreptoquinasa Republicas de Americas del Sur

EMIAT—European Myocardial Infarction Amiodarone Trial

EMIAT—European Myocardial Infarction Arrhythmia Trial

EMIP-FR—European Myocardial Infarction Project—Free Radicals

EMMA—Essai Multicentrique Medicaments vs Angioplastie

EMPAR—Enoxaparin Maxepa Prevention of Angioplasty Restenosis

EMS—European Multicenter Study

ENASA—Enoxaparin and/or Aspirin in Unstable Angina

ENCORE—Evaluation of Nifedipine and Cerivastatin on Recovery of Endothelial Function

ENOXART—Enoxaparin in Arterial Surgery

ENTICES—Enoxaparin and Ticlopidine after Elective Stenting

ENTIM—Etudes des Nouveaux Thrombolytiques dans Infarctus du Myocarde

EPAMSA—Estudio Piloto Argentino de Muerte Subita y Amiodarone

EPIC—Echo Persantine Italian Cooperative Study

EPIC—Evaluation of IIb/IIIa Platelet Receptor Antagonist 7E3 in Preventing Ischemic Complications

EPIDS—Early Post–Myocardial Infarction Intravenous Dipyridamole Study

EPILOG—Evaluation of Percutaneous Transluminal Coronary Angioplasty to Improve Long-Term Outcome by c7E3 GPIIb/IIIa Receptor Blockade

EPILOG Stent—Multicenter, Randomized Trial of Abciximab in Stenting and Comparison with Abciximab Plus Balloon

EPISTENT—Evaluation of IIb/IIIa Platelet Inhibitor for Stenting

EPPI—Etude de Prescription Post Infarctus

EPREDA—Essai Preeclampsie Dipyridamole Aspirine

EPSIM—Enquete de Prevention Secondaire de l'Infarctus du Myocarde

EQOL—Economics and Quality of Life Substudy of GUSTO

EQUIPP—Evaluation of Quinapril in Primary Practice

ERA—Enoxaparin Restenosis after Angioplasty

ERA—Estrogen Replacement and Atherosclerosis Study

ERASER—Evaluation of ReoPro and Stenting to Eliminate Restenosis

ERAYTIC—Etude dans la Maladie de Raynaud avec la Ticlopidine

ERNST—European Resuscitation Nimodipine Study

ESCALATE—Efegatran and Streptokinase to Canalize Arteries like Accelerated Tissue Plasminogen Activator

ESETCID—European Study of Epidemiology and Treatment of Cardiac Inflammatory Disease

ESPRIM—European Study Prevention Research of Infarct with Molsidomine

ESPRIT—Efficacy Safety Prospective Randomized Ibopamine Trial

ESPRIT—European and Australian Stroke Prevention in Reversible Ischemia Trial

ESPRIT—European Study of the Prevention of Reocclusion after Initial Thrombolysis

ESPS—European Stroke Prevention Study

ESSENCE—Efficacy Safety Subcutaneous Enoxaparin in Non–Q-Wave Coronary Events Study

EST—Early Stroke Trial

ESTIC—Estudio on Survival and Treatment in Insuficiencia Cardiaca in Spain

ETAMIN—Effects of Ticlopidine on Atherosclerosis Membri Inferii

ETCI—Etude Tanakan Claudication Intermittente

ETDRS—Early Treatment Diabetic Retinopathy Study

EUCLID—EURODIAB Controlled Trial of Lisinopril in Insulin-Dependent Diabetes Mellitus

EURAMIC—European Community Multicenter Study on Antioxidants, Myocardial Infarction, and Breast Cancer

EUROASPIRE—European Action on Secondary Prevention by Intervention to Reduce Events

EUROCARE—European Carvedilol Restenosis Trial

EUROPA—European Trial of Reduction of Cardiac Events with Perindopril in Stable Coronary Artery Disease

EVAS-IM—Etude Vaudois APSAC vs Streptokinase dans Infarctus du Myocarde

EWA—Estrogen Replacement for Women with Coronary Artery Disease

EWPHE—European Working Party on Hypertension in the Elderly

EXACT—Extended Release Adalat Canadian Trial

EXCEL—Expanded Clinical Evaluation of Lovastatin

EXCITE—Evaluation of Xemilofiban in Controlling Thrombotic Events

FACET—Flosequinan Angiotensin Converting Enzyme Inhibitor Trial

FACET—Fosinopril vs Amlodipine Cardiovascular Events Trial

FACT—Fraxiparine Angioplastie Coronaire Transluminale

FAMIS—Fosinopril in Acute Myocardial Infarction Study

FAMOUS—Fragmin Advanced Malignancy Outcome Study

FANTASTIC—Full Anticoagulation vs Aspirin Ticlopidine after Stent Implantation

FANTASTIC—Full Anticoagulation vs Ticlopidine plus Aspirin after Stent Implantation: A Randomized Multicenter European Study

FAP—Fibrinolytics vs Primary Angioplasty in Acute Myocardial Infarction

FAPIS—Flecainide and Propafenone Italian Study

FAPS—Felodipine Atherosclerosis Prevention Study

FAPS—French Aortic Plaques Study

FAST-MI—Field Ambulance Study of Thrombolysis in Myocardial Infarction

FATIMA—Fraxiparin Anticoagulant Therapy in Myocardial Infarction Study Amsterdam

FATS—Familial Atherosclerosis Treatment Study

FEMINA—Felodipine ER and Metoprolol in the Treatment of Patients with Stable Angina Pectoris

FEST—Fosinopril Efficacy/Safety Trial

FEST—Fosinopril on Exercise Tolerance Study

FHRS—Familial Hypercholesterolemia Regression Study

FIG—Flosequinan Investigator Group Study

FIPS—Frankfurt Isoptin Progression Study

FIRST—Flolan International Randomized Survival Trial

FISH—Finnish Isradipine Study in Hypertension

FISS—Fraxiparine in Stroke Study

FIT—Fibrinolytic Therapy Trialists Study

FLARE—Fluvastatin Angioplasty Restenosis Trial

FLEQUIN—Intravenous Flecainide Compared to Oral Quinidine

FLUENT—Fluvastatin Long-Term Extension Trial

FLVS—Fleurbaix Laventie Ville Sante Study

FMS—Finnish Multicenter Study of Doxazosin Therapy of Hypertension

FMT—Fragmin Multicenter Trial

FORT—Fish Oil Restenosis Trial

FRAMI—Fragnin in Acute Myocardial Infarction

FRAXIS—Fraxiparine in Ischemic Syndrome

FRIC—Fragmin in Unstable Coronary Artery Disease

FRISC—Fragmin during Instability in Coronary Artery Disease

FRISC II—Fast Revascularization during Instability in Coronary Artery Disease

FROST—Fibrinogen Receptor Occupancy Study

FTT—Fibrinolytic Therapy Trialists Study

GAIN—Glycine Antagonists in Neuroprotection

GAMIS—German-Austrian Myocardial Infarction Study

GARS—German-Austrian Reinfarction Study

GAUS—German Activator Urokinase Study

GAXS—German and Austrian Xamoterol Study

GDCMS—German Dilated Cardiomyopathy Study

GEART—Gemfibrozil Atherosclerosis Regression Trial

GELIA—German Experience with Low Intensity Anticoagulation

GEMICA—Grupo de Estudio Multicentrico de la Insuficiencia Coronaria en la Argentina

GEMT—German Eminase Multicenter Trial

GENOX—Groupe d'Etude de l'Enoxaparine Trial

GHAT—German Hip Arthroplasty Trial in Prevention of Deep Vein Thrombosis with Low Molecular Weight Heparin

GIFA—Gruppo Italiano di Farmavigilanza nell'Anziano

GIMA—Gallopamil e Ischemia Miocardica nell'Anziano

GIPSI—Gradual Inflation at Optimum Pressure vs Stent Implantation

GISSI—Gruppo Italiano per lo Studio della Streptochinasi nell' Infarto Miocardico

GISSI-2—Gruppo Italiano per lo Studio dello Sopravvivenza nell' Infarto Miocardico II

GISSI-3—Gruppo Italiano per lo Studio dello Sopravvivenza nell' Infarto Miocardico III

GISSI-APPI—GISSI-3 Angina precoce Post-Infarto

GISSI-EFRIM—Gruppo Italiano per lo Studio della Sopravvivenza nell'Infarto Epidemiologia dei Fttori di Rischio dell'Infarto Miocardico

GLANT—Group of Long-Term Antihypertensive Treatment Study

GMT—Goteborg Metoprolol Trial

GRAND—Glaxo Receptor Antagonist against Nottingham Deep Vein Thrombosis Study

GRAPE—Glycoprotein Receptor Antagonist Patency Evaluation

GRASP—Glaxo Restenosis and Symptoms Project

GREAT—Grampian Region Early Anistreplase Trial

GRECO—German Recombinant Plasminogen Activator Study

GRECO—German Study with Recombinant Tissue Plasminogen Activator in Coronary Occlusion

GUARANTEE—Global Unstable Angina Registry and Treatment Evaluation

GUARDIAN—GUARD During Ischemia Against Necrosis

GUSTO—Global Utilization of Streptokinase and Tissue Plasminogen Activator for Occluded Arteries

GUSTO-IIa—Global Use of Strategies to Open Occluded Arteries

GUSTO-IIb—Global Use of Strategies to Open Occluded Coronary Arteries in Acute Coronary Syndromes

GUSTO III—Global Use of Strategies to Open Occluded Coronary Arteries

GUSTO IV—Global Utilization of Streptokinase and Tissue Plasminogen Activator for Occluded Arteries

HALF—Homocysteine, Atherosclerosis, Lipids and Familial Hypercholesterolemia Study

HALT—Hypertension and Lipid Trial

HALT-MI—Hu23F2G Antiadhesion to Limit Cytotoxic Injury Following Acute Myocardial Infarction

HAMIT—Heparin in Acute Myocardial Infarction Trial

HANE—Hydrochlorothiazide, Atenolol, Nitrendipine, Enalapril Study

HAPI—Heparin as an Alternative to Promote Patency in Acute Myocardial Infarction

HAPI—Heparin after Percutaneous Intervention

HAPPHY—Heart Attack Primary Prevention in Hypertension

HARP—Harvard Atherosclerosis Reversibility Project

HART—Heparin Aspirin Reperfusion Trial

HART II—Heparin and Reperfusion Therapies

HAS—Hirulog Angioplasty Study

HAT—Heparin Associated Thrombocytopenia Study

HDFP—Hypertension Detection and Follow-Up Program

HDS—Hypertension in Diabetes Study

HEAP—Heparin in Early Patency Study

HEART—Healing and Early Afterload Reducing Therapy

HEART—Hyperlipidaemia, Epidemiology, Atherosclerosis, Risk Factor Trial

HELP—Heparin-Induced Extracorporeal Low-Density Lipoprotein Precipitation Treatment

HELP NSAID—Helicobacter Eradication for Lesion Prevention with Nonsteroidal Anti-Inflammatory Drugs

HELVETICA—Hirudin in a European Restenosis Prevention Trial vs Heparin Treatment in Percutaneous Transluminal Coronary Angioplasty Patients

HEMOSTAT—Hemostasis with Prostar XL vs Angioseal after Coronary Intervention Trial

HEP—Hypertension in the Elderly Persons Trial

HERO—Hirulog Early Reperfusion/Occlusion

HERS—Heart and Estrogen-Progestin Replacement Study

HHS—Helsinki Heart Study

HINT—Holland Interuniversity Nifedipine/Metoprolol Trial

HIPS—Heparin Delivery with the Infusasleeve Catheter Prior to Stent Implantation

HIPS—Heparin Infusion Prior to Stenting Trial

HIRMIT—High Risk Myocardial Ischemia Trial

HIS—Hemodilution in Stroke Study

HIS—Hormones in Stroke Study

HIS—Hungarian Isradipine Study

HIT—Hirudin for the Improvement of Thrombolysis

HIT—High-Density Lipoprotein Cholesterol Intervention Trial of the Department of Veterans Affairs

HIT-SK—Hirudin for Improvement of Thrombolysis in Combination with Streptokinase

HOPE—Heart Outcomes Prevention Evaluation Trial

HOT—Hypertension Optimal Treatment Study

HOT MI—Hyperbaric Oxygen and Thrombolysis in Myocardial Infarction

HRT—Hormone Replacement Trial

HSCSG—Hypertension Stroke Cooperative Study Group Trial

Hy-C—Hydralazine vs Captopril Trial

HYCAR—Hypertrophie Cardiaque Ramipril

HYPREN—Hypertension under Prazosin and Enalapril Study

HYSTENOX—Enoxaparin in Patients Following Hysterectomy

HYVET—Hypertension in the Very Elderly Trial

IAMA—Infection in Atherosclerosis and the Use of Macrolide Antibiotics

IARG—International Anticoagulant Review Group Study

IASSH—Italian Acute Stroke Study with Hemodilution

ICIN—Intracoronary Streptokinase Trial of the Interuniversity Cardiology Institute of the Netherlands

ICS—Iohexol Cooperative Study

ICSG—International Collaborative Study Group Trial with Early Use of Timolol in Acute Myocardial Infarction

ICUS—Intracoronary Ultrasound Study of Atherosclerosis Retardation in Transplanted Heart with Diltiazem

IDCS—Idiopathic Dilated Cardiomyopathy Study

IIHD—Israeli Ischemic Heart Disease Study

IIUK—Intraoperative Intraarterial Urokinase Study

IMAC—Intervention in Myocarditis and Acute Cardiomyopathy

IMAGE—International Metoprolol/Nifedipine Angina Exercise Trial

IMAGE—International Multicenter Angina Exercise Study

IMAGES—Intravenous Magnesium Efficacy in Stroke Trial

IMCT—International Multicentre Trial

IMEP—Investigation in Menopausal Women of the Effect of Estradiol and Progesterone on Cardiovascular Risk Factors

IMPACT—Integrelin to Manage Platelet Aggregation to Combat Thrombosis

IMPACT—Integrelin to Manage Platelet Aggregation to Prevent Coronary Thrombosis

IMPACT—International Mexiletine and Placebo Antiarrhythmic Coronary Trial

IMPACT-AMI—Integrelin to Minimize Platelet Aggregation and Prevent Coronary Thrombosis–Acute Myocardial Infarction

IMPACT-Stent —Integrelin to Minimize Platelet Aggregation and Coronary Thrombosis in Stenting

IMPACT II—Integrelin to Minimize Platelet Aggregation and Coronary Thrombosis II

IMPRESS—Intramural Low Molecular Weight Heparin for Prevention of Restenosis Study

INJECT—International Joint Efficacy Comparison of Thrombolytics Trial

INLINIS—Ireland-Netherlands Lisinopril-Nifedipine Study

INSIGHT—International Nifedipine-GITS Study Intervention as a Goal in Hypertension Treatment

INTACT—International Nifedipine Trial on Antiatherosclerotic Therapy

INTERCEPT—Infarction Trial of European Research Collaborators Evaluating Prognosis Postthrombolysis

INTIMA—Infusion of Tissue Plasminogen Activator in Myocardial Infarction at the Acute Phase

InTiME—Intravenous nPA for Treatment of Infarcting Myocardium Early

InTIME II—A Phase III Trial of Novel Bolus Thrombolytic Lanoteplase (nPA)

INVEST—International Verapamil SR/Trandolapril Study

IPO-V2—Indagine Policentrica Ospedaliera—Vessel 2

IPPHS—International Primary Pulmonary Hypertension Study

IRAS—Insulin Resistance Atherosclerosis Study

ISAM—Intravenous Streptokinase in Acute Myocardial Infarction

ISAR—Intracoronary Stenting and Antithrombotic Regimen Trial

ISCOAT—Italian Study on Complications of Oral Anticoagulant Therapy

ISG—Ibopamine Study Group Trial

ISIS—International Study of Infarct Survival

ISIS 4—Fourth International Study of Infarct Survival

ISLAND—Infarct Size Limitation: Acute N-acetylcysteine Defense Trial

IST—International Stroke Trial

ITALICS—Investigation by the Thoraxcenter of Antisense Given by Local Delivery and Assessed by Intravascular Ultrasound after Coronary Stenting

ITPASMT—International Tissue Plasminogen Activator/Streptokinase Mortality Trial

ITS—Israeli Thrombolytic Survey

JAMIS—Japanese Antiplatelet Myocardial Infarction Study

JaMSPUK—Japanese Multicenter Study for Pro-Urokinase

JETS—Japanese E5510 TIAA Study

JIMI—Japanese Intervention Trial in Myocardial Infarction

JLRCPS—Jerusalem Lipid Research Clinic Prevalence Study

KAMIT—Kentucky Acute Myocardial Infarction Trial

KAPS—Kuopio Atherosclerosis Prevention Study

KAT—Kuopio Angioplasty Gene Transfer Trial

KCSS—Keio Cooperative Stroke Study

KFC—Ketanserin for Carcinoid Trial

KFC—Ketanserin on Fibroblast Culture Study

KRIS—Kaunas-Rotterdam Intervention Study

KUMIS—Kumamoto University Myocardial Infarction Study

KYSMI—Kyoto Shiga Myocardial Infarction Study

LARA—Low Dose Aspirin Trial on Restenosis after Angioplasty

LART—Low-Density Lipoprotein Apheresis Angioplasty Restenosis Trial

LASAF—Low Quantities of Acetylsalicylic Acid in Atrial Fibrillation

LASAR—Local Alcohol and Stent Against Restenosis Trial

LASTLHY—Latin American Study of Lacidipine in Hypertension

LATE—Late Assessment of Thrombolytic Efficacy

LAVA—Leiden Artificial Valves and Anticoagulation Study

LBPS—Lubeck Blood Pressure Study

LCAS—Lipoprotein and Coronary Athlerosclerosis Study

LDHSPS—Low Dose Heparin Stroke Prevention Study

LET—Losartan Effectiveness and Tolerability Study

LEVEL—Lexxel vs Enalapril Study

LHS—Losartan Hemodynamic Study

LIDO—Levosimendan Infusion vs Dobutamine Study

LIFE—Losartan Intervention for Endpoint Reduction in Hypertension

LIFT—Late Intervention Following Thrombolysis

LIHPS—Local Delivery of Heparin in Stenting for Suboptimal Result of Threatened Closure Post–Percutaneous Transluminal Coronary Angioplasty Using the Local Med InfusaSleeve

LIMIT—Leicester Intravenous Magnesium Intervention Trial

LIMIT—Low Molecular Weight Heparin Delivered Intramurally to Inhibit Thrombosis and Restenosis

LIMIT-AMI—Double-blind, Placebo-Controlled, Multicenter Angiographic Trial of Rhumab CD18 in Acute Myocardial Infarction

LIMITS—Liquemin in Myocardial Infarction during Thrombolysis with Saruplase

LIPID—Long-term Intervention with Pravastatin in Ischemic Disease

LIPS—Lescol Interventional Prevention Study

LISA—Lescol in Severe Atherosclerosis

LIT—Lopressor Intervention Trial

LIVE—Left Ventricular Hypertrophy: Indapamide Vs Enalapril

LOCAT—Lopid Coronary Angiography Trial

LOMIR-MCT-IL—Lomir (Brand Name for Isradipine) Multicenter Study, Israel

LOT—Long-Term Outcome after Thrombolysis Study

LOTS—Long-Term Outcome after Thrombosis Study

LPS—Lovastatin Pravastatin Study

LQTS—Long QT Syndrome Study

LRC-CDPT—Lipid Research Clinics Coronary Drug Project Trial

LRC-CPPT—Lipid Research Clinics Coronary Primary Prevention Trial

LRT—Lovastatin Restenosis Trial

MAAS—Multicenter Antiatherosclerotic Study

MAAS—Multicentre Antiatheroma Study

MACH—Mortality Assessment in Congestive Heart Failure

MADAM—Moexipril as Antihypertensive Drug After Menopause

MAGIC—Magnesium in Coronaries

MAGICA—Magnesium in Cardiac Arrhythmias

MAPHY—Metoprolol Atherosclerosis Prevention in Hypertension

MARATHON—Medida de la Actividad Fisica y su Relacion Ambiental con Todoes los Lipidos en el Hombre

MARCATOR—Multicenter American Research Trial with Cilazapril after Angioplasty to Prevent Transluminal Coronary Obstruction and Restenosis

MARS—Monitored Atherosclerosis Regression Study

MASS—Medicine, Angioplasty or Surgery Study

MAST—Multicenter Acute Stroke Trial

MAST-E—Multicentre Acute Stroke Trial–Europe

MAST-I—Multicenter Acute Stroke Trial–Italy

MATE—Medicine vs Angioplasty for Thrombolytic Exclusions Trial

MATH—Modern Approach to Treatment of Hypertension Study

MATTIS—Multicenter Aspirin and Ticlopidine Trial after Intracoronary Stenting

MAVERIC—Midlands Trial of Empirical Amiodarone vs Electrophysiological Guided Intervention and Cardioverter Implant in Ventricular Arrhythmias

MDC—Metoprolol in Dilated Cardiomyopathy

MDC—Multicenter Dilated Cardiomyopathy Trial

MDPIT—Multicenter Diltiazem Post Infarction Trial

MED-TEP—Medical Treatment Effectiveness Program

MEHP—Metoprolol in Elderly Hypertensive Patients

MELODHY—Metoprolol Low Dose in Hypertension

MERCATOR—Multicenter European Research Trial with Cilazapril after Angioplasty to Prevent Transluminal Coronary Obstruction and Restenosis

MERIT-HF—Metoprolol Controlled-Release Randomised Intervention Trial in Heart Failure

MES—Minitran Efficacy Study

MEXIS—Metoprolol and Xamoterol Infarction Study

MHFT—Munich Mild Heart Failure Trial

MIAMI—Metoprolol in Acute Myocardial Infarction

MICOL—Multicenter Italian Study on Colesterolo

MICRO-HOPE—Microalbuminuria, Cardiovascular and Renal Outcomes in the Heart Outcomes Prevention Evaluation Trial

MIDAS—Multicenter Isradipine/Diuretic Atherosclerosis Study

MILESTONE—Multicenter Iloprost European Study on Endangeitis

MILIS—Multicenter Investigation of the Limitation of Infarct Size

MIMS—Migraine and Myocardial Ischemic Study

MINT—Myocardial Infarction with Novastan and Tissue Plasminogen Activator Study

MIRACL—Myocardial Ischemia Reduction with Aggressive Cholesterol Lowering

MIRSA—Multicenter International Randomized Study of Angina Pectoris

MISCHF—Management to Improve Survival in Congestive Heart Failure

MIST—Mibefradil Ischemia Suppression Trial

MIST—Multicenter Isradipine Salt Trial

MITRA—Maximal Individual Therapy in Acute Myocardial Infarction

MLCCHF—Multicenter Lisinopril Captopril Congestive Heart Failure Study

MMIRG—Multicenter Myocardial Ischemia Research Group Study

MMTT—Multicenter Myocarditis Treatment Trial

MOCHA—Multicenter Oral Carvedilol in Heart Failure Assessment

MOSES—Morbidity and Mortality after Stroke-Eprosartan vs Nitrendipine for Secondary Prevention

MPIP—Multicenter Post Infarction Program

MPRG—Multicenter Postinfarction Research Group

MRC—Medical Research Council Study of Mild Hypertension

MRC—Medical Research Council Trial of Treatment of Hypertension in Older Adults

MRC/BHF—Medical Research Council, British Heart Foundation Heart Protection Study

MRCOA—Medical Research Council Trial in Older Adults

MRFIT—Multiple Risk Factor Intervention Trial

MSHT—Mount Sinai Hypertension Trial

MSMI—Multicenter Study of Myocardial Ischemia

MSSMI—Multicenter Study on Silent Myocardial Ischemia

MTOP—Medical Treatment Outcome Project

MTT—Myocarditis Treatment Trial

MUST—Multicenter Stents Ticlopidine

MUST—Multicenter Ultrasound Study with Ticlid

MUSTT—Multicentre Unstable Tachycardia Trial

MUSTT—Multicenter Unsustained Tachycardia Trial

MVP—Multivitamins and Probucol Trial in Prevention of Restenosis Post Percutaneous Transluminal Coronary Angioplasty

NAMIS—Nifedipine Angina Myocardial Infarction Study

NASCET—North American Symptomatic Carotid Endarterectomy Trial

N-CAP—Nifedipine Gastrointestinal Therapeutic System Circadian Anti-ischemic Program

NEAT—Neurohormonal Effects in Acute Myocardial Infarction of Trandolapril

NEET—Nordic Enalapril Exercise Trial

NETWORK—NETWORK of General Practitioners and Hospital Physicians Involved in the Study of Low vs High Doses of Enalapril in Patients with Heart Failure

NEWDILTIL—New Diltiazem vs Tildiem

NGAST—Nimodipine German Austrian Stroke Trial

NHF—National Heart Foundation Trial

NHP—National Hypertension Project of Egypt

NHS—Nurses Health Study

NICOLE—Nisoldipine in Coronary Artery Disease in Leuven

NINDS-rtPA Stroke Study—National Institute of Neurological Disorders and Stroke Recombinant Tissue Plasminogen Activator Stroke Trial

NMS—Norwegian Multicenter Study

NNMT—Norwegian Nifedipine Multicenter Trial

NORDIL—Nordic Diltiazem Study

NORMALISE—Norvasc for Regression of Manifest Artherosclerotic Lesions by Intravascular Sonographic Evaluations

NPHDO—Nadroparin Post Hospital Discharge in Orthopedics

NPHS—Northwick Park Heart Study

NUAPS—National Unstable Angina Pectoris Study

OASIS-2—Organisation to Assess Strategies for Ischemic Syndromes

OAT—Ochanomizu Aspirin Trials

OAT—Open Artery Trial

OHS—Oslo Hypertension Study

OHT—Oslo Heart Trial

OIS—Oslo Ischemia Study

OPTIMAL—Optimal Therapy in Myocardial Infarction with the Angiotensin II Antagonist Losartan

OPTIME—Outcomes of a Prospective Trial of Intravenous Milrinone for Exacerbations of Chronic Heart Failure

OPTIME CHF—Outcomes of a Prospective Trial of Intravenous Milrinone for Exacerbations of Chronic Heart Failure

OPUS—Orbofiban in Patients with Unstable Coronary Syndromes

OPUS—Orbofiban Post Unstable Coronary Syndromes

OPUS—Optimal Angioplasty vs Primary Stenting

ORBIT—Oral Glycoprotein IIb/IIIa Receptor Blockade to Inhibit Thrombosis

OSCAR—Olive Oil Safflower Oil Canola Oil and Rapeseed Oil Dietary Study

OSIRIS—Optimization Study of Infarct Reperfusion Investigated by ST Monitoring

OST—Ottawa Stroke Trials

OURS—Oxford University Research Study

PACE—Prevention with Low-Dose Aspirin of Cardiovascular Disease in the Elderly

PACIFIC—Potential Angina Class Improvement from Myocardial Channels

PACK—Prevention of Atherosclerotic Complications with Ketanserin

PACT—Plasminogen Activator Angioplasty Compatibility Trial

PACT—Plasminogen Activator Coronary Angioplasty Trial

PACT—Prehospital Application of Coronary Thrombolysis

PACT—Pro-Urokinase in Acute Coronary Thrombosis

PAFIT—Paroxysmal Atrial Fibrillation Italian Trial

PAFT—Propafenone Atrial Fibrillation Trial

PAIMS—Plasminogen Activator Italian Multicenter Study

PAIS—Pravastatin in Acute Ischaemic Syndromes Study

PARADIGM—Platelet Aggregation Receptor Antagonist Dose Investigation for Reperfusion Gain in Myocardial Infarction

PARADISE—Platelet IIb/IIIa Antagonist for the Reduction of Acute Coronary Events Dose Investigation and Safety Evaluation Study

PARAGON—Platelet IIb/IIIa Antagonism for the Reduction of Acute Coronary Syndrome Events in a Global Organization Network

PARAT—Prevention of Arterial Restenosis Angiographic Trial

PARIS—Persantine Aspirin Reinfarction Study

PARK—Postangioplasty Restenosis Ketanserin

PARK—Prevention of Angioplasty Reocclusion with Ketanserin

PART—Prevention of Atherosclerosis with Ramipril Therapy

PART 2—Prevention of Atherosclerosis with Ramipril Therapy 2

PART—Probucol Angioplasty Restenosis Trial

PARTNER—Peripheral Arterial Disease Response to Taprostene with New Established Response Criteria

PAS—Polish Amiodarone Study

PASS—Piracetam in Acute Stroke Study

PASS—Practical Applicability of Saruplase Study

PATAF—Prevention of Arterial Thromboembolism in Nonvalvular Atrial Fibrillation Study

PATENT—Prourokinase and Tissue Plasminogen Activator Enhancement of Thrombolysis Trial

PATHS—Prevention and Treatment of Hypertension Study

PATS—Poststroke Antihypertensive Treatment Study

PATS—Prehospital Administration of Tissue Plasminogen Activator Study

PCVMETRA—Prevention CardioVasculaire en Medicine du Travail

PEACE—Prevention of Events with Angiotensin Converting Enzyme Inhibition Study

PECTE—Pulmonary Embolism Colfarit Trial in Elderly

PEP—Perindopril in Elderly Patients

PEPI—Postmenopausal Estrogen/Progestin Intervention

PERSPECTIVE—Perindopril's Prospective Effect on Coronary Atherosclerosis by Angiographical and Intravascular Ultrasound Evaluation

PHS—Physicians' Health Study

PHYLLIS—Plaque Hypertension Lipid Lowering Italian Study

PIAF—Pharmacological Intervention in Atrial Fibrillation Study

PICO—Pimobendan in Congestive Heart Failure

PILOT—Polish Intramural Low Molecular Weight Heparin Outpatient Stent Trial

PILOT—Preliminary Investigation of Local Therapy using Porous Percutaneous Transluminal Coronary Angioplasty Balloons and Low Molecular Weight Heparin

PLAC—Pravastatin Limitation of Atherosclerosis in the Coronary Arteries

PLAC-2—Pravastatin, Lipids and Atherosclerosis in the Carotid Arteries

PLM—Prevention of Mortality with Low Molecular Weight Heparin in Medical Patients

PLS—Postsurgery Logiparin Study

PMNSG—Pravastatin Multinational Study Group Trial

PMRG—Pimobendan Multicenter Research Group Study

PMS—Pravastatin Multinational Study

POLISH—a Trial by POLISH Investigators to Evaluation the Effect of Amiodarone on Mortality after Myocardial Infarction

Post CABG—Long-Term Follow-Up of the Post–Coronary Artery Bypass Graft Trial

PPP—Prospective Pravastatin Pooling Project

PQRST—Probucol Quantitative Regression Swedish Trial

PRACTICAL—Placebo Controlled Randomized Angiotensin Converting Enzyme Inhibition Comparative Trial in Cardiac Infarction and Left Ventricular Function

PRAIRE—Study of Survival after Thrombosis for Acute Myocardial Infarction by PRAIRE Cardiovascular Center, Springfield, Illinois

PRAISE—Prospective Randomized Controlled Clinical Trials

PRAISE II— Prospective Randomized Amlodipine Survival Evaluation

PREAMI—Perindopril and Remodelling in Elderly with Acute Myocardial Infarction

PRECISE—Prospective Randomized Evaluation of Carvedilol in Symptoms and Exercise

PREDICT—Prospective Randomized Evaluation of Diltiazem CD Trial

PREFACE—Pravatstatin Related Effects Following Angioplasty on Coronary Endothelium

PREMIS—Prehospital Myocardial Infarction Study

PRESERVE—Prospective Randomized Enalapril Study Evaluating Regression of Ventricular Enlargement

PRESTO—Prevention of Pestenosis with Tranilast and its outcomes– A placebo–controlled study

PREVENT—Prospective Randomized Evaluation of the Vascular Effects of Norvasc Trial

PRIME—Promotion of Reperfusion by Inhibition of Thrombin during Myocardial Infarction Evaluation

PRIME—Prospective Randomized Ibopamine Mortality Evaluation

PRIME—Prospective Randomized Study of Ibopamine on Mortality and Efficacy in Heart Failure

PRIMI—Prourokinase in Myocardial Infarction Trial

PRISM—Platelet Receptor Inhibition for Ischemic Stroke by Transesophageal Echocardiography

PRISM-PLUS—Platelet Receptor Inhibition for Ischemic Syndrome Management in Patients Limited by Unstable Signs and Symptoms

PRISTINE—Praxilene in Stroke Treatment in Northern Europe

PROACT—Prolyse in Acute Cerebral Thrombolytic Trial

PROACT—Prourokinase for Acute Cerebral Thromboembolism

PROACT-II—Recombinant prourokinase (rProUK) in Acute Cerebral Thromboembolism

PROFILE—Prospective Randomized Flosequinan Longevity Evaluation

PROGRESS—Perindopril Protection against Recurrent Stroke Study

PROLOG—Precursor to EPILOG Study

PROMISE—Prospective Randomized Milrinone Survival Evaluation

PROSPER—Prospective Study of Pravastatin in the Elderly at Risk

PROTECT—Perindopril Regression of Vascular Thickening European Community Trial

PROTECT—Prospective Reinfarction Outcomes in Thrombolytic Era Cardizem CD Trial

PROVED—Prospective Randomized Study of Ventricular Failure and the Efficacy of Digoxin

PSTAF—Pilsicainide Suppression Trial on Atrial Fibrillation

PURSUIT—Platelet IIb/IIIa in Unstable Angina: Receptor Suppression Using Integrelin Therapy

PURSUIT—Platelet IIb/IIIa Underpinning the Receptor for Suppression of Unstable Ischemia Trial

PUTS—Perindopril Therapeutic Safety Study

QHFT—Quinapril Heart Failure Trial

The information here is provided as guidance only. Prescribers should always consult the manufacturer's current prescribing information.

301

QUADS—Quinapril Australasian Dosing Study

QUASAR—Quinapril Anti-ischemia and Symptoms of Angina Reduction

QUIET—Quinapril Ischemic Event Trial

QUO VADIS—Quinapril on Vascular Ace and Determinants of Ischemia

RAAMI—Randomized Angiographic Trial of Alteplase in Myocardial Infarction

RAAMI—Rapid Administration of Alteplase in Myocardial Infarction

RAAS—Randomized Angiotensin II Receptor Antagonist, Angiotensin Converting Enzyme Inhibitor Study

RAAS—Renin-Angiotensin-Aldosterone System Trials

RACE—Ramipril Angiotensin Converting Enzyme Inhibition Study

RACE—Ramipril Cardioprotective Evaluation

RADIANCE—Randomized Assessment of Digoxin on Inhibitors of the Angiotensin Converting Enzyme

RAFT—Rhythmol-SR Atrial Fibrillation Trial

RALES—Randomized Aldactone Evaluation Study

RANTTAS—Randomized Trial of Tirilazad in Acute Stroke

RAPID—Recombinant Plasminogen Activator Angiographic Phase II International Dose Finding Study

RAPID 1—Reteplase Angiographic Phase II International Dose Finding Study

RAPID 2—Reteplase vs Alteplase Patency Investigation During Myocardial Infarction

RAPPORT—ReoPro in Acute Myocardial Infarction and Primary Percutaneous Transluminal Coronary Angioplasty Organization and Randomized Trial

RAPT—Ridogrel vs Aspirin Patency Trial

RAVES—Reduced Anticoagulation in Saphenous Vein Graft Stent Trial

RAVES—Reduced Anticoagulation Vein Graft Study

REACH—Research on Endothelin Antagonism in Chronic Heart Failure

REACT—Rapid Early Action for Coronary Treatment

REDUCE—Randomized Double Blind Unfractionated Heparin and Placebo Controlled Multicenter Trial

REDUCE—Restenosis Prevention after Percutaneous Transluminal Coronary Angioplasty. Early Administration of LMWH LU 47311 in a Double-blind Unfractionated Heparin and Placebo Controlled Evaluation

REFLECT I—Randomized Evaluation of Flosequinan on Exercise Tolerance—Initial Efficacy Trial

REFLECT II—Randomized Evaluation of Flosequinan on Exercise Tolerance—Dose Response Study

REFLEX—Randomized Evaluation of Flosequinan on Exercise Tolerance Study

REGRESS—Regression Growth Evaluation Statin Study

REIN—Ramipril Efficacy in Nephropathy Study

RENAAL—Reduction of Endpoints in Non–Insulin Dependent Diabetes Mellitus with Angiotensin II Antagonist Losartan

ReoMI—ReoPro in Myocardial Infarction

REPAIR—Reperfusion in Acute Infarction, Rotterdam

RESOLVD—Randomized Evaluation of Strategies for Left Ventricular Dysfunction

RESTORE—Randomized Efficacy Study of Tirofiban for Outcomes and Restenosis

RHEOTRIX—RHEOThRX vs Placebo for Infarct-Size Reduction

RIGHT—Cerivastatin Gemfibrozil Hyperlipidemia Treatment Study

RISC—Research on Instability in Coronary Artery Disease

RITA—Randomised Intervention Treatment of Angina

ROBUST—Recanalization of Occluded Bypass Graft with Prolonged Urokinase Infusion Site Trial

ROXIS—Roxithromycin Ischemic Syndromes

RRPCE—Reduction of Recurrence and Prevention of Cerebral Emboli

RUTH—Raloxifene Use for the Heart

SAFIRE D—Symptomatic Atrial Fibrillation Investigation and Randomized Evaluation of Dofetilide

SAHCS—Streptokinase Aspirin Heparin Collaborative Study

SALT—Swedish Aspirin in Low Dose Trial

SALTS—Strategic Alternatives with Ticlopidine in Stenting Study

SAMI—Streptokinase Angioplasty Myocardial Infarction Trial

SAMIT—Streptokinase Angioplasty Myocardial Infarction Trial

SAMPLE—Study on Ambulatory Monitoring of Pressure and Lisinopril Evaluation

SAPAT—Swedish Angina Pectoris Aspirin Trial

SAPPHIRE—Stanford Asian Pacific Program in Hypertension and Insulin Resistance

SAS—Scandinavian Angiopeptin Study

SASS—Sygen Acute Stroke Study

SAT—Saruplase Alteplase Trial

SATE—Safety Antiarrhythmic Trial Evaluation

SATT—Scottish Adjuvant Tamoxifen Trial

SAVE—Survival and Ventricular Enlargement Trial

SCAT—Simvastatin Enalapril Coronary Atherosclerosis Trial

SCATI—Studio sulla Calciparina nell'Angina e nella Trombosi Ventricolare nell'Infarto

SCD-HeFT—Sudden Cardic Death in Heart Failure: Trial of Prophylactic Amiodarone vs Implantable Defibrillator Therapy

SCIC—Sopravvivenza con Captopril nell'Insufficienza Cardiaca

SCIV—Subcutaneous vs Intravenous Heparin in Deep Venous Thrombosis

SEARCH—Study of the Effectiveness of Additional Reductions of Cholesterol and Homocysteine

SECURE—Study to Evaluate Carotid Ultrasound Changes with Ramipril and Vitamin E

SESAIR—Studio Epoorine Sottocutanea nell'Angina Instabile Refrattoria

SESAM—Study in Europe of Saruplase and Alteplase in Myocardial Infarction

SHAPE—Study of Heparin and Actilyse Processed Electronically

SHARP—Study of Heparin in Angioplasty Restenosis Prevention

SHELL—Systolic Hypertension in the Elderly: Long-Term Lacidipine Trial

SHEP—Systolic Hypertension in the Elderly Program

SHIPS—Shiga Pravastatin Study

SHOCK—Should We Emergently Revascularize Occluded Coronary Arteries for Cardiogenic Shock

SHP—Skaraborg Hypertension Project

SIAC—Studio Indobufene Angioplastica Coronarica

SIAM—Streptokinase in Acute Myocardial Infarction

SIMAP—Studio Italiano Multicentrico Angina Pectoris

SISAMI—Silent Ischemia in Survivors of Acute Myocardial Infarction

SISH—Study of Isolated Systolic Hypertension

SISTEMI—Southern Italian Study on Thrombolysis Early in Myocardial Infarction

SKDAMI—Streptokinase plus Desmopressin in Acute Myocardial Infarction

SLIP—Studio Lipidi Isoptin Press

SMART—Self Measurement for Assessment of the Response to Trandolapril

SMART—Study of Medicine vs Angioplasty Reperfusion Trial

SMARTT—Serum Markers, Acute Myocardial Infarction, and Rapid Treatment Trial

SMILE—Survival of Myocardial Infarction: Long-term Evaluation

SMOG—Studio Multicentrico Ospedaliero Gallopamil

SMS—Simvastatin Multicenter Study

SMT—Stockholm Metoprolol Trial

SnaP—Study of Sodium and Blood Pressure

SNAPE—Study Nicorandil Angina Pectoris Elderly

SOAR—Safety of Orbofiban in Acute Coronary Research

SOCRATES—Study of Coroanry Revascularization and Therapeutic Evaluations

SOLVD—Studies of Left Ventricular Dysfunction

SPAF—Stroke Prevention in Atrial Fibrillation

SPAF TEE—Stroke Prevention in Atrial Fibrillation III Transesophageal Echo Study

SPEED—Strategies for Patency Enhancement in the Emergency Department

SPI—Study of Perioperative Ischemic

SPIC—Studio Policentrico Italiano Cardiomiopatie

SPICE—Study of Patients Intolerant of Converting Enzyme Inhibitors

SPINAF—Stroke Prevention in Nonrheumatic Atrial Fibrillation

SPIR—Study of Perioperative Ischemia Research

SPIRIT—Salvage from Perindopril in Reperfused Infarction Trial

SPIRIT—Stroke Prevention in Reversible Ischemia Trial

SPRINT—Secondary Prevention Reinfarction Israeli Nifedipine Trial

SPRS—Sixty Plus Reinfarction Study

SPRT Sixty Plus Reinfarction Trial

SPS—Stockholm Prospective Study

SSSS—Scandinavian Simvastatin Survival Study

STAI—Studio della Ticlopidina nell'Angina Instabile

STAMP—Systemic Thrombolysis in Acute Myocardial Infarction with Prourokinase and Urokinase

STAR—Staphylokinase Recombinant Trial

STARC—Studio Trapidil vs Aspirin nella Restenosi Coronarica

STARS—Standard Treatment with Activase to Reverse Stroke

STARS—Stent Anticoagulation Restenosis Study

START—St. Thomas' Atherosclerosis Regression Trial

START—Saruplase and Taprostene Acute Reocclusion Trial

START—Study of Thrombolytic Therapy with Additional Response Following Taprostene

START—Study of Titration and Response to Tiazac

STARTS—Stent Antithrombotic Regimen Study

STAT—Stroke Treatment with Ancrod Trial

Stent-PAMI—Primary Angioplasty in Myocardial Infarction Trial

STEP—Study of Taprostene in Elective Percutaneous Transluminal Coronary Angioplasty

STEREO—Stents and ReoPro Trial

STILE—Surgery vs Thrombolysis for Ischemic Lower Extremity

STIMS—Swedish Ticlopidine Multicenter Study

STIPAS—Safety Study of Tirilazad Mesylate in Patients with Acute Ischemic Stroke

STONE—Shanghai Trial of Nifedipine in the Elderly

STOP-Hypertension—Swedish Trial in Old Patients with Hypertension

STOP-2—Swedish Trial in Old Patients with Hypertension

STRETCH—Symptoms Tolerability Response to Exercise Trial of Candesartan Cilexitil in Patients with Heart Failure

SUTAMI—Saruplase and Urokinase in Treatment of Acute Myocardial Infarction

SUVIMAX—Supplementation Vitamin Minerals and Antioxidant Trial

SVTS—Sotalol Ventricular Tachycardia Study

SWAT—Stroke Prevention with Warfarin or Aspirin Trial

SWIFT—Should we Intervene Following Thrombolysis?

SWISH—Swedish Isradipine Study in Hypertension

SWISSI—Swiss Interventional Study on Silent Ischemia

SWORD—Survival with Oral D-Sotalol

SYMPHONY—Sibrafiban versis Aspirin to Yield Maximum Protection from Ischemic Heart Events Post Acute Coronary Syndromes

SYST-CHIN—Systolic Hypertension in Elderly Chinese Trial

SYST-CHINA—Systolic Hypertension in Elderly Chinese Trial

SYST-EUR—Systolic Hypertension in Elderly in Europe Trial

TACIP—Triflusal, Aspirin, Cerebral Infarction Prevention

TACS—Thrombolysis and Angioplasty in Cardiogenic Shock

TACT—Ticlopidine Angioplastie Coronaire Transluminale

TACT—Ticlopidine Angioplasty Coronary Trial

TACT—Ticlopidine vs Placebo for Prevention of Acute Closure after Angioplasty Trial

TACTICS—Thrombolysis and Counterpulsation to Improve Cardiogenic Shock Survival

TACTICS TIMI-18—Treat Angina with Aggrastat and Determine Cost of Therapy with an Invasive or Conservative Strategy—Thrombolysis in Myocardial Infarction

TAIM—Trial of Antihypertensive Interventions and Management

TAIST—Tinzaparin in Acute Stroke Trial

TAMI—Thrombolysis and Angioplasty in Myocardial Infarction

TAPIRSS—Triflusal vs Aspirin for the Prevention of Infarction: a Randomized Stroke Study

TAPS—Tissue Plasminogen Activator APSAC Patency Study

TARGET—TANGIBLE-Safety of LDL-C Reduction with Atorvastatin vs Simvastatin in a Coronary Heart Disease Population

TASH—Transcoronary Ablation of Septum Hypertrophy Study

TASMAN—Thrombosis Anticoagulant Study Mediterranean Australia New Zealand

TASS—Ticlopidine Aspirin Stroke Study

TASTE—Ticlopidine Aspirin Stent Evaluation

TAUSA—Thrombolysis and Angioplasty in Unstable Angina

TCG—Thromboprophylaxis Collaborative Group Trial

TEAHAT—Thrombolysis Early in Acute Heart Attack Trial

TEAM—Thrombolytic Trial of Eminase in Acute Myocardial Infarction

TEMS—Trimetazidine European Multicentre Study

TESS—Tirilazud Efficacy Stroke Study

TEST—Timolol, Encainide, Sotalol Trial

THAMES—Tenormin in Hypertension and Myocardial Ischemia Epidemiological Survey

THAT—Thrombolysis in Acute Myocardial Infarction Trial

THEOPACE—Theophylline vs Pacemaker on the Symptoms and Complications of Sick Sinus Syndrome

THESEE—Tinzaparine ou Heparine Standard: Evaluations dans l'Embolie Pulmonaire

THIS—Tissue Plasminogen Activator Heparin Interaction Study

TIARA—Timolol en Infarto Agudo, Republica Argentina

TIBBS—Total Ischaemic Burden Bisoprolol Study

TIBET—Total Ischemic Burden European Trial

TICO—Thrombolysis in Coronary Occlusion

TIDES—Transdermal Intermittent Dosing Evaluation Study

TIM—Triflusal in Acute Myocardial Infarction

TIMAD—Ticlopidine in Microangiopathy of Diabetes

TIMED—Trial to Investigate the Effect of Morning vs Evening Dosing of Nisoldipine on Pharmacodynamics in Hypertensive Patients

TIMI—Thrombolysis in Myocardial Infarction

TIMI-7—Thrombin Inhibition in Myocardial ischemia Trial

TIMI-9—Thrombolysis and Thrombin Inhibition in Myocardial Infarction

TIMS—Tertatolol International Multicentre Study

TIPE—Thrombolysis in Pulmonary Embolism Study

TIPE—Thrombolysis in Peripheral Embolism Patient Study

TISS—Ticlopidine Indobufen Stroke Study

TITS—Tetrofosmin International Trial Study Group

TIVT—Thrombolysis in Deep Vein Thrombosis

TNT—Transderm-Nitro Trial

TOAST—Treatment of Acute Stroke Trial

TOAST—Trial of Org 10172 in Acute Stroke Treatment

TOHMS—Trial of Hypertensive Medications Study

TOHP—Trials of Hypertension Prevention

TOLC—Treatment of Low High-Density Lipoprotein Cholesterol Study

TOMHS Treatment of Mild Hypertension Study

TOP—Thrombolysis in Old Patients

TOPAS—Thrombolysis or Peripheral Arterial Surgery

TOPS—Treatment of Post-Thrombolytic Stenoses Study

TOPS—Thrombolysis in Old Patients Study

TOSCA—Total Occlusion Study of Canada

TOWARD—Toyama Warfarin Rational Dosage Study

TPASK—Tissue Plasminogen Activator vs Streptokinase Trial by the International Study Group

TPAT—Tissue Plasminogen Activtor Toronto Trial

TPI—Thrombolytic Predictive Instrument Project

TPT—Thrombosis Prevention Trial

TRACE—Trandolapril Cardiac Evaluation

TRAPIST—Trapadil vs Placebo to Prevent In-Stenting Intimal Hyperplasia

TREAT—Tranilast Restenosis Following Angioplasty Trial

TREND—Trial on Reversing Endothelial Dysfunction

TRENT—Trial of Early Nifedipine Treatment in Acute Myocardial Infarction

TRIC—Thrombolysis with Recombinant Tissue Plasminogen Activator during Instability in Coronary Artery Disease

TRIM—Thrombin Inhibition in Myocardial Ischemia

TROPHY—A Placebo Controlled Trial Assessing the Treatment Effects of Lisinopril vs Hydrochlorothiazide in Obese Patients with Hypertension

TROPHY—Treatment of Obese Patients with Hypertension

TROPHY—Trial of Preventing Hypertension

TRUST—Trial of United Kingdom for Stoke Treatment

TTATTS—Thrombolytic Therapy in Acute Thrombotic/Thromboembolic Stroke

TTOPP—Thrombolytic Therapy in an Older Patient Population

TUCC—Tissue Plasminogen Activator/Urokinase Comparisons in China

UD-AHF—UD-CG 115 BS in Acute Heart Failure Study

UKCSG—United Kingdom Collaborative Study Group Trial with Timolol

UKHAS—United Kingdom Heart Attack Study

UK in USA—Urokinase in Unstable Angina

UK-TIA—United Kingdom Transient Ischemic Attack Aspirin Trial

UNASEM—Unstable Angina Study using Eminase

UNRPCA—Use of Nicardipine to Retard the Progression of Coronary Atherosclerosis

UNSA—Unstable Angina Study

UPET—Urokinase Pulmonary Embolism Trial

URALMI—Urokinase and Alteplase in Myocardial Infarction

USIM—Urochinasi per via Sistemica nell'Infarto Miocardico

USPET—Urokinase Streptokinase Pulmonary Embolism Trial

USPHS—United States Physicians' Health Study

USPHS—United States Public Health Service Hospitals Intervention Trial in Mild Hypertension

UTOPIA—Utilization of Platelet Inhibition in Angina Trial

VACS—Veterans Administration Cooperative Study

VA-HIT—Veterans Affairs HDL Intervention Trial

Val-HeFT—Valsartan Heart Failure Trial

VALIENT—Valsartan in Acute Myocardial Infarction

VALUE—Valsartan Antihypertensive Long Term Use Evaluation

VAMI—Verapamil Acute Myocardial Infarction

VANQWISH—Veterans Affairs Non–Q-Wave Infarction Strategies in Hospital Study

VAS—Verapamil Angioplasty Study

VASPNAF—Veterans Administration Stroke Prevention in Nonrheumatic Atrial Fibrillation

VEGF—Vascular Endothelial Growth Factor Gene Therapy Study

VENUS—Very Early Nimodipine Use in Stroke Trial

VERAS—Verringerung der Restenoserate nach Angioplastie durch ein Somatostatin Analogon

VERDI—Verapamil vs Diuretic Trial

VERDICT—Verapamil Digoxin Cardioversion Trial

VEST—Vesnarinone Trial

VHAS—Verapamil Hypertension Atherosclerosis Study

V-HeFT—Veterans Administration Heart Failure Trial

V-HeFT II—Veterans Administration Heart Failure Trial II

V-HeFT II—Vasodilator Heart Failure Trial II

VISP—Vitamin Intervention for Stroke Prevention

VIVA—VEGF in Ischemia for Vascular Angiogenesis

VSG—Vesnarinone Study Group Trial

VT-MASS—Metoprolol and Sotalol for Sustained Ventricular Tachycardia

WAAT—Warfarin plus Aspirin vs Aspirin Trial

WAFUS—Warfarin Anticoagulation Follow up Study

WARIS—Warfarin Reinfarction Study

WARIS II—Warfarin Aspirin Reinfarction Study Norwegian

WARSS—Warfarin-Aspirin Recurrent Stroke Study

WASH—Warfarin Aspirin Study of Heart Failure

WASID—Warfarin-Aspirin Symptomatic Intracranial Disease Study

WATCH—Warfarin Antiplatelet Trial in Chronic Heart Failure

WAVE—Women's Angiographic Vitamin and Estrogen Trial

WELL-HEART—Women's Estrogen/Progestin and Lipid Lowering Hormone Atherosclerosis Regression Trial

WEST—Womens Estrogen for Stroke Trial

WHAT—Worcester Heart Attack Trial

WHI—Womens Health Initiative

WHIMS—Women's Health Initiative Memory Study

WHS—Womens Health Study

WHT—Warm Heart Trial

WOOFS—Warfarin Optimized Outpatient Follow up Study

WOSCOPS—West of Scotland Coronary Prevention Study

WWICT—Western Washington Intracoronary Streptokinase Trial

WWISK—Western Washington Intracoronary Streptokinase Trial

WWIST—Western Washington Intravenous Streptokinase Trial

WWIV—Western Washington Intravenous Streptokinase Trial

WWIVSK—Western Washington Intravenous Streptokinase Trial

WWSIMIT—Western Washington Streptokinase in Myocardial Infarction Trial

XISHF—Xamoterol in Severe Heart Failure Study

ZEST—Zocor Early Start Trial

ZWOLLE—A Trial from ZWOLLE, The Netherlands, Comparing Primary Coronary Angioplasty with Intravenous Streptokinase

Drugs	Pregnancy	Lactation	Pregnancy category
α-adrenergic antagonists			
Doxazosin	Weigh benefits vs risk	Breastfeeding not recommended; excretion in milk unknown	C
Phenoxybenzamine	Weigh benefits vs risk	Breastfeeding not recommended; excretion in milk unknown	C
Phentolamine	Weigh benefits vs risk	Breastfeeding not recommended; excretion in milk unknown	C
Prazosin	Weigh benefits vs risk	Breastfeed with caution; drug excreted in breast milk	C
Terazosin	Weigh benefits vs risk	Breastfeeding not recommended; excretion in milk unknown	C
α-adrenergic agonists			
Clonidine	Weigh benefits vs risk	Breastfeed with caution; drug excreted in breast milk	C
Guanabenz	Weigh benefits vs risk	Breastfeeding not recommended; excretion in milk unknown	C
Guanfacine	Use only if clearly indicated	Breastfeeding not recommended; excretion in milk unknown	B
Methyldopa	Weigh benefits vs risk	Breastfeed with caution; drug excreted in breast milk	B (IV), C (PO)
Angiotensin converting enzyme inhibitors			
Benazepril	Use of ACE inhibitors during the second and third trimesters of pregnancy has been associated with fetal and neonatal injury, including hypotension, neonatal skull hypoplasia, anuria, reversible or irreversible renal failure, and death	Breastfeeding not recommended; excretion in milk unknown	C (first trimester) D (second, third trimesters)
Captopril		Breastfeeding not recommended; drug excreted in breast milk	
Enalapril		Breastfeeding not recommended; drug excreted in breast milk	
Fosinopril		Breastfeeding not recommended; drug excreted in breast milk	
Lisinopril		Breastfeeding not recommended; excretion in milk unknown	
Moexipril		Breastfeeding not recommended; excretion in milk unknown	
Perindopril		Breastfeeding not recommended; excretion in milk unknown	
Quinapril		Breastfeeding not recommended; drug excreted in breast milk	
Ramipril		Breastfeeding not recommended; excretion in milk unknown	
Trandolapril		Breastfeeding not recommended; excretion in milk unknown	
Angiotensin II receptor blockers			
Candesartan	Use of medications that act directly on the renin angiotensin system during the second and third trimesters of pregnancy has been associated with fetal and neonatal injury, including hypotension, neonatal skull hypoplasia, anuria, reversible or irreversible renal failure, and death	Breastfeeding not recommended; excretion in milk unknown	C (first trimester) D (second, third trimesters)
Irbesartan		Breastfeeding not recommended; excretion in milk unknown	
Losartan		Breastfeeding not recommended; excretion in milk unknown	
Telmisartan		Breastfeeding not recommended; excretion in milk unknown	
Valsartan		Breastfeeding not recommended; excretion in milk unknown	
Antiarrhythmic agents			
Class IA			
Disopyramide	Weigh benefits vs risk	Breastfeeding not recommended; drug excreted in breast milk	C
Procainamide	Weigh benefits vs risk	Breastfeeding not recommended; drug excreted in breast milk	C
Quinidine	Weigh benefits vs risk	Breastfeeding not recommended; drug excreted in breast milk	C
Class IB			
Lidocaine	Use only if clearly indicated	Breastfeed with caution; drug excreted in breast milk	B
Mexiletine	Weigh benefits vs risk	Breastfeeding not recommended; drug excreted in breast milk	C
Tocainide	Weigh benefits vs risk	Breastfeeding not recommended; drug excreted in breast milk	C
Class IC			
Flecainide	Weigh benefits vs risk	Breastfeeding not recommended; drug excreted in breast milk	C

Drugs	Pregnancy	Lactation	Pregnancy category
Class IC (continued)			
Moricizine	Use only if clearly indicated	Breastfeeding not recommended; drug excreted in breast milk	B
Propafenone	Weigh benefits vs risk	Breastfeeding not recommended; excretion in milk unknown	C
Class II (β blockers)			
Acebutolol	Use only if clearly indicated	Breastfeeding not recommended; drug excreted in breast milk	B
Atenolol	Not recommended	Breastfeeding not recommended; drug excreted in breast milk	D
Betaxolol	Weigh benefits vs risk	Breastfeed with caution; drug excreted in breast milk	C
Bisoprolol	Weigh benefits vs risk	Breastfeeding not recommended; excretion in milk unknown	C
Carteolol	Weigh benefits vs risk	Breastfeeding not recommended; excretion in milk unknown	C
Carvedilol	Weigh benefits vs risk	Breastfeeding not recommended; excretion in milk unknown	C
Esmolol	Weigh benefits vs risk	Breastfeeding not recommended; excretion in milk unknown	C
Labetalol	Weigh benefits vs risk	Breastfeed with caution; drug excreted in breast milk	C
Metoprolol	Weigh benefits vs risk	Breastfeeding not recommended; drug excreted in breast milk	C
Nadolol	Weigh benefits vs risk	Breastfeed with caution; drug excreted in breast milk	C
Penbutolol	Weigh benefits vs risk	Breastfeeding not recommended; excretion in milk unknown	C
Pindolol	Use only if clearly indicated	Breastfeed with caution; drug excreted in breast milk	B
Propranolol	Weigh benefits vs risk	Breastfeed with caution; drug excreted in breast milk	C
Timolol	Weigh benefits vs risk	Breastfeed with caution; drug excreted in breast milk	C
Class III			
Amiodarone	Not recommended	Breastfeeding not recommended; drug excreted in breast milk	D
Bretylium	Weigh benefits vs risk	Breastfeeding not recommended; excretion in milk unknown	C
Dofetilide	Data not available	Breastfeeding not recommended; excretion in milk unknown	
Ibutilide	Weigh benefits vs risk	Breastfeeding not recommended; excretion in milk unknown	C
Sotalol	Use only if clearly indicated	Breastfeeding not recommended; drug excreted in breast milk	B
Class IV (calcium antagonists)*			
Amlodipine	Weigh benefits vs risk	Breastfeeding not recommended; excretion in milk unknown	C
Bepridil	Weigh benefits vs risk	Breastfeeding not recommended; drug excreted in breast milk	C
Diltiazem	Weigh benefits vs risk	Breastfeeding not recommended; drug excreted in breast milk	C
Felodipine	Weigh benefits vs risk	Breastfeeding not recommended; excretion in milk unknown	C
Isradipine	Weigh benefits vs risk	Breastfeeding not recommended; excretion in milk unknown	C
Nicardipine	Weigh benefits vs risk	Breastfeeding not recommended; excretion in milk unknown	C
Nifedipine	Weigh benefits vs risk	Breastfeeding not recommended; drug excreted in breast milk	C
Nimodipine	Weigh benefits vs risk	Breastfeeding not recommended; excretion in milk unknown	C
Nisoldipine	Weigh benefits vs risk	Breastfeeding not recommended; excretion in milk unknown	C
Verapamil	Weigh benefits vs risk	Breastfeeding not recommended; drug excreted in breast milk	C
Antithrombotic agents			
Anticoagulants			
Ardeparin	Weigh benefits vs risk	Breastfeeding not recommended; excretion in milk unknown	C
Dalteparin	Use only if clearly indicated	Breastfeeding not recommended; excretion in milk unknown	B
Danaparoid	Use only if clearly indicated	Breastfeeding not recommended; excretion in milk unknown	B
Enoxaparin	Use only if clearly indicated	Breastfeeding not recommended; excretion in milk unknown	B
Heparin	Weigh benefits vs risk	Not excreted in breast milk	C
Lepirudin	Use only if clearly indicated	Breastfeeding not recommended; excretion in milk unknown	B
Warfarin	Contraindicated	Breastfeeding not recommended; drug excreted in breast milk	X

Drugs	Pregnancy	Lactation	Pregnancy category
Antiplatelets			
Aspirin	Contraindicated in first trimester	Breastfeed with caution; drug excreted in breast milk	D
Abciximab	Weigh benefits vs risk	Breastfeeding not recommended; excretion in milk unknown	C
Clopidogrel	Use only if clearly indicated	Breastfeeding not recommended; excretion in milk unknown	B
Dipyridamole	Use only if clearly indicated	Breastfeed with caution; drug excreted in breast milk	B
Eptifibatide	Use only if clearly indicated	Breastfeeding not recommended; excretion in milk unknown	B
Ticlopidine	Use only if clearly indicated	Breastfeeding not recommended; excretion in milk unknown	B
Tirofiban	Use only if clearly indicated	Breastfeeding not recommended; excretion in milk unknown	B
Thrombolytics			
Alteplase (tPA)	Weigh benefits vs risk	Breastfeeding not recommended; excretion in milk unknown	C
Anistreplase	Weigh benefits vs risk	Breastfeeding not recommended; excretion in milk unknown	C
Reteplase	Weigh benefits vs risk	Breastfeeding not recommended; excretion in milk unknown	C
Streptokinase	Weigh benefits vs risk	Breastfeeding not recommended; excretion in milk unknown	C
Urokinase	Use only if clearly indicated	Breastfeeding not recommended; excretion in milk unknown	B
Diuretics			
Loop			
Bumetanide	Weigh benefits vs risk	Breastfeeding not recommended; excretion in milk unknown	C
Ethacrynic acid	Use only if clearly indicated	Breastfeeding not recommended; excretion in milk unknown	B
Furosemide	Weigh benefits vs risk	Breastfeeding not recommended; drug excreted in breast milk	C
Torsemide	Use only if clearly indicated	Breastfeeding not recommended; excretion in milk unknown	B
Thiazides			
Bendroflumethiazide	Weigh benefits vs risk	Breastfeed with caution; drug excreted in breast milk	C
Benzthiazide	Weigh benefits vs risk	Breastfeed with caution; drug excreted in breast milk	C
Chlorothiazide	Use only if clearly indicated	Breastfeed with caution; drug excreted in breast milk	B
Chlorthalidone	Use only if clearly indicated	Breastfeeding not recommended; drug excreted in breast milk	B
Hydrochlorothiazide	Use only if clearly indicated	Breastfeed with caution; drug excreted in breast milk	B
Hydroflumethiazide	Weigh benefits vs risk	Breastfeeding not recommended; drug excreted in breast milk	C
Indapamide	Use only if clearly indicated	Breastfeeding not recommended; drug excreted in breast milk	B
Methyclothiazide	Use only if clearly indicated	Breastfeeding not recommended; drug excreted in breast milk	B
Metolazone	Use only if clearly indicated	Breastfeeding not recommended; drug excreted in breast milk	B
Polythiazide	Weigh benefits vs risk	Breastfeed with caution; drug excreted in breast milk	C
Quinethiazide	Weigh benefits vs risk	Breastfeed with caution; drug excreted in breast milk	C
Trichlormethiazide	Weigh benefits vs risk	Breastfeed with caution; drug excreted in breast milk	C
Potassium sparing			
Amiloride	Use only if clearly indicated	Breastfeeding not recommended; excretion in milk unknown	B
Spironolactone	Weigh benefits vs risk	Breastfeeding not recommended; drug excreted in breast milk	C
Triamterene	Use only if clearly indicated	Breastfeeding not recommended; excretion in milk unknown	B
Inotropic and vasopressor agents			
Digoxin	Weigh benefits vs risk	Breastfeed with caution; drug excreted in breast milk	C
Amrinone	Weigh benefits vs risk	Breastfeeding not recommended; excretion in milk unknown	C
Milrinone	Weigh benefits vs risk	Breastfeeding not recommended; excretion in milk unknown	C
Dobutamine	Use only if clearly indicated	Breastfeeding not recommended; excretion in milk unknown	B
Dopamine	Weigh benefits vs risk	Breastfeeding not recommended; excretion in milk unknown	C

Drugs	Pregnancy	Lactation	Pregnancy category
Isoproterenol	Weigh benefits vs risk	Breastfeeding not recommended; excretion in milk unknown	C
Epinephrine	Weigh benefits vs risk	Breastfeed with caution; drug excreted in breast milk	C
Metaraminol	Weigh benefits vs risk	Breastfeeding not recommended; excretion in milk unknown	C
Methoxamine	Weigh benefits vs risk	Breastfeeding not recommended; excretion in milk unknown	C
Midodrine	Weigh benefits vs risk	Breastfeeding not recommended; excretion in milk unknown	C
Norepinephrine	Weigh benefits vs risk	Breastfeeding not recommended; excretion in milk unknown	C
Phenylephrine	Weigh benefits vs risk	Limited absorption in gastrointestinal tract; excretion in milk unknown	C
Lipid-lowering agents			
Bile acid sequestrants			
Cholestyramine	Weigh benefits vs risk	Breastfeed with caution; excretion in breast milk unknown	C
Colestipol	Weigh benefits vs risk	Breastfeed with caution; excretion in breast milk unknown	
Fibric acid derivatives			
Clofibrate	Weigh benefits vs risk	Breastfeeding not recommended; excretion in milk unknown	C
Fenofibrate	Weigh benefits vs risk	Breastfeeding not recommended; excretion in milk unknown	C
Gemfibrozil	Weigh benefits vs risk	Breastfeeding not recommended; excretion in milk unknown	C
Nicotinic acid	Weigh benefits vs risk	Breastfeed with caution; excretion in breast milk unknown	C
HMG-CoA reductase inhibitors			
Atorvastatin	Contraindicated	Breastfeeding not recommended; excretion in milk unknown	X
Cerivastatin	Contraindicated	Breastfeeding not recommended; drug excreted in breast milk	X
Fluvastatin	Contraindicated	Breastfeeding not recommended; drug excreted in breast milk	X
Lovastatin	Contraindicated	Breastfeeding not recommended; excretion in milk unknown	X
Pravastatin	Contraindicated	Breastfeeding not recommended; drug excreted in breast milk	X
Simvastatin	Contraindicated	Breastfeeding not recommended; excretion in milk unknown	X
Neuronal and ganglionic blockers			
Guanadrel	Use only if clearly indicated	Breastfeeding not recommended; excretion in milk unknown	B
Guanethidine	Weigh benefits vs risk	Breastfeeding not recommended; drug excreted in breast milk	C
Mecamylamine	Weigh benefits vs risk	Breastfeeding not recommended; excretion in milk unknown	C
Reserpine	Weigh benefits vs risk	Breastfeeding not recommended; drug excreted in breast milk	C
Trimethaphan	Not recommended	Breastfeeding not recommended; excretion in milk unknown	D
Vasodilators			
Cilostazol	Weigh benefits vs risk	Breastfeeding not recommended; excretion in milk unknown	C
Diazoxide	Weigh benefits vs risk	Breastfeeding not recommended; excretion in milk unknown	C
Epoprostenol	Use only if clearly indicated	Breastfeeding not recommended; excretion in milk unknown	B
Fenoldopam	Use only if clearly indicated	Breastfeeding not recommended; excretion in milk unknown	B
Hydralazine	Weigh benefits vs risk	Breastfeeding not recommended; drug excreted in breast milk	C
Isosorbide dinitrate	Weigh benefits vs risk	Breastfeeding not recommended; excretion in milk unknown	C
Isosorbide mononitrate	Weigh benefits vs risk	Breastfeeding not recommended; excretion in milk unknown	C
Isoxsuprine	Weigh benefits vs risk	Breastfeeding not recommended; excretion in milk unknown	C
Minoxidil	Weigh benefits vs risk	Breastfeeding not recommended; drug excreted in breast milk	C
Nitroglycerin	Weigh benefits vs risk	Breastfeeding not recommended; excretion in milk unknown	C
Nitroprusside	Weigh benefits vs risk	Breastfeeding not recommended; excretion in milk unknown	C
Papaverine	Weigh benefits vs risk	Breastfeeding not recommended; excretion in milk unknown	C
Pentoxifylline	Weigh benefits vs risk	Breastfeeding not recommended; drug excreted in breast milk	C
Tolazoline	Weigh benefits vs risk	Breastfeeding not recommended; excretion in milk unknown	C

The information here is provided as guidance only. Prescribers should always consult the manufacturer's current prescribing information.

309

*Only diltiazem and verapamil are indicated for arrhythmias.

†Pregnancy categories/US Food and Drug Administration Pregnancy Risk Classification:

B: Either animal reproduction studies have not demonstrated fetal risk or else they have not shown an adverse effect (other than a decrease in fertility). However, there are no controlled studies of pregnant women in the first trimester to confirm these findings and no evidence of risk in the later trimesters.

C: Either animal studies have revealed adverse effects (teratogenic or embryocidal) but there are no confirmatory studies in women, or studies in both animals and women are not available. Because of the potential risk to the fetus, drugs should be given only if justified by potentially greater benefits.

D: Evidence of human fetal risk is available. Despite the risk, benefits from use in pregnant women may be justifiable in select circumstances (eg, if the drug is needed in a life-threatening situation and no other safer, more acceptable drugs are effective). An appropriate warning statement will appear on the labeling.

X: Studies in animals and humans have demonstrated fetal abnormalities or evidence of risk based on human experience. Thus, the risk of drug use and consequent fetal harm outweigh any potential benefit, and the drug is contraindicated in pregnant women. An appropriate contraindication statement will appear on the labeling.

ACE—angiotensin converting enzyme; HMG CoA—hydroxymethylglutaryl coenzyme A; IV—intravenous; PO—by mouth.

Adapted from Ngo A, Frishman WH, Elkayam E: Cardiovascular pharmacotherapeutic considerations during pregnancy and lactation. In Cardiovascular Pharmacotherapeutics. Edited by Frishman WH, Sonnenblick EH. New York: McGraw Hill; 1997:1309.

APPENDIX III. DOSING RECOMMENDATIONS OF CARDIOVASCULAR DRUGS IN PATIENTS WITH HEPATIC DISEASE AND/OR CONGESTIVE HEART FAILURE

Drug	Cirrhosis	Congestive heart failure
α_1-Selective adrenergic antagonists (peripheral acting)		
Doxazosin	Usual dose with frequent monitoring	Usual dose with frequent monitoring
Phenoxybenzamine	Usual dose with frequent monitoring	Usual dose with frequent monitoring
Phentolamine	Usual dose with frequent monitoring	Usual dose with frequent monitoring
Prazosin	Usual dose with frequent monitoring	Usual dose with frequent monitoring
Terazosin	Usual dose with frequent monitoring	Usual dose with frequent monitoring
α-Adrenergic agonists (central acting)		
Clonidine	Usual dose with frequent monitoring	Usual dose with frequent monitoring
Guanabenz	Initiate with lower dose	Usual dose with frequent monitoring
Guanfacine	Initiate with lower dose	Usual dose with frequent monitoring
Methyldopa	Initiate with lower dose	Usual dose with frequent monitoring
Angiotensin converting enzyme inhibitors		
Benazepril	Usual dose with frequent monitoring	Usual dose with frequent monitoring
Captopril	Usual dose with frequent monitoring	Usual dose with frequent monitoring
Enalapril	Usual dose with frequent monitoring	Usual dose with frequent monitoring
Fosinopril	Usual dose with frequent monitoring	Usual dose with frequent monitoring
Lisinopril	Usual dose with frequent monitoring	Usual dose with frequent monitoring
Moexipril	Dose reduction may be necessary	Usual dose with frequent monitoring
Perindopril	Usual dose with frequent monitoring	Usual dose with frequent monitoring
Quinapril	Usual dose with frequent monitoring	Usual dose with frequent monitoring
Ramipril	Usual dose with frequent monitoring	Usual dose with frequent monitoring
Trandolapril	Initiate with lower dose	Usual dose with frequent monitoring
Angiotensin II receptor antagonists		
Candesartan	Usual dose with frequent monitoring	Usual dose with frequent monitoring
Irbesartan	Usual dose with frequent monitoring	Usual dose with frequent monitoring
Losartan	Initiate with lower dose	Usual dose with frequent monitoring
Telmisartan	Dose reduction may be necessary; consider alternative treatment	Dose reduction may be necessary
Valsartan	Usual dose with frequent monitoring	Usual dose with frequent monitoring
Antiarrhythmics		
Adenosine	Usual dose with frequent monitoring	Usual dose with frequent monitoring
Amiodarone	Usual dose with frequent monitoring	Usual dose with frequent monitoring
Atropine	Usual dose with frequent monitoring	Usual dose with frequent monitoring
Bretylium	Usual dose with frequent monitoring	Usual dose with frequent monitoring
Disopyramide	Initiate with lower dose	Dose reduction may be necessary
Dofetilide	Initiate with lower dose	Dose reduction may be necessary
Flecainide	Use lower dose or alternative treatment	Dose reduction may be necessary
Ibutilide	Usual dose with frequent monitoring	Usual dose with frequent monitoring
Lidocaine	Initiate with lower dose	Initiate with lower dose
Mexiletine	Initiate with lower dose	Initiate with lower dose
Moricizine	Use lower dose or alternative treatment	Dose reduction may be necessary
Procainamide	Dose reduction may be necessary	Dose reduction may be necessary

Drug	Cirrhosis	Congestive heart failure
Propafenone	Initiate with lower dose	Contraindicated in uncontrolled CHF
Quinidine	Initiate with lower dose	Initiate with lower dose
Sotalol	Usual dose with frequent monitoring	Contraindicated in uncontrolled CHF
Tocainide	Initiate with lower dose	Dose reduction may be necessary
Antithrombotics		
Anticoagulants		
Heparin	Dose reduction may be necessary	Usual dose with frequent monitoring
Warfarin	Initiate at lower dose	Dose reduction may be necessary
Ardeparin	Usual dose with frequent monitoring	Usual dose with frequent monitoring
Danaparoid	Usual dose with frequent monitoring	Usual dose with frequent monitoring
Enoxaparin	Usual dose with frequent monitoring	Usual dose with frequent monitoring
Dalteparin	Usual dose with frequent monitoring	Usual dose with frequent monitoring
Lepirudin	Usual dose with frequent monitoring	Usual dose with frequent monitoring
Antiplatelets		
Aspirin	Usual dose with frequent monitoring	Usual dose with frequent monitoring
Dipyridamole	Reduce dose with biliary obstruction	Usual dose with frequent monitoring
Ticlopidine	Contraindicated	Usual dose with frequent monitoring
Clopidogrel	Usual dose with frequent monitoring	Usual dose with frequent monitoring
Abciximab	Usual dose with frequent monitoring	Usual dose with frequent monitoring
Eptifibatide	Usual dose with frequent monitoring	Usual dose with frequent monitoring
Tirofiban	Initiate at lower dose	Usual dose with frequent monitoring
Thrombolytics		
Alteplase	Usual dose with frequent monitoring	Usual dose with frequent monitoring
Anistreplase	Dose reduction may be necessary	Usual dose with frequent monitoring
Streptokinase	Dose reduction may be necessary	Usual dose with frequent monitoring
Urokinase	Dose reduction may be necessary	Usual dose with frequent monitoring
Reteplase	Usual dose with frequent monitoring	Usual dose with frequent monitoring
β-Adrenergic blockers		
Nonselective		
Nadolol	Usual dose with frequent monitoring	Usual dose with frequent monitoring
Propranolol	Initiate with lower dose	Usual dose with frequent monitoring
Sotalol	Usual dose with frequent monitoring	Usual dose with frequent monitoring
Timolol	Initiate with lower dose	Usual dose with frequent monitoring
β_1-Selective		Usual dose with frequent monitoring
Atenolol	Usual dose with frequent monitoring	Usual dose with frequent monitoring
Betaxolol	Dose reduction may be necessary	Usual dose with frequent monitoring
Bisoprolol	Dose reduction may be necessary	Usual dose with frequent monitoring
Esmolol	Usual dose with frequent monitoring	Usual dose with frequent monitoring
Metoprolol	Dose reduction may be necessary	Usual dose with frequent monitoring

APPENDIX III. DOSING RECOMMENDATIONS OF CARDIOVASCULAR DRUGS IN PATIENTS WITH HEPATIC DISEASE AND/OR CONGESTIVE HEART FAILURE (CONTINUED)

Drug	Cirrhosis	Congestive heart failure
With ISA: nonselective		
Carteolol	Usual dose with frequent monitoring	Usual dose with frequent monitoring
Penbutolol	Dose reduction may be necessary	Usual dose with frequent monitoring
Pindolol	Dose reduction may be necessary	Usual dose with frequent monitoring
With ISA: β_1-selective		
Acebutolol	Usual dose with frequent monitoring	Usual dose with frequent monitoring
Dual acting		
Carvedilol	Initiate with lower dose	Initiate at lower dose; contraindicated in severely decompensated CHF
Labetalol	Dose reduction may be necessary	Usual dose with frequent monitoring
Calcium channel blockers		
Amlodipine	Initiate with lower dose	Usual dose with frequent monitoring
Bepridil	Dose reduction may be necessary	Contraindicated in uncompensated cardiac insufficiency
Diltiazem	Dose reduction may be necessary	Usual dose with frequent monitoring
Felodipine	Dose reduction may be necessary	Usual dose with frequent monitoring
Isradipine	Dose reduction may be necessary	Usual dose with frequent monitoring
Nicardipine	Initiate with lower dose	Usual dose with frequent monitoring
Nifedipine	Dose reduction may be necessary	Usual dose with frequent monitoring
Nimodipine	Initiate with lower dose	Usual dose with frequent monitoring
Nisoldipine	Initiate with lower dose	Usual dose with frequent monitoring
Verapamil	Initiate with lower dose	Avoid in patients with severe left ventricular dysfunction
Diuretics		
Loop		
Bumetanide	May precipitate hepatic coma; patients are usually diuretic resistant; dose reduction is probably not necessary	Usual dose with frequent monitoring
Ethacrynic Acid		
Furosemide		
Torsemide		
Thiazide		
Bendroflumethiazide	May precipitate hepatic coma; diuretic effect is decreased in patients with renal insufficiency (CrCl < 30 mL/min)	Usual dose with frequent monitoring
Benzthiazide		
Chlorothiazide		
Hydrochlorothiazide		
Hydroflumethiazide		
Methyclothiazide		
Metolazone		
Polythiazide		
Quinethazone		
Trichlormethiazide		
Indapamide	Dose reduction may be necessary	Usual dose with frequent monitoring

Drug	Cirrhosis	Congestive heart failure
K-sparing		
Amiloride	Dose reduction may be necessary	Usual dose with frequent monitoring
Spironolactone	Usual dose with frequent monitoring	Usual dose with frequent monitoring
Triamterene	Usual dose with frequent monitoring	Usual dose with frequent monitoring
Inotropic and vasopressor agents		
Amrinone	Dose reduction may be necessary	Usual dose with frequent monitoring
Digoxin, Dobutamine, Dopamine, Milrinone	Usual dose with frequent monitoring	Usual dose with frequent monitoring
Midodrine	Initiate at lower dose	Usual dose with frequent monitoring
Norepinephrine, Epinephrine, Isoproterenol, Metaraminol, Methoxamine, Phenylephrine	Usual dose with frequent monitoring	Usual dose with frequent monitoring
Lipid lowering agents		
Bile acid sequestrants		
Cholestyramine	Contraindicated in total biliary obstruction	Usual dose with frequent monitoring
Colestipol	Contraindicated in total biliary obstruction	Usual dose with frequent monitoring
Fibric acid derivatives		
Clofibrate	Contraindicated in clinically significant hepatic dysfunction	Usual dose with frequent monitoring
Fenofibrate	Contraindicated in hepatic dysfunction including primary biliary cirrhosis and patients with unexplained persistent transaminase elevation	Unknown
Gemfibrozil	Contraindicated in hepatic dysfunction including primary biliary cirrhosis	Unknown
HMG-CoA reductase inhibitors		
Atorvastatin, Cerivastatin, Fluvastatin, Lovastatin, Pravastatin, Simvastatin	Start at lowest dose and titrate cautiously; contraindicated in patients with active liver disease or unexplained persistent transaminase elevation	Usual dose with frequent monitoring
Nicotinic acid	Use with caution; contraindicated in patients with active liver disease or unexplained persistent transaminase elevation	Usual dose with frequent monitoring
Neuronal and ganglionic blockers		
Guanadrel	Usual dose with frequent monitoring	Contraindicated in frank CHF
Guanethidine	Dose reduction may be necessary	Contraindicated in frank CHF
Mecamylamine	Usual dose with frequent monitoring	Usual dose with frequent monitoring
Reserpine	Dose reduction may be necessary	Usual dose with frequent monitoring
Trimethaphan	Dose reduction may be necessary	Contraindicated in severe cardiac disease
Vasodilators		
Alprostadil	Usual dose with frequent monitoring	Usual dose with frequent monitoring
Cilostazol	Usual dose with frequent monitoring	Contraindicated
Diazoxide	Dose reduction may be necessary	Contraindicated in uncompensated CHF
Epoprostenol	Usual dose with frequent monitoring	Contraindicated in severe left ventricular systolic dysfunction
Fenoldopam	Usual dose with frequent monitoring	Usual dose with frequent monitoring
Hydralazine	Dose reduction may be necessary	Higher doses have been used
Isosorbide dinitrate	Use lower dose; avoid in severe hepatic impairment	Used in combination with hydralazine
Isosorbide mononitrate	Caution in severe hepatic impairment	Avoid in acute CHF

Drug	Cirrhosis	Congestive heart failure
Isoxsuprine	Dose reduction may be necessary	Usual dose with frequent monitoring
Minoxidil	Usual dose with frequent monitoring	Usual dose with frequent monitoring
Nitroglycerin	Dose reduction may be necessary; avoid in severe hepatic impairment	Usual dose with frequent monitoring
Sodium Nitroprusside	Initiate with lower dose	Usual dose with frequent monitoring
Papaverine	Dose reduction may be necessary	Usual dose with frequent monitoring
Pentoxifylline	Usual dose with frequent monitoring	Unknown
Sildenafil	Initiate with lower dose	Usual dose with frequent monitoring
Tolazoline	Unknown	Unknown

CHF—congestive heart failure; HMG-CoA—hydroxymethylglutaryl coenzyme A; ISA—intrinsic sympathomimetic activity.

Adapted from Frishman WH, Sokol SI: Cardiovascular drug therapy in patients with intrinsic hepatic disease and impaired hepatic function secondary to congestive heart failure. In Cardiovascular Pharmacotherapeutics. Edited by Frishman WH, Sonnenblick EH. New York: McGraw Hill, 1997:1561–1576.

APPENDIX IV. DOSE ADJUSTMENT IN PATIENTS WITH RENAL INSUFFICIENCY

Drug	Creatinine clearance 30 to 60 mL/min	Creatinine clearance less than 30 mL/min	Dialyzability (hemodialysis)
α-Adrenergic antagonists			
Doxazosin	Use usual dose	Use usual dose	No
Phenoxybenzamine	Use usual dose	Use usual dose	No
Phentolamine	Use usual dose	Use usual dose	No
Prazosin	Use usual dose	Start with low dose and titrate based on response	No
Terazocin	Use usual dose	Use usual dose	No
α₂-Adrenergic agonists			
Clonidine	Use usual dose	Start with low dose and titrate based on response	No
Guanabenz	Use usual dose	Use usual dose	Unknown
Guanfacine	Use usual dose	Start with low dose and titrate based on response	No
Methyldopa	Use usual dose	Start with low dose and titrate based on response	Yes
Angiotensin converting enzyme inhibitors			
Benazepril	Use usual dose	Start with low dose and titrate based on response	No†
Captopril	Start with low dose and titrate based on response	Start with low dose and titrate based on response	Yes
Enalapril	Use usual dose	Start with low dose and titrate based on response	Yes
Fosinopril	Use usual dose	Start with low dose and titrate based on response	No
Lisinopril	Use usual dose	Start with low dose and titrate based on response	Yes
Moexipril	For patients with CrCl of 40 mL/min or less, start with low dose and titrate based on response	Start with low dose and titrate based on response	Unknown
Perindopril	Start with low dose and titrate based on response	Start with low dose and increase dosing interval to every 48 h; titrate based on response. For patients with CrCl below 15 mL/min and on dialysis, give dose on the day of dialysis	Yes
Quinapril	Start with low dose and titrate based on response	Start with low dose and titrate based on response	No
Ramipril	For patients with CrCl less than 40 mL/min, start with low dose and titrate based on response	Start with low dose and titrate based on response. Up to a max of 5 mg/d	Unknown
Trandolapril	Use usual dose	Start with low dose and titrate based on response	Yes (trandolaprilat)
Angiotensin II receptor blockers			
Candesartan	Use usual dose	Start with low dose and titrate based on response	No
Irbesartan	Use usual dose	Use usual dose	No
Losartan	Use usual dose	Use usual dose	No
Telmisartan	Use usual dose	Use usual dose with caution	No

The information here is provided as guidance only. Prescribers should always consult the manufacturer's current prescribing information.

Drug	Creatinine clearance 30 to 60 mL/min	Creatinine clearance less than 30 mL/min	Dialyzability (hemodialysis)
Valsartan	Use usual dose	Use usual dose with caution	Unknown (probably no)
Antiarrhythmic agents			
Adenosine	Use usual dose	Use usual dose	No
Atropine	Use usual dose with caution	Use usual dose with caution	No
Class IA			
Disopyramide	Decrease loading dose by 25% to 50% Decrease maintenance dose by 25% or give 100 mg (nonsustained release) every 6 to 8 h	Decrease loading dose by 50% to 75% Decrease maintenance dose by 50% to 75% or give 100 mg (nonsustained release) every 12 to 24 h	No†
Procainamide	Increase dosing interval to every 4 to 6 h	Increase dosing interval to every 8 to 24 h	Yes (Give maintenance dose after dialysis or supplement with 250 mg post hemodialysis)
Quinidine	Use usual dose	Use usual dose with caution	Yes (Give maintenance dose after dialysis or supplement with 200 mg post hemodialysis)
Class IB			
Lidocaine	Use usual dose	Use usual dose with caution	No
Mexiletine	Use usual dose	Decrease 25% if CrCl is below 10 mL/min	No
Tocainide	Use usual dose	Decrease 25% to 50% or increase dosing interval to every 24 h	Yes (Give maintenance dose after dialysis or supplement with 25% of maintenance dose post hemodialysis)
Class IC			
Flecainide	Use usual dose	Initiate with 100 mg every 24 h or 50 mg every 12 h; titrate based on response	No
Moricizine	Use usual dose	Start with low dose and titrate based on response	Unknown
Propafenone	Use usual dose	Use usual dose with caution	No
Class II (β-adrenergic antagonists)			
Acebutolol	Decrease 50%	Decrease 75%	Yes (acebutolol and diacetolol)
Atenolol	Use usual dose with caution	Up to a max of 50 mg every 24 to 48 h	No
Betaxolol	Use usual dose with caution	Up to a max of 20 mg every 24 h	No
Bisoprolol	Use usual dose with caution	Start with low dose and titrate based on response	No
Carteolol	Increase dosing interval to every 48 h	Increase dosing interval to every 48 to 72 h	Unknown
Carvedilol	Use usual dose with caution	Start with low dose and titrate based on response	No
Esmolol	Use usual dose	Use usual dose	No
Labetalol	Use usual dose	Use usual dose	No
Metoprolol	Use usual dose	Use usual dose	No
Nadolol	Use usual dose with caution	Increase dosing interval to every 48 to 72 h	Yes
Penbutolol	Use usual dose	Use usual dose	No
Pindolol	Use usual dose	Use usual dose	Unknown

Drug	Creatinine clearance 30 to 60 mL/min	Creatinine clearance less than 30 mL/min	Dialyzability (hemodialysis)
Propranolol	Use usual dose	Use usual dose	No
Timolol	Use usual dose	Use usual dose	No
Class III			
Amiodarone	Use usual dose	Use usual dose	No
Bretylium	Decrease 50%	Decrease 50% to 75%	No
Dofetilide	Start with low dose and titrate based on response; specific dosing guidelines are lacking	Start with low dose and titrate based on response; specific dosing guidelines are lacking	Unknown
Ibutilide	Use usual dose	Use usual dose with caution	Unknown (probably no)
Sotalol	Increase dosing interval to every 24 h	Increase dosing interval to every 36 to 48 h; individualize dosage for patients with CrCl below 10 mL/min	Yes (Give maintenance dose after dialysis or supplement with 80 mg post hemodialysis)
Class IV (calcium antagonists*)			
Amlodipine	Use usual dose	Use usual dose with caution	No
Bepridil	Use usual dose	Use usual dose with caution	No
Diltiazem	Use usual dose	Use usual dose with caution	No
Felodipine	Use usual dose	Use usual dose	No
Isradipine	Use usual dose	Use usual dose with caution	No
Nicardipine	Use usual dose	Use usual dose; titrate dose carefully	No
Nifedipine	Use usual dose	Use usual dose	No
Nimodipine	Use usual dose	Use usual dose	No
Nisoldipine	Use usual dose	Use usual dose	No
Nitrendipine	Use usual dose	Use usual dose	No
Verapamil	Use usual dose	Use usual dose with caution	No
Antithrombotic agents			
Antiplatelet agents			
Abciximab	Use usual dose	Use usual dose with caution	No
Aspirin	Use usual dose	Use usual dose with caution	Yes
Clopidogrel	Use usual dose	Use usual dose	No
Dipyridamole	Use usual dose	Use usual dose	No
Eptifibatide	Use low dose if SCr is above 2 mg/dL	Contraindicated if SCr is above 4 mg/dL	Yes
Ticlopidine	Use usual dose	Use with caution; dose reduction may be required	No
Tirofiban	Use usual dose with caution	Decrease 50 %	Yes
Anticoagulants			
Ardeparin	Use usual dose	Use usual dose with caution	No
Dalteparin	Use usual dose	Use usual dose with caution	No
Danaparoid	Use usual dose	Use usual dose with caution if SCr is above 2 mg/dL	No
Enoxaparin	Use usual dose	Use with caution; dose reduction may be required (20% to 30%)	No
Heparin	Use usual dose	Use usual dose with caution	No

Drug	Creatinine clearance 30 to 60 mL/min	Creatinine clearance less than 30 mL/min	Dialyzability (hemodialysis)
Lepirudin	Bolus dose: 0.2 mg/kg; infusion rate 30% to 50% of usual dose	Bolus dose: 0.2 mg/kg; infusion rate: 15% of usual dose; contraindicated if SCr is above 6 mg/dL	Yes
Warfarin	Use usual dose	Use usual dose with caution	No
Thrombolytic agents			
Alteplase	Use usual dose with caution	Use usual dose with caution	No
Anistreplase	Use usual dose with caution	Use usual dose with caution	No
Reteplase	Use usual dose with caution	Use usual dose with caution	No
Streptokinase	Use usual dose with caution	Use usual dose with caution	No
Urokinase	Use usual dose with caution	Use usual dose with caution	No
Diuretics (contraindicated in anuric patients)			
Loop			
Bumetanide	Use usual dose	Use usual dose with caution	No
Ethacrynic acid	Use usual dose	Use usual dose with caution	No
Furosemide	Use usual dose	Use usual dose with caution	No
Torsemide	Use usual dose	Use usual dose with caution	No
Thiazide			
Chlorthalidone	Use usual dose	Ineffective	No
Hydrochlorothiazide and similar agents	Use usual dose	Ineffective	No
Indapamide	Use usual dose	Ineffective if CrCl below 15 mL/min	No
Metolazone	Use usual dose	Use usual dose	No
Potassium-sparing			
Amiloride	Use usual dose with caution	Contraindicated	Unknown
Spironolactone	Use usual dose with caution	Contraindicated	No
Triamterene	Use usual dose with caution	Contraindicated	Unknown
Inotropic and vasopressors agents			
Amrinone	Start with low dose and titrate based on response	Start with low dose and titrate based on response	No
Digoxin	Use usual dose and titrate based on response	Start with low dose, many patients only need a dose every 48 to 72 h (if loading dose is indicated, decrease 25%)	No
Milrinone	Decrease 25% to 50%; start with low dose and titrate based on response	Decrease 50% to 75%; start with low dose and titrate based on response	Unknown
Midodrine	Start with low dose and titrate based on response	Start with low dose and titrate based on response	Yes (midodrine and desglymidodrine)
Lipid-lowering agents			
Bile acid sequestrants			
Cholestyramine	Possibility of hyperchloremic acidosis is increased in patients with renal insufficiency; use usual dose with caution	Possibility of hyperchloremic acidosis is increased in patients with renal insufficiency; use usual dose with caution	
Colestipol	Possibility of hyperchloremic acidosis is increased in patients with renal insufficiency; use usual dose with caution	Possibility of hyperchloremic acidosis is increased in patients with renal insufficiency; use usual dose with caution	

The information here is provided as guidance only. Prescribers should always consult the manufacturer's current prescribing information.

Drug	Creatinine clearance 30 to 60 mL/min	Creatinine clearance lessthan 30 mL/min	Dialyzability (hemodialysis)
Fibric acid derivatives			
Clofibrate	Increase dosing interval to every 6 to 12 h	Increase dosing interval to every 12 to 24 hrs; avoid use if CrCl is below 10 mL/min	No
Fenofibrate	Start with low dose and titrate based on response	Start with low dose and titrate based on response	No
Gemfibrozil	Use usual dose with caution	Use usual dose with caution	No
HMG-CoA reductase inhibitors			
Atorvastatin	Use usual dose	Use usual dose	No
Cerivastatin	Start with low dose and titrate based on response	Start with low dose and titrate based on response	No
Fluvastatin	Use usual dose	Use usual dose with caution	No
Lovastatin	Use usual dose	Use usual dose with caution	No
Pravastatin	Use usual dose	Use usual dose with caution	No
Simvastatin	Use usual dose	Start with low dose and titrate based on response	No
Nicotinic Acid	Start with low dose and titrate based on response; use with caution	Start with low dose and titrate based on response; use with caution	Unknown
Neuronal and ganglionic blockers			
Guanadrel	Increase dosing interval to every 24 h; dosage increments should be made cautiously at intervals of 7 or more days	Increase dosing interval to every 48 h; dosage increments should be made cautiously at intervals of 14 days or more	Unknown (probably no)
Guanethidine	Start with low dose and titrate based on response	Start with low dose and titrate based on response; use with caution	Unknown
Mecamylamine	Start with low dose and titrate based on response	Start with low dose and titrate based on response; use with caution, if at all	Unknown
Reserpine	Use usual dose	Use usual dose with caution; avoid use if CrCl is below 10 mL/min	No
Trimethaphan	Start with low dose and titrate based on response	Start with low dose and titrate based on response; use with caution	Unknown
Vasodilators			
Alprostadil	Individualize dose	Individualize dose	Unknown
Cilostazol	Use usual dose	Use usual dose with caution; patients on hemodialysis have not been studied.	No
Diazoxide	Start with low dose and titrate based on response	Start with low dose and titrate based on response; use with caution	No
Epoprostenol	Individualize dose	Individualize dose	Unknown
Fenoldopam	Individualize dose	Individualize dose	Unknown
Hydralazine	Increase dosing interval to every 6 to 8 h	Increase dosing interval to every 8 to 24 h	No
Isosorbide dinitrate	Use usual dose	Start with low dose and titrate based on response; use with caution	Unknown
Isosorbide mononitrate	Use usual dose	Use usual dose with caution	No
Isoxsuprine	Start with low dose and titrate based on response	Start with low dose and titrate based on response; use with caution	Unknown
Minoxidil	Use usual dose	Start with low dose and titrate based on response	No
Nitroglycerin	Use usual dose	Use usual dose with caution	No

Drug	Creatinine clearance 30 to 60 mL/min	Creatinine clearance less than 30 mL/min	Dialyzability (hemodialysis)
Nitroprusside	Start with low dose and titrate based on response; use with caution	Start with low dose and titrate based on response; use with caution	Yes
Papaverine	Use usual dose	Use usual dose with caution	Unknown
Pentoxifylline	Use usual dose	Use usual dose with caution	Unknown
Sildenafil	Use usual dose	Start with low dose and titrate based on response	No
Tolazoline	Start with low dose and titrate based on response; use with caution. Specific dosing guidelines are lacking	Start with low dose and titrate based on response; use with caution; specific dosing guidelines are lacking	Unknown

* Only diltiazem and verapamil are indicated for arrhythmias.

†Hemodialysis does not remove appreciable amounts of this drug. However, dialysis may be considered in overdosed patients with severe renal impairment.

CrCl—creatinine clearance; HMG-CoA—hydroxymethylglutaryl coenzyme A; SCr—serum creatinine.

APPENDIX V

Drug	Evidence for efficacy in women	Considerations when treating women
Agents that Affect Blood Pressure		
Angiotensin converting enzyme inhibitors	Decreased mortality after MI*; decreased mortality in CHF*	Cough is 2 to 3 times greater in women; increased fetal abnormalities possible; present in breast milk
β-Blockers	Antihypertension: effective in preventing MI, CVA, and death in women*; decreases mortality after MI	Present in breast milk; blood levels of propranolol may be higher in men
Calcium blockers	Increased risk of MI in women*; increased effect of amlodipine in women in reducing blood pressure*	Edema may be more common in women; verapamil clearance may be greater in women than men; present in breast milk
Clonidine	No data about efficacy in women	Inability to achieve orgasm; possible decreased craving for tobacco more common in women
Thiazide diuretics	Decreased CVA, MI, death*	Decreased urinary calcium excretion; women have greater increase in risk of gout; acute pulmonary edema and allergic interstitial pneumonitis; excreted in breast milk
Guanethidine		Orthostatic hypotension more common in women
Hydralazine	Effective in hypertension in pregnancy and peripartum	SLE more common in women than men; present in breast milk
Methyldopa	Often preferred in pregnancy for treating hypertension	Painful breast enlargement; decreased libido
Nitrates	Decreased mortality after MI*	Potential for difference in metabolism in women
Angiotensin II receptor blockers		Increased fetal abnormalities possible
Antiarrhythmic agents		
Disopyramide	No data about efficacy in women	Complication of Torsade de Pointes more frequent in women*
Procainamide	No gender-specific data available	Drug-induced SLE more common in women
Quinidine	No gender-specific data available	Torsades more common in women; clearance may be faster in women; present in breast milk
Aspirin	Primary prevention: US Nurses' Cohort shows decreased MI†; Women's Health Initiative in progress† Secondary CAD Prevention: decreases reinfarction*	Higher rate of hemorrhagic stroke in women; Physician's Health Study showed increased risk of bleeding with aspirin; increased risk of bleeding at term in pregnancy; present in breast milk
Conjugated estrogens	Increases HDL-cholesterol, decreases total cholesterol and lipoproteins†; not effective after MI†	Need for progestin in women with intact uterus to prevent endometrial abnormalities
Hypolipidemic agents		
Colestipol	No effect on primary prevention*	
Clofibrate	Effective in secondary prevention in women*	
HMG-CoA reductase inhibitors	Primary and secondary prevention: possible efficacy in women*; decreases cholesterol and slows plaque progression without respect to gender†	Gastrointestinal side effects more common in women
Nicotine preparations	Gum equally effective in women*; patch effective in women*	Gum may suppress weight gain; not recommended in pregnancy

*Studies of efficacy in both men and women, with analysis by gender.

†Studies of efficacy in women

CAD—coronary artery disease; CHF—congestive heart failure; CVA—cerebrovascular accident; HDL—high-density lipoprotein; MI—myocardial infarction; SLE—systemic lupus erythematosus.

Adapted from Charney P, Meyer BR, Frishman WH, et al.: Gender, race and genetic issues in cardiovascular pharmacotherapy. In Cardiovascular Pharmacotherapeutics. Edited by Frishman WH, Sonnenblick EH. New York: McGraw Hill; 1997:1350–1351.

APPENDIX VI. PHARMACOKINETIC CHANGES, ROUTE(S) OF ELIMINATION, AND DOSAGE ADJUSTMENT OF SELECTED CARDIOVASCULAR DRUGS IN THE ELDERLY

Drug	Half-life	Volume of distribution	Clearance	Primary route(s) of elimination	Dosage adjustment
α-Adrenergic agonists (centrally and peripherally acting)					
Clonidine	—	—	—	Hepatic/renal	Initiate at lowest dose; titrate to response
Guanabenz	—	—	—	Hepatic	Initiate at lowest dose; titrate to response
Guanfacine	Increase	—	Decrease	Hepatic/renal	Initiate at lowest dose; titrate to response
Methyldopa	—	—	—	Hepatic	Initiate at lowest dose; titrate to response
Doxazosin	Increase	Increase	Increase*	Hepatic	Initiate at lowest dose; titrate to response
Prazosin	Increase	—	—	Hepatic	Initiate at lowest dose; titrate to response
Terazosin	Increase	—	—	Hepatic	Initiate at lowest dose; titrate to response
Angiotensin converting enzyme inhibitors					
Benazepril	Increase	—	Decrease	Renal	No adjustment needed
Captopril	NS	—	Decrease	Renal	Initiate at lowest dose; titrate to response
Enalapril	—	—	—	Renal	Initiate at lowest dose; titrate to response
Fosinopril	—	—	—	Hepatic/renal	No adjustment needed
Lisinopril	Increase	NS	Decrease	Renal	Initiate at lowest dose; titrate to response
Perindopril	—	—	Decrease	Renal	Initiate at lowest dose; titrate to response
Quinapril	—	—	—	Renal	Initiate at lowest dose; titrate to response
Ramipril	—	—	—	Renal	Initiate at lowest dose; titrate to response
Moexipril	—	—	—	Hepatic/renal	Initiate at lowest dose; titrate to response
Trandolapril	—	—	—	Hepatic/renal	No adjustment needed
Angiotensin II receptor blockers					
Candesartan	—	—	—	Hepatic/renal	No adjustment needed
Irbesartan	NS	—	—	Hepatic	No adjustment needed
Losartan	—	—	—	Hepatic	No adjustment needed
Telmisartan	—	—	—	Hepatic/biliary	No adjustment needed
Valsartan	Increase	—	—	Hepatic	No adjustment needed
Antiarrhythmic agents					
Class I					
Disopyramide	Increase	—	Decrease	Renal	Initiate at lowest dose; titrate to response
Flecainide	Increase	Increase	Decrease	Hepatic/renal	Initiate at lowest dose; titrate to response
Lidocaine	Increase	Increase	NS	Hepatic	Initiate at lowest dose; titrate to response
Mexilitine	—	—	—	Hepatic	Initiate at lowest dose; titrate to response
Moricizine	—	—	—	Hepatic	Initiate at lowest dose; titrate to response
Procainamide	—	—	Decrease	Renal	Initiate at lowest dose; titrate to response
Propafenone	—	—	—	Hepatic	Initiate at lowest dose; titrate to response
Quinidine	Increase	NS	Decrease	Hepatic	Initiate at lowest dose; titrate to response
Tocainide	Increase	—	Decrease	Hepatic/renal	Initiate at lowest dose; titrate to response
Class II (see β blockers)					
Class III					
Amiodarone	—	—	—	Hepatic/biliary	Initiate at lowest dose; titrate to response
Bretylium	—	—	—	Renal	Initiate at lowest dose; titrate to response
Dofetilide	—	—	—	Hepatic/renal	Initiate at lowest dose; titrate to response
Ibutilide	—	—	—	Hepatic	No adjustment needed

The information here is provided as guidance only. Prescribers should always consult the manufacturer's current prescribing information.

323

Drug	Half-life	Volume of distribution	Clearance	Primary route(s) of elimination	Dosage adjustment
Sotalol	—	—	—	Renal	Initiate at lowest dose; titrate to response
Class IV (see calcium channel blockers)					
Other antiarrhythmics					
Adenosine	—	—	—	Erythrocytes/vascular endothelial cells	No adjustment needed
Atropine	—	—	—	Hepatic/renal	Use usual dose with caution
Antithrombotics					
Anticoagulants					
Heparin	—	—	—	Hepatic/reticuloendothelial system	Use usual dose with caution
Ardeparin	—	—	—	Renal	Use usual dose with caution
Dalteparin	—	—	—	Renal	Use usual dose with caution
Enoxaparin	—	—	—	Renal	Use usual dose with caution
Danaparoid	NS	NS	NS	Renal	Use usual dose with caution
Lepirudin	Increase	—	Decrease	Renal	Adjust dose based on renal function
Warfarin	NS	NS	NS	Hepatic	Initiate at lowest dose; titrate to response
Antiplatelets					
Aspirin	—	—	Decrease	Hepatic/renal	Use usual dose with caution
Abciximab	—	—	—	Unknown	Use usual dose with caution
Clopidogrel	NS	—	—	Hepatic	Use usual dose with caution
Dipyridamole	—	—	—	Hepatic/biliary	Use usual dose with caution
Eptifibatide	—	—	—	Renal/plasma	Use usual dose with caution
Ticlopidine	—	—	Decrease	Hepatic	Use usual dose with caution
Tirofiban	Increase	—	Decrease	Hepatic	Use usual dose with caution
Thrombolytics					
Alteplase	—	—	—	Hepatic	Use usual dose with caution
Anistreplase	—	—	—	Unknown	Use usual dose with caution
Reteplase	—	—	—	Hepatic	Use usual dose with caution
Streptokinase	—	—	—	Circulating antibodies/reticuloendothelial system	Use usual dose with caution
Urokinase	—	—	—	Hepatic	Use usual dose with caution
β-Adrenergic blockers					
Nonselective without ISA					
Nadolol	NS	—	—	Renal	Initiate at lowest dose; titrate to response
Propranolol	Increase	NS	Decrease	Hepatic	Initiate at lowest dose; titrate to response
Timolol	—	—	—	Hepatic	Initiate at lowest dose; titrate to response
β₁-Selective					
Atenolol	Increase	NS	Decrease	Renal	Initiate at lowest dose; titrate to response
Betaxolol	—	—	—	Hepatic	Initiate at lowest dose; titrate to response
Bisoprolol	—	—	—	Hepatic/renal	Initiate at lowest dose; titrate to response
Esmolol	—	—	—	Erythrocytes	Use usual dose with caution
Metoprolol	NS	NS	NS	Hepatic	Initiate at lowest dose; titrate to response
Nonselective with ISA					
Acebutolol	Increase	Decrease	—	Hepatic/biliary	Initiate at lowest dose; titrate to response

Drug	Half-life	Volume of distribution	Clearance	Primary route(s) of elimination	Dosage adjustment
Carteolol	—	—	—	Renal	Initiate at lowest dose; titrate to response
Penbutolol	—	—	—	Hepatic	Use usual dose with caution
Pindolol	—	—	—	Hepatic/renal	Initiate at lowest dose; titrate to response
Dual acting					
Carvedilol	—	—	—	Hepatic/biliary	Initiate at lowest dose; titrate to response
Labetalol	—	—	NS	Hepatic	No adjustment needed
Calcium channel blockers					
Amlodipine	Increase	—	Decrease	Hepatic	Initiate at lowest dose; titrate to response
Bepridil	—	—	—	Hepatic	Use usual dose with caution
Diltiazem	Increase	NS	Decrease	Hepatic	Initiate at lowest dose; titrate to response
Felodipine	—	NS	Decrease	Hepatic	Initiate at lowest dose; titrate to response
Isradipine	—	—	—	Hepatic	Initiate at lowest dose; titrate to response
Nicardipine	NS	—	—	Hepatic	No adjustment needed
Nifedipine	Increase	NS	Decrease	Hepatic	Initiate at lowest dose; titrate to response
Nimodipine	—	—	—	Hepatic	Use usual dose with caution
Nisoldipine	—	—	—	Hepatic	Initiate at lowest dose; titrate to response
Verapamil	Increase	NS	Decrease	Hepatic	Initiate at lowest dose; titrate to response
Diuretics					
Loop					
Bumetanide	—	NS	—	Renal/hepatic	Initiate at lowest dose; titrate to response
Ethacrynic Acid	—	—	—	Hepatic	Initiate at lowest dose; titrate to response
Furosemide	Increase	NS	Decrease	Renal	Initiate at lowest dose; titrate to response
Torsemide	—	—	—	Hepatic	Initiate at lowest dose; titrate to response
Thiazides					
Bendroflumethiazide	—	—	—	Renal	Initiate at lowest dose; titrate to response
Benzthiazide	—	—	—	Unknown	Initiate at lowest dose; titrate to response
Chlorothiazide	—	—	—	Renal	Initiate at lowest dose; titrate to response
Chlorthalidone	—	—	—	Renal	Initiate at lowest dose; titrate to response
Hydrochlorothiazide	—	—	Decrease	Renal	Initiate at lowest dose; titrate to response
Hydroflumethiazide	—	—	—	Unknown	Initiate at lowest dose; titrate to response
Indapamide	—	—	—	Hepatic	Initiate at lowest dose; titrate to response
Methyclothiazide	—	—	—	Renal	Initiate at lowest dose; titrate to response
Metolazone	—	—	—	Renal	Initiate at lowest dose; titrate to response
Polythiazide	—	—	—	Unknown	Initiate at lowest dose; titrate to response
Quinethazone	—	—	—	Unknown	Initiate at lowest dose; titrate to response
Trichlormethiazide	—	—	—	Unknown	Initiate at lowest dose; titrate to response
Potassium sparing					
Amiloride	—	—	Decrease	Renal	Initiate at lowest dose; titrate to response
Spironolactone	—	—	—	Hepatic/biliary/renal	Initiate at lowest dose; titrate to response
Triamterene	Increase	—	—	Hepatic/renal	Initiate at lowest dose; titrate to response
Inotropic and vasopressor agents					
Amrinone	—	—	—	Hepatic/renal	Initiate at lowest dose; titrate to response

Drug	Half-life	Volume of distribution	Clearance	Primary route(s) of elimination	Dosage adjustment
Digoxin	Increase	Decrease	Decrease	Renal	Initiate at lowest dose; titrate to response
Dobutamine	—	—	—	Hepatic/tissue	Initiate at lowest dose; titrate to response
Dopamine	—	—	—	Renal/hepatic/plasma	Initiate at lowest dose; titrate to response
Epinephrine	—	—	—	Sympathetic nerve endings/plasma	Initiate at lowest dose; titrate to response
Isoproterenol	—	—	—	Renal	Initiate at lowest dose; titrate to response
Metaraminol	—	—	—	Unknown	Initiate at lowest dose; titrate to response
Methoxamine	—	—	—	Unknown	Initiate at lowest dose; titrate to response
Midodrine	—	—	—	Tissue/hepatic/renal	No adjustment necessary
Milrinone	—	—	—	Renal	Adjust based on renal function
Norepinephrine	—	—	—	Sympathetic nerve endings/plasma	Initiate at lowest dose; titrate to response
Phenylephrine	—	—	—	Hepatic/intestinal	Initiate at lowest dose; titrate to response
Lipid-lowering agents					
Bile acid sequestrants					
Cholestyramine	—	—	—	Not absorbed from GI tract	No adjustment needed
Colestipol	—	—	—	Not absorbed from GI tract	No adjustment needed
Fibric acid derivatives					
Clofibrate	—	—	—	Hepatic/renal	Adjust based on renal function
Fenofibrate	—	—	—	Renal	No adjustment necessary
Gemfibrozil	—	—	—	Hepatic/renal	No adjustment necessary
Nicotinic acid	—	—	—	Hepatic/renal	No adjustment necessary
HMG-CoA reductase inhibitors					
Atorvastatin	Increase	—	—	Hepatic/biliary	No adjustment necessary
Cerivastatin	—	—	—	Hepatic/fecal/renal	Adjust based on renal function
Fluvastatin	—	—	—	Hepatic	No adjustment necessary
Lovastatin	—	—	—	Hepatic/fecal	No adjustment necessary
Pravastatin	—	—	—	Hepatic	Initiate at lowest dose; titrate to response
Simvastatin	—	—	—	Hepatic/fecal	Initiate at lowest dose; titrate to response
Neuronal and ganglionic blockers					
Guanadrel	—	—	—	Hepatic/renal	Initiate at lowest dose; titrate to response
Guanethidine	—	—	—	Hepatic/renal	Initiate at lowest dose; titrate to response
Mecamylamine	—	—	—	Renal	Initiate at lowest dose; titrate to response
Reserpine	—	—	—	Hepatic/fecal	Initiate at lowest dose; titrate to response
Trimethaphan	—	—	—	Hepatic/renal	Initiate at lowest dose; titrate to response
Vasodilators					
Alprostadil	—	—	—	Pulmonary/renal	Initiate at lowest dose; titrate to response
Cilostazol	—	—	—	Hepatic/renal	No adjustment necessary
Diazoxide	—	—	—	Hepatic/renal	Initiate at lowest dose; titrate to response
Epoprostenol	—	—	—	Hepatic/renal	Use usual dose with caution
Fenoldopam	—	—	—	Hepatic	No adjustment necessary
Hydralazine	—	—	—	Hepatic	Initiate at lowest dose; titrate to response

Appendix VI. Pharmacokinetic Changes, Route(s) of Elimination, and Dosage Adjustment of Selected Cardiovascular Drugs in the Elderly

Drug	Half-life	Volume of distribution	Clearance	Primary route(s) of elimination	Dosage adjustment
Isosorbide dinitrate	—	—	—	Hepatic	Initiate at lowest dose; titrate to response
Isosorbide mononitrate	NS	—	NS	Hepatic	No adjustment necessary
Isoxsuprine	—	—	—	Renal	Initiate at lowest dose; titrate to response
Minoxidil	—	—	—	Hepatic	Initiate at lowest dose; titrate to response
Nitroglycerin	—	—	—	Hepatic	Initiate at lowest dose; titrate to response
Nitroprusside	—	—	—	Hepatic/renal/erythrocytes	Use usual dose with caution
Papaverine	—	—	—	Hepatic	Initiate at lowest dose; titrate to response
Pentoxifylline	—	—	Decrease	Hepatic/renal	Use usual dose with caution
Sildenafil	—	—	—	Hepatic/fecal	Initiate at lowest dose; titrate to response

*Increase in clearance is small compared to increase in volume of distribution.

GI—gastrointestinal; ISA—intrinsic sympathomimetic activity; NS—no significant change; ——no information or not relevant; HMG-CoA—hydroxymethylglutaryl coenzyme A.

The information here is provided as guidance only. Prescribers should always consult the manufacturer's current prescribing information.

333